To Sandy

With all good wishes

Andrew

Potassium in Cardiovascular and Renal Medicine

KIDNEY DISEASE

Editors

J. Stewart Cameron
Professor in Renal Medicine
Clinical Science Laboratories
Guy's Hospital
London, England

Richard J. Glassock
Chairman, Department of Medicine
UCLA School of Medicine and
Harbor-UCLA Medical Center
Torrance, California

Andrew Whelton
Associate Professor of Medicine
The Johns Hopkins University School of Medicine
Baltimore, Maryland

Volume 1 Proteinuria: An Integrated Review, *Amadeo J. Pesce and Martin Roy First*

Volume 2 The Aminoglycosides: Microbiology, Clinical Use, and Toxicology, *edited by Andrew Whelton and Harold C. Neu*

Volume 3 Hepatorenal Disorders, *S. P. Wilkinson*

Volume 4 Acute Renal Failure: Correlations Between Morphology and Function, *edited by Kim Solez and Andrew Whelton*

Volume 5 Renal Tubular Disorders: Pathophysiology, Diagnosis, and Management, *edited by Harvey C. Gonick and Vardaman M. Buckalew, Jr.*

Volume 6 Potassium in Cardiovascular and Renal Medicine: Arrhythmias, Myocardial Infarction, and Hypertension, *edited by Paul K. Whelton, Andrew Whelton, and W. Gordon Walker*

Volume 7 Kidney Transplant Rejection: Diagnosis and Treatment, *edited by G. Melville Williams, James Burdick, and Kim Solez*

Other Volumes in Preparation

Potassium in Cardiovascular and Renal Medicine

Arrhythmias, Myocardial Infarction, and Hypertension

edited by

PAUL K. WHELTON
The Johns Hopkins School
of Hygiene and Public Health
The Johns Hopkins University
School of Medicine
The Johns Hopkins Hospital
Baltimore, Maryland

ANDREW WHELTON   W. GORDON WALKER
The Johns Hopkins University
School of Medicine
The Johns Hopkins Hospital
Baltimore, Maryland

MARCEL DEKKER, INC.   New York • Basel

Library of Congress Cataloging in Publication Data

Main entry under title:

Potassium in cardiovascular and renal medicine.

(Kidney disease ; v. 6)
Based, in large part, on the proceedings of a meeting held at the Johns Hopkins University, Baltimore, Md., on June 7th and 8th, 1984.
Includes index.
1. Hypertension--Chemotherapy--Complications and sequelae--Congresses. 2. Diuretics--Side effects--Congresses. 3. Hypokalemia--Congresses. 4. Arrhythmia--Congresses. 5. Heart--Infarction--Congresses. 6. Potassium--Metabolism--Disorders--Congresses. I. Whelton, Paul K. (Paul Kieran). II. Whelton, Andrew. III. Walker, W. Gordon. IV. Series. [DNLM: 1. Arrhythmia--etiology--congresses. 2. Diuretics--adverse effects--congresses. 3. Hypertension--physiopathology--congresses. 4. Hypokalemia--physiopathology--congresses. 5. Myocardial Infarction--complications--congresses. 6. Potassium--physiology--congresses. W1 KI586R v.6 / WD 220 P859 1984]
RC685.H8P647 1986 616.1 85-29383
ISBN 0-8247-7376-4

Marcel Dekker, Inc.
270 Madison Avenue, New York, New York 10016

Current printing (last digit):
10 9 8 7 6 5 4 3 2 1

PRINTED IN THE UNITED STATES OF AMERICA

About the Series

This book is the sixth in a series of texts on nephrology intended to cover all aspects of that discipline. Nephrology has grown at a great rate over the past decade, and the available knowledge has outstripped the texts available. The discipline has, however, attained such maturity that a description of any one of its parts becomes more than ephemeral—or worse, outdated before it even appears. We aim to fill some of the many gaps that exist, not only for the specialist in nephrology, but also for the general physician interested in nephrology. In this description, we include the study and management of hypertension, since these two are interwoven at so many points. We welcome comments on the series as it evolves, or suggestions for topics that might be considered for future volumes.

J. Stewart Cameron
London, England

Richard J. Glassock
Torrance, California

Andrew Whelton
Baltimore, Maryland

Preface

Severe hypokalemia and hyperkalemia have been well recognized as important and, on occasion, life-threatening for at least four decades. Recent studies have suggested that modest deficits in body potassium content, as a result of either nutritional inadequacy or continued diuretic usage, may have important clinical implications as well. In many patients plasma potassium values fall within the range usually considered to be normal despite a body deficit of 100–300 mEq of potassium. Hypokalemia has been implicated in the precipitation of arrhythmias in patients with diuretic-treated essential hypertension and in the arrhythmias seen in patients with acute myocardial infarction. Following the demonstration that nutritional potassium deficits could play an important role in experimental hypertension, a number of studies have suggested that both potassium intake and total body potassium are abnormally low in patients with hypertension even before treatment is instituted. Correction of apparent deficiencies of body potassium through the use of potassium supplementation or potassium-sparing agents may not be hazard-free. Overzealous attention to potassium-replacement therapy in patients on maintenance diuretic treatment and in other hypokalemic states has been documented to be associated with a small but definite risk of death from hyperkalemia. Thus, both deficits and excesses of potassium have recently been demonstrated to be associated with health hazards not previously recognized.

Approximately 30 million individuals in the United States are on continuous diuretic therapy, and a comparable number of individuals have been estimated to have abnormally elevated blood pressure. Although there is considerable overlap between the two groups, it seems likely that about 40 million individuals in the U.S. have hypertension and/or are on continuous diuretic therapy. While these are only estimates, it is evident that a significant proportion of the total U.S. population may be at risk for the potential complications of disordered potassium metabolism. Adverse clinical consequences of a disturbance in potassium metabolism could thus represent a substantial public health hazard. Difference of opinion exists as to the relative importance of these issues and, in fact, some of the reports relating diuretic-induced potassium deficits to cardiac arrhythmia have led to considerable controversy.

This volume contains a collection of most of the significant contributions to the recent literature dealing with these important issues. The text, in large part, is based on the proceedings of a meeting held at The Johns Hopkins University, Baltimore, Maryland, on June 7th and 8th, 1984. A major justification for this publication is that it makes available in one volume most of the relevant data that bear on the clinical significance of mild and persistent disturbances in potassium homeostasis.

In planning for the symposium, we received advice and encouragement from many colleagues. We also received enthusiastic support from Dr. Edward Roccella, coordinator of the National Heart and Blood Pressure Education Program.

The assembly of participants from this country and abroad was achieved at considerable cost and would not have been possible without the educational grant support provided by several generous donors. We gratefully acknowledge the major educational grant in aid support provided by Ayerst Laboratories, Ciba-Geigy Corp., Hoffmann-La Roche, Inc., Merck Sharp & Dohme Inc., Merck Sharp & Dohme International, and Miles Laboratories Inc. We also acknowledge with gratitude the contributions of Dista Products of Eli Lilly & Co., Hoechst-Roussel Pharmaceuticals Inc., Lederle Laboratories, Revlon Health Care Group, Inc., A. H. Robins, Co., Sandoz Inc., Schering Corp., and E. R. Squibb & Sons.

This book is dedicated first to the clinical investigators who preceded us and who provided the elegant and quantitative description of potassium homeostasis that forms the background for virtually all the studies reported in this volume, and second to future investigators who will provide the solution to some of the problems and issues articulated in this volume.

Paul K. Whelton
Andrew Whelton
W. Gordon Walker

Contributors

Gerald S. Berenson, M.D.* Professor of Medicine, Chief, Section of Cardiology, and Director, Specialized Center of Research–Arteriosclerosis, Department of Medicine, Louisiana State University Medical Center, New Orleans, Louisiana

Christopher J. Bulpitt, M.D., M.Sc., F.R.C.P. Senior Lecturer, Department of Epidemiology, London School of Hygiene and Tropical Medicine, London, England

Warren D. Cooper, M.B., B.S., B.Sc.† Clinical Research Physician, Medical Department, Merck Sharp & Dohme Ltd., Hoddesdon, Hertfordshire, England

Cornelius J. Cronin, M.B., B.Ch., M.R.C.P.I. Honorary Research Fellow, Department of Clinical Pharmacology, University College London, London, England

Raffaele David, M.D.‡ Adjunct Associate Professor, Department of Pathology, University of Maryland School of Medicine, Baltimore, Maryland

Patricia J. Elmer, M.S., R.D.§ Research Associate, Division of Epidemiology, School of Public Health, University of Minnesota, Minneapolis, Minnesota

Gail C. Frank, R.D., Dr.P.H. Assistant Professor, Department of Medicine, Louisiana State University Medical Center, New Orleans, Louisiana

---

Current affiliation:
*Professor of Medicine, Chief, Section of Cardiology, and Director, National Research and Demonstration Center–Arteriosclerosis, Department of Medicine, Louisiana State University Medical Center, New Orleans, Louisiana
†Director of Medical Affairs, Medical Department, Merck Sharp & Dohme Ltd.
‡Head, Department of Pathology, Central Emek Hospital, Afula, Israel
§Research Associate, Division of Epidemiology, School of Public Health, University of Minnesota, and Division of Epidemiology, Disease Prevention, and Health Promotion, Minnesota Department of Health, Minneapolis, Minnesota

Edward D. Freis, M.D. Senior Medical Investigator, Hypertension Research, Veterans Administration Medical Center, and Professor, Department of Medicine, Georgetown University School of Medicine, Washington, D.C.

Gerhard Giebisch, M.D. Sterling Professor of Physiology, Department of Physiology, Yale University School of Medicine, New Haven, Connecticut

Ray W. Gifford, Jr., M.D. Vice-Chairman, Division of Medicine, The Cleveland Clinic Foundation, Cleveland, Ohio

John R. Gill, Jr., M.D. Chief of Service, Hypertension-Endocrine Branch, National Heart, Lung and Blood Institute, National Institutes of Health, Bethesda, Maryland

David A. Goodkin, M.D. Instructor, Renal Section, Department of Medicine, Temple University Health Sciences Center, Philadelphia, Pennsylvania

David Y. Graham, M.D. Professor of Medicine and Virology, Veterans Administration Medical Center and Baylor College of Medicine, Houston, Texas

George T. Griffing, M.D. Assistant Professor of Medicine, Department of Endocrinology and Metabolism, University Hospital and Boston University School of Medicine, Boston, Massachusetts

Richard H. Grimm, Jr., M.D., Ph.D. Assistant Professor, Division of Epidemiology, School of Public Health, University of Minnesota, Minneapolis, Minnesota

John T. Harrington, M.D. Chief, General Medicine Division, Department of Medicine, New England Medical Center Hospital, and Professor of Medicine, Tufts University School of Medicine, Boston, Massachusetts

O. Bryan Holland, M.D. Associate Professor, Department of Internal Medicine, University of Texas Medical Branch at Galveston, Galveston, Texas

John W. Hollifield, M.D. Director, Hypertension Center of Nashville, Nashville, Tennessee

Norman M. Kaplan, M.D. Professor, Department of Internal Medicine, University of Texas Southwestern Medical School and University of Texas Health Science Center at Dallas, Dallas, Texas

Kay-Tee Khaw, M.R.C.P., M.Sc. Wellcome Trust Research Fellow, Department of Family and Community Medicine, University of California–San Diego, La Jolla, California

James P. Knochel, M.D. Professor and Vice Chairman, Department of Internal Medicine University of Texas Southwestern Medical School, and Chief, Medical Service, Veterans Administration Medical Center, Dallas, Texas

Herbert G. Langford, M.D. Professor of Medicine and Chief, Endocrinology and Hypertension Division, Department of Medicine, University of Mississippi Medical Center, Jackson, Mississippi

Graham A. MacGregor, M.A., F.R.C.P. Senior Lecturer, Blood Pressure Unit, Department of Medicine, Charing Cross Hospital Medical School, London, England

Robert C. May, M.D. Research Fellow, Department of Medicine, Harvard Medical School, and Brigham and Women's Hospital, Boston, Massachusetts

James C. Melby, M.D. Head, Section of Endocrinology and Metabolism, University Hospital, and Professor, Departments of Medicine and Physiology, Boston University School of Medicine, Boston, Massachusetts

Wolfgang Johannes Mergner, M.D., Ph.D. Professor, Department of Pathology, University of Maryland School of Medicine, Baltimore, Maryland

William E. Mitch, M.D. Associate Professor, Department of Medicine, Harvard Medical School, and Brigham and Women's Hospital, Boston, Massachusetts

Trefor Owen Morgan, M.D., F.R.C.P. Professor, Department of Physiology, University of Melbourne, Melbourne, Victoria, Australia

Gilbert H. Mudge, M.D. Emeritus Professor, Departments of Pharmacology and Medicine, Dartmouth Medical School, Hanover, New Hampshire

Robert G. Narins, M.D. Professor of Medicine and Chief, Nephrology Section, Department of Medicine, Temple University Health Sciences Center, Philadelphia, Pennsylvania

James D. Neaton, Ph.D. Assistant Professor, Division of Biometry, School of Public Health, University of Minnesota, Minneapolis, Minnesota

Nga Nguyen, M.D. Resident, Department of Pathology, University of Maryland School of Medicine, Baltimore, Maryland

Jan Erik Nordrehaug, M.D.* Senior Registrar, Department of Medicine, Diakonissehjemmet Hospital, Bergen, Norway

Vasilios Papademetriou, M.D., D.Sc. Cardiology Fellow, Department of Cardiology, Veterans Administration Medical Center and Georgetown University School of Medicine, Washington, D.C.

Philip A. Poole-Wilson, M.D., F.R.C.P. Professor of Cardiology, Department of Cardiac Medicine, The Cardiothoracic Institute and National Heart Hospital, London, England

Current affiliation:
*Registrar, Department of Clinical Physiology, Haukeland Hospital and University of Bergen, Bergen, Norway

B. N. C. Prichard, M.B., M.Sc., F.R.C.P. Professor, Department of Clinical Pharmacology, School of Medicine, University College London, and Consultant Physician, Hypertension Clinic, University College Hospital, London, England

Ronald J. Prineas, M.B., B.S., Ph.D. Professor, Division of Epidemiology, School of Public Health, University of Minnesota, Minneapolis, Minnesota

Simon W. Rabkin, M.D., F.R.C.P.(C), F.A.C.C. Professor, Department of Medicine, University of British Columbia, Vancouver, British Columbia, Canada

John L. Reid, D.M., F.R.C.P. Regius Professor, Department of Materia Medica and Therapeutics, University of Glasgow, and Stobhill General Hospital, Glasgow, Scotland

Geoffrey Rose, D.M., D.Sc., F.R.C.P. Professor, Department of Epidemiology, London School of Hygiene and Tropical Medicine, London, England

Michael P. Ryan, B.Sc., Ph.D. Statutory Lecturer, Department of Pharmacology, University College Dublin, Blackrock, County Dublin, Ireland

Daniel G. Sapir, M.D. Associate Professor, Division of Nephrology, The Johns Hopkins University School of Medicine, and Chief, Department of Medicine, Wyman Park Health System Hospital, Baltimore, Maryland

Allan B. Schwartz, M.D. Professor of Medicine and Director, Nephrology Service B, Department of Medicine, Hahnemann University and Hahnemann University Hospital, Philadelphia, Pennsylvania

Marvin S. Segal, M.D. Clinical Associate Professor, Departments of Clinical Studies and Medicine, Mt. Sinai Hospital and University of Minnesota, Minneapolis, Minnesota

Roger Sherwin, M.B., B.Chir. Professor, Department of Epidemiology and Preventive Medicine, University of Maryland School of Medicine, Baltimore, Maryland

Richard J. Solomon, M.D. Associate Professor, Department of Medicine, Brown University Program in Medicine; Director, Division of Nephrology, Roger Williams General Hospital; and Chief, Renal-Hypertension Section, Veterans Administration Medical Center, Providence, Rhode Island

Richard L. Tannen, M.D. Professor, Department of Internal Medicine, and Director, Division of Nephrology, University of Michigan Medical School, Ann Arbor, Michigan

Louis Tobian, M.D. Professor, Department of Medicine, University of Minnesota School of Medicine, Minneapolis, Minnesota

Malcolm J. VandenBurg, B.Sc., M.B.B.S., M.R.C.P.* Director of Clinical Research, Medical Department, Merck Sharp & Dohme Ltd., Hoddesdon, Hertfordshire, England

Current affiliation:
*Director of Cardiovascular Research, Cardiac Unit, Oldchurch and Rush Green Hospitals, Romford, Essex, England

W. Gordon Walker, M.D. Chairman, Division of Nephrology, Director, Clinical Research Center, and Professor, Department of Medicine, The Johns Hopkins University School of Medicine and The Johns Hopkins Hospital, Baltimore, Maryland

Alan J. Watson, M.D. Assistant Professor, Renal Division, Department of Medicine, The Johns Hopkins University School of Medicine and The Johns Hopkins Hospital, Baltimore, Maryland

Andrew Whelton, M.D. Associate Professor, Department of Medicine, The Johns Hopkins University School of Medicine and The Johns Hopkins Hospital, Baltimore, Maryland

Paul K. Whelton, M.B., B.Ch., M.Sc. Associate Professor, Department of Epidemiology, The Johns Hopkins University School of Hygiene and Public Health; Associate Professor, Department of Medicine, The Johns Hopkins University School of Medicine; and Director, Outpatient Clinical Research Center, The Johns Hopkins Hospital, Baltimore, Maryland

Kenneth Zierler, M.D. Professor, Departments of Physiology and Medicine, The Johns Hopkins University School of Medicine, Baltimore, Maryland

Contents

PHYSIOLOGY AND PATHOLOGY OF HYPOKALEMIC DISORDERS

1

Physiology of Potassium Metabolism

GERHARD GIEBISCH
Yale University School of Medicine, New Haven, Connecticut

This chapter will survey the key factors responsible for the maintenance of potassium homeostasis. Three physiological processes are involved in setting overall potassium balance: *uptake* by the intestinal tract, *distribution* within the body such that a high cellular and a low extracellular concentration is maintained, and *excretion*, which is largely a function of the kidney. It is presently believed that the reabsorption of potassium ions across the intestinal epithelium is not subject to regulation. Of the other components of potassium homeostasis, we know most about the regulation of potassium partitioning between extracellular and cellular fluid (4), and about the mechanism and control of renal potassium excretion (10, 13, 14, 43). The colon is also an organ of potassium excretion, but its contribution to overall potassium balance is, however, limited.

ROLE OF POTASSIUM IN CELL FUNCTION

Potassium ions, as the most abundant cation in the cellular fluid compartment, play a key role in several important cell functions. The typical distribution of potassium (high intracellular and low extracellular concentration), together with the significant diffusion permeability of cells, provides the basis for the generation of the resting membrane potential and thus for the fundamental properties of excitation and contraction in nerve and muscle (29). As the cation with the highest concentration within cells, it also contributes significantly to the osmolality of the intracellular fluid. Accordingly, changes in the cell content of potassium are almost always associated with alterations of the cell volume, and the regulation of cell volume depends critically upon those factors that control the cell potassium content (30).

Changes in cell potassium have also long been known to lead to alterations in cell pH. A loss of potassium from cells is frequently associated with acidosis, a gain of potassium with alkalosis (1). Through this relationship between cell potassium and cell pH, potassium ions affect metabolic processes by their effect on cell pH.

The concentration of potassium ions in cells depends on the balance between *active* uptake from the extracellular fluid and *passive* leakage from the cell into the interstitium.

The active uptake of potassium ions is mediated by the ATPase-driven sodium–potassium exchange pump (10, 30). These pump sites are uniformly distributed on the cell surface of nonpolarized cells, such as muscle, nerve, and red blood cells, but their distribution in epithelial cells such as those lining the renal tubule is limited to the basolateral cell membrane.

Two general features of sodium–potassium exchange are of special interest. First, there is now abundant evidence that the sodium–potassium pump operates in an electrogenic fashion: the rate at which sodium ions are extruded from the cell exceeds the rate at which potassium ions are taken up. Thus, the activity of the electrogenic cation exchange contributes directly to the electrical negativity of renal tubule cells (28, 39). For instance, renal cell depolarization by ouabain or ambient temperature reduction, or cell hyperpolarization by mineralocorticoids includes a component of cell potential change directly related to an alteration of electrogenic pump activity (28, 39).

A second aspect of active, ATPase-driven sodium–potassium exchange has to do with the control of the passive potassium "leak" across cell membranes. Passive potassium movement plays an important role in the regulation of cell potassium since in the steady state the rate of *active* potassium uptake must be matched by an equal rate of *passive* potassium movement out of the cell (29). Recent evidence has shown that in a variety of cells, including epithelial preparations, changes in active pump rate are closely related to the passive leak component of potassium movement (41). In general, an increase of pump activity is associated with an increased potassium leak whereas a reduction of sodium–potassium exchange is matched by a decline of potassium permeability. Recent findings support the view that the generally observed constancy of intracellular potassium in the presence of large changes of transepithelial sodium transport depends critically upon appropriate adjustments of the basolateral potassium conductance (31, 41). By adjusting the potassium leak conductance to changes in active Na^+-K^+ exchange, cells in transporting epithelia such as the renal tubule can maintain cell potassium activity and cell volume within narrow limits *despite* dramatic changes in net sodium transport.

COMPONENTS OF POTASSIUM HOMEOSTASIS

Figure 1 shows the three routes of potassium transit during steady-state potassium balance: intestinal intake, distribution between fluid compartments, and excretion.

Internal distribution of potassium ions is determined by several factors, the most important of which are several hormones (aldosterone, epinephrine, and insulin) and the acid–base status of the body fluids (1, 4, 10, 13, 38).

The intracellular potassium pool, present largely in muscle, represents a large potential sink for potassium entering the extracellular fluid. The cellular potassium pool is large: 98% of the body's potassium is located intracellularly. Following addition of potassium to the extracellular fluid, activation of several factors as depicted in Figure 1 leads to a rapid and effective shift of potassium ions into the cell compartment. Uptake of potassium into tissues effectively prevents potentially dangerous fluctuation of the plasma potassium level and provides an important and highly significant defense mechanism for the extracellular potassium concentration (4).

The protective role of extrarenal mechanisms for the temporary storage of potassium is of particular relevance following either the acute addition of potassium to the extracellular fluid (gastrointestinal potassium uptake or intravenous administration), or the acute release of potassium from localized tissue stores (tissue damage, destruction of

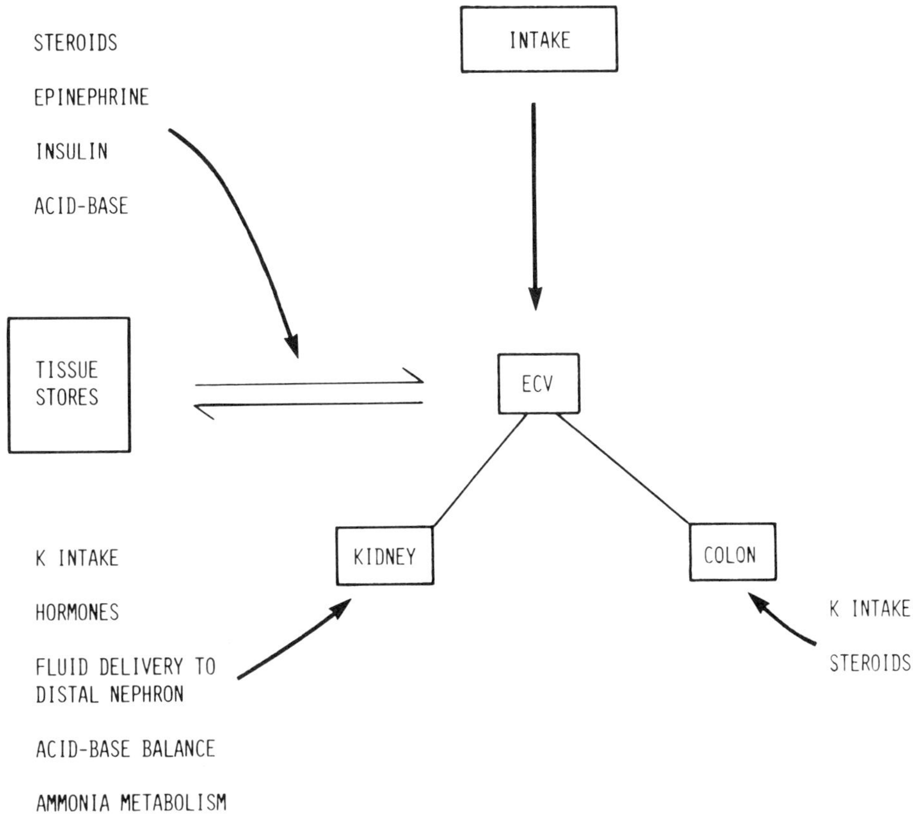

Figure 1 Components of potassium homeostasis. Potassium homeostasis depends on the matching of intake and excretion of potassium. Acute changes in the extracellular potassium concentration are minimized by an effective transfer system that shifts potassium in and out of large cellular tissue stores (4, 10, 13, 14).

blood cells, rigorous exercise). Should there be a deficiency of the hormonal mechanisms that augment transfer of potassium from the extracellular to the cellular compartment (lack of mineralocorticoids, catecholamines or insulin, administration of β-blockers). potassium levels in the blood may reach dangerously high levels, particularly if renal mechanisms of potassium excretion are compromised. Care must also be taken to use the plasma potassium level as an index of the body's total potassium pool since the plasma potassium level is determined not only by the ability of the kidney to maintain external balance, but also by the extrarenal factors just reviewed. These exert a very significant effect on the plasma potassium concentration by modulating the movement of potassium ions across cell membranes in tissue stores at a time when total body potassium has not changed.

Finally, it should be emphasized that the renal response to a given potassium load also depends on extrarenal factors. Renal excretion will be sharply attenuated if the potassium challenge is associated with the simultaneous administration of hormones (or alkali) that stimulate the deposition of potassium in tissue. Under these conditions, plasma potassium levels will be lower and renal excretion diminished proportionally (4). From this we conclude that the renal response to a potassium load is importantly modulated by the behavior and responsiveness of a complex extrarenal humoral system that regulates the internal distribution of this ion.

Whereas the internal potassium balance is of great significance in preventing large fluctuations of the plasma potassium level following acute changes in extracellular potassium, balance depends ultimately upon adequate renal mechanisms of potassium excretion. Figure 1 also summarizes the key factors that affect real potassium excretion. Since the colonic epithelium does not play a major role in safeguarding the external potassium balance, we shall focus in the following sections on the renal mechanisms that underly tubular potassium transport and on the factors that regulate urinary potassium excretion.

TRANSPORT OF POTASSIUM IONS ALONG THE NEPHRON

Based on a classic series of clearance studies, Berliner et al. (3) and Mudge et al. (32) had postulated that the excretion of potassium into the urine depends essentially on a "distal" secretory system. Their evidence rested on the observation that changes in glomerular filtration rate, and thus in the filtered load of potassium ions, do not play a major role in potassium excretion.

Free-flow micropuncture studies in a variety of mammalian species have confirmed the view of an important distal tubular control site of potassium regulation. Figure 2 summarizes results from rat micropuncture studies in conditions of potassium conservation (top) following dietary restriction of potassium, and during conditions in which the potassium content in the diet was either normal (10% excretion) or sharply elevated (150%) by the administration of an acute potassium load to animals that had also received a high-potassium diet for several weeks (13, 14, 43).

It is apparent from Figure 2 that most of the filtered potassium load is reabsorbed along the proximal tubule (80%) and along the thick ascending limb of Henle's loop (10%). When potassium ions are avidly conserved (top panel of Fig. 2), further potassium reabsorption takes place along the superficial distal tubule and the collecting ducts. The situation is strikingly different when the potassium content in the diet is either normal or when potassium excretion is further stimulated: potassium secretion can then be shown to be activated. It is now well-established that, with the exception of potassium conservation, potassium secretion along the late distal tubule and along the cortical collection tubule largely accounts for urinary potassium secretion. These tubular sites of potassium secretion are also those that respond to most of the factors known to regulate potassium secretion (8, 9, 13, 14, 16, 28, 43, 45).

Investigation of transport events beyond these sites of potassium secretion has shown that potassium ions may escape from the tubular lumen to be reabsorbed further downstream along the medullary portions of the collecting tubule (23). Such reabsorption occurs by diffusion from the lumen of the collecting ducts into the interstitium of the papilla (23, 47). The concentration of potassium ions in the collecting tubules is maintained at very high levels due to distal potassium secretion and continuous water reabsorption; this provides an adequate driving force for passive exit into the interstitium of the renal papilla and the lumen of Henle's loop.

Figure 3 provides further insight into the tubular handling of potassium ions by including information on juxtamedullary nephrons (23). Fluid samples from the hairpin bend of the loop in the exposed papilla from rodents have shown that the amount of potassium delivered to the end of the descending limb of the loop of Henle about equals the amount of potassium filtered across the glomerulus. If we assume that the proximal

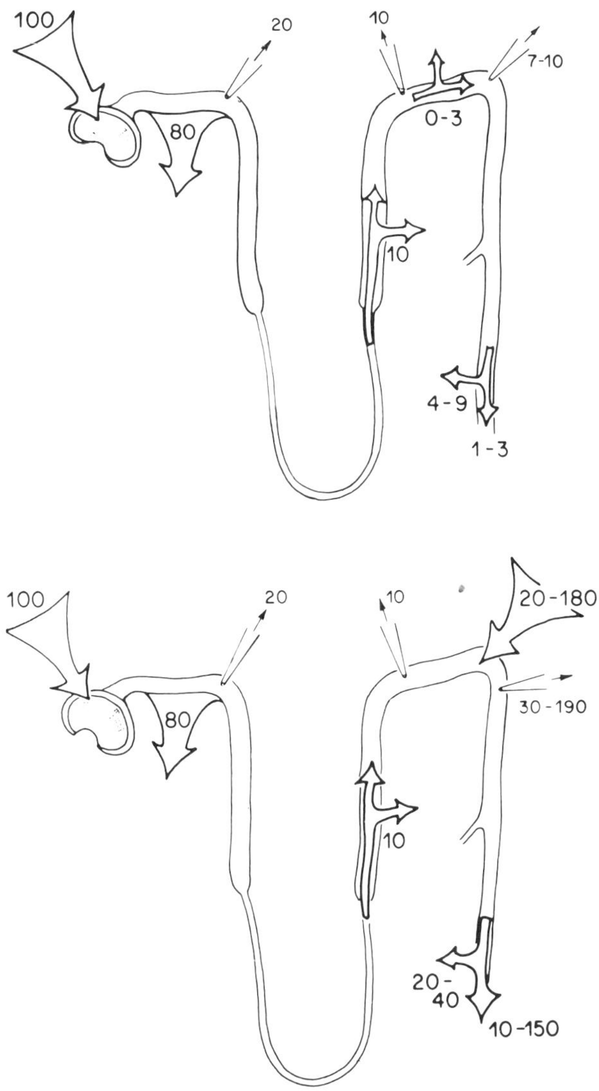

Figure 2 Potassium transport across the mammalian superficial tubule. Top: Condition of potassium conservation. Bottom: Condition of normal or elevated potassium excretion. (From Ref. 43.)

convoluted tubule of these juxtamedullary nephrons reabsorbs potassium similar to its superficial counterparts, it is clear that entry of potassium ions must have occurred into the pars recta and/or into the thin descending limb of Henle's loop (23, 47). This added potassium most likely originates in the medullary collecting duct where, as pointed out above, potassium reabsorption may occur. Several aspects of this process of potassium recycling have been discussed (23). However, its possible involvement in pathological states remains to be explored.

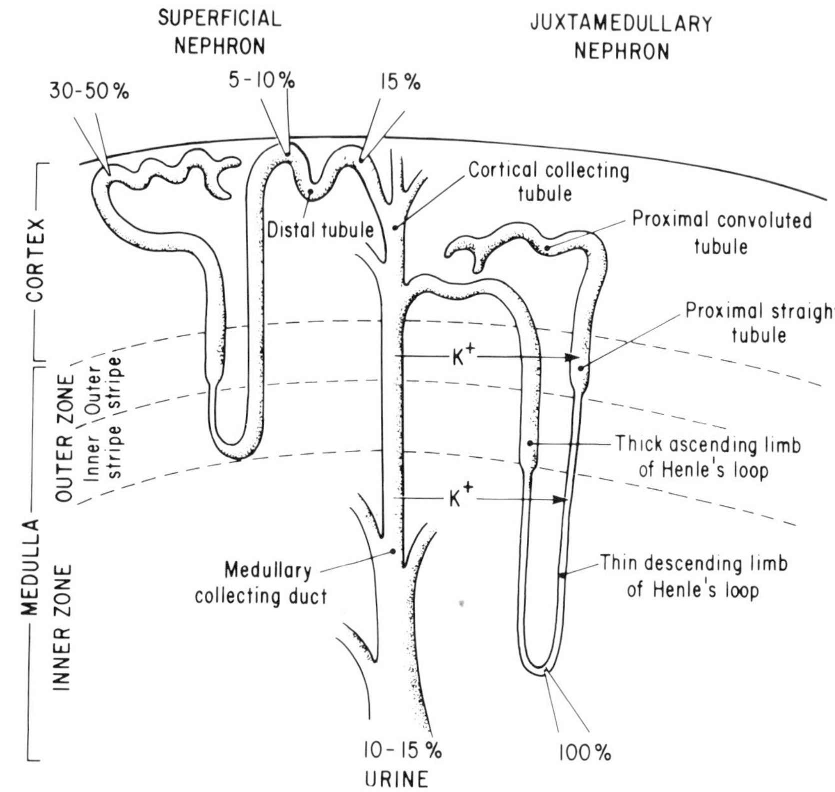

Figure 3 Sites of potassium handling by superficial and juxtamedullary nephrons. A representative superficial and juxtamedullary nephron is shown, with typical values of fractional delivery of K (% of filtered load) at the sites accessible to micropuncture (animal on normal potassium diet). The arrows in the juxtamedullary nephrons indicate the pathways for recycling of potassium within the medulla. (Adapted from Ref. 10.)

CELL MECHANISMS OF POTASSIUM TRANSPORT

Proximal Tubule

The proximal convoluted and straight tubule are the main nephron sites of potassium reabsorption. Figure 4 summarizes the known components of the two transport pathways: one through proximal tubule cells and one between cells.

Measurements of intracellular potassium activities together with values for the electrical cell potentials indicate that potassium ions are actively taken up across both the luminal and the peritubular cell membrane (6, 7). Since the absolute potassium permeability of the luminal cell membrane is less than that of the peritubular cell membrane, most of the potassium ions, pumped actively into the cell either via a luminal or a peritubular transport mechanism, will leave the cell across the peritubular cell membrane. The latter is also the site of the ATPase-driven sodium-potassium pump. Little is known about the features of the luminal potassium pump. In particular, it is not known whether it is involved in any counter- or cotransportation and what its metabolic source of energy might be.

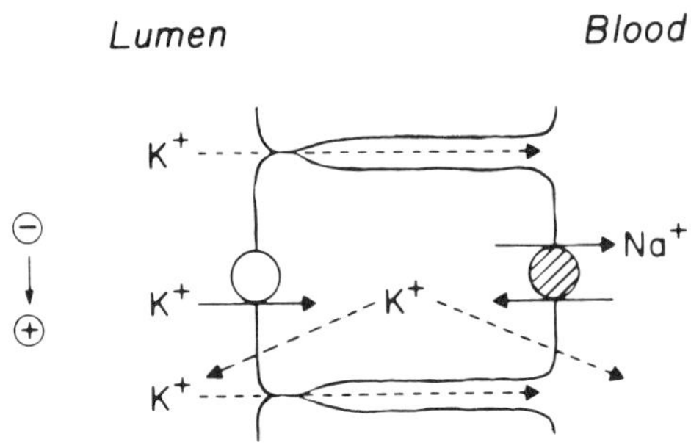

Figure 4 Cell model of proximal tubule cell. Broken arrows indicate passive movement, solid arrows indicate active transport. Note transition from lumen-negative (early proximal tubule) to lumen-positive (late proximal tubule) transepithelial voltage. (From Ref. 10.)

As indicated in Figure 4, an additional, intercellular transport route has also been identified. Two driving forces act to promote proximal tubular potassium transport by this intercellular route. The first is the lumen-positive electrical potential difference that exists in later portions of the proximal convoluted tubule. This transepithelial potential provides a significant driving force that acts to drive potassium from lumen to the interstitial fluid. In view of the low electrical resistance of the intercellular shunt pathway, it is virtually certain that such passively reabsorbed potassium moves largely through the intercellular shunt pathway. A second passive driving force promoting proximal potassium reabsorption is bulk fluid movement, secondary to active sodium transport. Evidence in support of such a mechanism is the observation that changing the rate, or even the direction, of fluid movement across the proximal tubular epithelium by imposing transepithelial osmotic gradients has significant and similar effects on potassium transport. That such a mechanism of entrainement (solvents-drag) of potassium is of physiological importance is implied by observations that maneuvers that lower proximal tubular fluid transport (such as extracellular volume expansion or mannitol administration) have similar inhibitory effects upon potassium reabsorption.

Loop of Henle

As pointed out above, available evidence suggests that the thin descending limb of Henle's loop is a nephron site of potassium entry into the lumen. Given the measured potassium permeability of this nephron segment and the increase of interstitial potassium concentration along the corticomedullary axis, potassion ions would be passively "secreted" into this portion of Henle's loop, particularly in juxtamedullary nephrons with long loops. We have already pointed out that this net entry of potassium ions represents a key component of medullary recycling of potassium in the renal medulla (23, 33, 47).

Considerable advances have recently been made in our understanding of the mechanism of tubular potassium transport in the thick ascending limb of Henle (17, 19). Results based on studies on isolated, perfused segments of either the rabbit (17) or mouse (19) thick ascending limb in vitro, or of the diluting segment of the early distal tubule of Amphiuma (33) provide strong evidence that potassium ions are reabsorbed by a cotransport mechanism involving sodium and chloride ions.

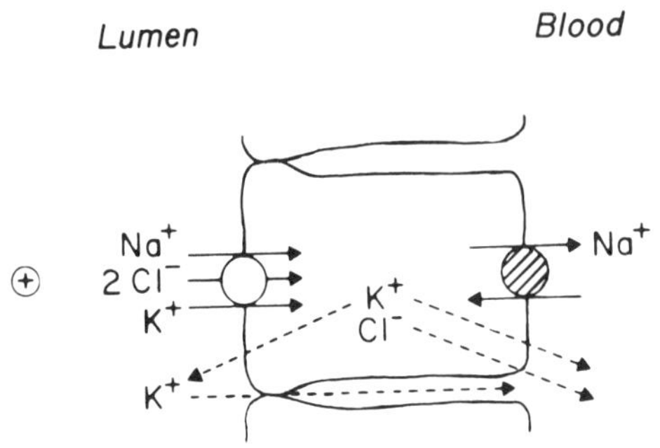

Figure 5 Cell model of the thick ascending limb and early distal tubule. (Adapted from Refs. 17, 33.)

Figure 5 summarizes relevant features of the potassium transport system across the thick ascending limb of Henle's loop (17) and the amphibian diluting segment (33). The model is based on extensive studies of net fluxes, transepithelial and intracellular potential recordings, and intracellular measurements of the activities of the cotransported ion species. The following transport components are important. The primary driving force for net potassium reabsorption via the Na^+, K^+, 2 Cl^-cotransporter is active, ATPase-driven sodium extrusion across the peritubular cell membrane. This pump activity is responsible for the generation of the steep sodium gradient across the luminal cell membrane; it thus provides the main energy source for the coupled, electrically neutral entry of Na^+,K^+, and 2 Cl^-across the luminal cell membrane.

Distinctive features of the cell model summarized in Figure 5 are a conductive pathway for potassium ions in the luminal cell membrane and finite chloride and potassium permeabilities in the peritubular cell membrane (17, 33). These selective passive ion permeabilities of the luminal (high K permeability) and the peritubular cell membrane (chloride and potassium permeability) are probably largely responsible for the lumen-positive electrical potential across this tubule segment (17).

Several implications of this transport model deserve mention. Interference with the activity of the luminal cotransport system, either by administration of loop diuretics, such as furosemide, or replacement of luminal chloride with bicarbonate (metabolic alkalosis), have been shown to lower net potassium reabsorption. Indeed, furosemide administration or complete replacement of luminal chloride with a nontransported anion species may result in the appearance of net potassium secretion because the passive leak of potassium ions from cell to lumen is no longer opposed by the reabsorptive cotransport system (10, 33). The luminal potassium conductance is subject to modification by several factors. It has been found to be increased by adaptation to high potassium intake (33) and by vasopressin (19). The luminal potassium conductance has been found to be reduced by acidification (44).

The high potassium conductance also plays a key role in the process of luminal sodium chloride entry. The high luminal potassium permeability permits extensive recycling of potassium ions back into the tubular lumen to sustain cotransport with sodium chloride (17, 18). Rapid exchange of luminal and cellular potassium is essential for sodium chloride transport since the sodium chloride concentration in the lumen exceeds significantly that of potassium. Hence, potassium ions would quickly disappear were it not for reentry from the cell pool across the luminal cell membrane.

Distal Tubule and Cortical Collecting Tubule

Two cell types line the epithelium of these two tubule segments that are largely responsible for potassium secretion: the principal cell and the intercalated cell (25, 42, 45, 46). We shall present evidence below that principal cells are most likely the cell type that secretes potassium ions.

A simple cell schema of a principal cell is shown in Figure 6. Similarly to other body cells, principal cells have a peritubular active pump, a mechanism that exchanges potassium for sodium ions. It is driven by ATPase and has been shown to operate in an electrogenic fashion, particularly when stimulated by adrenal steroids (28, 40). This active mechanism of potassium uptake has been shown to be stimulated by alkalosis, by a rise in plasma potassium, and by mineralocorticoids (13, 28, 40).

Two membrane properties within the luminal cell membrane of principal cells are of significance for potassium secretion. The first is a high potassium permeability in the luminal cell membrane that permits potassium ions to diffuse along a favorable electrochemical potential gradient from the tubule cell into the lumen. The second is the significant apical membrane permeability to sodium ions. This permeability plays a significant role in potassium secretion since it generates the lumen-negative potential that drives potassium ions from the interstitium into the lumen. Given the direction of the sodium concentration gradient from lumen (high) to cell (low), the negative electrical potential across this cell membrane is reduced by sodium movement such that unequal electrical polarization of the tubule cell results. This generates the lumen-negative transepithelial potential difference (13).

The potassium permeability of the luminal cell membrane has been found to be increased by mineralocorticoids (28), by tubule fluid acidification, and by perfusion of the lumen with barium-containing solutions (35-37). One potassium-conductive pathway has recently been further analyzed by application of the patch-clamp technique to cells of the isolated mammalian collecting duct (22). An interesting feature was, besides its marked barium sensitivity, the significant activation by increasing the cytoplasmic calcium activity.

To complete the description of the cellular transport mechanisms that reside within the distal nephron, we must mention the existence of a transport mechanism responsible for active potassium reabsorption (13). It is most likely activated by potassium depletion. Morphological evidence, discussed below, strongly suggests that it is located in the luminal cell membrane of intercalated cells (46).

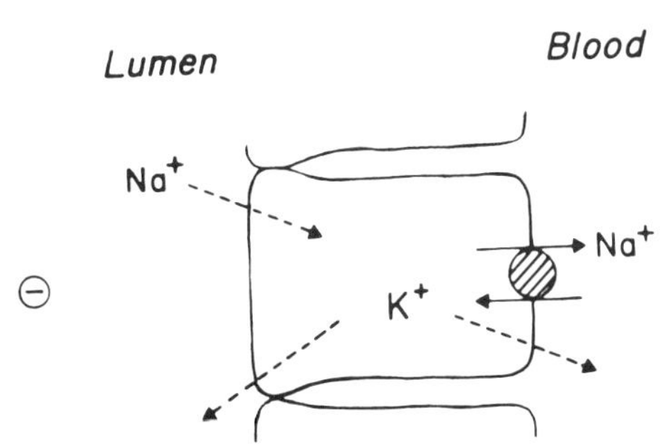

Figure 6 Cell model of the principal cell of the initial and cortical collecting tubule. (From Refs. 28, 35.)

MORPHOLOGICAL CONSIDERATIONS OF CELL HETEROGENEITY

Figure 7 provides a schematic overview of the cell types found in the mammalian distal tubule and collecting duct. Interest in the morphological behavior of the cells lining these portions of the nephron has arisen because their morphological heterogeneity has significant functional correlates with respect to distal tubule potassium transport (13, 14, 25, 42-46).

As is apparent from Figure 7, the distal tubule is divided into three segments, and a total of four cell types have been identified. The first segment, the distal convoluted tubule (DCT) is made up exclusively of a distal cell population. It is the "early distal tubule" as identified in micropuncture experiments. It is followed by a shorter connecting tubule (CNT in Fig. 7). This transitional segment is lined by two cell types: connecting tubule cells and intercalated cells. The latter have luminal microplicae, apical vesicles, and basal mitochondria. The third segment, (the "late" distal tubule in micropuncture studies), is referred to as the initial collecting tubule (ICT) and consists of two cell types, the intercalated cell, described above, and the principal cell. Principal cells have a smooth luminal cell surface, shallow basolateral infoldings, and lack cytoplasmic vesicles. We note from inspection of Figure 7 that the cortical collecting tubule, located below the kidney surface, is also characterized by the presence of intercalacted and principal cells.

The morphological heterogeneity just described has functional implications. Potassium secretion occurs only along the connecting tubule and the initial and cortical collecting tubule (43). Following stimulation of "distal" tubular potassium secretion, only principal cells undergo significant fine structural alterations (25, 42). This consists of a dramatic increase of the basolateral membrane area in principal cells that line both the initial and the cortical collecting tubule. These cell-specific structural changes are consistent with the interpretation that principal cells are the cell type that secretes potassium and that baso-

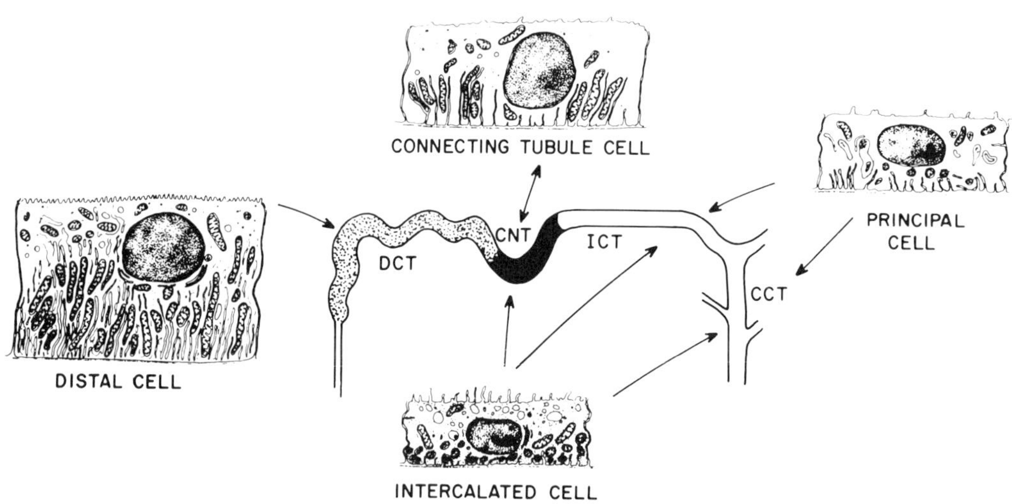

Figure 7 Schematic presentation of the superficial distal nephron of the rat. Note four distinct cell types. DCT, distal convoluted tubule; CNT, connecting tubule; ICT, initial collecting tubule; CCT, cortical collecting tubule. (From Ref. 42.)

lateral cell membrane amplification and the ATPase-driven active Na^+-K^+ pump are stimulated by factors that increase potassium secretion. This view is supported by segmental analysis of ATPase activity in the same collecting duct segments that show basolateral membrane amplification. ATPase activity was shown to correlate well with the selective increase of the basolateral surface area in the collecting tubules of animals whose potassium secretion was stimulated by a high-potassium diet (24).

The role of adrenal steroids in the modulation of cell morphology has shown that these hormones participate importantly in the regulation of the basolateral surface of principal cells. Figure 8 summarizes results of a series of experiments in which adrenalectomized rats were kept on a fixed potassium intake. Morphometric results of principal cells were then compared in animals receiving known amounts of aldosterone. A significant reduction of the basolateral surface area occurred after adrenalectomy, and a very significant increase after the level of circulating aldosterone was elevated (45). Dexamethasone had no morphological effects. Thus it is safe to conclude that the modulation of the basolateral membrane area of principal cells is controlled by mineralocorticoids.

In contrast to those very marked morphological changes observed in principal cells, no significant alterations in basolateral membrane area occur in intercalated cells during stimulation of potassium secretion. However, stimulation of tubular potassium conservation following reduction of potassium intake has been shown to lead both to an increase in the surface area of the luminal membrane area and to insertion of rod-shaped particles (46). It has been proposed that these particles originate from the vesicular pool located below the surface of the luminal cell membrane of intercalated cells, because morphometric studies demonstrated that the pool is significantly reduced at the time of increased

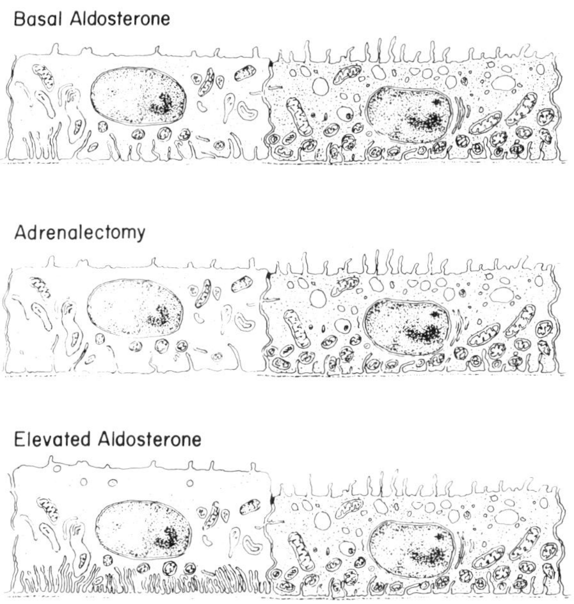

Figure 8 Schematic presentation of effects of variations of aldosterone levels on the morphology of principal and intercalated cells. Principal cells (left) show aldosterone-dependent basolateral membrane amplification. Intercalated cells (right) are not affected. (From Ref. 45.)

appearance of the rod-shaped particles in the apical membrane (46). These newly inserted luminal particles correlate with the stimulation of potassium reabsorption. They may be the morphological equivalent of "potassium pumps" recruited into the apical membrane of intercalated cells during potassium conservation.

REGULATION OF POTASSIUM EXCRETION

Figure 9 summarizes the main factors that have been identified to affect potassium secretion in the distal tubule (10, 13). They have been grouped according to their main site of action into luminal and peritubular factors.

Of the factors acting from the tubule lumen, changes in flow rate are particularly important since it is well established that an increase in fluid delivery into the distal tubule enhances potassium secretion (12, 27). A fall in luminal sodium concentration, however, to levels below 35 mmol, has been shown in distal microperfusion studies to curtail potassium secretion (15). On the other hand, a fall of the luminal chloride concentration below the normal concentration range of 25-35 mmol stimulates distal potassium secretion (48). The electrical potential difference across the distal tubule is also of importance since the normal lumen-negative potential represents one of the driving forces from potassium entry into the tubule. A fall of the potential decreases net potassium secretion (11).

Two inhibitors which are not illustrated in Figure 9 affect potassium secretion from the lumen: the potassium-sparing diuretic amiloride (12, 34, 37), and barium (28, 35-37). Amiloride acts by blocking the sodium permeability of the luminal cell membrane, which leads to hyperpolarization of the luminal membrane of distal and collecting duct cells. This change in luminal potential decreases the electrochemical driving force for translocation of potassium ions from the tubule cell into the lumen. Addition of barium to the luminal fluid also decreases potassium secretion, but this effect is best explained by a direct blocking action of barium ions on potassium channels in the luminal cell membrane (22, 36).

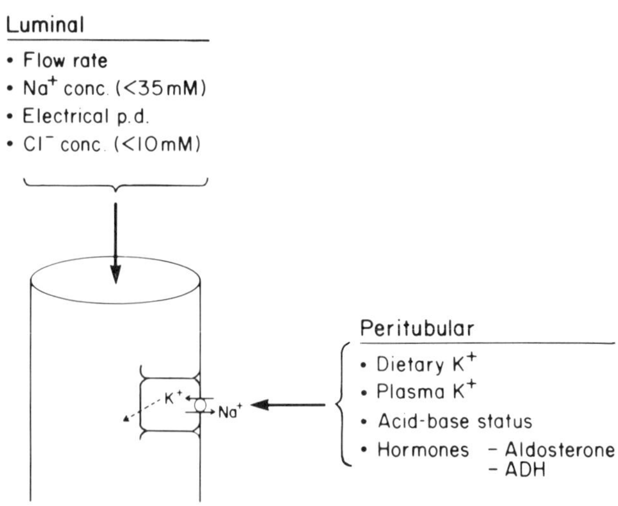

Figure 9 Factors influencing potassium secretion across the distal tubule. (From Ref. 10.)

The peritubular factors listed in Figure 9 include plasma constituents such as potassium and bicarbonate ions, and hormones such as aldosterone and antidiuretic hormone (ADH). Although these factors are represented as having a primary peritubular site of action, their ultimate effects on tubular potassium transport may include modulation of luminal membrane properties. It is known that a high dietary potassium intake (33), and an increase in cell pH (44), aldosterone (28, 40), and ADH (vasopressin) (9, 19) all increase the luminal potassium permeability.

INTERACTION AMONG FACTORS REGULATING POTASSIUM EXCRETION

The net effect of many systemic alterations on the urinary excretion of potassium frequently represents the results of several interacting factors. Of particular relevance is the marked effect of changes in flow rate of tubular fluid along the distal tubule that modifies the "intrinsic" response of the distal tubular secretory system to several primary influences on distal tubular potassium secretion. The final effect of such interactions may be to minimize the "direct" effect of the initial disturbance on potassium excretion. Alternatively, flow-mediated effects and the direct effect on distal tubular potassium transport may be additive and further stimulate potassium excretion.

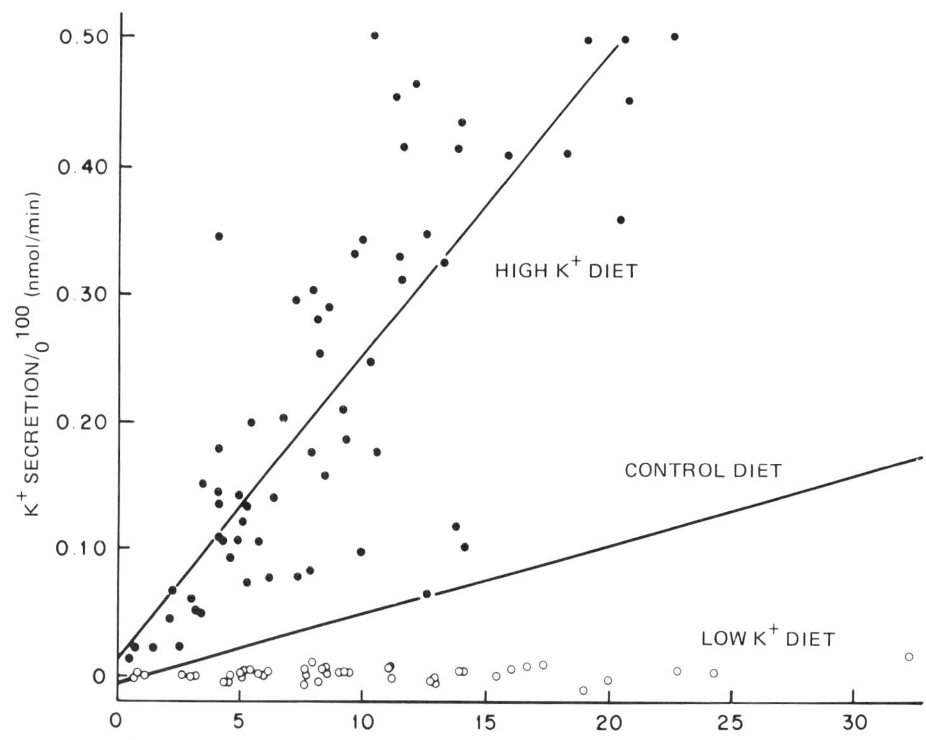

Figure 10 Relationship between distal tubular flow rate and potassium secretion. (From Ref. 27.)

Figure 10 summarizes the effects of augmenting distal tubular flow rate upon the secretion of potassium ions. The increase in flow rate along the distal tubule was achieved by progressive expansion of the extracellular fluid compartment by the infusion of isotonic saline (27). With enhanced delivery of fluid into the distal tubule, potassium secretion increased without reaching a transport maximum. However, for a given enhancement of distal tubular flow rate, the stimulation of potassium secretion was dependent on the dietary potassium content, and increased with a high-potassium diet.

Several diuretic agents increase potassium secretion by delivery of an increased fraction of the glomerular filtrate into the distal tubule (12). Such diuretics include mannitol, carbonic anhydrase inhibitors, loop diuretics such as furosemide, ethacrynic acid, and mercurials, and thiazide diuretics. Common to all of these is a site of action upstream of the late distal tubule (12).

The effect of mineralo- and glucocorticoids upon renal tubular potassium transport is also significantly modified by flow-related phenomena (9). Figure 11 summarizes the results of recent studies that addressed this problem by comparing the effects of several

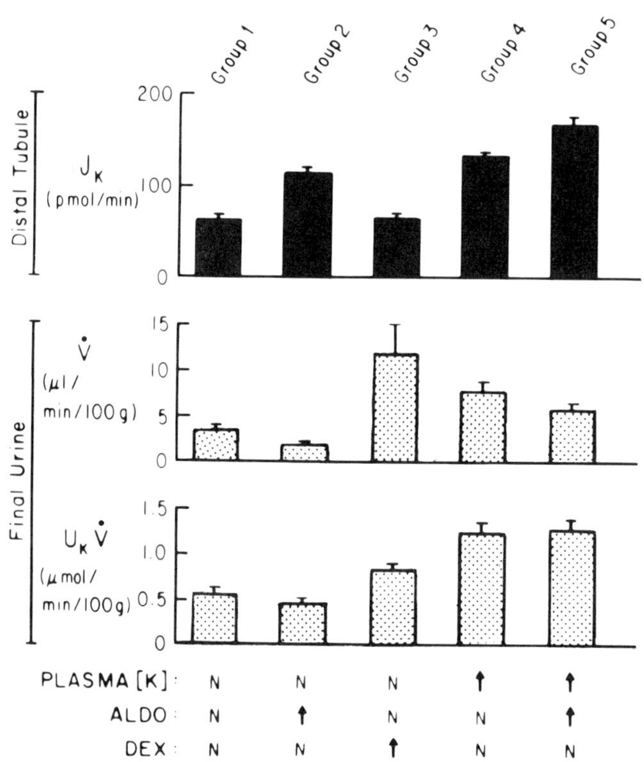

Figure 11 Comparison of distal tubular potassium secretion (J_K), urinary flow rate ($\dot{V}$), and urinary potassium excretion ($U_K \dot{V}$) during different hormone treatments. Potassium secretion by single distal tubules (J_K) was measured by microperfusion in vivo at a constant rate. Adrenalectomized rats were given basal replacement dosages of either aldosterone or dexamethasone, resulting in "normal" (*N*) hormone levels. Aldosterone or dexamethasone (or vehicle only) were infused acutely, resulting in elevated (↑) levels in the hormone. Plasma potassium was either "normal" (N), or elevated (↑) by acute KCl infusion. (From Ref. 9.)

variables upon the rate of *distal* tubular potassium secretion (J_K), when care was taken to keep distal tubular flow rate constant by pump perfusion (9). In the same series of experiments, urinary flow rate (V) and urinary potassium excretion ($U_K V$) were also evaluated. Experiments were done in "hormone-clamped" animals that were first adrenalectomized and then received either aldosterone on dexamethasone by osmotic minipumps for 1 week. In additional experiments, the plasma potassium level was also raised.

Several conclusions can be drawn from these experiments. Considering the effect of selectively increasing the plasma aldosterone level, it is apparent that distal tubular potassium secretion is markedly increased. However, urinary potassium excretion failed to be augmented. This can best be explained by the concurrent effect of aldosterone administration upon urine flow rate which was sharply reduced. Since urinary flow rate can safely be taken as a reasonable measure of distal flow rate, we conclude that the latter was reduced following stimulation of distal tubular sodium transport by aldosterone. In this experimental setting in which urine sodium output was initially quite low, the powerful effect of aldosterone upon flow rate thus opposes the direct stimulating effect of aldosterone upon distal tubular potassium transport.

The extent to which aldosterone affects kaliuresis depends strongly upon distal tubular flow rate. The latter is affected by the delivery of fluid into the distal tubule (see above). A high salt intake, infusion of sodium chloride, administration of diuretics, and expansion of the extracellular fluid volume all render the distal tubular secretory mechanism of potassium more sensitive to the action of aldosterone.

In contrast to these variable acute effects of aldosterone, chornic aldosterone administration usually stimulates potassium excretion. This is most likely due to a sequence of events that includes high aldosterone at a time of extracellular volume expansion, diminished proximal sodium and fluid reabsorption, and increased delivery of fluid into the distal tubule. Thus, variations in distal tubular flow rate are responsible for the great variability of kaliuresis that has been observed following administration of aldosterone.

Figure 11 also summarizes the effects of selectively increasing the level of the glucocorticoid dexamethasone. It is apparent that this hormone treatment does not directly affect distal tubular potassium secretion (J_K) when care is taken to keep tubular flow rate constant by microperfusion. Nevertheless, urinary excretion of potassium is sharply enhanced, an effect that coincides with the sharp increase in urine flow rate. Glucocorticoids are known to increase glomerular filtration rate and to decrease the distal tubular water permeability (21), factors that increase distal and urinary flow rate. The kaliuretic effect of glucocorticoids in low physiological dosages is thus not "direct" but due to high distal tubular flow rate (9). Through this effect, glucocorticoids play an important role in potassium homeostasis: they determine the sensitivity to "direct" distal stimuli by their potent modulation of the rate of flow past the site of potassium secretion.

Finally, Figure 11 demonstrates that acutely raising the plasma potassium concentration stimulates potassium excretion in the absence of changes of the aldosterone level (9). This effect is due to a direct effect on distal secretion (J_K) and on urine flow (V). Raising aldosterone acutely under these conditions (last column in Fig. 11) does not further increase potassium secretion. Again, the coincident fall in urinary flow rate may limit the display of the kaliuretic action of aldosterone action.

Figures 12 and 13 show how interaction of direct and flow-related effects on potassium excretion may serve to stabilize urinary potassium excretion during physiological fluctuations of water and sodium uptake.

Figure 12 provides evidence obtained from microperfusion studies in Brattleboro rats which are congenitally deficient in vasopressin (8). Distal tubules were microperfused in

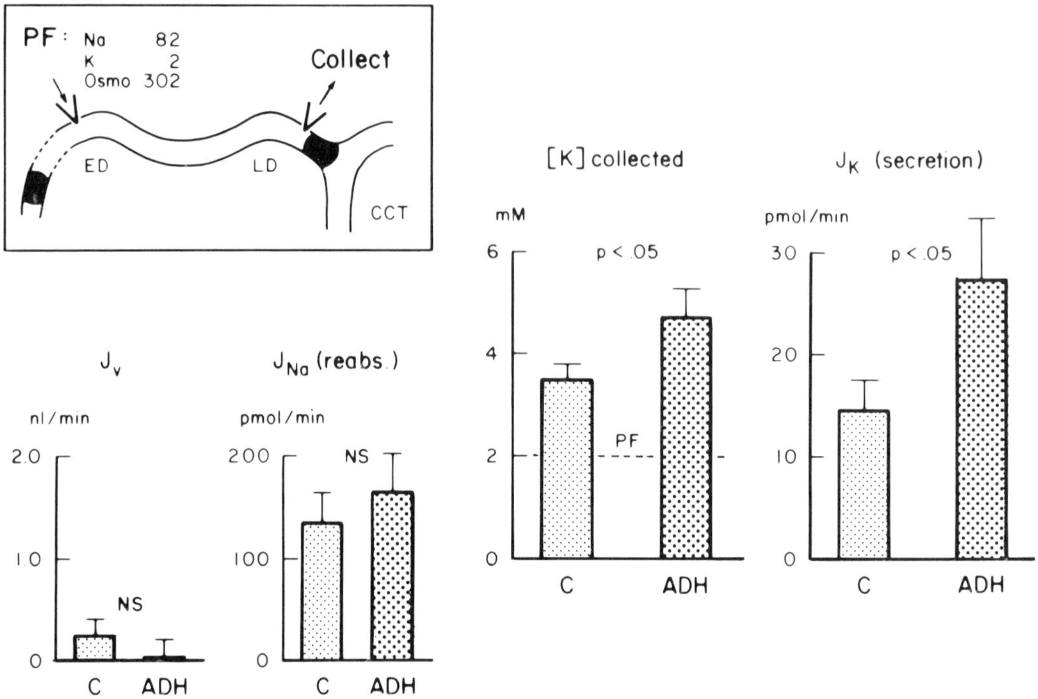

Figure 12 Microperfusion study of distal tubules in vasopressin-deficient (Brattleboro) rat. Left upper panel: Schematic presentation of microperfusion set-up. PF, perfusion fluid; ED, early distal; LD, late distal; CCT, cortical collecting tubule. Left lower panel: Absence of significant changes in fluid (J_V) and sodium (J_{Na}) transport following acute ADH. Right panel: Stimulation of distal potassium secretion (J_K) by ADH. (From Ref. 9.)

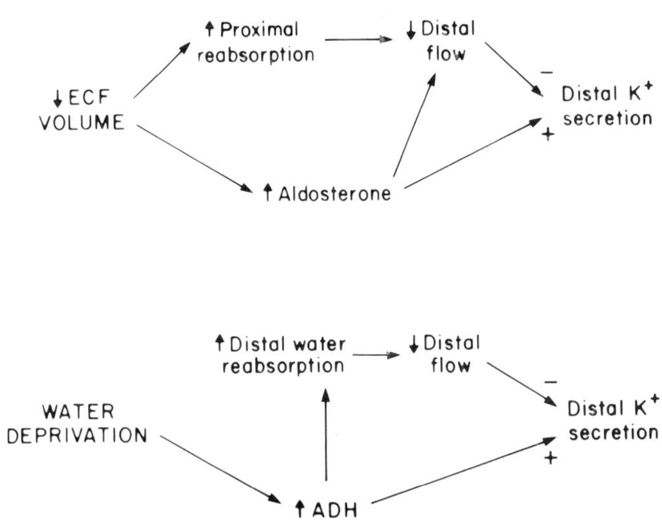

Figure 13 Interaction of factors regulating potassium excretion by the distal tubule during reduction of extracellular fluid (top) and water deprivation (bottom). (From Ref. 10.)

vivo at constant rate using isotonic solutions that would minimize changes in fluid movement following the systemic administration of vasopressin. Potassium transport in the distal tubule could thus be studied at constant flow rate. It is apparent that ADH had a direct stimulatory effect on distal potassium secretion as evidenced by the increase of potassium concentration in the collected perfusate and the similarly increased J_K. Supportive evidence for stimulation of potassium secretion in the thick ascending limb of Henle's loop (19) and the cortical collecting tubule of rats (Troutman and Schafer, personal communication) is also available. Vasopressin probably directly activates a potassium channel in the luminal membrane.

The described action of vasopressin (ADH) may have implications for the maintenance of potassium homeostasis during different states of water balance. Two mechanisms affecting potassium secretion along the distal tubule are activated following ADH release. The reduction in flow rate along the distal tubule following ADH release during hydropenia would tend to decrease potassium secretion. On the other hand, the direct effect of ADH on the distal tubule is to stimulate the secretory mechanism (see above). These opposing effects, summarized in Figure 13, may account for the finding that minimal alterations in potassium excretion are observed during water deprivation. Failure of potassium excretion to increase during water diuresis may again be a consequence of the interaction of two opposing factors: urine flow rate is high but ADH levels are low.

Pathophysiological implications of the direct stimulation by vasopressin of renal potassium secretion can also be documented. Potassium loss and hypokalemia are occasionally observed in the syndrome of inappropriate ADH secretion, a state of chronically elevated ADH levels (2). There are also reports of improvement of potassium tolerance by administration of vasopressin (20). Finally, loop diuretics may induce potassium loss, in addition to their direct tubular effects, also by acute stimulation of ADH release. This conclusion is based on the recent observation that the acute kaliuresis following furosemide administration is reduced if the diuretic is given during a water load rather than during water deprivation (26).

Figure 13 also depicts the possible sequence of events that dissociates, at least partially, the flow-induced fall of urinary potassium excretion following contraction of the extracellular fluid compartment. The key factors here involve the opposing effects of distal flow rate (low) and aldosterone levels (high) that tend to stabilize the rate of distal and urinary potassium excretion.

Direct and flow-related effects may also be additive. We already have mentioned acute hyperkalemia, in which the high plasma potassium level stimulates distal potassium secretion directly when urine flow rate is high (9). Another disturbance is that of metabolic alkalosis. When care is taken in distal microperfusion experiments to maintain constant flow rate, induction of systemic metabolic alkalosis stimulates distal tubular potassium secretion. At the same time, diminished fluid reabsorption along the thick ascending limb of Henle's loop due to high luminal bicarbonate levels and a low chloride concentration leads to increased fluid delivery, which is a potent factor that further stimulates potassium loss.

Finally, the kaliuretic effect of aldosterone will be enhanced when the rate of delivery of fluid to the potassium secretory system in the distal nephron is abnormally high. Thus, potassium loss following administration of diuretics is strongly affected by the state of the renin-angiotensin-aldosterone system, with potentiation of potassium loss by high aldosterone levels. Increased levels of aldosterone commonly associated with disorders of extracellular volume distribution (cardiac failure, nephrotic syndrome, cirrhosis) and a low salt intake are known to aggravate the loss of potassium following increased distal tubular flow rate that results from administration of diuretics.

ACKNOWLEDGMENT

Work in the author's laboratory was supported by NIH grant AM-17433.

REFERENCES

1. Adler, S. F. and Fraley, D.: Potassium and intracellular pH. *Kidney Int.* 11:433–442, 1977.
2. Bartter, F. C., and Schwartz, W. B.: The syndrome of inappropriate secretion of antidiuretic hormone. *Am. J. Med.* 42:790–806, 1967.
3. Berliner, R. W.: Renal mechanism for potassium excretion. *Harvey Lecture* 55:141–171, 1961.
4. Bia, M. J., and De Fronzo, R. A.: Extrarenal potassium homeostasis. *Am. J. Physiol.* 240:F257–F268, 1981.
5. Bomsztyk, K., and Wright, F. S.: Effects of transepithelial fluid flux on transepithelial voltage and transport of calcium, sodium, chloride and potassium by renal proximal tubule. *Kidney Int.* 21:269, 1982.
6. Cemerikic, D. A., Wilcox, C. S., and Giebisch, G.: Intracellular potential and K^+ activity in rat kidney proximal tubular cells in acidosis and K depletion. *J. Membrane Biol.* 69:159–165, 1982.
7. Edelman, A., Curci, S., Samazija, I., and Frömter, E.: Determination of intracellular K^+ activity in rat kidney proximal tubular cells. *Pflügers Arch.* 378:37–46, 1978.
8. Field, M. J., Stanton, B. A., and Giebisch, G.: Influence of ADH on renal potassium handling: a micropuncture and microfusion study. *Kidney Int.* 25:502–511, 1984.
9. Field, M. J., Stanton, B. A., and Giebisch, G.: Differential acute effects of aldosterone, dexamethasone and hyperkalemia on distal tubular potassium secretion in the rat kidney. *J. Clin. Invest.* 74:1792–1802, 1984.
10. Field, M. J., Berliner, R. W., and Giebisch, G.: Regulation of renal potassium metabolism. In *Clinical Disorders of Fluid and Electrolyte Metabolism*, edited by Maxwell, M., Kleeman, C., and Narins, R. G., New York, McGraw Hill, 1985, in press.
11. Garcia-Filho, E., Malnic, G., and Giebisch, G.: Effects of changes in electrical potential difference on tubular potassium transport. *Am. J. Physiol.* 238:F235–F246.
12. Giebisch, G.: Effects of diuretics on renal transport of potassium. In *Methods in Pharmacology*, Vol. 4A, edited by Martinez-Maldonado, M., New York, Plenum, 1976.
13. Giebisch, G.: Renal potassium transport. In *Membrane Transport in Biology*, Vol. IVA, edited by Giebisch, G., Tosteson, D. C., and Ussing, H. H., New York, Springer-Verlag, 1978, p. 215.
14. Giebisch, G., Malnic, G., and Berliner, R. W.: Renal transport and control of potassium excretion. In *The Kidney*, 2nd edition, edited by Brenner, B. M., and Rector, F. C., Jr., Philadelphia, W. B. Saunders, 1981, p. 408.
15. Good, D. W., Velázquez, H., and Wright, F. S.: Luminal influences on potassium secretion: low sodium concentration. *Am. J. Physiol.* 246:F609–F619, 1984.
16. Grantham, J. J., Burg, M. B., and Orloff, J.: The nature of transtubular Na and K transport in isolated rabbit collecting tubules. *J. Clin. Invest.* 49:1815–1826, 1970.
17. Greger, R., and Schlatter, E.: Properties of the basolateral membrane of the cortical thick ascending limb of Henle's loop of rabbit kidney. A model for secondary active chloride transport. *Pflügers Arch.* 396:325–334, 1983.

18. Greger, R., and Schlatter, E.: Presence of luminal K^+, a prerequisite for active NaCl transport in the cortical thick ascending limb of Henle's loop of rabbit kidney. *Pflügers Arch.* 392:92–94, 1981.
19. Hebert, S., and Andreoli, T.: Control of NaCl transport in the thick ascending limb. *Am. J. Physiol.* 246:F745–F756, 1984.
20. Hiatt, N., Miller, A., and Katayansgi, T.: Kaliuresis and diuresis after administration of antidiurestic hormone to hyperkalemic dogs. *Am. J. Physiol.* 228:1108–1112, 1975.
21. Hierholzer, K., and Lange, S.: The effects of adrenal steroids on renal function. In *MTP International Review of Science, Series I, Vol. 6, Kidney and Urinary Tract Physiology*, edited by K. Thurau, London, Baltimore, Butterworth–University Park Press, 1974, pp. 273–334.
22. Hunter, M., Lopes, A. G., Boulpaep, E. L., and Giebisch, G.: Single channel recordings of potassium-selective channels from cortical collecting tubule of rabbit. *Natl. Acad. Sci. USA* 81:4237–4239, 1984.
23. Jamison, R., Work, J., and Schafer, J.: New pathways for potassium transport in the kidney. *Am. J. Physiol.* 242:F297–F312, 1982.
24. Kaissling, B.: Structural aspects of adaptive changes in renal electrolyte excretion. *Am. J. Physiol.* 243:F211–F226, 1983.
25. Katz, A. I., Doucet, A., and Morel, F.: Na-K-ATPase activity along the rabbit, rat and mouse nephron. *Am. J. Physiol.* 237:F114–F120, 1979.
26. Kelly, R. A., Wilcos, C. S., Souney, P., and Mitch, W. E.: Effect of aldosterone and ADH on potassium excretion with furosemide. *Kidney Int.* 25:169, 1984.
27. Khuri, R. N., Strieder, N., Wiederholt, M., and Giebisch, G.: The effects of flow rate and potassium intake on distal tubular potassium transfer. *Am. J. Physiol.* 228: 1249–1261, 1975.
28. Koeppen, B. M., Biagi, B. A., and Giebisch, G.: Intracellular microelectrode characterization of the rabbit cortical collecting duct. *Am. J. Physiol.* 244:F35–F47, 1983.
29. Kuffler, S. W., Nichols, J. G., and Martin, A. R.: *From Neuron to Brain*, 2nd ed., Sunderland, Mass, Sinauer Associates, 1984.
30. Macknight, A. D. C., and Leaf, A.: Regulation of cellular volume. In *Physiology of Membrane Disorders*, edited by Andreoli, T. E., Hoffman, J. F., and Fanestil, D. D., New York, Plenum, 1978, p. 315.
31. Matsumura, Y., Cohen, B., Guggino, W. B., and Giebisch, G.: Regulation of the basolateral potassium conductance of the *Necturus* proximal tubule. *J. Membrane Biol.* 79:153–161, 1984.
32. Mudge, G. H., Ames, A., Foulks, J., and Gilman, A.: Effects of drugs on renal secretion of potassium in the dog. *Am. J. Physiol.* 161:151–158, 1950.
33. Oberleithner, H., Guggino, W., and Giebisch, G.: Potassium transport in the early distal tubule of Amphiuma. Effects of potassium adaptation. *Pflügers Arch.* 396: 185–191, 1983.
34. O'Neil, R., and Boulpaep, E.: Effect of amiloride on the apical cell membrane cation channels of a sodium-absorbing, potassium-secreting renal epithelium. *J. Membrane Biol.* 50:365–387, 1979.
35. O'Neil, R. G.: Potassium secretion by the cortical collecting tubule. *Fed. Proc.* 40: 2403–2407, 1981.
36. O'Neil, R. G.: Voltage-dependent interaction of barium and cesium with the potassium conductance of the cortical collecting duct apical cell membrane. *J. Membrane Biol.* 74:165, 1983.
37. O'Neil, R. G., and Sansom, S. C.: Characterization of apical membrane Na^+ and K^+ conductances of cortical collecting duct using microelectrode techniques. *Am. J. Physiol.* 247:F14–F24, 1984.
38. Rosa, R., Silva, P., Young, J., Landsberg, L., Brown, R., Rowe, J., and Epstein, F.:

Adrenergic modulation of extrarenal potassium disposal. *N. Engl. J. Med.* 302:431–434, 1980.
39. Sackin, H., and Boulpaep, E. L.: Rheogenic transport in the renal proximal tubule. *J. Gen. Physiol.* 82:819–851, 1983.
40. Sansom, S. C., and O'Neil, R. G.: Effects of mineralocorticoids on cellular conductive properties of the cortical collecting duct. *Fed. Proc.* 43:302, 1984.
41. Schultz, S. G.: Homocellular regulatory mechanisms in sodium-transporting epithelia: an extension of the Koefoed-Johnsen-Ussing model. In *Seminars in Nephrology*, Vol. II, edited by Kurtzman, N., New York, Grune and Stratton, 1982, pp. 343–347.
42. Stanton, B. A., Biemesderfer, D., Wade, J. B., and Giebisch, G.: Structural and functional study of the rat distal nephron: effects of potassium adaptation and depletion. *Kidney Int.* 19:36–48, 1981.
43. Stanton, B. A., and Giebisch, G.: Regulation of potassium homeostasis. In *Functional Regulation at the Cellular and Molecular Levels*, edited by R. A. Corradino, New York, Elsevier-North Holland, 1982, p. 259.
44. Stanton, B. A., Guggino, W. B., and Giebisch, G.: Acidification of the basolateral solution reduces potassium conductance of the apical membrane. *Fed. Proc.* 41:1006, 1982.
45. Stanton, B. A.: Role of adrenal hormones in regulating distal nephron structural and ion transport. *Fed. Proc.* 1985, in press.
46. Stetson, D., Wade, J., and Giebisch, G.: Morphological alterations in the rat medullary collecting duct following K^+ depletion. *Kidney Int.* 17:45–56, 1980.
47. Stokes, J. B.: Ion transport by the cortical and outer medullary collecting tubule. *Kidney Int.* 22:473–484, 1982.
48. Velazquez, H., Wright, F. S., and Good, D. W.: Luminal influences on potassium secretion: chloride replacement with sulfate. *Am. J. Physiol.* 242:F46–F55, 1982.

2

The Role of Magnesium in Potassium Deficiency

MICHAEL P. RYAN
University College Dublin, Blackrock, County Dublin, Ireland

The extracellular and intracellular compartments differ greatly in their ionic composition, especially with respect to sodium, chloride, calcium, potassium, and magnesium. Sodium, chloride, and calcium are found in much higher concentrations in the extracellular compartments, while potassium and magnesium are in much higher concentrations in the intracellular compartments. Magnesium is second only to potassium as the main intracellular cation. Evidence accumulated in the literature indicates close interrelationships in the metabolism of magnesium and potassium. In particular, evidence from both experimental animal studies and clinical observations shows that magnesium may play a very important role in potassium metabolism.

In this chapter, I will review the experimental and clinical evidence from my own laboratory and from others which support the following statements concerning the role of magnesium during potassium deficiency.

1. Magnesium deficiency results in decreased cell potassium.
2. Combined magnesium and potassium deficiencies result in greater loss of cell potassium than occur in simple potassium deficiency.
3. Uncorrected coexisting magnesium deficiency impairs repletion of cell potassium.

EXPERIMENTAL OBSERVATIONS

Magnesium Deficiency Results in Decreased Cell Potassium

Dietary restriction of magnesium in the rat has been the most widely used model of magnesium deficiency. Since Cotlove et al. (22) first detected in 1951 a significant loss of skeletal muscle potassium in magnesium-deficient rats, many workers (36,46,57,75,79,81, 139) have confirmed that magnesium deficiency results in loss of skeletal muscle potassium in rats. Loss of cell potassium has also been reported in cardiac tissue (81,97,112) and renal medulla (79) in rats. Reduced muscle potassium content during magnesium deficiency has also been shown in guinea pigs (51) and rabbits (1).

Table 1 Effect of Magnesium Deficiency on Cell Potassium in Ascites Tumor Cells Grown in vivo in Mice

Mice	Potassium (m mol/L cell H_2O)
Control (n = 7)	138 ± 3.0
Magnesium-deficient (n = 9)	112 ± 7.6
P value	<0.01

Source: Data from Ref. 104.

Many cell types appear to require magnesium for maintenance of normal cell potassium. Table 1 shows results from an in vivo experiment comparing the ability of ascites tumor cells to grow and maintain potassium levels in control mice and in magnesium-deficient mice (104). As can be seen in Table 1, there was a significant reduction in potassium in the ascites tumor cells taken from magnesium-deficient mice. Gunther et al. (55) reported that fetuses from pregnant rats fed magnesium-deficient diets had greatly reduced potassium and increased sodium contents. The cell potassium loss during magnesium deficiency is usually accompanied by a slight decrease in magnesium concentration and an increase in sodium and calcium concentrations. We have identified such electrolyte alterations in peripheral blood lymphocytes taken from magnesium-deficient rats (97). It is also interesting to note that cardiac muscle showed much more calcification than skeletal muscle during magnesium deficiency in rats (102).

Combined Magnesium and Potassium Deficiencies Result in Greater Losses of Cell Potassium than Occur in Simple Potassium Deficiency

Whang and Welt (139) first demonstrated that during potassium deficiency, the presence of coexisting magnesium deficiency accentuates the losses of potassium from skeletal muscle. We later (105) confirmed this finding for skeletal muscle and demonstrated that the same principle applied to cardiac muscle. The comparison of the effects of potassium deficiency and of coexisting magnesium and potassium deficiency on skeletal and cardiac muscle potassium is shown in Table 2.

Uncorrected Coexisting Magnesium Deficiency Impairs Repletion of Cell Potassium

Magnesium also plays a role in restoring potassium loss from skeletal muscle cells. Figure 1 shows results of an experiment by Ryan and Hingerty (99) which compared restoration

Table 2 Effect of Coexisting Magnesium Deficiency on Skeletal Muscle and Cardiac Muscle Potassium

	Muscle potassium (mmol/100g FFDS)	
	Skeletal	Cardiac
Potassium-deficient (n = 7)	38.3 ± 2.8	32.5 ± 0.9
Potassium- and magnesium-deficient (n = 5)	32.6 ± 1.7	30.9 ± 0.9
P value	< 0.005	< 0.01

Source: Data from Ref. 105.

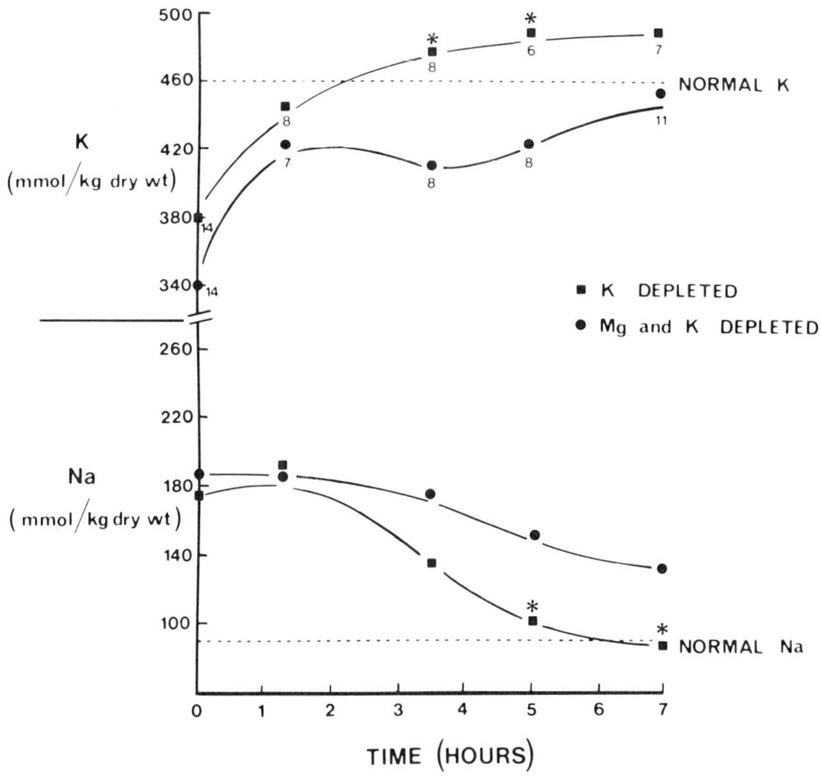

Figure 1 Comparison of skeletal muscle potassium and sodium restoration rates following intraperitoneal injection of KCl to potassium-depleted (■) and magnesium- and potassium-depleted (●) rats. (Data from Ref. 99.)

rates of rat muscle potassium and sodium in potassium-depleted rats and in combined magnesium- and potassium-depleted rats following intraperitoneal injection of KCl. It can be clearly seen from results shown in Figure 1 that within a few hours after intraperitoneal injection of KCl the potassium-depleted group had restored muscle potassium to normal values. While the extrusion of sodium was a slower process, the potassium-depleted group had restored muscle sodium to normal values by about 7 hr. In marked contrast, the combined magnesium- and potassium-depleted group did not restore either muscle potassium or sodium values after intraperitoneal injection of KCl. Whang et al. (134) reported that continuing magnesium deficiency retarded muscle potassium repletion following attempts to replete potassium by administration of oral KCl in rats.

Possible Mechanisms for Effects of Magnesium Deficiency on Cell Potassium

Indirect Effects

The mechanism(s) involved in the effects of magnesium deficiency on cell potassium have not been fully elucidated. A number of possibilities exist and are listed in Table 3.

Increased aldosterone secretion in magnesium-depleted rats has been reported (19,35). It has been suggested that this may account for the negative potassium balance in

Table 3 Possible Mechanisms for Effects of Magnesium Deficiency on Potassium Metabolism

Secondary effects
Alterations in renin–angiotensin–aldosterone system
Renal leakage of potassium
Associated electrolyte abnormalities, such as increased intracellular calcium
Direct effects
Increased membrane fluidity resulting in leaky membranes
Alteration of Na-K-ATPase activity
Impaired energy production

magnesium-deficient rats (47). While increased kaliuresis (137,139) has been reported in magnesium-depleted rats, this may reflect an "overflow" phenomenon due to the cells' inability to maintain normal potassium concentrations during magnesium deficiency. Carney et al. (20) used micropuncture techniques to investigate the effect of magnesium deficiency on renal tubular potassium transport in the rat. They found dietary magnesium restriction that reduced total-body magnesium by 30% did not alter renal potassium excretion despite a 10% reduction in total body potassium. These authors' conclusion supported Whang and Welt's hypothesis (139) that a reduction in cell potassium during magnesium deficiency in the presence of normal plasma potassium levels is a reflection of the cells' inability to maintain an appropriate potassium gradient.

Associated electrolyte abnormalities during magnesium deficiency in the rat include hypercalcemia (139) and increased muscle calcium (102,142). Hypercalcemia (39,40) and increased cell calcium (28,118) could result in potassium deficiency and interest has recently been shown in calcium-activated potassium channels in many cell systems.

Ryan and McKenna (100) studied the accumulation of cesium by tissues of magnesium-deficient rats. Cesium can compete with potassium for carrier sites but diffuses out of cells much more slowly than potassium through permeability channels. The finding of reduced cesium concentrations in red blood cells and soleus muscle of magnesium-deficient rats with similar plasma cesium concentrations in both the control and magnesium deficient group suggests a direct effect of magnesium deficiency on active potassium transport.

Direct Effects

Evidence from a number of in vitro systems indicates that lack of magnesium per se has an effect on ion transport. Some of the main systems investigated are listed in Table 4. Whang and Welt (139) demonstrated that in vitro perfusion of rat diaphragms with magnesium-free perfusate resulted in diminished muscle potassium. Arnold and Ryan (2) confirmed earlier in vivo findings of magnesium requirement for cellular potassium repletion, in demonstrating that isolated rat soleus muscle was unable to replete cell potassium in high-potassium-containing medium in the absence of magnesium. Work on ascites tumor cells in vitro has also confirmed a magnesium requirement for maintenance of cell potassium. Gunther (53) has discussed these findings in a broad review of the biochemistry and pathobiochemistry of magnesium. The possible mechanism for a direct effect of magnesium on cell potassium is shown in Table 3. Figure 2 illustrates the possible effects of magnesium on membrane potassium transport.

Table 4 Evidence from in vitro Studies Suggesting that Magnesium per se has an Effect on Ion Transport

In vitro system	Investigators	Reference
Rat diaphragm	Whang and Welt, 1963	139
Rat liver slices	Eshove and Van Rossum, 1963	38
Rat soleus muscle	Arnold and Ryan, 1973	2
E. coli	Gunther and Marisz, 1968	56
Ascites tumor cells	Gunther and Averdunk, 1970	54
Ascites tumor cells	Schilling et al., 1980	108
Rat interventricular septa	Shine and Douglas, 1974	116
Rabbit ventricle	Shine and Douglas, 1975	117
Human erythrocytes	Welt, 1964	132
	Dunn, 1974	29
	Flatman and Lew, 1979	41
	Flatman and Lew, 1983	42
	Ellory et al., 1983	37
Rabbit kidney Na-K-ATPase	Bonting et al., 1983	9
Barnacle muscle	Bittar and Chambers, 1984	8
Rabbit terminal ileum	Booth et al., 1984	12

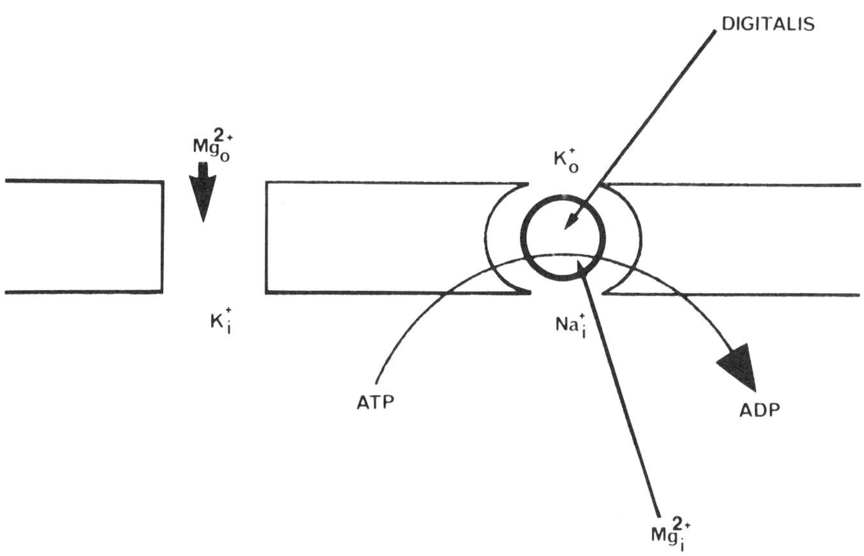

Figure 2 Schematic representation of a cell membrane shows possible sites of action of magnesium on potassium transport.

Binding of divalent cations to negatively charged groups (glycoproteins and/or phospholipids) decreases their mobility within the membrane and thus induces structural change. This results in decreased membrane fluidity and produces changes in electrokinetic behavior usually referred to as the zeta potential (110). Lack of magnesium could therefore have profound effects on membranes leading to loss of cell potassium. Schilling (108) showed that magnesium altered the surface (zeta) potential of ascites tumor cells and that resulted in altered cell potassium. Shine and Douglas (116) demonstrated that increased extracellular magnesium abruptly decreased ^{42}K efflux from isolated blood-perfused rat interventricular septa. In another publication the same authors (117) demonstrated that raising extracellular magnesium to 10 mmol could decrease the net ^{42}K loss induced by acetyl strophanthidin in rabbit septa without altering the depressed influx of ^{42}K produced by the glycoside. Shine (115) suggested that the effect of magnesium in reducing cell potassium losses during digitalis treatment arises from a direct effect of magnesium on potassium channels in the sarcolemmal membrane.

Magnesium has been established as an absolute requirement for the Na-K-ATPase or sodium pump as recently reviewed by Bonting et al. (9). Flatman and Lew (41) have produced evidence in intact human red blood cells that, at magnesium concentrations around the physiological range (10^{-4} - 10^{-3} mol/L), sodium/sodium exchange stays constant whereas sodium/potassium exchange increased linearly with increasing intracellular magnesium concentration. Ellory et al. (37) have recently clearly demonstrated that human red cell sodium and potassium transport is affected by altering magnesium concentrations. Magnesium was shown to have effects on the ouabain-sensitive (Na-K-ATPase component), the bumetanide-sensitive (Na-K co-transport), and residual (ouabain- and bumetanide-insensitive) routes of transport in human red blood cells (37).

CLINICAL OBSERVATIONS

Human Magnesium Depletion Results in Disturbed Potassium Metabolism

A number of investigators (30,58,95,114) have specifically investigated the effects of magnesium depletion on potassium metabolism in human subjects. Petersen (95) demonstrated reduced exchangeable potassium and magnesium in malabsorption and that correction of the magnesium in malabsorption and that correction of the magnesium deficiency resulted in enhanced potassium repletion. Dunn and Walser (30) demonstrated hypokalemia, alkalosis, and reduced muscle potassium content in a normal volunteer subjected to dietary magnesium restriction. Haijamae and MacDowell (58) investigated the distribution of magnesium, potassium, sodium, and calcium in the extracellular and intracellular compartments during magnesium depletion in primary hypomagnesemia in infancy. An interruption of magnesium substitution resulted in hypomagnesemia, hypokalemia, and hypocalcemia while intracellular potassium decreased and intracellular sodium increased. The most convincing evidence that magnesium depletion in human subjects produces disturbed potassium metabolism was produced by the report of Shils (114). He studied patients who had undergone radical surgery of the head and neck for treatment of carcinoma. Patients were fed magnesium-deficient diets via nasoesophageal tube. Magnesium depletion resulted in hypomagnesemia, hypocalcemia, and reduced total exchangeable potassium. Provision of additional KCl did not correct the hypokalemia or the reduced total exchangeable potassium. Magnesium repletion did, however, restore plasma and total ex-

Table 5 Clinical Conditions Associated with Concurrent Magnesium and Potassium Depletion

Gastrointestinal
Malnutrition
Malabsorption
Diarrhea
Primary hypomagnesemia
IV therapy without magnesium supplementation
Renal losses
Drug-induced: Diuretics, especially loop-blocking, gentamicin, cisplatin, alcohol
Postobstruction diuresis
Primary magnesium wasting
Aldosteronism

changeable potassium to normal levels even though the amount of potassium ingested was the same as during the period of magnesium depletion.

Clinical Conditions Associated with Concurrent Magnesium and Potassium Depletion

Both magnesium and potassium are usually acquired by absorption mainly from the upper gastrointestinal tract (77). Usually about 30% of ingested magnesium is absorbed, as documented by Parfitt and Kleerekoper (92). Both cations are primarily excreted by the kidneys and therefore these organs are extremely important in maintaining magnesium and potassium homeostasis. Table 5 lists some clinical conditions associated with concomitant magnesium and potassium depletion.

Deficiencies Associated with Gastrointestinal Tract Problems

In the presence of malabsorption, deficiencies of both magnesium and potassium have been demonstrated (4,10,76). Correction of the magnesium deficiency during malabsorption resulted in enhanced potassium repletion (95). Primary hypomagnesemia, or malabsorption of magnesium without other evidence of intestinal disease may also occur and is associated with other electrolyte disturbances especially hypocalcemia in infancy (49,90, 93,119, 122).

Postoperative patients who are maintained on intravenous therapy in the presence of extrarenal losses of magnesium and potassium, primarily gastrointestinal losses, are another group at risk for coexisting magnesium and potassium deficiencies (7,107). Patients with protein-calorie malnutrition have been shown to be deficient in both magnesium and potassium (18,89). Subsequent studies have suggested that supplemental magnesium significantly improves clinical response (16,17). Lim and Jacob (72) studied magnesium levels in tissues of seven patients with chronic diarrhea. Six patients were found to have reduced skeletal muscle magnesium and skeletal muscle potassium levels were low in four patients. Magnesium therapy alone restored skeletal potassium to normal in the two patients in whom this was reestimated.

In a study of the relationship between plasma and erythrocyte magnesium and potassium concentrations in obese subjects during 18-day fasts, Stewart and Fleming (121) reported that erythrocyte potassium concentration was decreased by between 5 and 9% in those patients who had a decreased plasma magnesium concentration. However, erythrocyte potassium levels did not fall in subjects who were given magnesium supplements. These workers interpreted their findings as indicating a possible effect of extracellular magnesium or some other correlate of magnesium supplementation on potassium distribution and transport between extracellular and intracellular compartments.

Deficiencies Associated with Renal Problems

Although Lim and Jacob (71) reported significantly reduced muscle magnesium in patients with chronic uremia, other workers (21,82) found normal or increased muscle magnesium values in such patients. Stewart and Fleming (120) studied the effect of varying dialysate magnesium concentrations on plasma and red blood cell magnesium and potassium concentrations during maintenance hemodialysis. These authors indicated that low-magnesium dialysis had advantages: it corrected hypermagnesemia and reduced red blood cell potassium to more normal values. This is further evidence for an effect of magnesium on potassium transport. However, red blood cell potassium may not be a good index of general cell potassium in patients with chronic renal failure (127).

Transient severe hypomagnesemia has been reported during the massive diuresis that sometimes follows relief of urinary tract obstruction or renal transplantation (83). Renal tubular acidosis may also cause magnesium deficiency (44). During the diuretic phase of acute tubular necrosis, marked loss of magnesium can occur in the urine and symptomatic magnesium deficiency may occur (44).

Intrinsic defects in the reabsorption of magnesium have been reported by several investigators (11,48,50,88,94,96). It is noteworthy that hypokalemia was usually an accompanying feature of this disorder. Hypomagnesemia also occurs in Bartter's syndrome (124).

Tubular dysfunction resulting in large urinary losses of magnesium has been produced by administration of gentamicin and other antibiotics (5,61,129,130). Cisplatin also causes tubular damage resulting in loss of magnesium (109). Again, in these situations, potassium disturbances usually accompany the renal magnesium wasting.

It is well established that alcohol enhances the urinary excretion of magnesium; the diminished intake of food by alcoholic patients is also an important factor contributing to depletion of both magnesium and potassium (43,45). Hypomagnesemia (in 60%) and hypokalemia (in 30%) have been reported in a series of 44 patients entering the hospital with acute alcoholism (80). Flink has reviewed the evidence establishing magnesium deficiency in this condition (44). Muscle biopsy specimens have shown coexisting magnesium and potassium deficiencies (67,70). The possibility therefore exists that intracellular potassium depletion in alcoholic patients may be contributed to by coexisting magnesium deficiency. Whang et al. (135) have shown that some alcoholic patients present with refractory potassium depletion in the presence of coexisting magnesium depletion. After magnesium replacement therapy, both the hypomagmesemia and hypokalemia were corrected.

Both magnesium and potassium are affected by aldosteronism. Increased urinary losses of these cations in primary hyperaldosteronism may account in many cases for the coexisting magnesium and potassium depletion (62,78). Some studies indicate that aldosterone does not have a direct effect on magnesium reabsorption but that sodium-linked magnesium reabsorption is reduced in the proximal tubule and Henle's loop by the chronic extracellular fluid volume expansion seen in hyperaldosteronism (83). Urinary magnesium excretion was reduced by spironolactone in patients with aldosteronism

(62,73). However, these were unlikely to be direct effects on renal magnesium handling. Devane and Ryan (24) could not detect any change in clearance of magnesium following acute administration of potassium-canrenoate during furosemide diuresis in rats.

Some diuretics may exert effects on magnesium indirectly through activation of the renin-angiotensin-aldosterone system. The effects of diuretics or their contribution to possible coexisting magnesium and potassium deficiencies are discussed below.

Role of Magnesium during Potassium Deficiency in Cardiovascular Disease

Diuretic Treatment

The effects of diuretics on renal magnesium excretion have been recently reviewed (24, 84,125). Agents such as acetazolamide, acting in the proximal tubule, appear to have only minor effects (6). Agents causing extracellular fluid volume depletion, such as mannitol, have been shown to enhance magnesium reabsorption from the proximal tubule (140). On the other hand agents which cause extracellular fluid expansion, such as saline infusion, have been shown to depress tubular reabsorption of magnesium (85). The effects of mineralocorticoids have been discussed above.

Diuretics acting in Henle's loop cause major losses of magnesium. Large urinary losses of magnesium have been shown to occur with the loop-blocking diuretics including mercurials, furosemide, and ethacrynic acid (24,84,125). These findings are compatible with studies in rats citing the loop of Henle as the major site of magnesium reabsorption (14). It is estimated that 50-60% of filtered magnesium is reabsorbed at this site.

In contrast to loop-blocking diuretics, thiazide diuretics cause less alteration in magnesium excretion. The acute administration of thiazides to dogs (34) or rats (24) did not increase magnesium clearance. The effects of thiazides on magnesium excretion in humans are variable (86). Long-term studies with thiazides have suggested that these agents promote some urinary magnesium wasting (60,91,123,128). Thiazides may produce indirect effects on magnesium excretion, possibly mediated through altered aldosterone levels.

The potassium-sparing diuretics amiloride and triamterene are used mainly in association with more effective diuretics in attempts to reduce urinary potassium excretion. Some recent studies indicate that these agents may also exert magnesium-sparing effects (24-27,59,101,103). A dosage-dependent action of amiloride in reducing magnesium clearance during furosemide diuresis in rats has been demonstrated by Devane and Ryan (27). The effects of amiloride on magnesium and potassium metabolism in patients with congestive heart failure are discussed below.

Congestive Heart Failure

Magnesium deficiency has been reported in cardiac failure and its role in cardiac disorders has been reviewed (15,65). Muscle magnesium has been shown to be reduced in heart failure (64,68,126). We have investigated magnesium and potassium metabolism and the effects of amiloride in patients with congestive heart failure (103). The results of plasma electrolyte measurements are shown in Figure 3. Patients with congestive heart failure had significantly reduced plasma potassium levels, but plasma magnesium was not significantly reduced compared to control subjects. Lymphocyte electrolyte analysis revealed significant intracellular depletion of both potassium and magnesium (Fig. 4). It should be noted that even though these patients were being treated with potassium supplements, a significant intracellular depletion of potassium could be demonstrated.

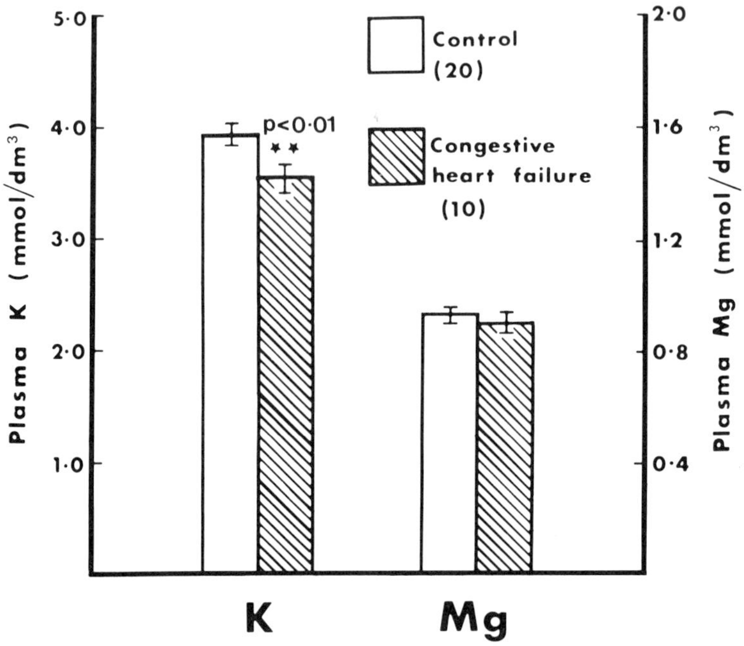

Figure 3 Plasma magnesium and potassium concentrations in control subjects and in patients with congestive heart failure. Ref. 103.)

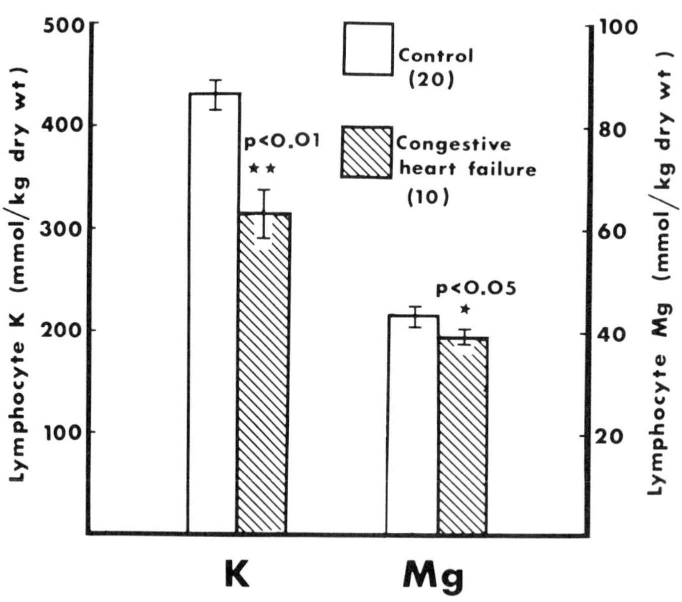

Figure 4 Lymphocyte magnesium and potassium concentrations in control subjects and in patients with congestive heart failure. (Data adapted from Ref. 103.)

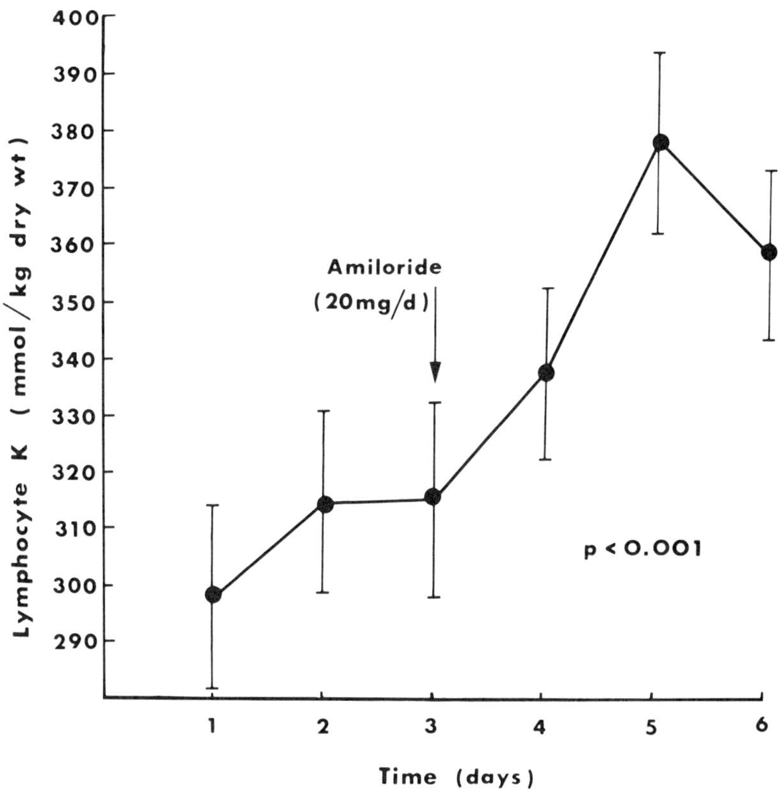

Figure 5 The effects of amiloride on lymphocyte potassium in patients with congestive heart failure. (Data from Ref. 103.)

Administration of amiloride (20 mg/day) reduced urinary excretion of both magnesium and potassium and also increased plasma magnesium and potassium (103). The magnesium- and potassium-sparing properties of amiloride were also reflected in increased lymphocyte potassium (Fig. 5) and increased lymphocyte magnesium (Fig. 6). Correction of the intracellular magnesium depletion may have had beneficial effects on potassium metabolism.

Magnesium Requirement for Potassium Repletion

During investigation of the effects of amiloride on magnesium metabolism in congestive heart failure, we (23) found that a patient with extremely high rates of aldosterone excretion and persistently low plasma magnesium had reduced lymphocyte magnesium and potassium levels. Amiloride did not correct the intracellular magnesium and potassium depletion in this patient. However, administration of $MgSO_4$ either intravenously or intramuscularly produced significant increases in both lymphocyte magnesium and potassium. Dyckner and Wester (31-33) have, with the use of muscle biopsy techniques, demonstrated a key role of magnesium in restoring intracellular potassium concentrations in cardiac patients treated with diuretics. They also demonstrated that the magnesium-induced restoration of normal potassium concentrations was important in the control of arrhythmias. A

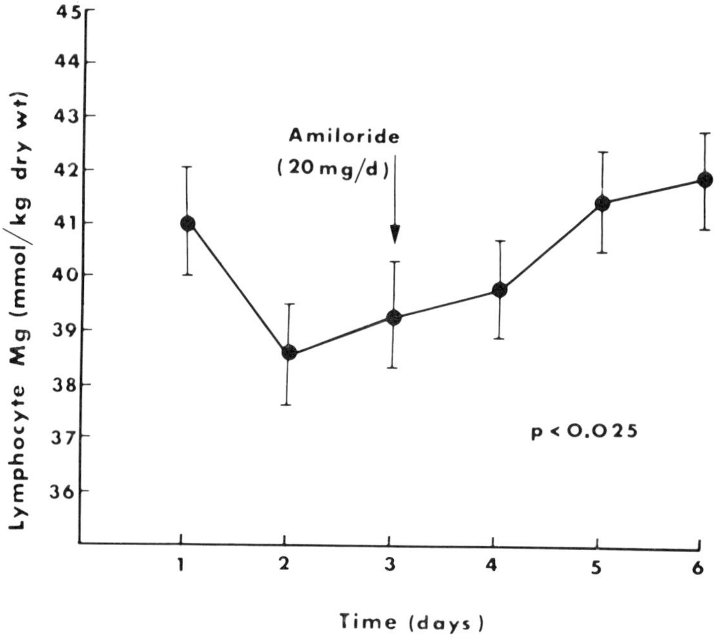

Figure 6 The effects of amiloride on lymphocyte magnesium in patients with congestive heart failure. (Data from Ref. 103.)

number of other cases have been documented in which coexisting magnesium and potassium depletion was resistant to potassium supplementation unless the magnesium deficiency was identified and corrected (3,52,74,87,131). Ryan and Whang have reviewed the interrelationships in the metabolism of magnesium and potassium (106).

Magnesium-Digitalis Arrhythmias

Evidence for a magnesium deficiency in the pathogenesis of cardiovascular disease and arrhythmias including digitalis-toxic arrhythmias has been reviewed (63,111). The authors have also reviewed the successful use of magnesium to treat arrhythmias including digitalis-toxic arrhythmias. As can be seen from Figure 2, there are a number of possible mechanisms for magnesium to exert beneficial effects during digitalis-toxic arrhythmias. As well as affecting potassium transport, magnesium may directly affect the binding of digitalis. Recently, we have demonstrated that lowered magnesium levels in vitro enhance the binding of digoxin to red blood cell membranes from human subjects (98).

Incidence of Hypomagnesemia in Hospitalized Patients: Association with Hypokalemia

Table 6 lists some observations on the incidence of hypomagnesemia in hospitalized patients. The incidence of hypomagnesemia ranges between 7 and 11% (133,141). Two groups of workers (13,136) showed a remarkably high (40%) incidence of hypokalemia in association with hypomagnesemia. In samples sent for digoxin assay, Whang et al. (138) detected a 19% incidence of hypomagnesemia and a 9% incidence of hypokalemia. They interpreted these findings as indicating that physicians were more aware of dangers of

Table 6 Incidence of Hypomagnesemia in Hospitalized Patients

Condition	Incidence (%)	Author	Reference
Hypomagnesemia (<0.62 mmol/L)	7	Whang et al., 1980	133
	11	Wong et al., 1983	141
Association with hypokalemia	42	Whang et al., 1978	136
(<3.5 mmol/L)	38	Boyd et al., 1983	13
In samples sent for digoxin assay			
Hypomagnesemia	19	Whang et al., 1979	138
Hypokalemia	9	Whang et al., 1979	138

hypokalemia than of hypomagnesemia and were more expert in avoiding hypokalemia. In any case, the very high incidence of hypomagnesemia in this group indicates that more attention should be given to this problem.

Diuretic treatment is probably the main cause of concomitant magnesium and potassium depletion. Many workers have documented the depletion of magnesium and potassium after treatment with diuretics, especially loop-blocking diuretics (33,66,69,103,113).

Potassium depletion, which is resistant to conventional potassium replacement therapy, may in many cases be due to an underlying concomitant but undetected magnesium deficiency. I have reviewed the evidence from both experimental and clinical observations which indicates that magnesium can play a pivotal role in both potassium depletion and repletion. Magnesium metabolism should be investigated in patients with disturbed potassium metabolism.

ACKNOWLEDGMENTS

The author acknowledges the stimulation obtained from many colleagues in working on the investigations described here: D. H. Hingerty, Honor Smyth, Olive Arnold, R. Whang, W. Yamalis, P. Mc Kenna, M. F. Ryan, T. B. Counihan, J. Devane, and Loretta Thornton.

Many of the studies reported here were supported by the Medical Research Council of Ireland.

Thanks are also due to Grainne Furlong for typing the manuscript.

REFERENCES

1. Aikawa, J. K., and David, A. P.: ^{28}Mg studies in magnesium deficient animals. *Ann. N.Y. Acad. Sci.* 162:744–757, 1969.
2. Arnold, O. F., and Ryan, M. P.: The effect of magnesium on potassium transport in isolated rat soleus muscle. In *Proceedings of the First International Symposium on Magnesium Deficit; Human Pathology*, edited by Durlac, J., Vittel, France, 1973, pp. 63–66.
3. Baehler, R. W., Work, J., Kotchen, T. A., McMorrow, G., and Guthrie, G.: Studies in the pathogenesis of Bartter's syndrome. *Am. J. Med.* 69:933–938, 1980.
4. Balint, J. A., and Hirschowitz, B. I.: Hypomagnesemia with tetany in non-tropical sprue. *N. Engl. J. Med.* 265:631–633, 1961.
5. Bar, R. S., Wilson, H. E., and Mazzaferri, E. L.: Hypomagnesemic hypocalcemia secondary to renal magnesium wasting. *Ann. Intern. Med.* 82: 646–649, 1975.
6. Barker, E. S., Elkinton, J. R., and Clark, J. K.: Studies on the renal excretion of magnesium in man. *J. Clin. Invest.* 38:1733–1745, 1959.

7. Barnes, B. A.: Magnesium conservation: a study of surgical patients. *Ann. N.Y. Acad. Sci.* 162:786–801, 1969.
8. Bittar, E. E., and Chambers, G.: The importance of external magnesium in the sensitivity of the sodium efflux to injected cyclic AMP: the barnacle muscle fibre as a preparation. *Comp. Biochem. Physiol.* 77A:573–575, 1984.
9. Bonting, S. L., Stewarts, H. G. P., Peters, W. H. M., Schaurmansstekhoven, F. M. A. H., and De Pont, J. J. H. H. M.: Magnesium-induced conformational changes in Na-K-ATPase. *Curr. Top. Membranes Transp.* 19:403–424, 1983.
10. Booth, C. C., Hanna, S., Babouris, N., and Mac Intyre, I.: Evidence of hypomagnesemia in intestinal malabsorption. *Br. Med. J.* 2:141–144, 1963.
11. Booth, B. E., and Johnson, A.: Hypomagnesemia due to renal tubular defect in reabsorption of magnesium. *J. Pediatr.* 85:350–354, 1974.
12. Booth, I. W., Milla, P. J., and Harries, J. T.: The effects of magnesium on ion transport in short circuited rabbit terminal ileum. *Clin. Sci.* 66:465–471, 1984.
13. Boyd, J. C., Bruns, D. E., and Wills, M. R.: Frequency of hypomagnesemia in hypokalemic states. *Clin. Chem.* 29:178–179, 1983.
14. Brunett, M. G., Vigneault, N., and Carriere, S.: Micropuncture study of magnesium transport along the nephrom in the young rat. *Am. J. Physiol.* 227:891, 1974.
15. Burch, G. E., and Giles, T. D.: The importance of magnesium deficiency in cardiovascular disease. *Am. Heart J.* 94:649, 1977.
16. Caddell, J. L.: Studies in protein-calorie malnutrition 11. Double-blind clinical trial to assess magnesium therapy. *N. Engl. J. Med.* 276:535–540, 1967.
17. Caddell, J. L.: Magnesium deficiency in protein-calorie malnutrition: a follow-up study. *Ann. N.Y. Acad. Sci.* 162:874–890, 1969.
18. Caddell, J. L., and Goddard, D. R.: Studies in protein-calorie malnutrition. I. Clinical evidence for magnesium deficiency. *N. Engl. J. Med.* 276:533–535, 1967.
19. Cantin, M.: Relationship of juxtaglomerular apparatus and adrenal cortex to biochemical and extracellular fluid volume changes in magnesium deficiency. *Lab. Invest.* 22:558–588, 1970.
20. Carney, S. L., Wong, N. L. M., and Dirks, J. H.: Effects of magnesium deficiency and excess on renal tubular potassium transport in the rat. *Clin. Sci.* 60:549–554, 1981.
21. Contiguglia, S. R., Alfrey, A. C., Miller, N., and Butkus, D.: Total body magnesium excess in chronic renal failure. *Lancet* 1:1300–1302, 1972.
22. Cotlove, E., Holliday, M. A., Schwartz, R. A., and Wallace, W. M.: Effects of electrolyte depletion and acid-base disturbances on muscle cations. *Am. J. Physiol.* 167: 665–667, 1951.
23. Counihan, T. B., Halley, E., Ryan, M. F., and Ryan, M. P.: The effect of magnesium sulphate administration on lymphocyte magnesium and potassium in a patient with congestive heart failure (abstr.). *Ir. J. Med. Sci.* 147:331, 1978.
24. Devane, J., and Ryan, M. P.: Diuretics and magnesium excretion. *Magnesium Bull.* 3:122–123, 1981.
25. Devane, J., and Ryan, M. P.: The effects of amiloride and triamterene on urinary magnesium excretion in conscious saline-loaded rats. *Br. J. Pharmacol.* 72:285–289, 1981.
26. Devane, J., and Ryan, M. P.: Evidence for a magnesium-sparing action by amiloride during renal clearance studies in rats. *Br. J. Pharmacol.* 79:891–896, 1983.
27. Devane, J., and Ryan, M. P.: Dose-dependant reduction in renal magnesium clearance by amiloride during a frusemide-induced diuresis in rats. *Br. J. Pharmacol.* 80:421–428.
28. Dunham, E. T., and Glynn, I. M.: Adenosinetriphosphatase activity and the active movements of alkali metal ions. *J. Physiol.* 156:274–293, 1961.
29. Dunn, M. J.: Red blood cell calcium and magnesium: effects upon sodium and

potassium transport and cellular morphology. *Biochem. Biophys. Acta* 352:97, 1974.

30. Dunn, M. J., and Walser, M.: Magnesium depletion in normal man. *Metabolism* 15: 884–895, 1966.
31. Dyckner, T., and Wester, P. O.: The relation between extra and intracellular electrolytes in patients with hypokalemia and/or diuretic treatment. *Acta Med. Scand.* 204:269, 1978.
32. Dyckner, T., and Wester, P. O.: Ventricular extrasystoles and intracellular electrolytes before and after potassium and magnesium infusion in patients on diuretic treatment. *Am. Heart J.* 97:12, 1979.
33. Dyckner, T., and Wester, P. O.: Extra and intracellular potassium, magnesium, diuretics and arrhythmias. In *Potassium–Its Biologic Significance*, edited by Whang, R., Boca Raton, C.R.C. Press, 1983, pp. 137–154.
34. Eknoyan, G., Suki, W. N., and Martinez-Maldonado, M.: Effect of diuretics on urinary excretion of phosphate, calcium and magnesium in thyroparathyroidectomized dogs. *J. Lab. Clin. Med.* 76:257, 1970.
35. Elin, R. L., Armstrong, W. D., and Singer, L.: Adrenal gland factors in magnesium-deficient rats. *Proc. Soc. Exp. Biol. Med.* 134:542–547, 1970.
36. Elin, R. L., Armstrong, W. D., and Singer, L.: Body fluid electrolyte composition of chronically magnesium-deficient and control rats. *Am. J. Physiol.* 220:543–548, 1971.
37. Ellory, J. C., Flatman, P. W., and Stewart, G. W.: Inhibition of red cell sodium and potassium transport by divalent cations. *J. Physiol.* 340:1–17, 1983.
38. Elshove, A., and von Rossum, G. D. V.: Net movements of sodium and potassium and their relations to respiration, in slices of rat liver incubated in vitro. *J. Physiol. (Lond)* 168:531, 1963.
39. Ferris, T. F., Kashgarian, H., Levitin, H., and Epstein, F. H.: Renal tubular acidosis and renal potassium-wasting acquired as a result of hypercalcemic nephropathy. *N. Engl. J. Med.* 265:924–928, 1961.
40. Ferris, T. F., Levitin, H., Phillips, E. T., and Epstein, F. H.: Renal potassium wasting induced by vitamin D. *J. Clin. Invest.* 41:1212–1229.
41. Flatman, P. W., and Lew, V. L.: The magnesium-dependence of sodium/potassium and sodium/sodium exchange mediated by the sodium pump in intact human red cells. *J. Physiol.* 287:33, 1979.
42. Flatman, P. W., and Lew, V. L.: Magnesium dependence of sodium pump mediated sodium transport in intact human red cells. *Curr. Top. Membranes Transp.* 19:653–657, 1983.
43. Flink, E. B.: Magnesium deficiency syndrome in man. *JAMA* 160:1406–1409, 1956.
44. Flink, E. B.: Magnesium deficiency: etiology and clinical spectrum. *Acta Med. Scand.* [*suppl.*] 647:125, 1981.
45. Flink, E. B., Stutzman, F. L., Anderson, A. R., Konig, T., and Fraser, R.: Magnesium deficiency after prolonged parenteral fluid administration and after chronic alcoholism complicated by delirium tremens. *J. Lab. Clin. Med.* 43:169–183, 1954.
46. Forbes, R. M.: Effects of magnesium, potassium and sodium nutriture on mineral composition of selected tissues of the albino rat. *J. Nutr.* 88:403–410, 1966.
47. Francisco, L. L., and Dibona, G. F.: Mechanism of negative potassium balance in the magnesium deficient rat (abstr.). *Kidney Int.* 16:852, 1979.
48. Freeman, R. M., and Pearson, E.: Hypomagnesemia of unknown etiology. *Am. J. Med.* 41:645–656, 1966.
49. Friedman, M., Gatcher, G., and Watson, L.: Primary hypomagnesaemia with secondary hypocalcaemia in an infant. *Lancet* 1:703–705, 1967.

50. Gitelman, H. J., Graham, J. B., and Welt, L. G.: A familial disorder characterized by hypokalemia and hypomagnesemia. *Ann. N.Y. Acad. Sci.* 162:856–864, 1969.
51. Grace, N. D., and O'Dell, B. L.: Effects of magnesium deficiency on the distribution of water and cations in the muscle of the guinea pig. *J. Nutr.* 100:45–50, 1970.
52. Gullner, H. G., Gill, J. R. Jr., Bartter, F. C.: Correction of hypokalemia by magnesium repletion in familial hypokalemic alkalosis with tubulopathy. *Am. J. Med.* 71:578–582, 1981.
53. Gunther, T.: Biochemistry and pathobiochemistry of magnesium. *Magnesium Bull.* 3:91–101, 1981.
54. Gunther, T., and Averdunk, R.: K-transport und Stoffwechsel von Mg-arm gewachsenen Yoshida-ascites-tumorzeller. *Z. Klin. Chem. Klin. Biochem.* 8:621–625, 1970.
55. Gunther, T., Dorn, F., and Merker, H. J.: Embryo toxic effects produced by magnesium deficiency in rats. *Z. Klin. Chem. Klin. Biochem.* 11:87–92, 1973.
56. Gunther, T., and Marisz, P.: Uber den K-transport bei Mg-arm gewachsen zellen von E. Coli. *Z. Naturforsch.* 23:334–338, 1968.
57. Gunther, T.: Wasser und Electrolytverteilung in einigen organen von Mg-arm ernahrten ratten. *Z. Klin. Chem. Klin. Biochem.* 8:65–68, 1970.
58. Haijamae, H., and Mac Dowall, I. G.: Distribution of divalent cations at the cellular level during primary hypomagnesemia in infancy. *Acta Paediatr. Scand.* 61: 591–596, 1972.
59. Hanze, S., and Seyberth, H.: Untersuchungen zur Wirkung und Triamteren auf die renale Magnesium-und Calciumausscheidung. *Klin. Wochenschr.* 45:313, 1967.
60. Higgins, B. A., Nassin, J. R., Collins, J., and Hilb, A.: The effect of bendrofluazide on urine calcium excretion. *Clin. Sci.* 27:459–462, 1964.
61. Holmes, A. M., Hesling, C. M., and Wilson, T. M.: Drug induced secondary aldosteronism in patients with pulmonary tuberculosis. *Q. J. Med.* 39:299, 1969.
62. Horton, R., and Biglieri, E. G.: Effects of aldosterone on the metabolism of magnesium. *J. Clin. Endocrinol. Metab.* 22:1187, 1962.
63. Iseri, L. T.: Potassium, magnesium and digitalis toxicity. In *Potassium: Its Biologic significance*, edited by Whang, R., Boca Raton, C.R.C. Press, 1983, pp. 125–136.
64. Iseri, L. T., Alexander, L. C., Mc Caughey, R. S., Boyle, A. J., and Myers, G. B.: Water and electrolyte content of cardiac and skeletal muscle in heart failure and myocardial infarction. *Am. Heart. J.* 43:215, 1952.
65. Iseri, L. T., Freed, J. R., and Bures, A. R.: Magnesium deficiency and cardiac disorders. *Am. J. Med.* 58:837, 1975.
66. Jackson, C. E., and Meier, D. W.: Routine serum magnesium analysis. Correlation with clinical state in 5,100 patients. *Ann. Intern. Med.* 69:743–748, 1968.
67. Jones, J. E., Shane, S. R., Jacobs, W. H., and Flink, E. B.: Magnesium balance studies in chronic alcoholism. *Ann. N.Y. Acad. Sci.* 162:934–946, 1969.
68. Lim, P., and Jacob, E.: Magnesium in patients on long-term diuretic therapy for heart failure. *Br. Med. J.* 3:620, 1970.
69. Lim, P., and Jacob, E.: Magnesium deficiency in patients on long-term diuretic therapy for heart failure. *Br. Med. J.* 111:620–622, 1972.
70. Lim, P., and Jacob, E.: Magnesium status of alcoholic patients. *Metabolism* 21: 1045–1051, 1972.
71. Lim, P., and Jacob, E.: Magnesium status in chronic uremic patients. *Nephron* 9: 300–307, 1972.
72. Lim, P., and Jacob, E.: Tissue magnesium level in chronic diarrhoea. *J. Lab. Clin. Med.* 80:313–321, 1972.
73. Lim, P., and Jacob, E.: Magnesium-saving property of an aldosterone antagonist in the treatment of oedema of liver cirrhosis. *Br. Med. J.* 1:755, 1978.
74. Lipner, A.: Symptomatic magnesium deficiency after small intestinal bypass for obesity. *Br. Med. J.* 1:148, 1977.

75. Mac INtyre, I., and Davidsson, D.: The production of secondary potassium depletion, sodium retention, nephrocalcinosis and hypercalcaemia by magnesium deficiency. *Biochem. J.* 70:456–462, 1958.
76. MacIntyre, I., Hanna, S., Booth, C. C., and Reed, A. E.: Intracellular magnesium deficiency in man. *Clin. Sci.* 20:297–305, 1961.
77. Mac Intyre, I., and Robinson, C. J.: Magnesium and the gut: experimental and clinical observations. *Ann. N.Y. Acad. Sci.* 162, 865–873, 1969.
78. Mader, L. T., and Iseri, L. T.: Spontaneous hypopotassemia, hypomagnesemia, alkalosis and tetany due to hypersecretion of corticosterone-like mineralcorticoid. *Am. J. Med.* 19:976–988, 1975.
79. Manitius, A., and Epstein, F. H.: Some observations on the influence of a magnesium-deficient diet on rats, with special reference to renal concentration ability, *J. Lab. Clin. Invest.* 42:208–215, 1963.
80. Martin, H. E., McCuskey, C. Jr., and Tupikova, N.: Electrolyte disturbance in acute alcoholism. *Am. J. Clin. Nutr.* 7:191–196, 1959.
81. Martindale, L., and Heaton, F. W.: Magnesium deficiency in the adult rat. *Biochem. J.* 92:119–126, 1964.
82. Mashio, G., Campanacei, L., Mioni, G., Bazzato, G., Brushi, E., Riz, G., and Gionfronceschi, G.: Acqua ed elettroliti tessutali nell'uremia cronica. *Minerva Nephrol.* 16:41, 1969.
83. Massry, S. G. Pharmacology of magnesium. *Annu. Rev. Pharmacol. Toxicol.* 17:67–82, 1977.
84. Massry, S. G.: Role of hormonal and non-hormonal factors in the control of renal handling of magnesium. *Magnesium Bull.* 3:277, 1981.
85. Massry, S. G., Coburn, J. W., Chapman, L. W., and Kleeman, C. R.: Effect of NaCl infusion on urinary calcium and magnesium during reduction in their filtered loads. *Am. J. Physiol.* 213:1218–1244, 1967.
86. Mc Collister, R. J., Prasad, A. S., Doe, R. P., and Flink, E. B.: Normal renal magnesium clearance and the effect of water loading, chlorothiazide and ethanol on magnesium excretion. *J. Lab. Clin. Med.* 52:928, 1958.
87. Medalle, R., Waterhouse, C.: A magnesium-deficient patient presneting with hypocalcemia and hyperphosphatemia. *Ann. Intern. Med.* 79:76–79, 1973.
88. Michelis, M. F., Drash, A. L., Linarelli, G., De Rubertis, F. R., and Davis, B. B.: Decreased bicarbonate threshold and renal magnesium wasting in a sibship with distal tubular acidosis (evaluation of the pathophysiologic role of parathyroid hormone). *Metabolism* 21:905–920, 1972.
89. Montgomery, R. D.: Magnesium metabolism in infantile protein malnutrition. *Lancet* 2:74–76, 1960.
90. Mordio, S., Donath, A., Macago, F., and Gatti, R.: Chronic hypomagnesemia with magnesium-dependent hypocalcemia. *Acta Paediatr. Scand.* 60:441–448, 1971.
91. Parfitt, A. M.: The interactions of thiazide diuretics with parathyroid hormone and Vit. D. Studies in patients with hypoparathyroidism. *J. Clin. Invest.* 51:1879–1888, 1972.
92. Parfitt, M. A., and Kleerekoper, M.: The divalent ion homeostatic system–physiology and metabolism of calcium phosphorus, magnesium and bone. In *Clinical Disorders of Fluid and Electrolytes Metabolism*, edited by Maxwell, M. H., and Kleeman, C. R., New York, McGraw-Hill, 1980, pp. 269–368.
93. Paunier, L., Radde, I. C., Kosh, S. W., Conen, P. E., and Fraser, D.: Primary hypomagnesemia with secondary hypocalcemia in an infant. *Pediatrics* 41:385–402, 1968.
94. Paunier, L., and Sizonenko, P. C.: Asymptomatic chronic hypomagnesemia and hypokalemia in a child: cell membrane disease? *J. Pediatr.* 88:51–55, 1976.
95. Petersen, V. P.: Potassium and magnesium turnover in magnesium deficiency. *Acta Med. Scand.* 174:595–604, 1963.

96. Runeberg, L., Collan, Y., Jokinen, E. J., Lahdevirta, J., and Aro, A.: Hypomagnesemia due to renal disease of unknown etiology. *Am. J. Med.* 59:873–881, 1975.
97. Ryan, M. F., and Ryan, M. P.: Lymphocyte electrolyte alterations during magnesium deficiency in the rat (abstr.). *Ir. J. Med. Sci.* 148:108, 1979.
98. Ryan, M. F., and Ryan, M. P.: The effects of magnesium on the binding of ^{3}H-digoxin to membranes of intact human red blood cells (abstr.). *Ir. J. Med. Sci.* 12: 219, 1983.
99. Ryan, M. P., and Hingerty, D.: Effects of magnesium deficiency on restoration of potassium and sodium levels in potassium-depleted muscle. *Ir. J. Med. Sci.* 2:137–140, 1969.
100. Ryan, M. P., and Mc Kenna, P.: Caesium accumulation in vivo by tissues of magnesium-deficient rats. In *Magnesium in Health and Disease,* edited by Cantin, M., and Seelig, M., New York, Spectrum Publications, 1980, pp. 105–111.
101. Ryan, M. P., and Phillips, O.: Diuretic-induced calcium and magnesium excretion in the rat (abstr.). *Ir. J. Med. Sci.* 146, 303, 1977.
102. Ryan, M. P., and Ryan, M. F.: Muscle calcium accumulation during magnesium deficiency in the rat. *Biochem. Soc. Trans.* 5:1744, 1977.
103. Ryan, M. P., Ryan, M. F., and Counihan, T. B.: The effect of diuretics on lymphocyte magnesium and potassium. *Acta. Med. Scand.* [*Suppl.*] 647:153–161, 1981.
104. Ryan, M. P., Smyth, H., and Hingerty, D.: Effects of magnesium and potassium deficiencies on composition and growth of ascites tumour cells *in vivo. Life Sci.* 8: 485–494, 1969.
105. Ryan, M. P., Whang, R., and Yamalis, W.: Effect of magnesium deficiency on cardiac and skeletal muscle potassium during dietary potassium restriction. *Proc. Soc. Exp. Biol. Med.* 143:1045–1047, 1973.
106. Ryan, M. P., and Whang, R.: Interrelationships between potassium and magnesium. In *Potassium: Its Biological Significance,* edited by Whang, R., Boca Raton, CRC Press, 1983, pp. 97–107.
107. Sawyer, R. B., Drew, M. A., Gesink, M. H., and Sawyer, K. C.: Postoperative magnesium metabolism. *Arch. Surg.* 100:343–348, 1970.
108. Schilling, K., Bornig, H., Comme, G., and Hoppe, H.: *Acta. Biol. Med.* 38:1101–1114, 1979.
109. Schilsky, R. L., and Anderson, T.: Hypomagnesemia and renal magnesium wasting in patients receiving cisplatin. *Ann. Intern. Med.* 90:929–931, 1970.
110. Seaman, G. V. F.: Electrokinetic behaviour of red cells. In *The Red Blood Cell,* 2nd Ed. Vol 11, edited by Surgenor, D. M., London, Academic Press, 1975, pp. 1135–1229.
111. Seelig, M. S.: *Magnesium Deficiency in the Pathogenesis of Disease–Early Roots of Cardiovascular, Skeletal, and Renal Abnormalities.* New York, Plenum, 1980.
112. Seta, K., Hellerstein, E. E., and Vitale, J. J.: Myocardium and plasma electrolytes in dietary magnesium and potassium deficiency in the rat. *J. Nutr.* 87:179–188, 1965.
113. Sheehan, J. and White, A.: Diuretic-associated hypomagnesemia. *Br. Med. J.* 285: 1157–1159, 1982.
114. Shils, M. E.: Experimental human magnesium depletion. *Medicine* 48:61–85, 1969.
115. Shine, K. I.: Myocardial effects of magnesium. *Am. J. Physiol.* 237:H413, 1979.
116. Shine, K. I., and Douglas, A. M.: Magnesium effects on ionic exchange and mechanical function in rat ventricle. *Am. J. Physiol.* 227:317–324, 1974.
117. Shine, K. I., and Douglas, A. M.: Magnesium effect on rabbit ventricle. *Am. J. Physiol.* 228:1545, 1975.
118. Skou, J. C.: The influence of some cations on adenosine triphphosphatase from peripheral nerves. *Biochem. Biophys. Acta* 23:394–401, 1957.

119. Smales, O. R. C.: Primary infantile hypomagnesaemia. *Proc. R. Soc. Med.* 67:759–762, 1974.
120. Stewart, W. K., and Fleming, L. W.: The effect of dialysate magnesium on plasma and erythrocyte magnesium and potassium concentrations during maintenance hemodialysis. *Nephron* 10:222–231, 1973.
121. Stewart, W. K., and Fleming, L. W.: Relationship between plasma and erythrocyte magnesium and potassium concentrations in fasting obese subjects. *Metabolism* 22:535, 1973.
122. Stromme, J. H.: Familial hypomagnesemia. Biochemical, histological and hereditary aspects studied in two brothers. *Acta Paediatr. Scand.* 58:433–444, 1969.
123. Sullivan, J. M., Dluhy, R. G., Wacker, W. E. C., Soloman, H. S., Williams, G. H., and Somata, J. K.: Interrelationships among thiazide diuretics and calcium, magnesium, sodium and potassium balance in normal and hypertensive man. *J. Clin. Pharmacol.* 530–543, 1978.
124. Sutherland, L. E., Hartroft, P., Balis, J. U., Baily, J. D., and Lynch, M. J.: Bartter's syndrome: A report of four cases, including three in one sibship, with comparative histologic evaluation of the juxtaglomerular apparatuses and glomeruli. *Acta Paediatr. Scand.* [*Suppl.*] 201, 1970.
125. Sutton, R. A. L., and Dirks, J. H.: Renal handling of calcium, phosphate and magnesium. In *The Kidney,* 2nd ed., edited by Brenner, B. M., and Rector, F. C., Philadelphia, W.B. Saunders, 1981.
126. Szezepanski, I.: Electrolytes within cells of skeletal muscle and myocardium in congestive heart failure. *Polish Med. J.* 5:13, 1967.
127. Thornton, L., Ryan, M. P., Counihan, T. B., and Donohoe, J.: Plasma and lymphocyte potassium and magnesium in chronic renal failure patients on maintenance haemodialysis. *Ir. J. Med. Sci.* 152:219–220, 1983.
128. Wacker, W. E. C.: The effect of hydrochlorothiazide on magnesium excretion. *J. Clin. Invest.* 40:1086–1087, 1961.
129. Watson, A., Coffey, L., Keogh, B., and Mc Cann, S. R.: Severe hypomagnesaemia and hypocalcaemia following gentamicin therapy. *Ir. Med. J.* 76:381–383, 1983.
130. Watson, A. J. S., Watson, M. M. R., and Keogh, J. A. B.: Metabolic abnormalities associated with tobramycin therapy. *Ir. J. Med. Sci.* 153:96–99, 1984.
131. Webb, S., and Schade, D. S.: Hypomagnesemia as a cause of persistent hypokalemia. *JAMA* 233:23–24, 1975.
132. Welt, L. G.: Experimental magnesium depletion. *Yale J. Biol. Med.* 36:325–349, 1964.
133. Whang, R., Aikawa, J. K., and Hamiter, T.: Routine serum Mg determination—an unrecognized need. In *Magnesium in Health and Disease,* edited by Cantin, M., and Seeling, M., New York, Spectrum Publications, 1980, p. 1.
134. Whang, R., Morosi, H. J., Rodgers, D., and Reyes, R.: The influence of continuing magnesium deficiency on muscle K repletion. *J. Lab. Clin. Med.* 70:895–902, 1967.
135. Whang, R., Oei, T. O., Aikawa, J. K., Ryan, M. P., Watanabe, A., Chrysant, S. G., and Fryer, A.: Magnesium and potassium interrelationships: experimental and clinical. *Acta Med. Scand.* [*Suppl.*] 647, 139, 1981.
136. Whang, R., Oei, T. O., and Hamiter, T.: Frequency of hypomagnesemia associated with hypokalemia in hospitalized patients (abstr.). *Am. J. Clin. Pathol.* 71:610, 1979.
137. Whang, R., Ryan, M. P., and Yamalis, W.: Increased urinary output of ^{42}K during magnesium deficiency in the rat (abstr.). American Society for Nephrology, 6th annual meeting, 113, 1973.
138. Whang, R., Watanabe, A., and Oei, T.: Routine serum magnesium determinations in digitalized patients (abstr.). *Clin. Chem.* 25:1139, 1979.

139. Whang, R., and Welt, L. G.: Observations in experimental magnesium depletion. *J. Clin. Invest.* 42:305–313, 1963.
140. Wong, N. L. M., Quamme, G. A., Sutton, R. A. L., and Dirks, J. H.: The effect of mannitol on divalent ion transport in the kidney. *J. Lab. Clin. Med.* 94:683, 1979.
141. Wong, E. T., Rude, R. K., Singer, F. R., and Shaw, S. T. Jr.: A high prevalance of hypomagnesemia in hospitalized patients. *Am. J. Clin. Pathol.* 79:348–352, 1983.
142. Woodward, D. L., and Reed, D. J.: Effects of magnesium deficiency on electrolyte distribution in the rabbit. *Am. J. Physiol.* 217:1477–1482, 1969.

3

Differential Diagnosis of Hypokalemia

NORMAN M. KAPLAN
University of Texas Southwestern Medical School and University of Texas Health Science Center at Dallas, Dallas, Texas

Hypokalemia is common; it is often seen in the hospital as an acute epiphenomenon to stress and in the outpatient setting as a chronic accompaniment to diuretic therapy (Table 1). A low blood potassium level is particularly common because potassium conservation is relatively ineffectual and because the highly effective ways that have evolved to protect against diet-induced hyperkalemia may be inappropriately activated by a number of recently introduced medical therapies. Moreover, the major shift from a high-potassium-low-sodium diet ingested by our ancestors over many thousands of years to the relatively low-potassium-high-sodium diet that most people in the industrialized world have been ingesting over the last few hundred years has made us increasingly susceptible to hypokalemia.

Since the physiology of potassium metabolism has been discussed by Dr. Giebisch in Chapter 1, this chapter will focus on the clinical circumstances wherein physiology is disturbed enough to induce hypokalemia.

For this presentation, hypokalemia will be defined as a serum potassium level below 3.5 mmol/L, although many of the series to be reviewed use a level of 3.2 or even 3.0.

CLINICAL CIRCUMSTANCES

Hospitalized Patients

Hypokalemia may be found in as many as 30% of hospitalized patients and in up to 50% of those with an acute illness (26). Many of these instances will be transient, induced by a multitude of mechanisms that shift potassium out of blood and into cells. In Morgan and Young's series of 70 unselected hospitalized patients with plasma potassium levels at or below 2.8 mmol/L, an acute illness was present in 45; of these, 26 had a medical disorder and in 20 of these detailed information was available. Of these 20, no apparent cause could be identified in 11; they had probably experienced cellular shifts. Without potassium supplements, serum potassium levels rose back to normal spontaneously in many of these patients.

Table 1 Causes of Hypokalemia

Cellular shifts
Rapid changes in cell mass
Alkalosis
Hormones: insulin, beta-agonists
Periodic paralysis
Decreased intake: starvation
Increased loss
Gastrointestinal
Vomiting and drainage
Diarrhea and laxatives
Sweat
Renal
Diuretic therapy
Osmotic diuresis
Primary renal disease
Metabolic alkalosis (subsequent to acid loss)
Adrenocortical hormone excess

An even more severely hypokalemic group of hospitalized patients was identified by Lawson et al. (23) in a 3-year survey of 58,167 patients in hospitals in Glasgow. They found a plasma potassium level below 2.0 mmol/L in 73 patients and a level between 2.0 and 2.4 in 472, an overall incidence of such severe hypokalemia of 1%. Older women made up the majority of these patients, probably reflecting their lower dietary intake of potassium and their more common use of laxatives. Mortality was 30% in these groups compared to 8% in age- and sex-matched normokalemic patients.

The apparent causes of the hypokalemia below 2.0 mmol/L in 64 of the 73 patients in whom data were available are shown in Table 2. Drugs were involved in one-third of the cases, with diuretics the most common. In many of the other two-thirds, little or no potassium had been taken by mouth or in intravenous fluids. Excessive GI losses were responsible for 14% whereas renal wastage was involved in 12%. Acute leukemia was the diagnosis in 13%.

Table 2 Apparent Cause of Hypokalemia in 64 Patients With $K+ < 2$ mmol/L

Drug therapy	% of patients	Other causes	% of patients
Diuretics	16	Intravenous fluids with little K+	17
Insulin injection	5	Gastrointestinal losses	14
Peptic ulcer therapy	5	Acute leukemia	13
Clindamycin	3	Insufficient dietary potassium intake	9
Corticotropin	2	Secondary aldosteronism	6
Polystyrene sodium sulfonate	2	Urinary K+ losses from renal diseases	6
(Peritoneal dialysis)	2	Burns	2

Source: Ref. 23.

Immediate attention may need to be given to the profound hypokalemia that occurs in hospitalized patients as a result of stress-induced surges in catecholamines which then promote cellular shifts of potassium. This phenomenon is particularly likely in patients with inadequate dietary potassium intake or who are being treated with potassium-wasting drugs.

Let us consider in more detail some of the major causes of hypokalemia that are likely to be encountered in hospitalized patients, following the outline shown in Table 1.

Cellular Shifts

Rapid changes in cell mass: As observed in 13% of the patients reported by Lawson et al. (23) (Table 2), profound hypokalemia may be seen in patients with leukemia, particularly the acute myeloid form (2). This may reflect renal tubular loss of potassium (13) but a major component is probably the uptake of potassium into leukemic cells, both in vivo and in vitro (2).

A similar transfer of potassium may occur into the rapidly expanding red cell mass of patients early in the course of treatment for megaloblastic anemia and, possibly, severe iron-deficiency anemia (22). Yet another situation wherein potassium may rapidly enter cells is with the transfusion of freshly washed red blood cells.

Alkalosis: As Drs. Goodkin and Narins discuss in Chapter 5, alkalosis from whatever cause will result in potassium entering cells and will increase renal excretion of potassium (38). With hyperventilation, for every 10% reduction in arterial carbon dioxide tension, the serum potassium falls 0.5 mmol/L (12). The anxiety associated with painful venipuncture may be enough to induce a significant respiratory alkalosis and lower the serum K+. On the other hand, even a short period of forearm exercise, as an aid to venipuncture, may bring enough potassium out of cells to induce spuriously high levels (8).

Acid loss, as from vomiting, will lead to hypokalemia, less from the external loss of potassium in the gastrointestinal fluid than from the shift of potassium into cells and even more from the increase in renal potassium excretion that accompanies the metabolic alkalosis.

Hormones: Insulin and catecholamines have well-defined roles in the control of internal potassium balance and mineralocorticoids are largely responsible for the degree of external potassium losses (36). The role of mineralocorticoid role is covered in the section "Renal losses." Other hormones, such as glucagon and growth hormone, seem to play minimal, ancillary roles.

Insulin causes a dosage-related fall in plasma potassium that is progressive. Even small increments in plasma insulin stimulate cellular potassium uptake (11). Insulin-induced hypoglycemia causes hypokalemia both by the primary effect of insulin and the secondary, counterregulatory stimulation of epinephrine (29).

As defined by Dr. Reid (Chapter 15), stress-induced rises in epinephrine may cause the transfer of enough potassium into cells to lower the serum potassium level by as much as 1.0 mmol/L (37). In addition to being responsible for much of the transient hypokalemia seen during acute illness (26), this may serve as a major inciter of ventricular arrhythmias. The superimposition of such precipitous falls in serum potassium in patients with preexisting hypokalemia induced by high dosages of diuretics may explain the higher rates of coronary mortality, mostly sudden deaths, in the Oslo and MRFIT trials (19), an issue discussed by Dr. Sherwin (Chapter 22).

Beta$_2$-adrenergic agonists are being used increasingly to treat asthma and to inhibit uterine contractions in preterm labor. When administered either as intravenous or oral preparations they may induce serious arrhythmias, at least in part by their hypokalemic action (4,24).

A number of other drugs may induce hypokalemia by renal mechanisms, as discussed later.

Hypokalemic periodic paralysis: This exotic disease, discussed by Dr. Zierler in Chapter 10, is usually associated with marked movement of potassium out of blood into muscle.

Decreased Intake

Patients hospitalized for various chronic diseases often have not been able to eat adequate amounts of food to maintain total body potassium stores in the face of continued losses of potassium into the urine (6). When superimposed upon the usual fall in total body potassium with advancing age that likely reflects a lower dietary intake of potassium even in healthy elderly people (20), it is easy to see why even short periods of increased external losses and decreased intake of potassium with intravenous fluids could be so often associated with significant hypokalemia (23) (Table 2).

By itself, starvation is an infrequent cause of hypokalemia. However, decreased intake is likely involved in the common finding of hypokalemia in patients with chronic alcohol abuse and other debilitating illnesses (30). Alcohol abusers, with multiple reasons for hypokalemia, may be particularly vulnerable to arrhythmias during the stresses of alcohol withdrawal (40).

Rarely, clay ingestion may bind enough potassium to decrease intake to the point of hypokalemia (16).

Increased Losses

Significant hypokalemia may occur quickly if the losses of potassium through the gastrointestinal or renal tract are profound and persistent. The causes of hypokalemia listed in Table 1 are usually of a more chronic nature and moderate degree, and seen most frequently in outpatients.

Gastrointestinal losses: Excessive GI losses are usually fairly obvious but some patients may deny their surreptitious self-induced vomiting or laxative addiction. Severe hypokalemia is particularly common with laxative abuse (35), the most common cause of chronic secretory diarrhea.

More fulminant diarrhea with even more profound hypokalemia usually accompanies the pancreatic cholera syndrome associated with islet cell tumors or hyperplasia (39).

Sweating: Intense physical activity in hot climates can produce 10-12 L of sweat which may contain as much as 9 mmol/L of potassium, leading to a decrease in total body potassium content. With the marked shrinkage of fluid volume, secondary aldosteronism may also engender increased wastage of potassium both through the sweat glands and the urine. If body fluid deficits are replenished with sodium chloride and water, the propensity to potassium wastage may be even greater (21).

Renal losses (Table 3): These causes of hypokalemia encompass the most common causes for more chronic hypokalemia; diuretic therapy is by far the leading mechanism. Most of these causes are seen in outpatients.

Among hospitalized patients, an osmotic diuresis may sweep out large amounts of potassium, as in patients with poorly controlled diabetes. When diabetic ketoacidosis super-

Table 3 Causes of Renal Loss of Potassium

Diuretic therapy
Osmotic diuresis: glucose, nonreabsorbable anions
Primary renal disease
Renal tubular acidosis
Fanconi's syndrome
K+ wasting renal disease
With hypomagnesemia
With Na+ conservation
Metabolic alkalosis
Adrenocortical hormone excess
Exogenous cortisol
Cushing's syndrome
Primary aldosteronism
Excess DOC or other mineralocorticoid
Secondary aldosteronism
Accelerated hypertension
Renovascular hypertension
Renin-secreting tumor
Hypercalcemia

venes, the acidosis usually raises the serum potassium level initially and hypokalemia usually appears only during the course of effective therapy. However, hypokalemia may be present at the onset, implying severe total body depletion from both GI and renal losses (1).

Perhaps an even more common mechanism for acute hypokalemia is the osmotic diuresis induced by the use of large amounts of antibiotics, such as penicillin, carbenicillin, and nafcillin, which are excreted as nonreabsorbable anion (9,25). The large quantity of nonreabsorbable anion obligates the excretion of large amounts of cations, and potassium is usually a major portion (10).

Other antibiotics, including gentamicin, outdated tetracycline, and amphotericin B, may cause hypokalemia by increasing urinary excretion of potassium secondary to their nephrotoxicity, thus interfering with renal tubular handling of potassium.

Of the remaining renal causes of hypokalemia, those caused by adrenocortical hormone excess may also be encountered among hospitalized patients. Six of the 64 patients with profound hypokalemia in Lawson et al.'s series (Table 2) had secondary aldosteronism, which could reflect renal ischemia, as in accelerated hypertension, or shrunken intravascular fluid volume, as in cirrhosis with ascites.

In addition, the use of high dosages of glucocorticoids with some mineralocorticoid activity (cortisone or prednisone), may induce hypokalemia (5), as may the repetitive use of corticotrophin (27).

Lastly, a number of intrinsic renal diseases may be associated with hypokalemia. Patients with renal failure who are on hemodialysis (41) or peritoneal dialysis (33) may develop severe hypokalemia, either in association with the rapid correction of metabolic acidosis or in the presence of poor intake and increased GI losses. Without reaching end-stage renal disease, patients with either renal interstitial fibrosis (31) or renal tubular acidosis (15) may have profound potassium losses. As described by Dr. Gill in Chapter 9, profound potassium-wasting nephropathy is the hallmark of Bartter's syndrome.

Table 4 Factors Increasing Renal Potassium Losses

Factor	Clinical condition
Increased Na+ delivery to distal tubule	Diuretics High sodium intake
Mineralocorticoid excess	Diuretics Aldosteronism
Increased urine flow rate	Diuretics Osmotic loads
Increased non-reabsorbable anion delivery to distal tubule	Carbenicillin
Alkalosis	Vomiting
Increased bicarbonate exertion	Vomiting Renal tubular acidosis

Hypercalcemia: Hypercalcemia may interfere with tubular handing of potassium (14) and hypokalemia was found in 32% of 103 hypercalcemic patients (3). The potential hazard of worsening the hypokalemia by the administration of intensive saline and furosemide therapy to lower the serum calcium level should be recognized.

These and the other clinical conditions in which renal wastage of potassium occurs may involve a number of mechanisms (Table 4). Often more than one is involved in a given patient.

Outpatients

Of the various causes for hypokalemia shown in Table 1, those occurring in outpatients are so much more frequent that they demand most attention. Of the various causes for

Table 5 Hypokalemia Secondary to Drugs

- Increased transfer into cells
  - Insulin
  - Catecholamines
  - Alkali
  - Treatment of megaloblastic anemia
  - Transfusion of washed RBCs
- Increased GI losses: laxatives
- Increased renal losses
  - Diuretic
  - Mineralocorticoids
    - Cortisol, prednisone
    - Glycyrrhizinic acid (licorice)
    - Levodopa (increases aldosterone)
  - Anionic loads: carbenicillin
  - Osmotic loads: mannitol, glucose
  - Nephrotoxins
    - Aminoglycosides
    - Tetracylcine, outdated
    - Amphotericin B

hypokalemia among outpatients, chronic diuretic therapy of hypertension is almost certainly the most common. With as estimated 103 million prescriptions for diuretics written in 1981 and the multiple ways that diuretics may increase renal potassium loss (Table 4), it should be no surprise that "diuretic-induced"will prove to be the most likely diagnosis for hypokalemia, particularly among hypertensive patients. More details on this topic are provided by Drs. Mudge (Chapter 16) and Whelton (Chapter 17).

Hypokalemia Secondary to Drugs (7)

Before we focus on diuretics, it is useful to review the various ways by which drugs may lead to hypokalemia (Table 5). Most of these have been discussed earlier in this chapter.

From 10 to 30% of hypertensive patients given a daily dose of a diuretic will develop hypokalemia. In Sandor's series of 158 well-nourished English hypertensive patients, all under age 65, with no edema and receiving no concomitant digitalis therapy, 29% had a plasma K+ below 3.4 after 2 years of daily diuretic therapy (34). The frequency and severity of hypokalemia with diuretic therapy depend upon the dosage and duration of diuretic action, with less hypokalemia seen with smaller dosages of short- to intermediate-duration diuretics (18).

DIFFERENTIAL DIAGNOSIS

In both inpatients or outpatients, the cause of hypokalemia should be identified so that it can corrected and recurrences prevented. As noted in the series of hospitalized hypokemic patients reviewed by Morgan and Young (26), no apparent cause can be found in a considerable portion of acutely ill patients, though stress-induced, catecholamine-mediated transfer of potassium into cells is likely in many.

For those who are hypertensive and hypokalemic, the possibility of primary aldosteronism must be considered if the hypokalemia is not provoked by prior diuretic therapy or other recognizable causes. However, that diagnosis will apply to only a very small percentage, probably no more than 0.1%. The flow diagram for the differential diagnosis of hypertensives with hypokalemia (Fig. 1) starts with the simple determination of urinary potassium excretion (17). Though it may be difficult to collect a full 24-hr specimen before administration of potassium supolements to those who are severely hypokalemic and acutely ill, the following measures should be feasible in outpatients with asymptomatic hypokalemia:

1. All diuretics, potassium sparers, and supplements should be stopped for at least 4 days along with drugs known to increase potassium excretion.
2. The patient should be on an unrestricted sodium intake, at least 100 mmol/day.
3. A 24-hr urine specimen should be analyzed for Na+, K+, and creatinine.
4. The plasma K+ level must remain below 3.5 mmol/L; those who are normokalemic presumably will excrete whatever they ingest if they are in a balanced state. Under these circumstances, the presence of more than 30 mmol/day potassium in the 24-hr urine is strongly suggestive of either primary or, more likely, secondary aldosteronism or another of the renal causes (17).

As emphasized by Parker et al. (28), patients who are hypokalemic, hypochloremic, and alkalotic can be assessed with a 24-hr urine specimen measured for potassium and chloride content.

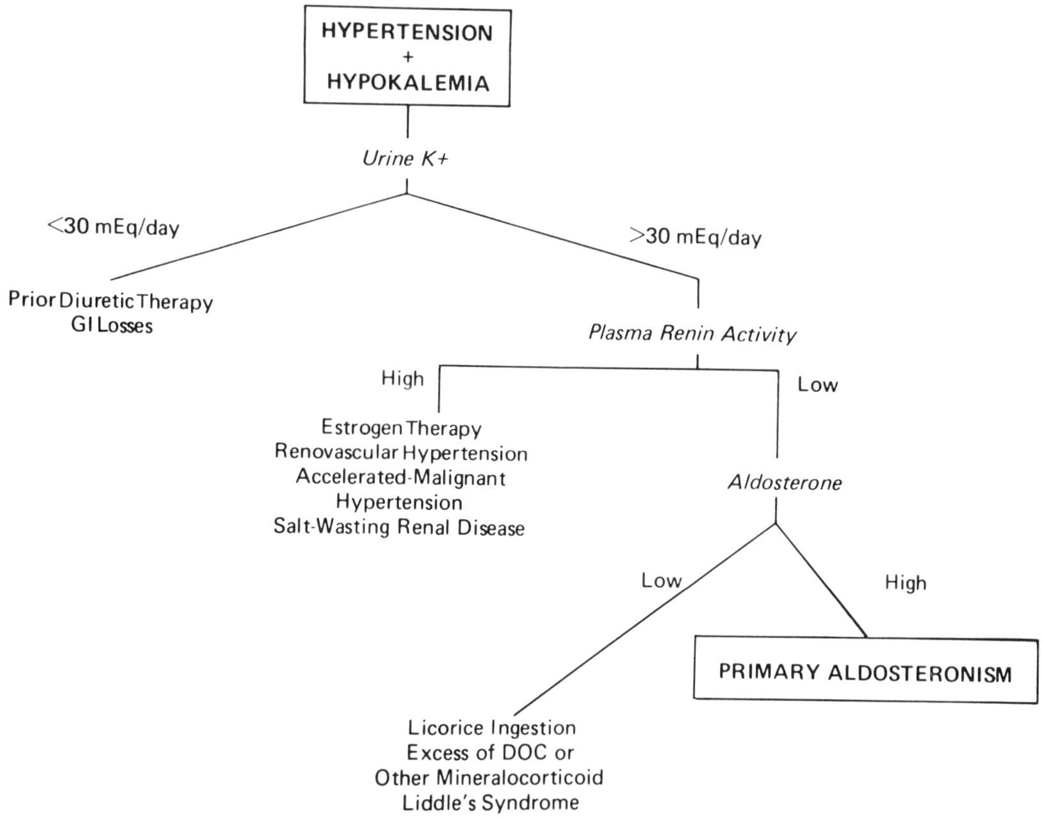

Figure 1 Flow diagram for the differential diagnosis of hypertension with hypokalemia. (From Ref. 18.)

With a careful history and the performance of the simple, though often hard-to-collect, 24-hr urine potassium measurement, the specific cause for most cases of hypokalemia should be identified. Additional studies, including measurement of blood gases and other constituents, renin and aldosterone assays, additional tests of renal function, and some detective work to identify surreptitious diuretic or laxative intake may be needed (32).

The search will usually be successful and well worth the effort. Hypokalemia is both common and potentially harmful. Once its cause is recognized, it should be both correctable and preventable.

REFERENCES

1. Abramson, E., and Arky, R.: Diabetic acidosis with initial hypokalemia. *JAMA* 196: 401–403, 1966.
2. Adams, P. C., Woodhouse, K. W., Adela, M., and Parnham, A.: Exaggerated hypokalemia in acute myeloid leukaemia. *Br. Med. J.* 282:1034–1035, 1981.
3. Aldinger, K. A., and Samaan, N. A.: Hypokalemia and hypercalcemia: prevalence and significance in treatment. *Ann. Intern. Med.* 87:571–573, 1977.
4. Al-Hillawi, A. H., Hayward, R., and Johnson, N. M.: Incidence of cardiac arrhythmias in patients taking slow release salbutamol and slow release terbutaline for asthma. *Br. Med. J.* 288:367, 1984.

5. Bagshawe, K. D., Curtin, J. R., and Garnett, E. S.: Effect of prolonged hydrocortisone administration on potassium metabolism. *Lancet* 1:18–21, 1965.
6. Black, D. A. K., and Milne, M. D.: Experimental potassium depletion in man. *Clin. Sci.* 11:397–415, 1952.
7. Brass, E. P., and Thompson, W. L.: Drug-induced electrolyte abnormalities. *Drugs* 24:207–228, 1982.
8. Broome, T. P., and Holt, J. M.: Venous stasis and forearm exercise during venipuncture as sources of error in plasma electrolyte determinations. *Can. Med. Assoc. J.* 90:1105–1107, 1964.
9. Brunner, F. P., and Frick, P. G.: Hypokalaemia, metabolic alkalosis, and hypernatraemia due to "massive" sodium penicillin therapy. *Br. Med. J.* 4:550–552, 1968.
10. Clapp, J. R., Rector, F. C., and Seldin, D. W.: Effects of unabsorbed anions on proximal and distal transtubular potentials in rats. *Am. J. Physiol.* 202:781–786, 1962.
11. DeFronzo, R. A., Felig, P., Ferrannini, E., and Wahren, J.: Effect of graded doses of insulin on splanchnic and peripheral potassium metabolism in man. *Am. J. Physiol.* 238:E421–E427, 1980.
12. Edwards, R., Winnie, A. P., and Ramamurthy, S.: Acute hypocapneic hypokalemia: an iatrogenic anesthetic complication. *Anesth. Analg.* 56:786–792, 1977.
13. Evans, J. J., and Bozdech, M. J.: Hypokalemia in nonblastic chronic myelogenous leukemia. *Arch. Intern. Med.* 141:784–787, 1981.
14. Ferris, T., Kashgarian, M., Levitin, H., Brandt, I., and Epstein, F. H.: Renal tubular acidosis and renal potassium wasting acquired as a result of hypercalcemic nephropathy. *N. Engl. J. Med.* 265:924–928, 1961.
15. Gill, J. R., Bell, N. H., and Bartter, F. C.: Impaired conservation of sodium and potassium in renal tubular acidosis and its correction by buffer anions. *Clin. Sci.* 33: 577–592, 1967.
16. Gonzalez, J. J., Owens, W., Ungaro, P. C., Werk, E. E., and Wentz, P. W.: Clay ingestion: a rare cause of hypokalemia. *Ann. Intern. Med.* 97:65–66, 1982.
17. Kaplan, N. M.: Hypokalemia in the hypertensive patient with observations on the incidence of primary aldosteronism. *Ann. Intern. Med.* 66:1079–1090, 1967.
18. Kaplan, N. M.: *Clinical Hypertension*, 3rd ed. Baltimore, Williams & Wilkins, 1982, p. 306.
19. Kaplan, N. M.: New approaches to the therapy of mild hypertension. *Am. J. Cardiol.* 51:621–627, 1983.
20. Kirkland, J. L., Lye, M., Levy, D. W., and Banerjee, A. K.: Patterns of urine flow and electrolyte excretion in healthy elderly people. *Br. Med. J.* 287:1665–1667, 1983.
21. Knochel, J. P.: Environmental heat illness: an eclectic review. *Arch. Intern. Med.* 133:841–864, 1974.
22. Lawson, D. H., Murray, R. M., Parker, J. L. W., and Hay, G.: Hypokalemia in megaloblastic anemias. *Lancet* 2:588–590, 1970.
23. Lawson, D. H., Henry, D. A., Lowe, J. M., Gray, J. M. B., and Morgan, H. G.: Severe hypokalemia in hospitalized patients. *Arch. Intern. Med.* 139:978–980, 1979.
24. Leitch, A. G., Clancy, L. J., Costello, J. F., and Flenley, D. C.: Effect of intravenous infusion of salbutamol on ventilatory response to carbon dioxide and hypoxia and on heart rate and plasma potassium in normal men. *Br. Med. J.* 1:365–367, 1976.
25. Mohr, J. A., Clark, R. M., Waack, T. C., and Whang, R.: Nafcillin-associated hypokalemia. *JAMA* 242:544, 1979.
26. Morgan, D. B., and Young, R. M.: Acute transient hypokalemia: new interpretation of a common event. *Lancet* 2:751–752, 1982.
27. Nuki, G., Boddy, K., Kennedy, A. C., King, P., Duncan, A. M., and Buchanan, W. W.: Potassium metabolism in patients with rheumatoid arthritis: effects of treatment

with depot tetracosactrin, spironolactone, and oral supplements of potassium chloride. *Ann. Rheum. Dis.* 34:506–514, 1975.
28. Parker, M. S., Oster, J. R., Perez, G. O., and Taylor, A. L.: Chronic hypokalemia and alkalosis. *Arch. Intern. Med.* 140:1336–1137, 1980.
29. Petersen, K.-G., Schluter, K. J., and Kerp, L.: Regulation of serum potassium during insulin-induced hypoglycemia. *Diabetes* 31:615–617, 1982.
30. Podolsky, S., Zimmerman, H. J., Burrows, B. A., Cardarelli, J. A., and Pattavina, C. G.: Potassium depletion in hepatic cirrhosis: a reversible cause of impaired growth-hormone and insulin response to stimulation. *N. Engl. J. Med.* 288:644–648, 1973.
31. Potter, W. Z., Trygstad, C. W., Helmer, O. M., Nance, W. E., and Judson, W. E.: Familial hypokalemia associated with renal interstitial fibrosis. *Am. J. Med.* 57: 971–977, 1974.
32. Rodman, J. S., and Reidenberg, M. M.: Symptomatic hypokalemia resulting from surreptitious diuretic ingestion. *JAMA* 246:1687–1689, 1981.
33. Rostand, S. G.: Profound hypokalemia in continuous ambulatory peritoneal dialysis. *Arch. Intern. Med.* 143:377–378, 1983.
34. Sandor, F. F., Pickens, P. T., and Crallan, J.: Variations of plasma potassium concentrations during long-term treatment of hypertension with diuretics without potassium supplements. *Br. Med. J.* 284:711–715, 1982.
35. Schwartz, W. B., and Relman, A. S.: Metabolic and renal studies in chronic potassium depletion resulting from overuse of laxatives. *J. Clin. Invest.* 32:258–271, 1953.
36. Sterns, R. H., Cox, M., Feig, P. U., and Singer, I.: Internal potassium balance and the control of the plasma potassium concentration. *Medicine* 60:339–354, 1981.
37. Struthers, A. D., Whitesmith, R., and Reid, J. L.: Prior thiazide diuretic treatment increases adrenaline-induced hypokalemia. *Lancet* 1:1358–1360, 1983.
38. Turino, G. M., Goldring, R. M., and Heinemann, H. O.: Renal response to mechanical ventilation in patients with chronic hypercapnia. *Am. J. Med.* 56:151–161, 1974.
39. Verner, J. V., and Morrison, A. B.: Endocrine pancreatic islet disease with diarrhea. Report of a case due to diffuse hyperplasia of nonbeta islet tissue with a review of 54 additional cases. *Arch. Intern. Med.* 133:492–497, 1974.
40. Vetter, W. R., Cohn, L. H., and Reichgott, M.: Hypokalemia and electrocardiographic abnormalities during acute alcohol withdrawal. *Arch. Intern. Med.* 120: 536–541, 1967.
41. Wiegand, C. F., Davin, T. D., Raij, L., and Kjellstrand, C. M.: Severe hypokalemia induced by hemodialysis. *Arch. Intern. Med.* 141:167–170, 1981.

4

Alterations in the Renin-Aldosterone System by Diuretics and Converting Enzyme Inhibitors

JAMES C. MELBY and GEORGE T. GRIFFING
University Hospital and Boston University School of Medicine, Boston, Massachusetts

Diuretics are fundamental to many of the clinical therapeutic regimens for hypertension and edema. These agents are not free of side effects and invariably produce potassium wastage and often hypokalemia (21). Although the cumulative effects of diuretics in the treatment of hypertension and edema are beneficial, many potentially harmful effects are associated with diuretic-induced hypokalemia, including increased ventrical ectopy, intestinal ileus, myopathy, digoxin toxicity, reversible renal tubular damage, the precipitation of type II diabetes mellitus, and hyposomatotropism (10,12,15,27,33,34).

Hypokalemia in hypertensive patients is a particularly common medical problem since diuretics are the mainstay of antihypertensive therapy. Hypokalemia can be difficult to correct since current treatments have serious limitations. Present therapy is limited to potassium supplementation with potassium salts or potassium-sparing diuretics, such as spironolactone and triamterene. Unfortunately, potassium salts are unpalatable, induce gastric and intestinal irritation (1,28), and may be ineffective in restoring potassium balance (18). Spironolactone, which requires the presence of aldosterone excess to be maximally effective, has a long latent period and sometimes requires potassium supplementation (32). Also, therapy with the drug is complicated by untoward effects in up to 20% of patients (8). Adverse reactions include gastrointestinal irritation, menstrual irregularities, gynecomastia, and hypogonadism in men (6,8,16).

Two mechanisms have been proposed to explain diuretic-induced hypokalemia: (a) increased delivery of sodium to distal tubular sodium-potassium exchange sites and (b) secondary hyperaldosteronism. Dietary sodium restriction has been advocated to prevent excess sodium delivery to renal distal tubular sodium-potassium exchange sites, thus reducing diuretic-induced kaliuresis (22,29). Although this theory is modestly successful, it prevents only about 50% of diuretic-induced potassium depletion. Furthermore, severe sodium restriction leads to secondary hyperaldosteronism and can attenuate the efficacy of diuretics in treating hypertension (2).

AMILORIDE THERAPY IN HYPERALDOSTERONISM

Diuretic-induced secondary hyperaldosteronism is mimicked by two disease states: primary aldosteronism and Bartter's syndrome. Like diuretic-induced hypokalemia, the hypokalemia of these disorders is due to hyperaldosteronism. Previous medical therapy for primary Bartter's syndrome has been limited to potassium supplements and potassium-sparing diuretics such as spironolactone or triamterene. Amiloride (N-amidino-3,5-diamino-6-chloropyraxinamide hydrochloride dihydrate) is a new potassium-sparing diuretic which offers significant advantages over previous therapy for hypokalemia. Amiloride acts on distal renal tubular cells to reduce the urinary excretion of potassium, while augmenting the excretion of sodium and chloride. This drug is a significant advancement in the treatment of hypokalemia since it is more potent than either spironolactone or triamterene and has fewer side effects (19,23).

Correction of hypokalemia is generally associated with changes in both renin and aldosterone secretion. Potassium repletion augments aldosterone production by direct zona glomerulosa stimulation (5,9). It also inhibits renin secretion by direct effects on the juxtaglomerulosa, independent or aldosterone (16,17). Potassium repletion induced by amiloride should produce similar renin-aldosterone responses, but these effects have not been systemically studied in either primary aldosteronism or secondary hyperaldosteronism. Amiloride was prospectively evaluated by us in hypokalemic patients with either primary hyperaldosteronism (PH) (10 patients) or Bartter's syndrome (BS) (5 patients).

Vital Signs

The systolic and diastolic blood pressure fell significantly in primary hyperaldosteronism following institution of amiloride therapy (171/112 vs. 150/97). Blood pressure remained unchanged in Bartter's syndrome (116/80 vs. 117/71) (see Fig. 1). The values of the remainder of the vital signs were unremarkable.

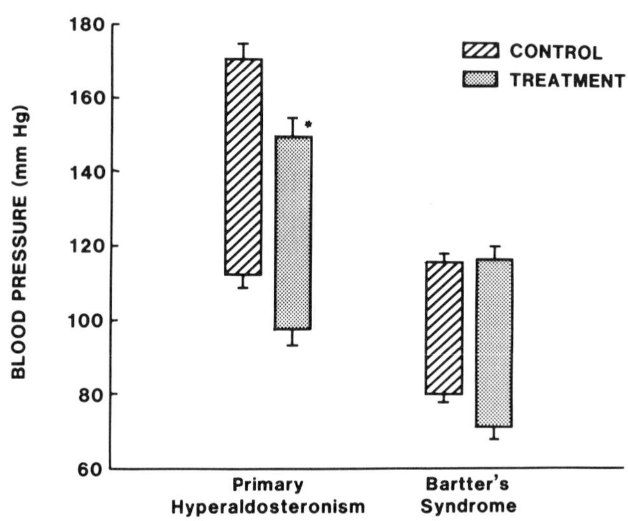

Figure 1 Changes in blood pressure before and after amiloride therapy in primary hyperaldosteronism and Bartter's syndrome (*$p < 0.05$ comparing control and treatment periods).

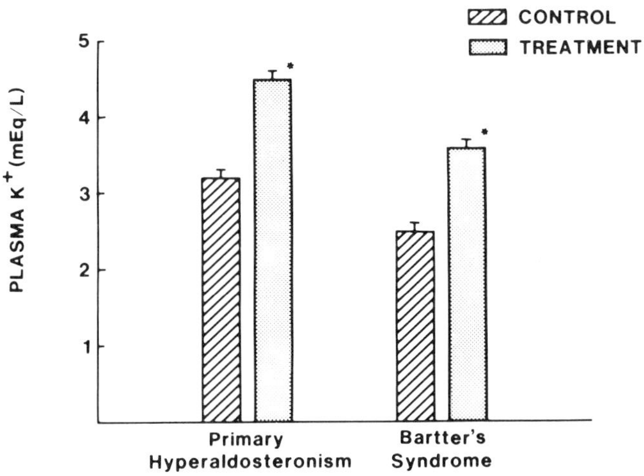

Figure 2 Changes in plasma potassium before and after amiloride therapy in primary hyperaldosteronism and Bartter's syndrome (*p < 0.05 compared to control period).

Plasma Potassium

Following several weeks of amiloride therapy, plasma potassium levels increased in patients with both primary hyperaldosteronism and Bartter's syndrome. The amiloride-induced plasma potassium increment was greater in those with primary hyperaldosteronism (3.2 vs. 4.5) than Bartter's syndrome (2.5 vs. 3.6 mEq/L) (see Fig. 2).

Plasma Renin Activity

The ambulatory plasma renin activity (PRA) following amiloride therapy declined in Bartter's syndrome (25.3 ± 1.9 vs. 11.9 ± 0.4), but increased in primary hyperaldosteronism (0.39 ± 0.18 vs. 2.21 ± 0.35) (see Fig. 3). In Bartter's syndrome, the decline in PRA occurred in 4 of 5 patients, and in primary hyperaldosteronism the rise in PRA occurred in all 10 patients.

Plasma Aldosterone

The plasma aldosterone level rose in both primary hyperaldosteronism (28.4 ± 1.8 vs. 54.3 ± 2.9 ng/dl) and Bartter's syndrome (19.5 ± 1.5 vs. 38.0 ± 3.0 ng/dl) during amiloride therapy (see Fig. 4). This increase occurred in 7 of 10 patients with primary hyperaldosteronism and in all 5 patients with Bartter's syndrome.

Summary

The results of this study demonstrate that amiloride therapy can improve the hypokalemia associated with either primary or secondary hyperaldosteronism. Furthermore, amiloride therapy is associated with changes in plasma renin activity and plasma aldosterone that cannot be explained by correction of the hypokalemia alone.

In Bartter's syndrome, the plasma renin activity fell, and the plasma aldosterone increased during amiloride therapy. These effects can be explained by potassium repletion, since potassium is known to stimulate aldosterone secretion directly and suppress renin

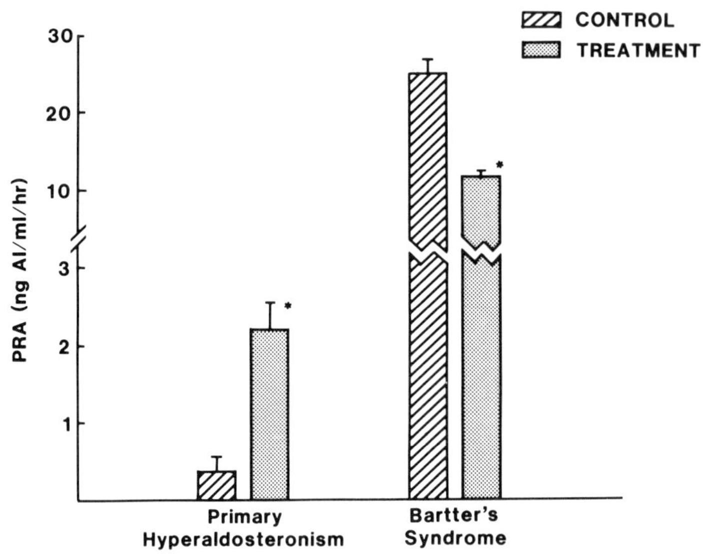

Figure 3 Changes in plasma renin activity (PRA) before and after amiloride therapy in primary hyperaldosteronism and Bartter's syndrome (*$p < 0.05$ compared to control).

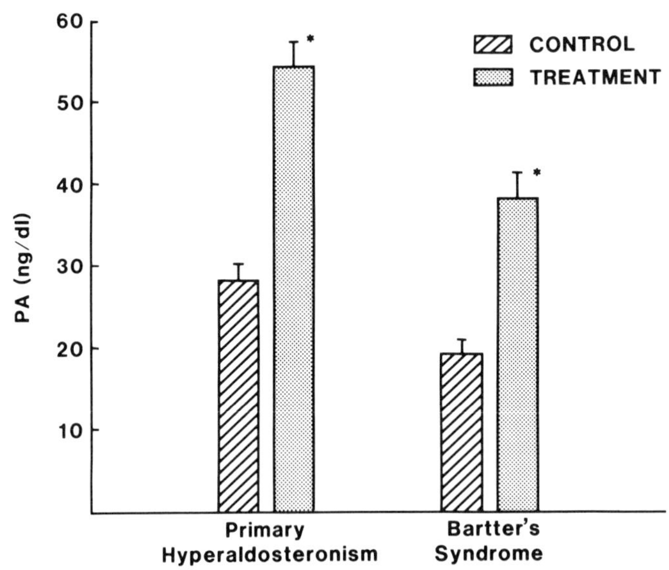

Figure 4 Plasma aldosterone (PRA) before and after amiloride therapy in primary hyperaldosteronism and Bartter's syndrome (*$p < 0.05$ compared to control).

production. Although these patients received concomitant potassium supplements and indomethacin, this treatment is unlikely to influence the results since the dosage schedule remained constant throughout the study. Furthermore, two of the five patients not receiving concomitant therapy demonstrated similar results.

In primary hyperaldosteronism, an increase in both plasma aldosterone and plasma renin activity was observed following amiloride therapy. The plasma aldosterone increment was greater than that in Bartter's syndrome, possibly due to the combined effects of renin and aldosterone stimulation. The rise in plasma aldosterone, as well as the rise in plasma potassium, should further suppress the plasma renin activity in this group of patients. The plasma renin activity in primary hyperaldosteronism, however, significantly increased following amiloride therapy. The plasma renin increment cannot be explained by concomitant antihypertensive medication, since this therapy remained constant throughout the study. Furthermore, three patients with primary hyperaldosteronism not receiving concomitant therapy had identical increments in plasma potassium, renin, and aldosterone levels. It is also unlikely that the decrease in blood pressure had a significant influence on plasma renin activity, since renin secretion is not activated by blood pressure changes in the high or normal range.

The results of the present study have both practical and theoretical implications. Despite an increase in aldosterone, amiloride therapy is effective in correcting potassium depletion in both primary and secondary hyperaldosteronism. An aldosterone antagonist, such as spironolactone, could act synergistically with amiloride in treating patients with severe or refractory hypokalemia. The aldosterone antagonist would theoretically prevent any additional urinary potassium wastage due to amiloride-induced hyperaldosteronism. Furthermore, a renin antagonist, such as a converting enzyme inhibitor, may potentiate the weak antihypertensive effects of amiloride in primary hyperaldosteronism. Since amiloride induces renin secretion, pharmacological interruption of the renin–angiotensin system could prevent any angiotensin-II-dependent vasoconstriction. In some instances, increased renin secretion in primary hyperaldosteronism could be beneficial. Amiloride therapy prior to adrenal surgery for an aldosterone-producing adenoma could theoretically stimulate recovery of the contralateral suppressed zona glomerulosa and prevent postoperative hypoaldosteronism.

In conclusion, amiloride therapy is efficacious in correcting the hypokalemia of both primary hyperaldosteronism and Bartter's syndrome. This is associated with a rise in plasma aldosterone in both disorders, but plasma renin activity decreases in Bartter's syndrome and increases in primary hyperaldosteronism. The amiloride-induced potassium repletion in this study probably explains the reinin suppression and aldosterone production observed in Bartter's syndrome. The increase in both renin and aldosterone in amiloride-treated primary hyperaldosteronism, however, may be evidence for a direct activation of the renin–angiotensin system or, alternatively, due to the mild natriuretic effects of amiloride.

PREVENTION OF DIURETIC-INDUCED SECONDARY HYPERALDOSTERONISM AND HYPOKALEMIA BY A NEW ANGIOTENSIN-CONVERTING ENZYME INHIBITOR (MK-421)

This study prospectively evaluated the prevention of diuretic-induced secondary hyperaldosteronism and hypokalemia by an angiotensin converting enzyme inhibitor (MK-421).

Of the angiotensin-converting enzyme inhibitors, captopril, currently the only approved drug of this class in the United States, is effective but has a high incidence of drug-related side-effects (4,13). Recently, a new group of non-sulfhydryl-converting enzyme inhibitors has been introduced for clinical investigation (26). Their unique structure (5) should theoretically prevent many of the sulfhydryl-related side effects produced by captopril. One of these agents, MK-421 [ethyl-ester-N-(S)-1-(ethoxycarbonyl)-3-(phenyl-propyl)-L-alanyl-L-proline], is more potent and has a longer duration of action than captopril (3,6).

Eighteen normal subjects were randomized into three groups for this study: (a) HCTZ group: HCTZ 50 mg/day; (b) MK-421 group: MK-421 10 mg/day; (c) HCTZ + MK-421 group: HCTZ 50 mg/day plus MK-421 10 mg/day.

Vital Signs

Only a few significant changes occurred in the vital signs during the treatment period. The upright (4-hr) blood pressure tended to decrease during the treatment period in each of the groups, but this was only significant in the MK-421 group at Day 28 compared to control (110/62 vs 118/76 mmHg). In addition, the upright heart rate tended to rise during the treatment period in each of the groups, but it was significantly elevated in only the HCTZ group at day 28 compared to control (98 vs. 86 beats/min). The body weight decreased significantly at day 7 in both the HCTZ group (4 lbs) and the HCTZ + MK-421 group (5 lbs). At Day 28, the HCTZ + MK-421 group had the greatest weight loss (3 lbs), although this was not statistically significant.

Plasma Renin Activity

The upright (4-hr) PRA rose in all three groups during the initial treatment period, as seen in Figure 5. The HCTZ group's PRA rose significantly throughout the study; however, the MK-421 group's PRA had a similar but greater rise at day 7, and again a slight fall at day 28. The HCTZ + MK-421 group PRA had the greatest PRA increment at day 7 and a subsequent fall at day 28.

Plasma Aldosterone

The only significant changes in upright (4-hr) PA occurred in the HCTZ group, as seen in Figure 5. The HCTZ group's supine and upright PA increased to the highest level at day 7 and then fell slightly at day 28. The MK-421 group's supine and upright PA tended to decrease both at days 7 and 28, but this was only significant at day 7. The HCTZ + MK-421 group had a significant rise in supine, but not upright, PA at day 7 and a subsequent fall at day 28.

Aldosterone Secretion Rate

The changes in aldosterone secretion rate (ASR) during the study can be seen in Figure 6. The HCTZ group had a dramatic increase in ASR at day 7, which then declined but remained elevated nearly twofold at day 28. The MK-421 group's ASR did not change at day 7 but decreased significantly at day 28. The HCTZ + MK-421 groups' ASR increased significantly at day 7, but it then decreased to nearly control levels at day 28.

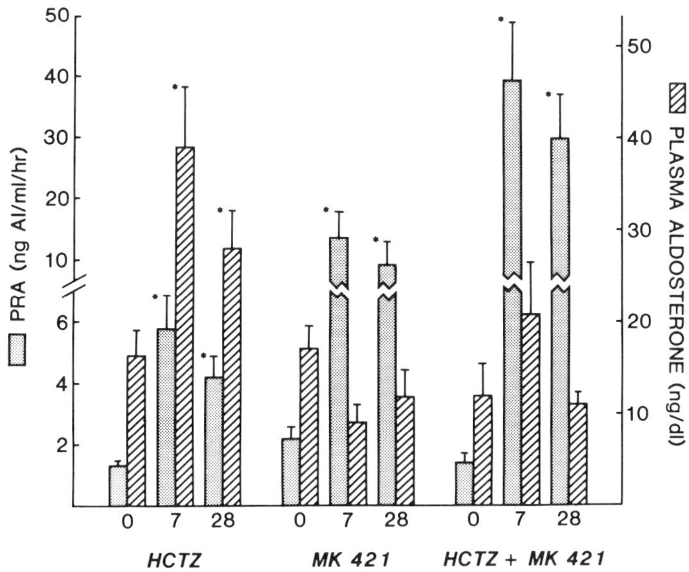

Figure 5 Plasma renin activity (PRA) and aldosterone measurements on days 0, 7, and 28 in the HCTZ group, MK-421 group, and HCTZ + MK-421 group (*$p < 0.05$ compared to control).

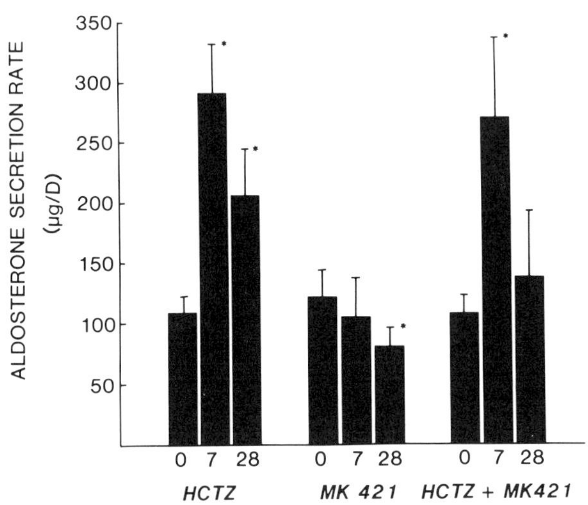

Figure 6 Aldosterone secretion rates on days 0, 7, and 28 in HCTZ group, MK-421 group, and HCTZ + MK-421 group (*$p < 0.05$ compared to control).

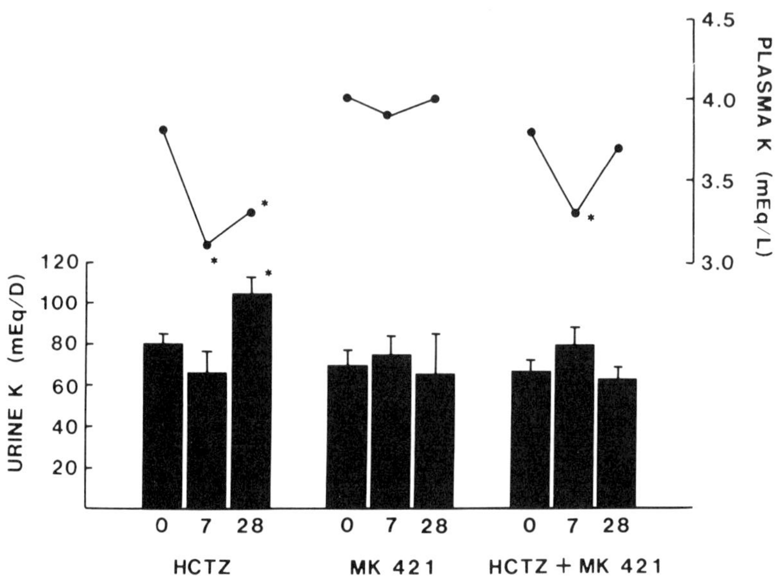

Figure 7 Urine and plasma potassium measurements on days 0, 7, and 28 in the HCTZ group, MK-421 group, and HCTZ + MK-421 group (*$p < 0.05$ compared to control).

Plasma and Urinary Electrolytes

Changes in the plasma and urinary potassium (K) and sodium (Na) levels during this study are seen in Figures 3 and 4. The HCTZ group had a significant fall in plasma K at day 7, which persisted to day 28 (see Figure 7). The HCTZ group's urinary K was unchanged at day 7 but did increase at day 28. The MK-421 group's plasma K did not change at either day 7 or day 28. The HCTZ + MK-421 groups' plasma K, however, fell at day 7 but returned to control levels at day 28 (see Figure 7). The HCTZ + MK-421 groups' urinary K rose slightly, but not significantly, at day 7 and decreased to nearly control values at day 28.

The HCTZ group's plasma Na did not change significantly at either day 7 or day 28 (see Figure 8). The HCTZ group's urinary Na remained unchanged at day 7 but tended to increase, although not significantly, at day 28. The MK-421 group's plasma Na remained nearly constant at day 7 and day 28 (see Fig. 4). Likewise, the MK-421 group's urinary Na demonstrated no significant changes at day 7 or day 28. The HCTZ + MK-421 group's plasma Na fell at day 7 but rose to nearly control values at day 28 (see Figure 8). The HCTZ + MK-421 group's urinary Na remained unchanged at day 7 but increased significantly at day 28.

Clinical Observations

In general, the subjects tolerated each of the drug regimens in this study with few, if any, adverse effects. On day 7, one patient in the HCTZ group complained of light-headedness and had mild orthostatic hypotension, hypokalemic electrocardiographic changes, and a plasma K of 3.0 mEq/L. These symptoms resolved without specific therapy and without a return of the plasma K to normal. Between days 6 and 8 of the study, three patients in

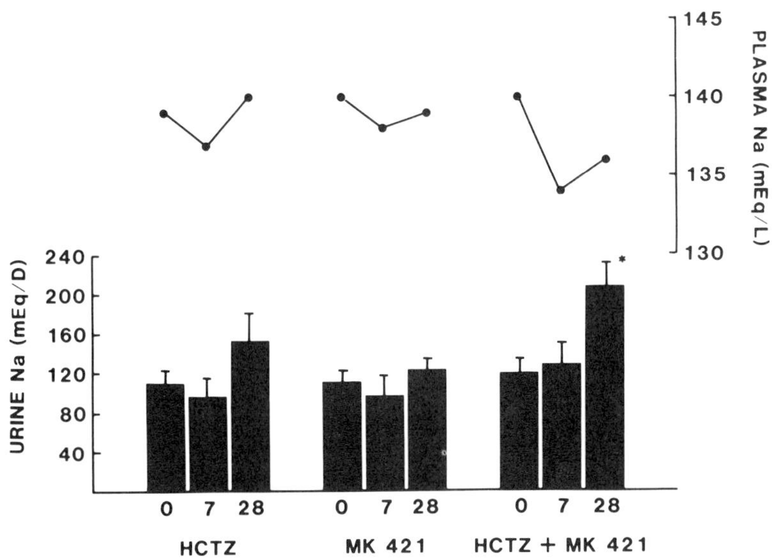

Figure 8 Urine and plasma sodium determinations on days 0, 7, and 28 in the HCTZ group, MK-421 group, and HCTZ + MK-421 group (*p < compared to control).

the HCTZ + MK-421 group developed similar symptoms. They complained of nausea and light-headedness without significant orthostatic hypotension. Two of the three HCTZ + MK-421 group patients had hypokalemia (3.3 and 2.8 mEq/L) and hypokalemic electrocardiographic changes, but the other patient had a normal plasma K (3.7 mEq/L) and electrocardiographic findings. The HCTZ + MK-421 group subject with the lowest plasma K (2.8 mEq/L) and the highest ASR (499 μg/day) withdrew from the study at day 12; the other two subjects had rapid and complete resolution of symptoms.

Discussion

This study demonstrates a delayed but effective prevention of diuretic-induced secondary hyperaldosteronism and hypokalemia by a new converting enzyme inhibitor, MK-421. Furthermore, a parallel promotion of natriuresis by MK-421 was not seen with diuretic therapy alone.

Diuretic therapy in the HCTZ group produced a rapid and dramatic secondary hyperaldosteronism by 7 days. This was manifest by a two and one-half times increase in aldosterone secretion rate and corresponding hypokalemia. One of the six patients in this group developed adverse symptoms and electrocardiographic changes related to the hypokalemia. The lack of a significant kaliuresis at Day 7 is difficult to reconcile, although early potassium wastage could have occurred prior to Day 7. The diminished kaliuresis with continuous diuretic therapy may reflect secondary alterations in renal blood flow, one of the major determinants of renal potassium secretion (7).

The HCTZ group had a reduction in diuretic-induced secondary hyperaldosteronism at day 28 of the study. The attenuation of secondary hyperaldosteronism on day 28 is probably related to increased dietary sodium intake since these patients were on an ad libitum sodium diet, their weights returned to nearly prestudy levels, and a urinary sodium surfeit was present.

The MK-421 group demonstrated MK-421's blockade of the renin–aldosterone system. The hyperreninism during angiotensin-converting enzyme inhibitor therapy is believed to be caused by the loss of feedback inhibition of angiotensin-II on renin secretion at the juxtaglomerular apparatus (16). The fact that the aldosterone secretion rate did not decrease at day 7 indicates that there was only a partial blockade of the renin–aldosterone axis. A more complete interruption of this axis would be expected to lower aldosterone secretion and perhaps further increase renin.

On day 28, however, the aldosterone secretion declined but the PRA also declined proportionally. This reduction in aldosterone secretion is probably not due to a more complete angiotensin-converting enzyme inhibition since this would be expected to elevate renin further. Instead, since PRA measures both renin and its substrate, angiotensinogen, a fall in renin substrate could offset the rise in renin, resulting in a lower PRA. Renin substrate levels have been demonstrated to decline during converting enzyme inhibitor therapy (30), and this has been explained by the loss of angiotensin-II's positive feedback response on hepatic synthesis of angiotensinogen (24). Therefore, prolonged converting enzyme inhibitor therapy could result in a decline in angiotensinogen levels and a more effective blockade of the renin–aldosterone system.

The HCTZ + MK-421 group demonstrated a relatively unopposed diuretic-induced secondary hyperaldosteronism and hypokalemia at day 7, comparable to the HCTZ group. During this initial period, three of the six subjects in the HCTZ + MK-421 group experienced adverse hypokalemic symptoms, prompting one subject to discontinue the study. Following 4 weeks of treatment, however, this group no longer had either hyperaldosteronism or hypokalemia.

The prevention of diuretic-induced secondary hyperaldosteronism in the HCTZ + MK-421 group at the fourth week could be a sum of the effects observed in the HCTZ group and the MK-421 group over the same time period. The HCTZ group demonstrated diminished diuretic-induced secondary hyperaldosteronism and the MK-421 group showed a lowering of aldosterone secretion over the course of 4 weeks. The ultimate balance between hydrochlorthiazide and MK-421 therapy at 4 weeks was a negation of the diuretic-induced secondary hyperaldosteronism and hypokalemia.

The natriuresis in the HCTZ + MK-421 group at Day 28 is an important and perhaps therapeutically beneficial observation. A natriuretic effect has been previously described with converting enzyme inhibitor therapy alone, and this is probably caused by an associated renal vasodilatation (11,20). This was also observed in the MK-421 group at day 28, when a fall in aldosterone secretion corresponded with a slight increase in urine sodium. Chronic diuretic therapy alone, as seen in the HCTZ group, results in less sodium wastage compared to the HCTZ + MK-421 group, as evidenced by less natriuresis and less total body weight loss. Although this could be related to a greater salt intake in the HCTZ group, it is more likely to be due to hyperaldosteronism since both groups had similar access to dietary sodium during this period. The natriuresis in the HCTZ + MK-421 group most likely reflects diuretic-induced sodium wastage unimpeded by secondary hyperaldosteronism. The natriuresis observed in the HCTZ + MK-421 group is often clinically desirable and could enhance the therapeutic efficacy of diuretics in the treatment of high blood pressure and states of fluid retention.

It is also significant that the natriuresis in the HCTZ + MK-421 group at 28 days did not result in significant kaliuresis or hypokalemia. The two primary causes of diuretic-induced hypokalemia include either excess sodium delivery to the renal tubule or secondary hyperaldosteronism. The fact that potassium depletion did not occur in the

HCTZ + MK-421 group in the face of natriuresis and blunting of diuretic-induced secondary hyperaldosteronism indicates that secondary hyperaldosteronism is the more important mechanism mediating diuretic-induced hypokalemia.

Caution, however, must be used in assessing the clinical significance of these results. The subjects in this study were normotensive, healthy volunteers taking no other medications. The effects of the drugs studied in this report could have quite different results when used to treat patients receiving other drug therapy or with certain diseases. For example, patients with hypertension or with edema-forming states usually have reduced renal blood flow and altered adrenal and vascular sensitivity to angiotensin-II (35). These factors could ultimately affect the therapeutic results of diuretics, converting enzyme inhibitors, or both. In addition, the present observations were restricted to 28 days of therapy, and the results of prolonged therapy can only be extrapolated.

In conclusion, these results demonstrate a delayed but effective prevention of diuretic-induced secondary hyperaldosteronism by a new converting enzyme inhibitor, MK-421, following 28 days of therapy. Furthermore, this was accompanied by a sustained natriuresis without a kaliuresis, establishing the importance of aldosterone in the medication of diuretic-induced hypokalemia. Therefore, interruption of the renin–aldosterone system by converting enzyme inhibitors, such as MK-421, can provide rational therapy directed at the underlying cause of diuretic-induced hypokalemia. These drugs promise to provide useful adjunctive therapy in patients treated with diuretics.

ACKNOWLEDGMENTS

This work was supported by Grants-in-Aid 1-R23-HL31049, RR-53-NIH, 5-PO-HL18318, 5-RO1-AM12027, 5-P32-HL07224, and 1-T30-AM21683 SCOR from the National Institutes of Health.

Dr. Griffing is the recipient of a New Investigator Research Award from the NIH (1-R23-HL31049).

REFERENCES

1. Boley, S. J., Allec, A. C., Shultz, L., and Schwartz, S.: Potassium-induced lesions of the small bowel. I. Clinical aspects. II. Pathology and pathogenesis. *JAMA* 193:997–1001, 1965.
2. Bourgoignie, J. J., Catanzaro, F. J., and Perry, H. M.: Renin-angiotensin–aldosterone system during chronic thiazide therapy of benign hypertension. *Circulation* 37:27–35, 1968.
3. Brunner, D. B., Desponds, G., Billaz, J., Keller, I., Ferber, F., Gavras, H., Brunner, H. R., and Schelling, J. L.: Effect of a new angiotensin-converting enzyme inhibitor, MK-421, and its lysine analogue on the components of the renin system in healthy subjects. *Br. J. Clin. Pharmacol.* 11:461–467, 1981.
4. Captopril: benefits and risks in severe hypertension (Editorial). *Lancet* 2:129–131, 1980.
5. Davis, J. O., Urquhart, J., Higgins, J. T. Jr., Capser, A., and Cavanaugh, E.: The effects of alterations of plasma sodium and potassium concentration on aldosterone secretion. *J. Clin. Invest.* 42:497, 1963.
6. Gavras, H., Waeber, B., Gavras, I., Biollaz, J., Brunner, H. R., and Davies, R. O.: Antihypertensive effect of a new oral angiotensin-converting enzyme inhibitor, "MK-421." *Lancet* 2:543–547, 1981.

7. Good, G. W., and Wright, F. S.: Luminal influence on potassium secretion: sodium concentration on fluid flow rate. *Am. J. Physiol.* 236:192-205, 1979.
8. Greenblatt, D. J., and Loch-Weser, J.: Adverse reactions to spironolactone. A report from the Boston Collaborate Drug Surveillance Program. *JAMA* 225:40–43, 1973.
9. Himathongkam, T., Dluhy, R. L., and Williams, G. H.: Potassium–aldosterone–renin interrelationships. *J. Clin. Endocrinol. Metab.* 41:153, 1975.
10. Holland, O. B., Nickson, J. V., and Kuhnert, L.: Diuretic-induced ventricular ectopic activity. *Am. J. Med.* 70:762–768, 1981.
11. Hollenberg, N. K., Swartz, S. L., Passan, D. R., and Williams, G. H.: Increased glomerular filtration rate after converting-enzyme inhibition in essential hypertension. *N. Engl. J. Med.* 301:9–12, 1979.
12. Hollifield, J. W., and Slaton, P. E.: Thiazide diuretics, hypokalemia and cardiac arythmias. *Acta Med. Scand. (Suppl.)* 647:67–73, 1981.
13. Hoorntje, S. J., Weening, J. J., The, T. H., Kallenberg, C. G. M., Donkar, A. J. M., and Hoedemaeker, P. J.: Immune-complex glomerulopathy in patients treated with captopril. *Lancet* 1:1212–1214, 1980.
14. Huffman, D. H., Kampmann, J. P., Hignite, C. E., and Azarnoff, D. L.: Gynecomastia induced by normal males by spironolactone. *Clin. Pharmacol. Ther.* 24:465–473, 1978.
15. Kameyma, M.: Hypokalemia myopathy caused by a long-term administration of thiazide preparation. *Clin. Neurol.* 17:162–169, 1977.
16. Kono, T., Ikeda, F., Oscko, F., Imura, H., and Endo, J.: Suppression of captopril-induced increase in plasma renin activity by des-asp^1-ileu^8-angiotensin II in man. *J. Clin. Endocrinol. Metab.* 52:354–358, 1981.
17. Landmann-Suter, R., and Struyvenberg, A.: Initial potassium loss and hypokalemia during chlorthaladone administration in patients with essential hypertension: The influence of dietary sodium restriction. *Eur. J. Clin. Invest.* 8:155–164, 1978.
18. Leemhuis, M. P., Van Damme, K. J., and Stuyvenberg, A.: Effects of chlorthalidone on serum and total body potassium in hypertensive patients. *Acta Med. Scand.* 200: 37–45, 1976.
19. McKenna, T. J., Donohoe, J. F., Brien, T. G., Healy, J. J., Canning, B. St. J., and Muldowney, F. P.: Potassium-sparing agents during diuretic therapy in hypertension. *Br. Med. J.* 2:739–741, 1971.
20. Mimran, A., Brunner, H. R., Turini, G. A., Waeber, G., and Brunner, D. V.: Effect of captopril on renal vascular tone in patients with essential hypertension. *Clin. Sci.* 57:421–423, 1979.
21. Morgan, D. B., and Davidson, C.: Hypokalemia and diuretics: An analysis of publications. *Br. Med. J.* 280:905–908, 1980.
22. Morgan, T., and Myers, J.: Potassium maintenance, potassium supplements, or potassium sparing agents. *Acta Med. Scand.* 647:117–123, 1981.
23. Multicnetric Diuretic Cooperative Study Group: Multiclinic comparison of amiliride, hydrochlorthiazide and hydrochlorthiazide plus amiloride in essential hypertension. *Arch. Intern. Med.* 141:482–486, 1981.
24. Nasjletti, A., and Masson, C. M. B.: Stimulation of angiotensin formation by renin and angiotensin. *Proc. Soc. Exp. Biol. Med.* 142:307-310, 1973.
25. NIH Conference: Spironolactone and endocrine dysfunction. *Ann. Intern. Med.* 85: 630–636, 1976.
26. Patchett, A. A., Harris, E., Tristram, E. W., et al: A new class of angiotensin-converting enzyme inhibitors. *Nature* 288:280–283, 1980.
27. Podolsky, S., and Melby, J. C.: Improvement of growth hormone response to stimulation in primary aldosteronism and correction of potassium deficiency. *Metabolism* 25:1027–1032, 1976.

28. Raf, L. E.: Enteric-coated potassium chloride tablets and ulcer of the small intestine. *Acta Clin. Scand.* 374(6):82, 1967.
29. Ran, C. V. S., Garrett, B. N., and Kaplan, N. M.: Moderate sodium restriction and various diuretics in the treatment of hypertension. *Arch. Intern. Med.* 242:1015–1019, 1981.
30. Rasmussen, S., Nielsen, M. D., and Giese, J.: Captopril combined with thiazide lowers renin substrate concentration: Implications for methodology in renin assays. *Clin. Sci.* 60:591–593, 1981.
31. Rose, L. I., Underwood, R. H., Newmark, S. R., Kisch, E. S., and Williams, G. H.: Pathophysiology of spironolactone-induced gynecomastia. *Ann. Intern. Med.* 87: 398–403, 1977.
32. Rosse, E. J.: Importance of potassium supplementation during the use of spironolactone and thiazide diuretics. *Br. Med. J.* 1:1508–1510, 1961.
33. Schwartz, W. B., and Relman, A. S.: Effects of electrolyte disorders on renal structure and function. *N. Engl. J. Med.* 276:383–389, 1967.
34. Wales, J. K., Krees, S. V., Grant, A. M., Viktora, J. K., and Wolff, F. W.: Structure-activity relationships of benzothiazine compounds as hyperglycemic agents. *J. Pharmacol. Exp. Ther.* 164:421–432, 1968.
35. Williams, G. H., and Hollenberg, N. K.: Accentuated vascular and endocrine response to SQ20881 in hypertension. *N. Engl. J. Med.* 297:184–188, 1977.

5

Quantitation of Serum Potassium Changes During Acute Acid-Base Disturbances

DAVID A. GOODKIN and ROBERT G. NARINS
Temple University Health Sciences Center, Philadelphia, Pennsylvania

For more than 50 years physicians have recognized a correlation between blood pH and serum potassium concentration. Acidosis causes hyperkalemia while alkalosis tends to result in hypokalemia. Burnell et al. were the first to study this interaction in humans (11). Based on their observations of five subjects treated for various acid-base disturbances, they concluded that serum potassium concentration changed by 0.6 mEq/L for every 0.1 unit change in extracellular pH. This rule of thumb gradually achieved the status of "conventional wisdom."

However, careful review of the considerable body of literature that has since amassed on this subject reveals that no single formula accurately projects the change in serum potassium concentration for all acid-base disturbances. In fact, it has proven most difficult to quantitate reproducibly the serum potassium alteration induced by any of the acid-base disorders.

In this chapter we will consider the interstudy variability in findings and discuss the various chemical and hormonal forces that influence blood potassium levels. We will stress the fact that many of the modifiers of serum potassium are changed during spontaneous or experimentally induced acid-base disturbances and that these changes confound interpretations of potassium-acid-base interactions. The effects of specific acid-base perturbations on serum potassium concentration will be examined and we will also demonstrate the importance of comparing changes in serum potassium levels to changes in blood hydrogen ion concentration, rather than to changes in blood pH.

INTERSTUDY VARIABILITY OF CHANGES IN SERUM POTASSIUM CONCENTRATION DURING ACUTE ACID-BASE DISTURBANCES

Figures 1-4 demonstrate the dramatic differences reported for the serum potassium concentration changes induced by acute acid-base disturbances. Figures 1 and 3 plot the mEq/L increases in serum potassium, factored for ΔpH, during metabolic and respiratory acidoses. Figure 3 excludes those studies of experimentally induced acute respiratory acidosis that employed grossly nonphysiological fractions of inspired CO_2. Figures 2 and 4 plot the mEq/L decreases in serum potassium concentration observed per 0.1 unit increase in pH, during metabolic and respiratory alkaloses. Table 1 summarizes the ranges of these effects on serum potassium, as well as the means (the value from each experiment was weighted according to the number of subjects) for each of the primary acid-base disturbances. Clearly, independent investigators report quite disparate findings after studying the same acid-base changes. In all likelihood, the variables that have confounded these experiments also serve to modify potassium balance in patients with spontaneous acid-base derangements. Thus, it is worthwhile to outline these important influences, before drawing conclusions regarding the effects of the specific acid-base disorders.

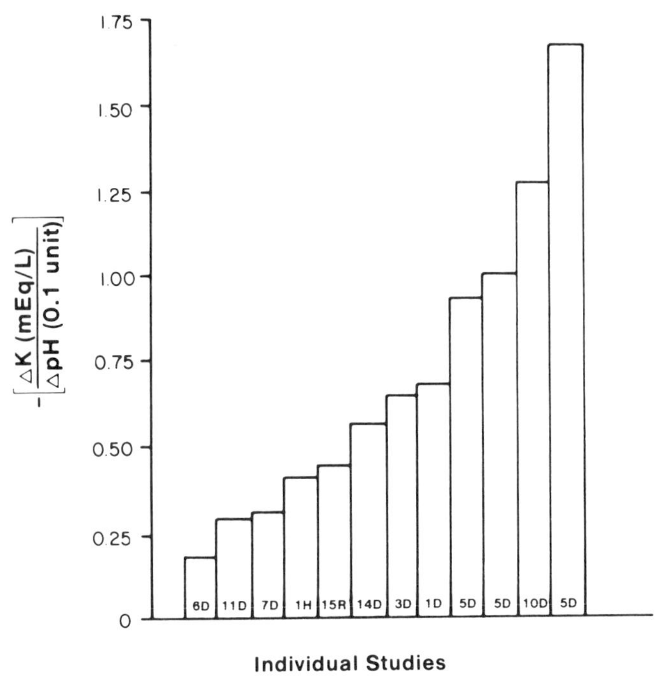

Figure 1 Effect of acute mineral acid infusion on serum potassium concentration, per 0.1 unit change in pH. Each bar represents a separate experiment. Numerals indicate number of subjects; letters indicate species (D, dog; H, human; r, rabbit). (Data from Ref. 3.)

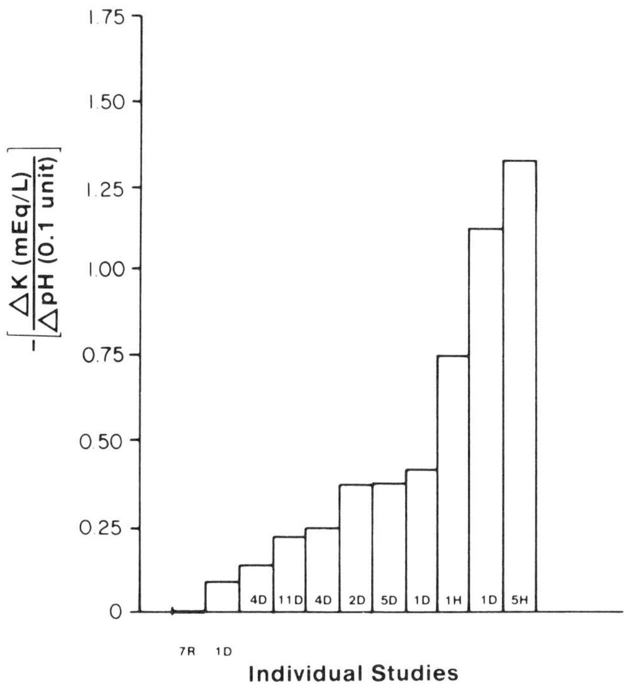

Figure 2 Effect of acute alkali infusion on serum potassium concentration, per 0.1 unit change in pH. Each bar represents a separate experiment. Numerals indicate the number of subjects and the letters indicate the species (D, dog; H, human; R, rabbit). (Data from Ref. 3.)

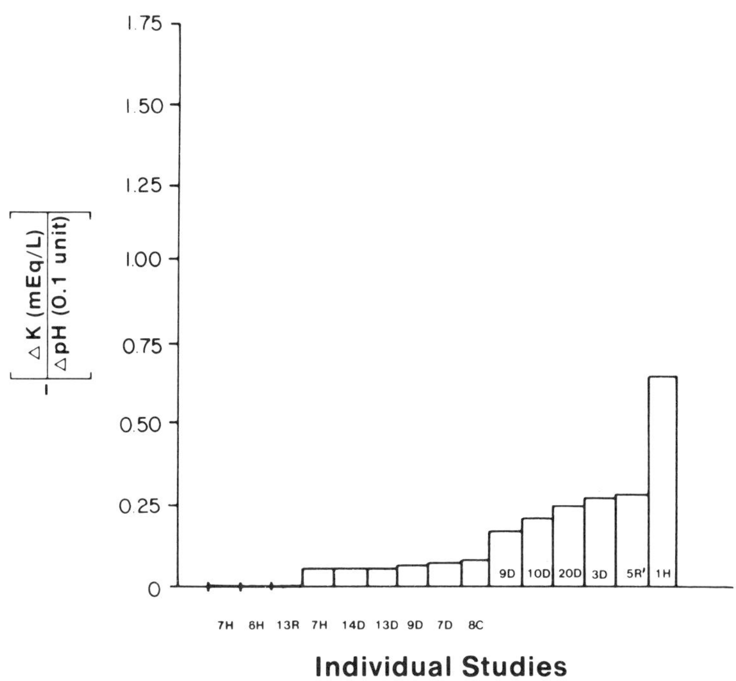

Figure 3 Effect of acute respiratory acidosis on serum potassium concentration, per 0.1 unit change in pH. Each bar represents a separate experiment. Numerals indicate the number of subjects and the letters indicate the species (D, dog; H, human; R, rabbit; C, cat; R′, rat). (Data from Ref. 3.)

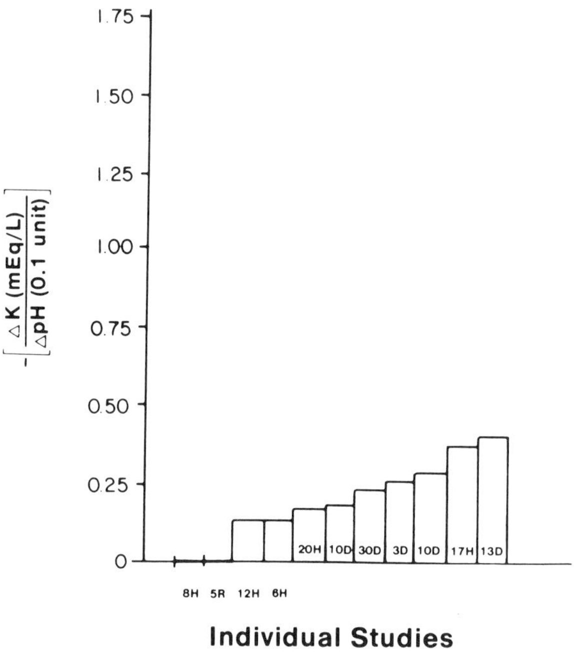

Figure 4 Effect of acute respiratory alkalosis on serum potassium concentration, per 0.1 unit change in pH. Each bar represents a separate experiment. Numerals indicate the number of subjects and the letters indicate the species (D, dog; H, human; R, rabbit). (Data from Ref. 3.)

Table 1 Summary of the Effects of Acute Acid-Base Changes on Serum Potassium Concentration

Acute pathological condition	Range $-[\Delta K^+/\Delta\ 0.1\ pH]$ (mEq/L)	Mean $-[\Delta K^+/\Delta\ 0.1\ pH]$ (mEq/L)
Metabolic acidosis (due to mineral acids)	0.17 - 1.67	0.66
Metabolic alkalosis	0.00 - 1.33	0.37
Respiratory acidosis	0.00 - 0.63	0.12
Respiratory alkalosis	0.00 - 0.41	0.22

FACTORS THAT MAY CONFOUND THE STUDY OF ACUTE ACID-BASE EFFECTS ON SERUM POTASSIUM CONCENTRATION

Potassium homeostasis may be altered by a host of influences distinct from the blood pH. Table 2 lists those factors relevant to the studies under consideration. A complete review of the factors that may play upon the serum potassium concentration, including entities not germane to the present discussion (e.g., periodic paralysis), is provided in Chapters 1 and 3.

Hormonal Variables

The catecholamines, insulin, and aldosterone each influence the serum potassium concentration. Review of numerous studies of catecholamines has demonstrated that β-adrenergic agonists prompt a shift of potassium from the extracellular fluid (ECF) to the intracellular fluid (ICF), while α-adrenergic agonists tend to increase the serum potassium concentration, by impairing its cellular uptake (62). Several recent reports reinforce the validity of these observations regarding the dual control of internal potassium balance by adrenergic activity (10,21,43,55).

Circulating insulin also prompts movement of potassium into cells, particularly into the liver and skeletal muscle. Insulinopenia induces an increase in basal serum potassium concentration and impairs tolerance to potassium challenges (15-17,30). In fact, insulin is commonly administered to treat severe hyperkalemia acutely.

Aldosterone, of course, stimulates the distal renal tubules to secrete potassium. It may also lower the serum potassium concentration by altering internal potassium balance, that is, by enhancing muscle uptake of the cation (2,4). In addition, data are beginning to suggest strongly that glucocorticoid hormones play a far greater role in potassium handling than has been appreciated previously (7).

There is no reason to expect that serum catecholamine, insulin, and adrenocortical hormone concentrations were similar among the hundreds of subjects included in the reported studies of acute acid-base effects on serum potassium concentration. In fact, considering the varying species and experimental protocols utilized (e.g., anesthetized or awake, nephrectomized or intact, etc.), it is more likely that the hormone levels were quite heterogeneous. Thus, confounding variables were likely introduced.

Table 2 Potentially Confounding Variables in the Study of Acid-Base Effects on Serum Potassium Concentration

Modifiers of internal K^+ balance	Modifiers of external K^+ balance
Hormones	Urinary losses
Catecholamines	Aldosterone
Insulin	Urine flow rate
Aldosterone	Acid-base status
Duration of acid-base changes	Distal Na^+ delivery
Serum $[HCO_3^-]$	Gastrointestinal losses
ECF osmolarity	
ECF volume	
Muscle relaxants	
FIO_2	

Table 3 Effects of Acute Acid-Base Changes on Hormonal Control of the Serum Potassium Concentration

	Effects of acidosis		Effects of alkalosis	
Hormone	Hormone secretion	Target organ response	Hormone secretion	Target organ response
Catecholamines	↑	↓ (?)	?	?
Insulin	↑	no effect (DKA)*	↓	?
Aldosterone	↑	↓	↓	↑

*See text for details

Further complicating the interpretation of acid-base vs. hormonal effects upon the serum potassium concentration is the possibility that a change in blood pH alters the secretion of the hormones and/or modifies the responses of their target organs. Table 3 summarizes the data that is now available concerning these phenomena. Metabolic and respiratory acidoses both stimulate the release of catecholamines, especially epinephrine (45,46). Acidemia also depresses the myocardial and arteriolar responses to catecholamines (42). Perhaps adrenergically stimulated cellular potassium uptake is impaired as well, though this has not yet been studied. Insulin release by isolated rat pancreatic islet cells significantly increases, in a linear fashion, when HCl lowers the extracellular pH from 7.8 to 7.0 (32). On the other hand, insulin-mediated potassium uptake is normal during diabetic ketoacidosis in humans (DeFronzo, R.A.; personal communication), though the effects of other acid-base disorders on this insulin function are unknown. Isolated rat adrenal cortical cells decrease their aldosterone production in response to either metabolic acidosis or alkalosis (28). The in vivo effect of lactic acidosis in the dog, however, is to increase plasma aldosterone levels (51). This apparent discrepancy is readily explained by the observation that plasma renin activity and ACTH concentration also increased during acidosis in the dogs, and presumably mediated the increase in aldosterone. Acidosis inhibits aldosterone-mediated renal potassium excretion (38), whereas alkalosis is likely to be stimulatory (40).

In conclusion, the disparities in type and severity of acid-base disturbance among the experiments depicted in Figures 1-4 certainly may have further diversified the hormonal influences on potassium balance from study to study, and thereby increased the variability of the results.

Duration of Acid-Base Change

The total change in serum potassium concentration induced by an acute acid-base disturbance is not attained instantly. For example, 1-4 hr elapse following an experimental acid infusion before the serum potassium concentration stabilizes (56,57,59) and at least 2 hr are required for the $\Delta K/\Delta pH$ ratio to become constant (59). Figure 5 illustrates the typical evolution of serum potassium, HCO_3^-, and pH changes elicited by the brief infusion of mineral acid into a dog. It is noteworthy that the serum potassium concentration does not reach its zenith coincident with the 45-min nadirs of serum HCO_3^- and pH, but continues to rise. This is suggestive of a relationship of the change in serum potassium concentration to the intracellular buffering process, which also takes approximately 2 hr to reach completion (56). We will expand upon this concept below. The duration of the

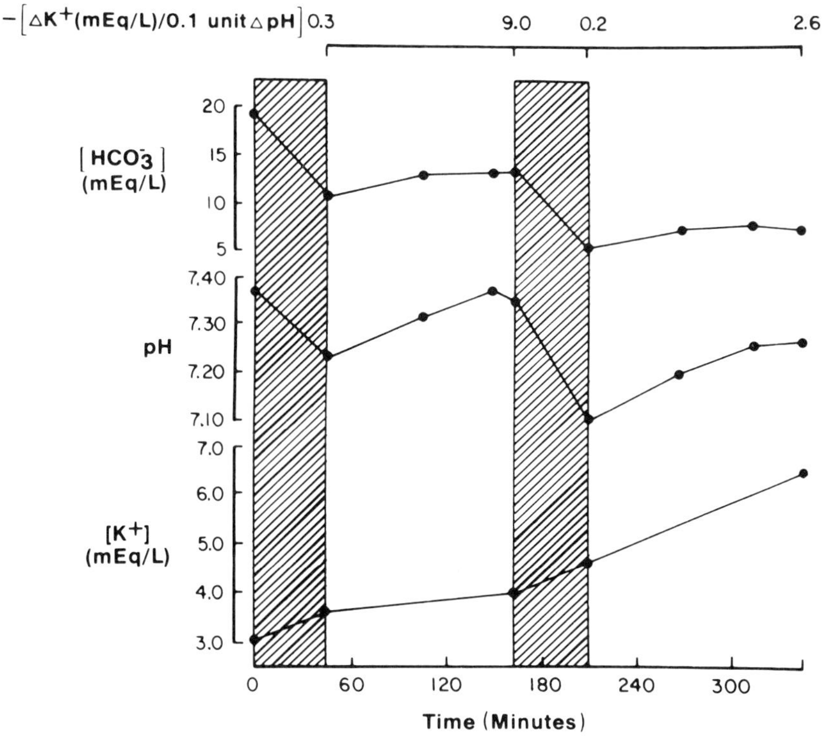

Figure 5 Chronology of the effects of acute HCl infusion on serum potassium, HCO_3^-, and pH in the dog. Shaded areas represent two 45-min infusions of 3.5 mEq/kg of HCl. (From Ref. 62. Data from Ref. 56.)

studies included in Figures 1-4 ranged from 6 min to 18 hr, which must account for some of the discordance of the data.

Serum HCO_3^- Concentration

Experimental evidence shows that serum HCO_3^- concentration, independent of ECF pH, affects the serum potassium concentration in rats (24), dogs (36), and humans (25). Specifically, infusion of sodium bicarbonate, while the PCO_2 is adjusted to maintain the pH at a constant level, decreases the serum potassium concentration. Conversely, HCl infusion under isohydric conditions increases the serum potassium concentration. Urinary potassium losses during these studies were of insufficient magnitude to account for the changes in serum potassium concentration. It appears that transcellular HCO_3^- equilibration concomitantly alters transcellular potassium distribution, probably because shifts of HCO_3^- create electrochemical gradients favoring the movement of cations such as potassium in the same direction. A single study, using dogs, failed to demonstrate such a relationship (59). However, in this case the serum potassium concentration was measured within only 45 min of the maximal change in serum HCO_3^- concentration. This probably was not too short an experimental period since the three investigations which found the effect measured the serum potassium concentration 1-6 hr after the full change in HCO_3^- concentration (24,25,36).

ECF Osmolarity

Increases in serum tonicity tend to increase the serum potassium concentration, under isohydric conditions (39,44). Efflux of water from cells in response to an increase in the ECF osmolarity would be expected to increase the intracellular potassium concentration. Thus, a gradient favoring traffic of potassium from the ICF to the ECF would be established. Additionally the bulk flow of water out of cells carries potassium with it. Experimental infusion of acidic or alkaline solutions of varying *tonicity* may thereby obfuscate the role of the acid-base change.

ECF Volume

The methods employed by the studies depicted in Figures 1 through 4 most likely resulted in highly variable states of ECF volume. For example, only some of the animals were nephrectomized, only some of the patients were anesthetized, and the experimental infusions differed greatly in rate and content. Resulting disparities in ECF volume would be expected to dilute serum potassium concentration variably.

Muscle Relaxants

The muscle relaxant succinylcholine is often administered during anesthesia to paralyze subjects. Muscular ionic permeability is increased by this drug, and patients undergoing elective surgical procedures showed a mean rise in serum potassium concentration of 0.6 mEq/L (41). In select situations (e.g., profound burns or trauma), this agent may precipitate hyperkalemia of lethal severity. At least one of the teams investigating the effects of acid-base disturbances on the serum potassium concentration unfortunately included succinylcholine in their protocol (59). Thus, another potentially confounding variable was introduced.

Fraction of Inspired Oxygen

Fraley and Adler report that ventilation of a rat, using 100% oxygen for 2½ hr, leads to a 1.2 mEq/L increase in the serum potassium concentration (24). No such change is elicited by ventilation with room air or 30% oxygen. This observation raises some doubt regarding the findings of the acute respiratory acidosis studies which used high fractions of inspired oxygen. The hyperkalemic effect allegedly induced by elevations of the FIO_2 remains controversial (3).

Urinary Losses

Increases in circulating aldosterone (see above), urinary flow rate, and distal tubular sodium delivery all increase urinary potassium excretion. Nonuniformity of these factors from study to study could certainly have splayed the resulting serum potassium levels. For example, the infusion of hypertonic sodium solutions during some, but not all, of the experiments would be expected to have variably augmented the urinary potassium losses.

Acid-base status also bears a direct role in determining urinary potassium excretion. Acute metabolic or respiratory acidosis reduces distal tubular potassium secretion in the rat (despite rises in serum potassium concentration), whereas either variety of alkalosis enhances distal potassium secretion (despite a fall in serum potassium) (40). Intracellular potassium in the distal tubule of rats, measured isotopically, shows a significant decrease during acidemia (18). Exchange of distal intracellular potassium for hydrogen ions is probably the predominant mechanism mediating acute acid-base influences on urinary potassium excretion. The work of Mahnensmith et al. supports this contention (38). They found that acute metabolic acidemia inhibits urinary potassium excretion by humans, without a change in plasma aldosterone concentration or sodium delivery to the distal tubule. As will be discussed below, flux of potassium between the ICF and ECF resulting from changes in ECF hydrogen ion concentration is the crucial determinant of changes in the serum potassium concentration, as well as an influence upon the rate of urinary potassium excretion.

It should be noted that a single study of isolated rabbit collecting tubules cites a decrease in luminal pH per se as inhibitory to potassium secretion (8).

How might the effects of acute acid-base changes on urinary potassium excretion confound the overall study of effects on serum potassium concentration? Mahnensmith et al. (38) found that urinary potassium excretion reached a minimum 100 min after an infusion of NH_4Cl, but gradually rose over the next 4 hr. Since the reported investigations of acid-base effects varied markedly in duration, the magnitude of the contribution of altered urinary potassium excretion must also have varied. Indeed, studies of anephric animals demonstrated greater increments in serum potassium concentration in metabolic acidosis and lesser decrements in metabolic alkalosis (34,53,63,64).

Gastrointestinal Losses

Figures 1 and 2 include several studies in which humans with preexisting metabolic acid-base disorders underwent therapeutic interventions, and the changes in serum potassium concentration were noted. However, the causes of these primary metabolic disturbances were not provided. If vomiting and diarrhea were among the underlying conditions, then the potentially confounding variable of gastrointestinal potassium loss must be considered. Gastric fluid contains only 10-20 mEq/L potassium (27,67). Although persistent vomiting may lead to metabolic alkalosis, renal potassium losses, and hypokalemia, it is highly unlikely that quantitatively significant potassium losses occurred due to emesis during the relatively brief experimental periods. Diarrhea can greatly increase fecal loss of potassium, which is normally less than 16 mEq/day (13). Thus, it is possible that diarrheal potassium losses exaggerated the decreases in serum potassium concentration induced by alkali infusion in a minority of the patients with preexisting metabolic acidosis.

EFFECTS OF THE INDIVIDUAL ACID-BASE DISTURBANCES ON SERUM POTASSIUM CONCENTRATION

In light of the differences in species studied (a veritable menagerie) and experimental designs employed, and of the confounding variables we have discussed, it is understandable that the results of the studies plotted in Figures 1-4 ranged to the extent shown in Table 1. While precise, predictable quantitation of the effects of acute acid-base changes on the serum potassium concentration is not feasible based on the available data, several important generalizations merit discussion. Firstly, the acidoses consistently increase the serum potassium concentration, while the alkaloses decrease it, regardless of the metabolic or respiratory origin of the perturbation. Secondly, the metabolic disorders engender greater changes than do their respiratory counterparts, as demonstrated by the mean values in Table 1. While it initially would appear that mineral metabolic acidosis is a more potent influence upon serum potassium concentration than metabolic alkalosis, careful scrutiny proves this supposition invalid.

pH vs. Hydrogen Ion Concentration

Review of the literature shows that investigators have uniformly chosen to consider the changes observed in serum potassium concentration in relation to the changes in pH. However, it is important to recall that the curvilinear relationship between pH and $[H^+]$ dictates that an increase of one pH unit denotes a decrease in $[H^+]$ which is smaller than the increase in $[H^+]$ denoted by a one pH unit decrease (47).

Table 4 elucidates this point. The normal blood $[H^+]$ equals 40 nEq/L, which corresponds to a pH of 7.40. Note that changes in pH of equal magnitude (0.30 unit), but opposite direction, denote unequal changes in $[H^+]$: an increase of 40 nEq/L with acidemia, but a decrease of only 20 nEq/L with alkalemia. In order to compare accurately the effects of acidosis and alkalosis upon serum potassium concentration, it is necessary to examine changes of equal magnitude in blood $[H^+]$. The last column in Table 4 lists the increases in serum potassium concentration per 10 nEq/L increase in $[H^+]$ during acidosis, and the decreases in serum potassium concentration per 10 nEq/L decrease in $[H^+]$ during alkalosis. Comparison of these data with those listed in the sixth column, which reiterates the potassium changes per 0.1 unit change in pH, clarifies certain misconceptions. Other authors have noted that acute metabolic acidosis exerts a greater effect on serum potassium concentration than does acute metabolic alkalosis (3,62). In fact, the two conditions alter serum potassium concentration to an almost identical degree, when considered per change in $[H^+]$. The metabolic disorders are again shown to be stronger influences upon potassium than are their respiratory counterparts. Finally, it emerges that acute respiratory alkalosis decreases the serum potassium concentration to a greater extent than the negligible increase in potassium concentration brought about by acute respiratory acidosis. Figure 6 illustrates these relative relationships. (This figure is *not* intended as a predictive guide to exact changes anticipated in serum potassium concentration, but only to demonstrate relative differences among the disorders.)

Role of Cellular Anion Permeability in Potassium Redistribution

We have not yet explored the major means by which acid-base alterations change the serum potassium concentration. Urinary and gastrointestinal losses of potassium contribute to changes in serum potassium (particularly during metabolic alkalosis), but acid-base effects have been demonstrated in the absence of significant changes in external potassium balance. Likewise, acid-base effects on serum potassium modulators such as catecholamines, insulin, and aldosterone, or the isohydric HCO_3^- effect described earlier, are of small magnitude and not likely to account for the changes seen in serum potassium concentration following acid-base disturbances. The experimental data strongly suggest that transcellular exchange of potassium and hydrogen ions underlies most of these changes. There is no ready formula to calculate the exact extent of the potassium/hydrogen exchange which occurs during these disorders. However, convincing evidence exists to show that qualitative differences in the transcellular redistribution of potassium which follows acute acid-base disturbances can be explained on the basis of the varying cellular permeability of different anions.

Table 4 Changes in Serum $[K^+]$ during Acute Acid-Base Disorders: Factored by Δ pH and $\Delta[H^+]$

	Examples of acidemia and alkalemia				ΔK^+ (Derived from reported data)		
Acute acid-base disorder	pH	H^+ (nEq/L)	ΔpH	$\Delta[H^+]$	ΔK^+(mEq/L)	$-(\Delta K^+/\Delta 0.1$ pH)	($\Delta K^+/\Delta 10$ nEq/L H^+)
Metabolic acidosis (mineral acid)	7.10	80	-0.30	+40	+1.98	0.66	0.50
Metabolic alkalosis	7.70	20	+0.30	-20	-1.11	0.37	0.56
Respiratory acidosis	7.10	80	-0.30	+40	+0.36	0.12	0.09
Respiratory alkalosis	7.70	20	+0.30	-20	-0.66	0.22	0.33

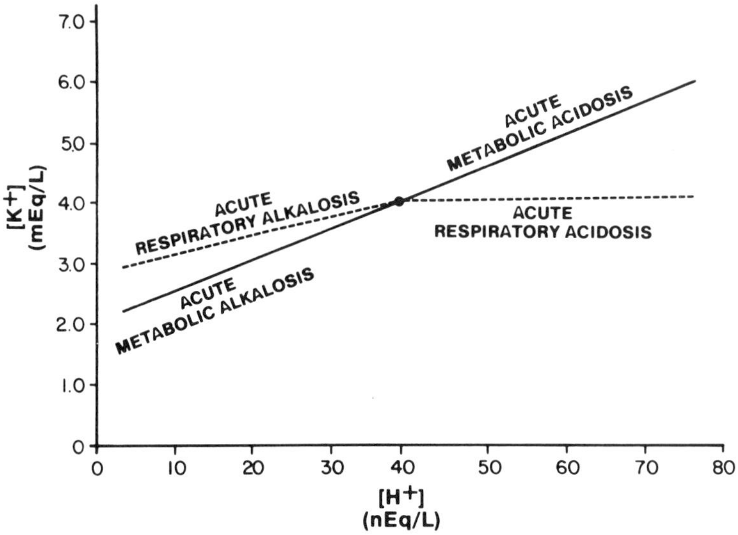

Figure 6 Serum potassium concentration as a function of serum hydrogen ion concentration (as predicted by the relations shown in Table 4). This plot is intended to aid in the comparison of the four primary disorders; it should *not* be used for absolute prediction of the serum potassium concentration.

Our discussion to this point has excluded acute organic metabolic acidosis, nor is this state included among the studies shown in Figure 1. In contrast to the acute mineral metabolic acidoses, the organic acidoses, in fact, do not induce significant increases in the serum potassium concentration. This has been documented by infusing animals with lactic acid (49,50,65), acetic acid (65), β-hydroxybutyric acid (50), and methylmalonic acid (50). Seizure-induced lactic acidosis in rats also fails to increase the serum potassium concentration (66). Figure 7 shows results typical of the infusion studies, from Perez et al. (52). Note that the dogs infused with HCl or NH_4Cl showed significant increases in their serum potassium concentration, whereas the serum potassium concentration following lactic or methylmalonic acid infusion was unchanged or diminished. Series describing patients with organic acidoses have also demonstrated the lack of an associated increase in the serum potassium concentration. These have included observations during lactic acidosis (26,48), alcoholic ketoacidosis (14,26,33,37), and methanol-induced acidosis (52). Rogers and Wachenfeld first proposed an explanation for the differing effects on potassium of mineral and organic acidoses (54). During mineral acidosis, hydrogen ions enter cells, leaving an inorganic anion (usually chloride) behind in the ECF, thus creating an electrochemical gradient favoring the egress of intracellular potassium. On the other hand, the easy entry of organic anions into the ICF, accompanying the hydrogen ions during an organic acidosis, would provide no stimulus for potassium to leave the cell and increase the serum concentration. These authors based this proposal on their observations of the effects of several acids on potassium movement from the rat hemidiaphragm (54). Hydrochloric acid displaced intracellular potassium, but lactic acid and β-hydroxybutyric acid did not. Figure 8 diagrams the crucial role of anion permeability in determining the impact of an acidosis upon transcellular redistribution of potassium.

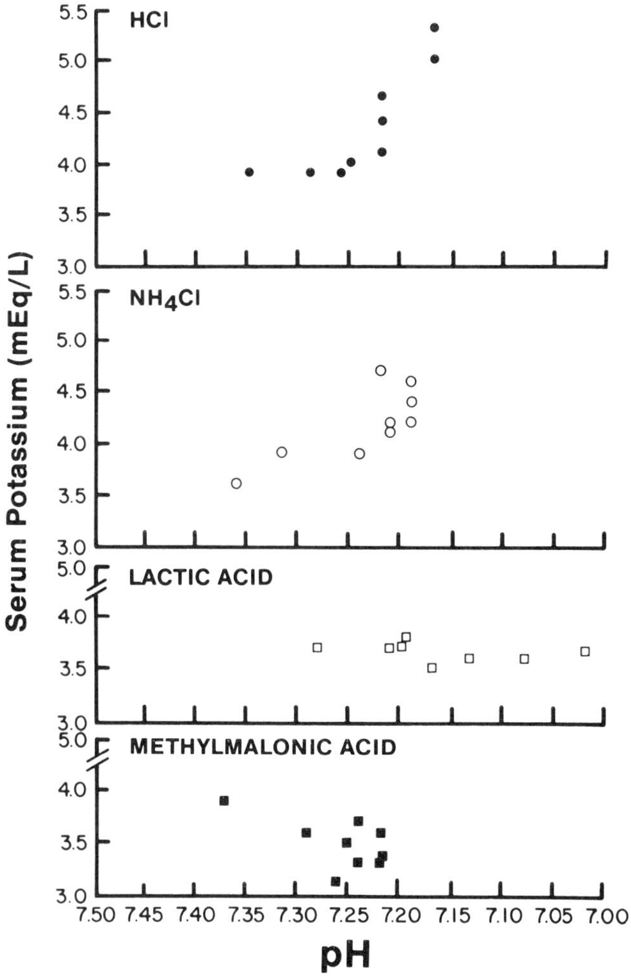

Figure 7 Mineral acid infusions (HCl, NH_4Cl) in the dog increase the serum potassium concentration, but organic acid infusions (la^tic, methylmalonic) do not. (From Ref. 52.)

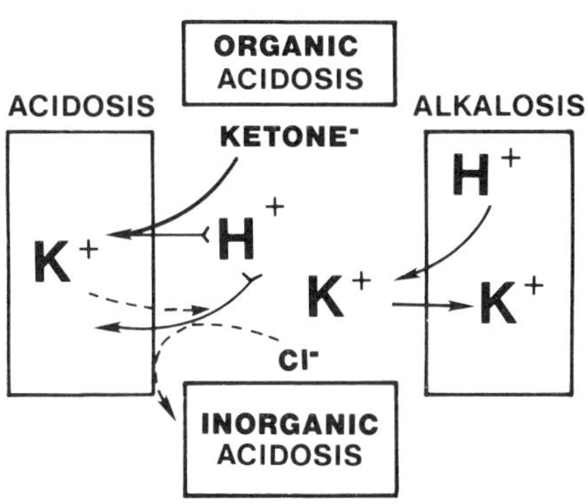

Figure 8 Effect of acid anion on the transcellular distribution of potassium. The reduced cellular penetration of inorganic anions (e.g., Cl^-), compared with that of organic anions, establishes electrical gradients favoring extracellular potassium entry. See text for details.

Diabetic ketoacidosis is an entity distinct from the other organic acidoses. In this setting, insulinopenia, hypertonicity, ECF volume contraction, and other unique factors contribute to the hyperkalemia frequently encountered. Rational assessment of the isolated acid-base effect on the serum potassium concentration is not possible.

As shown earlier, the decrease in serum potassium concentration elicited by an acute metabolic alkalosis is of equivalent magnitude to the increase in serum potassium induced by a mineral acidosis. When hydrogen ions leave the cells in response to the alkalemic change, they are largely titrated from proteins which cannot readily traverse the cell membrane. These impermeable anions then entice the serum potassium cations to enter the ICF, again indicating the important role of anion permeability.

The changes in arterial PCO_2 that occur during acute respiratory acid-base changes are rapidly reflected by similar changes in the intracellular PCO_2. Carbon dioxide enters cells and immediately forms carbonic acid, the ionization of which in turn generates H^+ and HCO_3^-. Thus, unlike mineral acid acidoses, in respiratory acidosis the cell interior is provided with both cation (H^+) and anion (HCO_3^-). This lack of transcellular charge separation minimizes the extracellular movement of potassium.

The situation is even more complex during respiratory alkalosis. Here, we would again expect the movement of CO_2 (this time from ICF to ECF) to engender *no* gradient for potassium movement. However, the compensatory response to respiratory alkalosis (i.e., hypobicarbonatemia) entails the movement of intracellular hydrogen ions into the ECF, which in turn produces an electrochemical gradient favoring the intracellular movement of potassium. This mechanism might account for the greater effect of acute respiratory alkalosis in lowering serum potassium concentration than the negligible effect of acute respiratory acidosis in increasing the serum potassium concentration.

REFERENCES

1. Abrams, W. B., Lewis, D. W., and Bellet, S.: The effect of acidosis and alkalosis on the plasma potassium concentration and the electrocardiogram of normal and potassium depleted dogs. *Am. J. Med. Sci.* 222:506-515, 1951.
2. Adler, S.: An extrarenal action of aldosterone on mammalian skeletal muscle. *Am. J. Physiol.* 218:616-621, 1970.
3. Adrogué, H. J., and Madias, N. E.: Changes in plasma potassium concentration during acute acid-base disturbances. *Am. J. Med.* 71:456-467, 1981.
4. Alexander, E. A., and Levinsky, N. G.: An extrarenal mechanism of potassium adaptation. *J. Clin. Invest.* 47:740-748, 1968.
5. Anderson, R. J., Rose, C. E., Jr., Berns, A. S., Erickson, A. L., and Arnold, P. E.: Mechanism of effect of hypercapnic acidosis on renin secretion in the dog. *Am. J. Physiol.* 238:F119-F125, 1980.
6. Arbus, G. S., Herbert, L. A., Levesque, P. R., Elsten, B. E., and Schwartz, W. B.: Characterization and clinical application of the "significance band" for acute respiratory alkalosis. *N. Engl. J. Med.* 280:117-123, 1969.
7. Bastl, C. P., and Marver, D.: The mechanism of action of aldosterone and glucocorticoids and their effects on fluid-electrolyte metabolism:review of ongoing and emerging controversies. In *Controversies in Nephrology and Hypertension*, edited by Narins, R. G., New York, Churchill Livingstone, 1984, pp. 579-605.
8. Boudry, J. F., Stoner, L. C., and Burg, M. B.: Effect of acid lumen pH on potassium transport in renal cortical collecting tubules. *Am. J. Physiol.* 230:239-244, 1976.
9. Brackett, N. C., Cohen, J. J., and Schwartz, W. B.: Carbon dioxide titration curve of normal man. *N. Engl. J. Med.* 272:6-12, 1965.

10. Brown, M. J., Brown, D. C., and Murphy, M. B.: Hypokalemia from $beta_2$-receptor stimulation by circulating epinephrine. *N. Engl. J. Med.* 309:1450–1451, 1983.
11. Burnell, J. M., Villamil, M. F., Uyeno, B. T., and Scribner, B. H.: The effect in humans of extracellular pH change on the relationship between serum potassium concentration and intracellular potassium. *J. Clin. Invest.* 35:935–939, 1956.
12. Cohen, J. J., Brackett, N. C., and Schwartz, W. B.: The nature of the carbon dioxide titration curve in the normal dog. *J. Clin. Invest.* 43:777–786, 1964.
13. Cohen, J. J., Gennari, F. J., and Harrington, J. T.: Disorders of potassium balance. In *The Kidney* (2nd ed.), Vol. 1, edited by Brenner, B. M., and Rector, F. C., Jr., Philadelphia, W. B. Saunders, 1981, p. 918.
14. Cooperman, M. T., Davidoff, F., Spark, R., and Pallotta, J.: Clinical studies of alcoholic ketoacidosis. *Diabetes* 23:433–439, 1974.
15. DeFronzo, R. A., Felig, P., Ferrannini, E., and Wahren, J.: Effects of graded doses of insulin on splanchnic and peripheral potassium metabolism in man. *Am. J. Physiol.* 238:E421–E427, 1980.
16. DeFronzo, R. A., Lee, R., Jones, A., and Bia, M.: Effect of insulinopenia and adrenal hormone deficiency on acute potassium tolerance. *Kidney Int.* 17:586–594, 1980.
17. DeFronzo, R. A., Sherwin, R. S., Dillingham, M., Hendler, R., Tamborlane, W. V., and Felig, P.: Influence of basal insulin and glucogon secretion on potassium and sodium metabolism. *J. Clin. Invest.* 61:472–479, 1978.
18. DeMello-Aires, M., Giebisch, G., and Malnic, G.: Kinetics of potassium transport across single distal tubules of rat kidney. *J. Physiol. (London)* 232:47–70, 1973.
19. Edwards, R., Winnie, A. P., and Ramamurthy, S.: Acute hypocapneic hypokalemia: An iatrogenic anesthetic complication. *Anesth. Analg. (Cleve)* 56:786–792, 1977.
20. Elkinton, J. R., Singer, R. B., Barker, E. S., and Clark, J. K.: Effects in man of acute experimental respiratory alkalosis and acidosis on ionic transfers in the total body fluids. *J. Clin. Invest.* 34:1671–1690, 1955.
21. Epstein, F. H., and Rosa, R. M.: Adrenergic control of serum potassium. *N. Engl. J. Med.* 309:1450–1451, 1983.
22. Fenn, W. O., and Asano, T.: Effects of carbon dioxide inhalation on potassium liberation from the liver. *Am. J. Physiol.* 185:567–576, 1956.
23. Finsterer, U., Luhr, H. G., and Wirth, A. E.: Effects of acute hypercapnia and hypocapnia on plasma and red cell potassium, blood lactate and base excess in man during anesthesia. *Acta Anaesthesiol. Scand.* 22:353–366, 1978.
24. Fraley, D. S., and Adler, S.: Isohydric regulation of plasma potassium by bicarbonate in the rat. *Kidney Int.* 9:333–343, 1976.
25. Fraley, D. S., and Adler, S.: Correction of hyperkalemia by bicarbonate despite constant blood pH. *Kidney Int.* 12:354–360, 1977.
26. Fulop, M.: Serum potassium in lactic acidosis and ketoacidosis. *N. Engl. J. Med.* 300:1087–1089, 1979.
27. Gardbiam, J. R., and Hobsley, M.: The electrolytes of alkaline human gastric juice. *Clin. Sci.* 39:77–87, 1970.
28. Gilchrist, M., Kem, D. C., and Washburn, D.: The effect of acidosis and alkalosis on in vitro aldosterone production. *Metabolism* 32:697–700, 1983.
29. Gledhill, N., Beirne, G. J., and Dempsey, J. A.: Renal response to short-term hypocapnia in man. *Kidney Int.* 8:376–386, 1975.
30. Goldfarb, S., Cox, M., Singer, I., and Goldberg, M.: Acute hyperkalemia induced by hyperglycemia: hormonal mechanisms. *Ann. Intern. Med.* 84:426–432, 1976.
31. Held, D. R., and Steiner, C. A.: Effect of acute respiratory acidosis on arterial plasma osmolality. *Respir. Physiol.* 12:25–35, 1971.
32. Hutton, S. C., Sener, A., Herchuelz, A., Valverde, I., Boschero, A. C., and Malaisse, W. J.: The stimulus-secretion coupling of glucose-induced insulin release. XLII. Ef-

fects of extracellular pH on insulin release: their dependency on nutrient concentration. *Horm. Metab. Res.* 12:294–299, 1980.

33. Jenkins, D. W., Eckel, R. E., and Craig, J. W.: Alcoholic ketoacidosis. *JAMA* 217: 177–183, 1971.
34. Keating, R. E., Weichselbaum, T. E., Alanis, M., Margraf, H. W., and Elman, R.: The movement of potassium during experimental acidosis and alkalosis in the nephrectomized dog. *Surg. Gynecol. Obstet.* 96:323–330, 1953.
35. Kilburn, K. H.: Movements of potassium during acute respiratory acidosis and recovery. *J. Appl. Physiol.* 21:679–684, 1965.
36. Kim, W. G., and Brown, E. B.: Potassium transfer with constant extracellular pH. *J. Lab. Clin. Med.* 71:678–875, 1968.
37. Levy, L. J., Duga, J., Girgis, M., and Gordon, E. E.: Ketoacidosis associated with alcoholism in non-diabetic subjects. *Ann. Intern. Med.* 78:213–219, 1973.
38. Mahnensmith, R., Thier, S. O., Cooke, R., Broadus, A., and DeFronzo, R. A.: Effect of acute metabolic acidemia on renal electrolyte transport in man. *Metabolism* 28:831–842, 1979.
39. Makoff, D. L., DaSilva, J. A., and Rosenbaum, B. J.: On the mechanism of hyperkalaemia due to hyperosmotic expansion with saline or mannitol. *Clin. Sci.* 41:383–393, 1971.
40. Malnic, G., De Mello Aires, M., and Giebisch, G.: Potassium transport across renal distal tubules during acid–base disturbances. *Am. J. Physiol.* 221:1192–1208, 1971.
41. Mazze, R. I., Escue, H. M., and Houston, J. B.: Hyperkalemia and cardiovascular collapse following administration of succinylcholine to the traumatized patient. *Anesthesiology* 31:540–547, 1969.
42. Mitchell, S. M., Wildenthal, K., and Johnson, R. L., Jr.: The effects of acid–base disturbances on cardiovascular and pulmonary function. *Kidney Int.* 1:375–389, 1972.
43. Montoliu, J., Martinez-Vea, A., Lopez-Pedret, J., and Revert, L.: Hypokalemia from $beta_2$-receptor stimulation by epinephrine. *N. Engl. J. Med.* 310:1329–1330, 1984.
44. Moreno, M., Murphy, C., and Goldsmith, C.: Increase in serum potassium resulting from the administration of hypertonic mannitol and other solutions. *J. Lab. Clin. Med.* 73:291–298, 1969.
45. Morris, M. E., and Millar, R. A.: Blood pH/plasma catecholamine relationships: nonrespiratory acidosis. *Br. J. Anaesthesiol.* 34:682–689, 1962.
46. Nahas, G. G., Zagury, D., Milhand, A., Manger, W. M., and Pappas, G. D.: Acidemia and catecholamine output of the isolated canine adrenal gland. *Am. J. Physiol.* 213: 1186–1192, 1967.
47. Narins, R. G., and Emmett, M.: Simple and mixed acid–base disorders: A practical approach. *Medicine* 59:161–187, 1980.
48. Orringer, C. E., Eustace, J. C., Wunsch, C. D., and Gardner, L. B.: Natural history of lactic acidosis after grand-mal seizures: a model for the study of an anion-gap acidosis not associated with hyperkalemia. *N. Engl. J. Med.* 297:796–799, 1977.
49. Oster, J. R., Perez, G. O., Castro, A., and Vaamonde, C. A.: Plasma potassium response to acute metabolic acidosis induced by mineral and nonmineral acids. *Mineral Electrolyte Metab.* 4:28–36, 1980.
50. Oster, J. R., Perez, G. O., and Vaamonde, C. A.: Relationship between blood pH and potassium and phosphorous during acute metabolic acidosis. *Am. J. Physiol.* 235: F345–351, 1978.
51. Perez, G. O., Kem, D. C., Oster, J. R., and Vaamonde, C. A.: Effect of acute metabolic acidosis on the renin–aldosterone system: Mechanism of increase in plasma aldosterone in dogs infused with lactic acid. *J. Lab. Clin. Med.* 96:371–378, 1980.

52. Perez, G. O., Oster, J. R., and Vaamonde, C. A.: Serum potassium concentration in acidemic states. *Nephron* 27:233-243, 1981.
53. Poole-Wilson, P. A., and Cameron, I. R.: Intracellular pH and K^+ of cardiac and skeletal muscle in acidosis and alkalosis. *Am. J. Physiol.* 229:1305-1310, 1975.
54. Rogers, T. A., and Wachenfeld, A. E.: Effect of physiologic acids on electrolytes in rat diaphragm. *Am. J. Physiol.* 193:623-626, 1958.
55. Rosa, R. M., Gervine, E. V., Silva, P., Brown, R. S., and Epstein, F. H.: Alpha-adrenergic modulation of potassium homeostasis (abstr.). *Clin. Res.* 32:460A, 1984.
56. Schwartz, W. B., Orning, K. J., and Porter, R.: The internal distribution of hydrogen ions with varying degrees of metabolic acidosis. *J. Clin. Invest.* 36:373-382, 1957.
57. Scribner, B. H., Fremont-Smith, K., and Burnell, J. M.: The effect of acute respiratory acidosis on the internal equilibrium of potassium. *J. Clin. Invest.* 34:1276-1285, 1955.
58. Siggaard Anderson, O.: Acute experimental acid-base disturbances in dogs. *Scand. J. Clin. Lab. Invest.* 66 [suppl] :1-20, 1962.
59. Simmons, D. H., and Avedon, M.: Acid-base alterations and plasma potassium concentration. *Am. J. Physiol.* 197:319-326, 1959.
60. Spurr, G. B., and Lambert, H.: Cardiac and skeletal muscle electrolytes in acute respiratory alkalemia and acidemia. *J. Appl. Physiol.* 15:459-464, 1960.
61. Spurr, G. B., and Liu, C. T.: Intra- and extracellular K^+ concentrations of cardiac and skeletal muscle during acute respiratory acid-base alterations. *Am. J. Med. Sci.* 252:413-418, 1966.
62. Sterns, R. H., Cox, M., Feig, P. U., and Singer, I.: Internal balance and the control of the plasma potassium concentration. *Medicine* 60:339-354, 1981.
63. Swan, R. C., Axelrod, D. R., Seip, M., and Pitts, R. F.: Distribution of sodium bicarbonate infused into nephrectomized dogs. *J. Clin. Invest.* 34:1795-1801, 1955.
64. Swan, R. C., and Pitts, R. F.: Neutralization of infused acid by nephrectomized dogs. *J. Clin. Invest.* 34:205-212, 1955.
65. Tobin, R. B.: Varying role of extracellular electrolytes in metabolic acidosis and alkalosis. *Am. J. Physiol.* 195:685-692, 1958.
66. Ward, J. R., and Call, L. S.: Changes in blood chemistry in rats following electrically-induced seizures. *Proc. Soc. Exp. Biol. Med.* 70:381-382, 1949.
67. Witten, T. A., and Bickel, J. G.: Potassium in gastric juice. *Gastroenterology* 59: 330-332, 1970.

6

Balance, Distribution, and Reference Ranges of Potassium Throughout the Body

ALLAN B. SCHWARTZ
Hahnemann University and Hahnemann University Hospital, Philadelphia, Pennsylvania

NORMAL RANGE

The normal range of laboratory values for serum potassium is variable. In most laboratories, the lower limit of normal varies from 3.5 to 3.8 mEq/L, and the upper limit of normal varies from 5.0 to 5.5 mEq/L. Some of the variance relates to a higher standard for serum samples compared to plasma samples. The wide range of low-grade symptoms with respect to abnormal potassium levels leads to some of the variability of "normal" potassium values. Even different analysis techniques may result in different normal potassium standards. Flame photometry results are consistently 0.2–0.3 mEq/L higher than newer autoanalyzer techniques. Thus, *serum* potassium determined by flame photometry may be 0.5 mEq/L greater than *plasma* potassium values determined by autoanalyzer from the same patient.

VARIABILITY OF SYMPTOMS

There is great variability of symptoms of "low-grade" hypokalemia and hyperkalemia. Vague, subtle complaints such as muscle fatigue and weakness may be confused and ignored between 3.5 and 3.0 mEq/L and between 5.5 and 6.0 mEq/L. Overt symptoms of potassium imbalance are more prevalent at values less than 3.0 mEq/L and greater than 6.0 mEq/L (34).

SAMPLING

Sampling blood without proper care may lead to spurious values for serum potassium. Excessive use of a tourniquet above the venipuncture site will result in tissue hypoxia and potassium leaching from tissue into serum. Muscle exercise below the tourniquet, such as with fist pumping, will allow potassium release from the muscle into serum. Whole blood left in a red-topped tube too long before separating serum will result in red cell lysis and potassium leak into the serum. Extremely elevated cell counts such as with erythrocytosis, leukemia, and primary thrombocytosis, may result in spurious hyperkalemia. Respiratory alkalinity due to pain and/or hyperventilation immediately prior to blood sampling may move potassium into the cells and hence reduce serum potassium levels.

Heparinized tubes allow collection of plasma rather than serum. Plasma potassium concentrations may be about 0.3 mEq/L lower than serum.

EXTRACELLULAR/INTRACELLULAR POTASSIUM DISTRIBUTION

Most often the serum potassium level reflects the status of the total body potassium. However, at any given time the extracellular fluid potassium level may be under the influence or control of such factors that can cause the serum potassium level to be quite disparate from the intracellular potassium level and total body potassium.

Potassium makes up only a small amount of the total extracellular electrolyte content. The extracellular fluid sodium concentration is approximately 140 mEq/L; in contrast, the potassium level is only about 4 mEq/L. Potassium is the dominant intracellular fluid cation with concentrations ranging from 130 to 150 and as high as 160 mEq/L. Sodium, on the other hand, is only 10-15 mEq/L in intracellular fluid. Sodium is the dominant extracellular cation; potassium is the dominant intracellular cation (35).

The division of sodium and potassium is dependent on the cell membrane energy consuming Na-K-ATPase pump. Sodium is constantly being pumped from the intracellular fluid, thus creating a relative electronegativity, or electrochemical gradient, down which potassium moves to enter and remain in the cell. The active pumping action removes sodium from the intracellular fluid; potassium entering the cell is a passive function.

Extracellular potassium represents only 1.5 to 2% of the total body potassium. Thus, the value obtained for serum potassium may not be representative of the quantity of total body potassium.

Within the physiological milieu of intracellular-extracellular potassium balancing forces, there is culmination of a finite regulation of (ICF K^+)/(ECF K^+) ratio to effect a proper cell membrane potential for normal nerve and muscle electrical physiology (36).

The total body potassium level varies between 3,200 and 3,800 mEq. Figure 1 shows an average total body potassium model at about 3,600 mEq.

The greatest amount of potassium is present within cells. The intracellular potassium pool is distributed among many tissues, predominantly in muscle (3,000 mEq). Most of this is found in skeletal muscle, with the remainder in cardiac and smooth muscle. The liver contains about 200 mEq of potassium, while the mass of red blood cells contain about 235 mEq. It will immediately be clear that rapid potassium releases will occur with muscle trauma. Patients involved in severe accidents, or those with crush injuries or burns, incur damage to or destruction of large muscle groups. These masses of cells are tremendously large sources of potassium. As the integrity of the muscle cell membrane is lost, potassium is released into the extracellular environment very rapidly. If the patient also has simultaneous acute renal failure, he or she loses renal potassium excreting capability. Without the ability to excrete the added extracellular potassium rapidly, and with trauma to skeletal muscle rapidly releasing 40-80 mEq of potassium, lethal hyperkalemia can occur.

Red blood cells are also a substantial source of potassium. A unit of mismatched blood undergoing rapid hemolysis can release up to 40 mEq potassium into the extracellular fluid fairly rapidly.

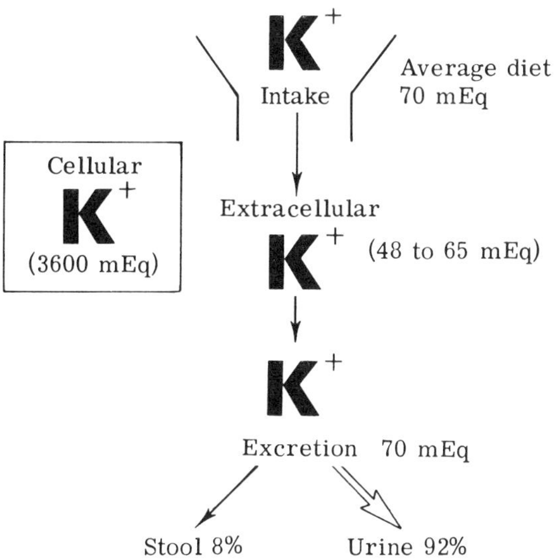

Figure 1 Model of total body potassium distribution and balance of intake and excretion. (From Schwartz, A. B., and Lyons, H.: *Acid-Base and Electrolyte Balance*, New York, Grune & Stratton, 1977, p. 205.)

Table 1 Potassium Content of Various Body Fluids

	mEq/L
Saliva	20–30
Gastric juice	5–15
Bile	5–12
Pancreatic	
Jejunal	2–10
Ileal	3–10
Cecal	5–45
Feces	50–120
Diarrhea	20–120
Diaphoresis	5–10

Source: Adapted from Mudge, G. H., and Welt, L. G.: Agents affecting volume and composition of body fluids. In *The Pharmacologic Basis of Therapeutics* (5th ed.), edited by Goodman, L. S., and Gilman, A. G., New York, Macmillan, 1975. Copyright 1975 by Macmillan Publishing Co., Inc.

Potassium content of transcellular body fluids is normally not of significance, since continuous secretion and reabsorption of enteric fluids results in no net changes. However, in disease states, losses of body fluids, if not recognized and replaced promptly, may cause great deficits of potassium (Table 1).

REGULATORS OF POTASSIUM DISTRIBUTION AND BALANCE

The daily homeostatic mechanisms of potassium balance are closely related to renal tubular function, sodium conservation, hydrogen ion balance, bicarbonate metabolism, chloride handling, glucose and insulin metabolism, tonicity of serum, prostaglandin action, renin-angiotensin-aldosterone balance, and adrenergic activity (Table 2).

Well-accepted extrarenal hormonal and neural mechanisms affecting intracellular-extracellular potassium balance include insulin, beta-adrenergic agonists, and the sympathetic nervous system.

The role of aldosterone as a mediator of renal tubular potassium secretion is well accepted, however, the possibility of an extrarenal modulation of potassium across cell membrane has been the subject of discussion.

Prostaglandins have been shown to stimulate renin synthesis and release from renal juxtaglomerular cells. This action of prostaglandin allows renin in turn to activate the angiotensin I-angiotensin II-aldosterone axis to bring about secretion of potassium from the renal distal tubular-collecting duct.

Acidosis

The association of acidosis and hyperkalemia has been appreciated for decades. In 1956, Scribner described a relationship between the degree of acidosis and resultant hyperkalemia (11,37).

Table 2 Factors Regulating Potassium Balance

Intake
Total body content
Sodium balance
Acid-base balance
Prostaglandins
Renin
Angiotensin
Aldosterone
Insulin
Thyroid
Sympathetic nervous system
Andrnergic activity
G.I. status: vomiting, diarrhea
Renal excretory capacity
Drugs

However, the conclusion that a change of 0.1 pH unit was associated with an increase of serum potassium of 0.6 mEq/L has not withstood years of clinical comparisons. First, the range of potassium change was 0.4-1.2 mEq/L for every 0.1 pH lowering. Second, the severity of hyperkalemia varies significantly between inorganic mineral acid acidosis and organic acid acidosis with the hyperkalemia usually being more prompt and more severe in the inorganic mineral acidosis (16). Third, *alkalosis*-induced hypokalemia follows trends but no proportionate rules.

Acidosis, whether metabolic or respiratory, causes hyperkalemia by shifting potassium into cells. Alkalosis, whether metabolic or respiratory, causes hypokalemia by shifting potassium out of cells.

Beta-2 Adrenergic Receptor Stimulation

This can cause a shift of extracellular potassium into skeletal muscle resulting in a decrease of the serum potassium. This adrenergic activity response of beta-2 variety is not shared by beta-1 receptors. The beta-2 adrenergic hypokalemia effect is mediated via activation of cell membrane adenylate cyclase which results in sodium-potassium-ATPase activation and pumping of sodium out of cells and potassium movement into cells. The sympathetic nervous system appears to be active in regulating potassium distribution. Experimental chemical sympathectomy with 6-hydroxy-dopamine reduces potassium tolerance in animals (38).

An increase of circulating epinephrine concentration of 15-30 times by infusion caused hypokalemia by a specific beta-2 receptor effect different from other epinephrine actions (8). Brown et al. questioned whether a dangerous hypokalemia may result from adrenergic and circulating epinephrine surge immediately following myocardial infarction.

Hypokalemia has been noted in stress associated with hyperadrenergic situations including acute myocardial infarction (31) and severe head trauma (12). Hypokalemia induced by adrenalin infusion has been shown to be aggravated by thiazide diuretic pretreatment (40).

Beta-adrenergic receptor agonists, especially those with a beta-2 adrenergic specificity, have been shown acutely to lower serum potassium presumably by acutely shifting potassium from the extracellular fluid to the intracellular compartment, similarly to the effect of epinephrine (23).

Hypokalemia was noted in a patient given intravenous terbutaline for the management of premature labor and in 18 other patients. Serum potassium returned to normal range within approximately 30 min following discontinuation of the terbutaline infusion (26).

Inhalation bronchodilator therapy with beta agonists may lower serum levels of potassium acutely (39). Exercise hyperkalemia is relieved by the alpha-adrenergic antagonist, phentolamine. Beta blockade with propranolol aggravates postexercise hyperkalemia by impairing cellular uptake of potassium ordinarily under the influence of beta-2 adrenergic receptor activity (47).

Hypokalemic periodic paralysis associated with hyperthyroidism, thought to be related to excessive beta-adrenergic stimulation, is appropriately effectively treated with the beta blocker, propranolol (48).

Beta-blocker therapy for hypertension has been associated with increases of serum potassium. Earlier investigation indicated the beta blocker inhibition of the renin-angiotensin-aldosterone system as cause of mild potassium elevation (5,10).

Later, using pindolol, a nonselective beta-adrenergic blocker with intrinsic sympathomimetic activity, an increase of serum potassium was noted despite a simultaneous reduction in renin activity (46).

In 1980, Traub and others noted that urinary excretion of potassium was not reduced during beta-adrenergic blockade at the same time that serum potassium was increased. The implication was that the elevation of serum potassium was a result of cationic shift from intracellular to extracellular fluid (44).

Pretreatment with beta blockers prevented the expected epinephrine-selective decrease of serum potassium induced by the beta-adrenergic agonist. The epinephrine-stimulated potassium entry into the skeletal muscle intracellular fluid compartment was effectively blocked by adrenergic beta blockade (20).

The extrarenal intracellular–extracellular potassium-modulating effect of the beta-adrenergic agonist epinephrine (15) is in turn effectively antagonized by the extrarenal effect of beta-adrenergic blockers.

Insulin

Insulin lowers serum potassium by moving potassium into cells (32). Hyperkalemia has been shown to stimulate pancreatic release of insulin (19). This insulin in turn moves potassium into cells. The resultant decrease of serum potassium removes the stimulus to the pancreatic islet cells and insulin secretion decreases to complete the cycle.

A glucose load given to an insulin-deficient diabetic patient will not cause potassium to move into cells, and may be associated with hyperkalemia (45).

An increase of potassium concentration from 4 to 8 mEq/L in isolated perfusion of pancreas directly results in an increase of insulin release without the influence of glucose.

Acute infusion of potassium is tolerated better in the dog with intact pancreas than in the pancreatectomized dog. Pancreatic insulin release protected against great increases in serum potassium after potassium chloride loading when compared to a pancreatectomized animal model without insulin release (30).

The insulin regulation of extracellular potassium concentration may represent a vestige of a primitive feedback system. A teleological explanation could be applied to the potassium–insulin relationship. The need to prevent sudden bursts of hyperkalemia from primitive high-potassium diets could have led to a functional insulin release which in turn could rapidly shift extracellular potassium safely into cells.

Glucagon

Glucagon causes release of intracellular potassium from the liver into the hepatic venous blood. However, myocardial potassium uptake is simultaneously increased by glucagon (6).

Hyperosmolar Infusion

Hyperosmolar infusions may pull potassium from the intracellular fluid compartment causing serious hyperkalemia. This has been described in diabetic patients with aldosterone deficiency (17), and with normal aldosterone levels (2).

Aldosterone

Potassium infusion into the isolated adrenal artery of the hypophysectomized and nephrectomized dog caused a prompt increase in aldosterone secretion. In their classic study of 1963, Davis et al. demonstrated that increased potassium concentration delivered to the adrenal zona glomerulosa resulted in a stimulation of aldosterone synthesis and secretion in the absence of ACTH and renin-angiotensin activity (14).

Thus, potassium is its own regulator of aldosterone which in turn moderates extracellular potassium concentration by stimulating renal secretion and excretion of the excess potassium.

This physiological sequence was later confirmed in investigation in humans. Potassium loading resulted in simultaneous stimulation of urinary aldosterone excretion, increased urinary potassium excretion, and reduced urinary sodium excretion. The potassium loading also suppressed plasma renin activity simultaneously (9).

Normally, as progressive loss of nephrons occurs in chronic renal disease, there is an adaptive process of potassium handling by the remaining functional nephrons that prevents hyperkalemia. This adaptation undoubtedly depends on a normal potassium-adrenal-renal axis. As little as one-sixth the number of normal nephrons may increase their potassium secretory capacity, each six times, to maintain potassium intake and output balance. The remnant kidney has been shown to quadruple its potassium excretion within 1 day and hextuple its potassium excretion by 7 days following removal of the contralateral normal kidney (7).

The expected increase of fractional excretion of potassium that occurs as an adaptive response to chronic renal failure did not occur in diabetic patients with hyperaldosteronism and chronic renal failure. After potassium loading, the maximal values of serum potassium were higher, and the fractional excretion of potassium lower in those diabetic hypoaldosterone patients (29).

Hyperkalemic, hyperchloremic metabolic acidosis has been noted in nondiabetic patients with only mild to moderate renal insufficiency arising as a consequence of aldosterone deficiency or tubular unresponsiveness to aldosterone (3).

In another series of hyperkalemic patients with mild to moderate chronic renal insufficiency, it was found that the deficiency of aldosterone contributed significantly to the hyperkalemia. In most (83%) of these patients, the hypoaldosteronism was accounted for by deficient renal secretion of renin (33).

Although the action of aldosterone in facilitating kaliuresis to protect against hyperkalemia is well-known, the role of an extrarenal effect of aldosterone on potassium balance has been challenged (1,2,13,25).

To determine the absence or presence of an extrarenal effect of aldosterone on potassium distribution, we studied anephric patients before and during a period of aldosterone administration, 0.5 mg twice daily for 7 days. The tolerance of the anephric patients to doses of 25-37.5 mEq of potassium citrate was no different in control studies than in high-dosage aldosterone study periods. We could not demonstrate an increased rate of movement of potassium from the extracellular fluid compartment to the intracellular fluid compartment upon challenge with a potassium load during aldosterone administration (28).

Prostaglandins

Prostaglandins, especially the prostacyclin metabolite (PGI_2), play a vital role in mediating renin secretion and release from the juxtaglomerular cells of the kidney, and thus serve to regulate potassium balance.

Low urinary PGE_2 levels have been noted in patients with hyporeninemic hypoaldosteronism (41).

Investigational prostaglandin administration has resulted in an increase of renin in a patient with hyporeninemia and hypoaldosteronism (21)

It has been suggested that prostaglandins participate in the conversion of inactive or prorenin to active renin. Two separate mechanisms may stimulate renin release: (a) beta adrenergic receptor on the juxtaglomerular (JG) cell, and (b) prostaglandin receptors on the JG cell (24,27).

Prostaglandin synthetase inhibitors inhibit renin release and thus produce a syndrome of hyporenin-hypoaldosterone-related inhibition of renal potassium excretion. Hyperkalemia and suppressed renin and aldosterone due to the prostaglandin synthetase inhibitor indomethacin have been reported in a patient with normal renal function (18) and in a patient with glomerulonephritis (42).

The angiotensin-converting enzyme (ACE) inhibitor interferes with the normal feedback mechanism of the renin-angiotensin-aldosterone axis necessary for proper renal tubular potassium secretion and potassium homeostasis. ACE inhibitors block the formation of angiotensin II and thus limit the stimulation of adrenal aldosterone synthesis. Reduced renal potassium secretion and hyperkalemia have been reported in azotemic patients receiving the ACE inhibitor, captopril, in association with reduced aldosterone (43). Enalapril, a newer ACE inhibitor, has also been implicated in a hyperkalemic complication (4). Angiotensin-converting enzyme inhibition therapy with captopril has been used to raise the low level of potassium in patients with Bartter's syndrome (22).

SUMMARY

The effect of insulin moving potassium into cells and aldosterone stimulating secretion and excretion of potassium from the renal distal tubule collecting duct serve as dual collaborative hormonal systems that protect against hyperkalemia. One disease state, diabetes with insulin deficiency and hyporenin-hypoaldosteronism, couples abnormalities of these two potassium regulatory mechanisms to cause dangerous hyperkalemia baseline. Adding to this vulnerable hyperkalemia baseline is the frequency of moderate renal insufficiency in chronic diabetic nephropathy. The patient with this triad of causes of hyperkalemia could easily experience the added hyperkalemic effect of one of today's modern pharmacologic agents; beta-adrenergic blockers for arrhythmia, nonsteroidal antiinflammatory drugs for arthritis, angiotensin-converting enzyme inhibitors for hypertension, potassium-sparing distal tubule collecting duct diuretics for edema, heparin anticoagulant, or succinylcholine anesthesia. The potential is lethal unless we have the knowledge and awareness to avoid such a hazard.

REFERENCES

1. Alexander, E. A., and Levinsky, N. G.: An extrarenal mechanism of potassium adaptation. *J. Clin. Invest.* 47:740–748, 1968.
2. Ammon, R. A., May, R. S., and Nightingale, S. D.: Glucose-induced hyperkalemia with normal aldosterone levels. *Ann. Intern. Med.* 89:349–351, 1978.
3. Arruda, J. A., Bottle, D. C., Sehy, J. T., Roseman, M. D., Baronowski, R. L., and Kurtzman, N. A.: Hyperkalemia and renal insufficiency: Role of selective aldosterone deficiency and tubular unresponsiveness to aldosterone. *Am. J. Nephrol.* 1:160–167, 1981.
4. Barnes, J. N., Davies, E. S., and Gent, C. B.: Rash, eosinophilia, and hyperkalemia associated with enalapril. *Lancet* 2:41–42, 1983.

5. Berglund, G., Anderson, O., Larsson, O., and Wilhelmsen, L.: Antihypertensive effect and side-effects of bendroflumethazide and propranolol. *Acta Med. Scand.* 199: 499-506, 1976.
6. Bianco, J. A., Shanahan, A., Osteimer, G. W., Guyton, R. A., Powell, W. J. Jr., and Daggett, W. M.: Effects of glucagon on myocardial oxygen consumption and potassium balance. *Am. J. Physiol.* 221:626-631, 1971.
7. Bricker, N. S., Schultze, R. G., Taggart, D. D., Shapiro, H., Pennell, J. P., and Coglar, S.: On the adaptation in potassium excretion associated with nephron reduction in the dog. *J. Clin. Invest.* 50:1061-1068, 1971.
8. Brown, M. J., Brown, D. C., and Murphy, M. B.: Hypokalemia from Beta-2 receptor stimulation by circulating epinephrine. *N. Engl. J. Med.* 309:1414-1419, 1983.
9. Brunner, H. R., Baer, L., Sealey, J. E., Ledingham, J. G. G., and Laragh, J. H.: The influence of potassium administration and of potassium deprivation on plasma renin in normal and hypertensive subjects. *J. Clin. Invest.* 49:2128-2138, 1970.
10. Buhler, F. R., Laragh, J. H., Baer, L., et al.: Propranolol inhibition of renin secretion. *N. Engl. J. Med.* 287:1209-1213, 1972.
11. Burnell, J. M., Villamil, M. F., Uyeno, B. T., and Scribner, B.: The effects in humans of extracellular pH change on the relationship between serum potassium concentration and intracellular potassium. *J. Clin. Invest.* 35:935-939, 1956.
12. Conci, F., Procaccio, F., and Boselli, L.: Hypokalemia from $beta_2$-receptor stimulation by epinephrine. Letter to the Editor. *N. Engl. J. Med.* 310:1329, 1983.
13. Cox, M., Sterns, R. H., and Singer, I.: The defense against hyperkalemia: The roles of insulin and aldosteronism. *N. Engl. J. Med.* 299:525-532, 1978.
14. Davis, J. O., Urquhart, J., and Higgins, J. T. Jr.: The effects of alterations of plasma sodium and potassium concentration on aldosterone secretion. *J. Clin. Invest.* 42: 597-608, 1963.
15. Epstein, F. H., and Rosa, R. M.: Adrenergic control of serum potassium. Editorial. *N. Engl. J. Med.* 309:1450-1451, 1983.
16. Fulop, M.: Serum potassium in lactic acidosis and ketoacidosis. *N. Engl. J. Med.* 300:1087-1089, 1979.
17. Goldfarb, S., Cox, M., Singer, I., and Goldberg, M.: Acute hyperkalemia induced by hyperglycemia: hormonal mechanisms. *Ann. Intern. Med.* 84:426-432, 1976.
18. Goldszer, R. C., Rosner, M. J., Simons, W. M., Schwartz, A. B., and Coodley, E. L.: Hyperkalemia associated with Indomethacin. *Arch. Intern. Med.* 141:802-804, 1981.
19. Grodsky, G. M., and Bennet, L. L.: Cation requirements for insulin secretion in the isolated perfused pancreas. *Diabetes* 15:910-913, 1966.
20. Grossi, A. O., DiLew, W. F., Cingolani, H. E., and Blesa, E. S.: Adrenergic beta blockade and changes in plasma potassium following epinephrine administration. *Eur. J. Pharmacol.* 15:209-213, 1971.
21. Hahn, J., Zipser, R., Zia, P., Tuch, M., Golub, M., and Horton R.: Induction of renin release by exogenous prostaglandins in hyporeninemic hypoaldosteronism. *Prostaglandins* 20:15-23, 1980.
22. Hene, R. J., Koomans, H. A., Baer, P., Mees, E. J. D.: Long-term treatment of Bartter's syndrome with captopril. *Br. Med. J.* 285:695, 1982.
23. Hurlbert, B. J., Edelman, J. D., and David, K.: Serum potassium levels during and after terbutaline. *Anesth. Analg. (Cleve.)* 60:723-725, 1981.
24. Keeton, T. K., and Campbell, W. B.: The pharmacologic alteration of renin release. *Pharmacol. Rev.* 32:91-227, 1980.
25. Knockel, J. P., and Wluli, M. G.: The role of aldosterone in renal physiology. *Arch. Intern. Med.* 131:876-884, 1973.

26. Moravec, M. A., and Hurlbert, B. J.: Hypokalemia associated with terbutaline administration in obstetrical patients. *Anesth. Analg. (Cleve.)* 59:917-920, 1980.
27. Oates, J., Whorton, R., Gerkins, J., Banch, R., Hollifield, J., and Frolich, J.: The participation of prostaglandins in control of renin release. *Fed. Proc.* 38:72-74, 1979.
28. Onesti, G., Schwartz, A. B., Persoff, M., Swartz, C., and Brest, A. N.: Aldosterone in anephric man. *Am. Soc. Nephrol. Abstract* II:48, 1968.
29. Perez, G. O., Lespier, L., Knowles, R., Oster, J. R., and Vaamonde, C. A.: Potassium homeostasis in chronic diabetes mellitus. *Arch. Intern. Med.* 137:1018-1022, 1977.
30. Pettit, G. W., and Vich, R. L.: Contribution of pancreatic insulin to extrarenal potassium homeostasis: a two-compartment model. *Am. J. Physiol.* 276:319-324, 1974.
31. Rolton, J., Simpson, E., Donnelly, T., and Rodger, J. C.: Plasma potassium in acute myocardial infarction (abstract). *Eur. Heart J.*, 2 Suppl., A:21, 1981.
32. Santeusanio, F., Faloona, G. F., Knochel, J. P. et al.: Evidence for a role of endogenous insulin and glucagon in the regulation of potassium homeostasis. *J. Lab. Clin. Med.* 81:809-817, 1973.
33. Schambelan, M., Sebastian, A., and Biglieri, E. G.: Prevalence, pathogenesis and functional significance of aldosterone in hyperkalemic patients with chronic renal insufficiency. *Kidney Int.* 17:89-101, 1980.
34. Schwartz, A. B.: Diuretic-induced hypokalemia. *Am. Fam. Physician* 11:101-104, 1975.
35. Schwartz, A. B.: Normal potassium balance. In *Acid-Base and Electrolyte Balance.* Edited by Schwartz, A. B., Lyons, H., New York, Grune & Stratton, 1977, pp. 203-212.
36. Schwartz, A. B.: Potassium-related cardiac arrhythmias and their treatment. *Angiology* 29:194-205, 1978.
37. Scribner, B. H., Bremont-Smith, K., and Burnell, J. M.: The effect of acute respiratory acidosis on the internal equilibrium of potassium. *J. Clin. Invest.* 34:1277-1285, 1955.
38. Silva, P., and Stokes, K.: Sympathetic system in potassium homeostasis. *Am. J. Physiol.* 241:F151-155, 1981.
39. Smith, S. R., and Kendall, M. J.: Inhaled bronchodilators and hypokalemia (Letter). *Lancet* 2:21B, 1983.
40. Struthers, A. D., Whitesmith, R., and Reed, J. C.: Prior thiazide treatment increases adrenaline-induced hypokalemia. *Lancet* 1:1358-1361, 1983.
41. Tan, S. Y., Antonipillai, I., and Mulrow, P. J.: Inactive renin and prostaglandin E_2 production in hyporeninemic hypoaldosteronism. *J. Clin. Endocrinol. Metab.* 51:849, 1980.
42. Tan, S. Y., Shapiro, R., Franco, R., Stockard, H., and Mulrow, P. J.: Indomethacin-induced prostaglandin inhibition with hyperkalemia. A reversible cause of hyporeninemic hypoaldosteronism. *Ann. Intern. Med.* 90:783-785, 1979.
43. Textor, S. C., Bravo, E. L., Fouad, F. M., and Tarazi, R. C.: Hyperkalemia in azotemic patients during angiotension-converting enzyme inhibition and aldosterone reduction with Captopril. *Am. J. Med.* 73:719-725, 1982.
44. Traub, Y. M., Robinson, M., Rosenfeld, J. B., and Treuherz, S.: Elevation of serum potassium during beta blockade: absence of relationship to the renin-aldosterone system. *Clin. Pharmacol. Ther.* 26:765-768, 1980.
45. Viberti, G. C.: Glucose-induced hyperkalemia: a hazard for diabetecs? *Lancet* 1:690-691, 1978.
46. Weber, M. A., Stokes, G. S., and Gain, J. M.: Comparison of the effects on renin release of beta adrenergic antagonists with differing properties. *J. Clin. Invest.* 54:1413-1419, 1974.

47. Williams, M., Gervino, E., Rosa, R. et al.: Modulation of the hyperkalemia of exercise by catecholamines (abstract). *Proc. Am. Soc. Nephrol.* 185A, 1983.
48. Young, R. T. T., and Tse, T. F.: Thyrotoxic periodic paralysis: effect of propranolol. *Am. J. Med.* 57:584–590, 1974.

7

Clinical Effects of Potassium Deficiency on Skeletal Muscle

JAMES P. KNOCHEL
University of Texas Southwestern Medical School and Veterans Administration Medical Center, Dallas, Texas

The major fraction of potassium in the body is located in skeletal muscle. Although the concentration of potassium in intracellular water of normal muscle cells is tightly regulated at about 150 mEq/L, we have learned that the muscle potassium pool is labile. Thus, in the event of deficiency, skeletal muscle readily gives up potassium ions. In early deficiency, potassium content may remain normal in vital organs such as the kidney (4), heart (17,21,37), liver (4,39), or brain (17). Although potassium content of these tissues may decline as the deficiency worsens (5), that of the heart appears to remain essentially normal. Skeletal muscle is consistently the first tissue to become deficient, apparently becomes more deficient than other tissues, and, because of its bulk, accounts for the majority of the deficit.

It is well-appreciated that acute potassium deficiency may cause more pronounced symptoms and greater morbidity than an equal degree of potassium deficiency that develops over a long period of time. In cases of long-standing deficiencies of any major intracellular ion, such as potassium or phosphate, an orderly shrinkage of cellular mass occurs, meaning a loss of protein and other major constituents from the cell, in an apparent a tempt to maintain a relatively normal intracellular milieu. For this reason, while a total deficit of potassium might approach 30 or 40% of original total body stores, if one expresses potassium content in terms of tissue protein, it is often found to be only modestly deficient. For such reasons, the gold standard to express potassium deficiency is the K/N ratio. In health, this ratio is about 3 mEq K/g N. Muscle most consistently reflects total body stores of potassium and accordingly, it is the tissue of choice for analysis. Since fat free, dry muscle powder is more easily measured than nitrogen and is about 85% protein by weight, it is acceptable to express muscle potassium content as mEq/100 g fat-free dry weight.

Maintenance of a high potassium concentration gradient between the inside and the outside of muscle cells is critically important for a variety of reasons. Among these are regulation of enzyme activity (27), protein synthesis, insulin release, electrical conduction, control of cellular volume, and regulation of muscle blood flow.

Although a large number of enzymes specifically require potassium ions for their activity, whether their activity would be substantially altered by a minor decline in intracellular potassium concentration from 150 to 130 mEq/L has not been clearly established. Concentrations between 100 and 150 mEq/L intracellular water are common in clinical potassium deficiency. Thus, in most studies, it has only been determined that enzyme activity is absent when potassium concentration is zero or fully active when potassium concentration is 150 mEq/L or more. To muddle the issue further, when potassium deficiency becomes moderately severe, there is an accumulation of sodium and hydrogen ions in sufficient concentration to affect activity of enzymes. Consequently, effects ascribed to potassium deficiency could conceivably result from a change of sodium concentration or pH. In addition, the accumulation of sodium ions that apparently always occurs in association with a major loss of potassium from cytoplasm (21,38) may indirectly facilitate entry of calcium ions (54). Calcium, in turn, may exert profound effects upon cellular function and metabolism. For example, decreasing the sodium gradient between the outside and the inside of the cell can reduce the normal sodium/calcium exchange and in turn, permit accumulation of calcium inside the cell (10). Calcium may thus attain a sufficient concentration to activate phospholipase that in turn may injure the cellular membrane (12) or activate neutral proteases inside the cell which may subsequently decompose myofibrillar protein (44). It seems apparent that the biochemical effects of potassium deficiency are not necessarily due to deficiency of potassium ions alone, but rather to a constellation of abnormalities that appear in association with potassium deficiency.

ROLES OF DIFFERENTIAL ION PERMEABILITY OF THE MUSCLE CELL AND ION TRANSPORT IN MAINTENANCE OF INTRACELLULAR POTASSIUM CONCENTRATION

The resting potential difference across the sarcolemmal membrane of muscle cells is essentially a potassium diffusion potential. If one directly measures the resting membrane potential of a normal muscle cell in vivo, the value obtained averages about -90 mV, the cell interior being negative. The value of an electrical force that precisely stops net movement of an ion through a membrane is termed its equilibrium or diffusion potential. This potential is expressed mathematically by the Nernst equation, $E_m = -61.5 \log Ki/Ko$.

In our own studies (8), direct measurements of skeletal muscle membrane potential in healthy subjects using Ling electrodes yield values that average -90.8 ± 0.9 mV. Although this value is essentially the same as the equilibrium potential for potassium and chloride, it deviates greatly from the diffusion potential for sodium ions. That the equilibrium potential for sodium predicted from the Nernst equation is vastly different from the measured membrane potential reflects active sodium transport from the cell or relatively low passive sodium conductivity of the membrane.

Maintenance of an electrical potential difference across the cellular membrane requires active ion transport. In the mammalian cell, the key event maintaining this potential difference is sodium transport from the cell. Because of the sodium pump, the cell membrane is effectively "impermeable" to sodium ions. As rapidly as sodium ions passively enter the cell down its electrochemical gradient, the sodium pump transports it back out, against its electrochemical gradient. This critical step has several important effects. First, by the pump's removing the positively charged sodium ion at a rate exceeding that at which potassium ions enter the cell, electronegativity is generated (51), thereby favoring potassium retention in the cytoplasm. Second, the electronegativity excludes chloride. Third, transport of sodium and the resulting distribution of solutes establish powerful osmotic forces by which cellular volume is regulated (40). That active transport and the related metabolism are critical to maintenance of ion gradients across the cell membrane becomes obvious if one inhibits transport by cold or certain metabolic inhibitors. Thereby, the electrical and ionic gradients for sodium, potassium, and chloride disappear and subsequently reappear when these inhibitory factors are removed (1). The magnesium-dependent, sodium, K-activated ATPase, the ion pump, is oriented in the cell membrane such that the portion activated by sodium ions is inside the cell and that portion activated by potassium is outside the cell (50). The enzyme requires both sodium and potassium to hydrolyze ATP.

Studies conducted in human erythrocytes have shown that the ion pump removes 3 moles of sodium from the cell for each 2 moles of potassium that enter, and in the process 1 mole of ATP is hydrolyzed (15,49). It is assumed that the same relationship prevails in skeletal muscle. If three potassium ions entered the cell for each three sodium ions pumped out, then the pump would be electrically neutral in the sense that there would be no net transfer of electrical charge. On the other hand, the pump appears to be electrogenic, (pumping more sodium ions out than potassium ions in), and in the process an electrical potential is generated.

Besides the differential permeability of the muscle cell membrane to sodium and potassium ions, and the maintenance of a high intracellular electronegativity by the electrogenic sodium pump, a third property of the membrane also helps to maintain a high intracellular concentration of potassium ions. Hodgkin and Katz (20) showed that potassium ions enter the muscle cell 160 times more easily than they leave. This bidirectional difference of potassium conductance has been termed anomalous rectification.

MEMBRANE POTENTIAL IN HYPOKALEMIA AND POTASSIUM DEFICIENCY

As predicted by the Nernst equation, a normal cell will become electrically hyperpolarized if the intracellular concentration of potassium ions remains normal while the extracellular concentration of potassium is reduced. This response has been adequately demonstrated in several animal species (8) as well as humans (46). Even in potassium deficiency, the fractional reduction of extracellular potassium is much more extensive than the fractional reduction of intracellular potassium concentration. Thus the Ki/Ko ratio becomes elevated and as a result, the cell becomes electrically hyperpolarized. In humans and dogs, when potassium deficiency is relatively long-standing or becomes more severe, there is apparently some alteration in the properties of the plasma cell membrane or the sodium pump itself so that the resting membrane potential of the cell falls to much lower values than predicted from the prevailing Ki/Ko ratio (8). This does not occur in the rat even in the presence of advanced potassium deficiency in skeletal muscle. At this time, the measured membrane potential becomes predictable by the Goldman constant field equation, provided one assumes that a slight increase in sodium conductance has occurred as a result of potassium deficiency (8). Table 1 gives data for these observations in dogs and rats with early and late potassium deficiency. The observation that the muscle cell hyperpolarization persists in the severely potassium-deficient rat suggests an important species difference, possibly based upon some fundamental difference in electrical properties of the sarcolemmal membrane or the sodium pump. In dogs, and presumably humans, the

Table 1 Effects of K Deficiency in the Rat and Dog

		$[K]^o$ (mEq/L)	$[K]^i$ (mEq/L)	$[Na]^i$ (mEq/L)	$E_m{}^G$ (-mV)	$E_m{}^M$ (-mV)	CK (IU/L)
Rat	Control	4.3	159	10.5	88.6	89.1	6
	K-deficient	1.5	97	58	92.1	94.9	5
Dog	Control	4.1	142	8.4	86.6	90.1	8
	K-deficient early	2.4	120	18.7	93.6	92.4	8
	K-deficient late	1.6	104	33.5	94.8	54.8	45

The superscripts ^{o} and ^{i} refer to concentrations outside and inside cells, respectively. The symbols $E_m{}^G$ and $E_m{}^M$ represent membrane potentials predicted from the Goldman equation and those measured directly with Ling electrodes. Creatine kinase (CK) activity, based upon Sigma International Units, ranges between 5 and 10 IU/L in normal animals.

severe muscular weakness that eventually occurs during the course of potassium deficiency appears to coincide with the decline of resting membrane potential (8,34). Similarly, at this time the activity of creatine kinase begins to rise in serum, suggesting that the enzyme is leaking from injured muscle cells. Inferential evidence suggests that depolarization of skeletal muscle observed in advanced potassium deficiency is the result of increased sodium permeability (19,25). A higher sodium permeability would increase the entry rate of sodium ions into cells so that the net coupling between sodium efflux and potassium influx would become reduced and thereby membrane potential would become depolarized.

Akaike recently published some interesting observations on rats with severe potassium deficiency (2). He noted that in early potassium deficiency there occurs a rapid fall in serum potassium to a level of 1.6 mEq/L and, thereafter, serum potassium concentration tends to stabilize in that range. He then showed that interruption of the spinal cord or motor nerve at a level above the muscle innervation or administration of the α-adrenergic receptor blocker phentolamine resulted in a sudden uptake of potassium from the extracellular fluid. Despite severe hypokalemia, the muscle potassium deficit was subsequently corrected. Ouabain prevented this response. He proposed that the α-adrenergic nervous system becomes activated in potassium deficiency, and in turn depresses activity of the sodium-potassium pump in skeletal muscle to prevent continued progression of hypokalemia. He also proposed that skeletal muscle must have α-adrenergic receptors responsive to norepinephrine, probably released from peripheral nerves. Since muscle becomes depleted of potassium in animals fed a potassium-deficient diet, while more vital organs such as brain, liver, heart and kidney may not become depleted, (4,5,17,21,37,39), Akaike proposed that sympathetic activation in the CNS might be responsible for this critical function. It is perhaps noteworthy that catecholamine levels are elevated in the plasma of potassium-deficient rats (16).

In advanced potassium deficiency, the gain of sodium and chloride in the cell exceeds the loss of potassium. Since a net increase in osmotically active particles occurs in the cell (40), potassium-deficient muscle cells generally become swollen (23). Almost all studies of experimental potassium deficiency in humans have demonstrated salt and water retention during potassium depletion. These abnormalities are reversible upon restoration of potassium balance.

RELATIONSHIP BETWEEN MUSCLE POTASSIUM STORES, EXERCISE HYPERKALEMIA, AND BLOOD FLOW DURING EXERCISE

In 1941, Dawes showed that intraarterial infusion of potassium chloride increased muscle blood flow and suggested that potassium ions might be released during exercise from the intracellular to the extracellular space and act there by dilating the muscle vessels (13). Since that time, a number of investigators have obtained evidence strongly supporting this hypothesis. Kjellmer (28), using the cat hind limb preparation, showed that during maximum exercise, potassium concentration in interstitial fluid of the gastrocnemius muscle rose two to four times more than the rise observed simultaneously in venous plasma potassium concentration. This concentration in interstitial fluid corresponded very closely to that observed in venous plasma, (20 mEq/L), when maximum blood flow was induced by intraarterial infusion of KCl solutions. The marked rise in interstitial potassium concentration during muscle contraction has recently been demonstrated in humans with the aid of potassium-sensitive liquid ion-exchange electrodes (53).

Studies were conducted in our laboratory to determine if muscle potassium release during exercise could possibly be impaired and thereby implicate ischemia as a cause of muscle cell necrosis or rhabdomyolysis in potassium-deficient human subjects following strenuous physical exertion (38). This hypothesis was examined by comparing the effect of electrically stimulated exercise on muscle blood flow, potassium release, and histologic characteristics of the intact gracilis muscle preparation in normal and potassium-depleted dogs. In normal dogs, muscle blood flow and potassium release rose sharply during exercise. In contrast, muscle blood flow and potassium release were markedly subnormal in

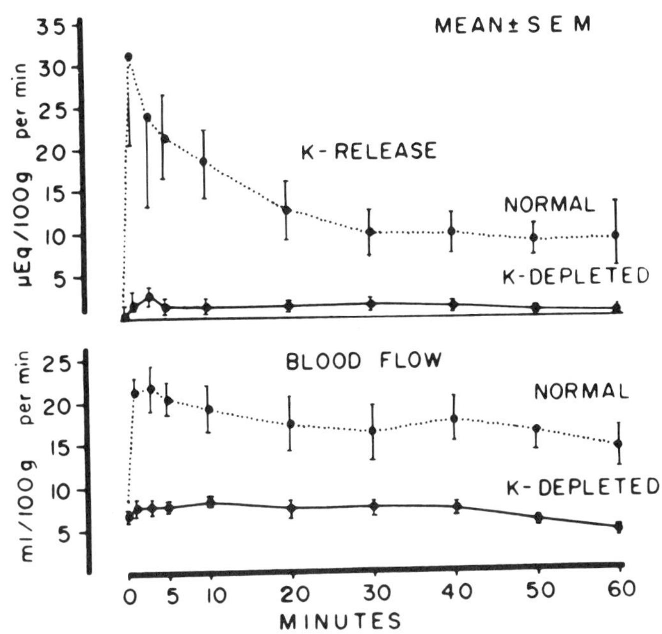

Figure 1 Effect of exercise on potassium release and blood flow from gracilis muscle of normal and potassium-depleted dogs (mean ± SEM). (From Ref. 38.)

depleted dogs despite brisk muscular contractions. These observations are illustrated in Figure 1. Although minor histologic changes were sometimes observed in nonexercised potassium-depleted muscle, frank rhabdomyolysis occurred in each potassium-depleted animal after exercise. We believe that these findings support the hypothesis that ischemia may be implicated as a mechanism of rhabdomyolysis with exercise in potassium deficiency.

MUSCLE GLYCOGEN METABOLISM IN POTASSIUM DEFICIENCY

Impaired energy production as a result of deranged glycolysis is a well-known cause of acute exertional rhabdomyolysis. Classic examples of these defects include myophosphorylase deficiency (McArdles syndrome) or phosphofructokinase deficiency (Tarui's syndrome). Under the anaerobic conditions of intense exercise, production of ATP sufficient to sustain vital functions of the contracting muscle cell becomes almost exclusively dependent on metabolism of glycogen to lactic acid. Although never proved in humans, substantial evidence suggests that severe, long-standing potassium deficiency in several animal species impairs not only glycogen formation but also glycogen utilization. Gardner and his associates studied rats with long-standing potassium deficiency and observed a marked reduction in muscle glycogen content (14). Several other investigators had already shown that potassium ions are necessary for synthesis of glycogen in vitro (18,52).

Several investigators have shown that in very early potassium deficiency, perhaps coinciding with that period of time when cellular hyperpolarization prevails and before intracellular sodium rises, muscle glycogen may in fact become abnormally elevated (14). With prolonged potassium deficiency, perhaps coinciding with that period of time when muscle cells become depolarized and when intracellular sodium increases, a decline in muscle glycogen content occurs. Losert and his associates (42) have suggested that it is not potassium deficiency per se that impairs glycogen metabolism, but that the accumulation of sodium ions inside the cell in advanced potassium deficiency is responsible for their observation that phosphorylase phosphatase activity declines. Inhibition of this enzyme reduces the rate of conversion of active glycogen phosphorylase A into the inactive glycogen phosphorylase B. The net effect of this abnormality could be responsible for decreased glycogen storage. Unfortunately, studies have never been conducted to determine the precise effect of lowering potassium concentration in the cell from a normal value of approximately 150 mEq/L to values that prevail in clinical potassium deficiency. The only studies reported have shown that glycogen is not synthesized in the absence of potassium but is when muscle is incubated in the presence of 0.15 mol KCl.

A major criticism of the studies examining glycogen metabolism in potassium-deficient animals is the possible implication of simultaneous starvation. Potassium deficiency in the experimental animal causes anorexia. The resulting decreased food intake may severely reduce the normal rate of growth in rats and may result in weight loss in dogs. Thus, caloric restriction and partial starvation could cause a substantial reduction in glycogen storage in muscle.

Muscle glycogen content is substantially lower, 0.1 g/dg wet weight, in normal rat muscle than it is in normal dogs. Muscle glycogen content in dog skeletal muscle is almost identical to that of humans: about 1.0 g/dg wet weight. In our studies, measures were taken to assure a normal intake of calories and other nutrients by gavage feeding during induction of potassium deficiency. Despite this precaution, both rats and dogs showed a marked reduction of muscle glycogen content after prolonged potassium depletion.

An interesting aspect of muscle glycogen metabolism is the "supercompensation phenomenon," described by Bergstrom and Hultman (7). If a normal subject performs exhaustive exercise, muscle glycogen content falls to zero. If one then measures muscle glycogen content in the exercised muscle over the succeeding 5 days, it may increase up to five times above normal. Competitive runners have taken advantage of this phenomenon by running themselves to the point of exhaustion 2 or 3 days before a competitive event ("glycogen unloading"), followed by ingestion of a high-carbohydrate diet ("carbohydrate loading") to increase muscle glycogen so that endurance may be prolonged. We have examined the effects of potassium deficiency on glycogen supercompensation (9). In healthy, potassium-replete dogs ingesting a normal carbohydrate intake, electrical stimulation of one leg for 2½ hr leads to complete disappearance of glycogen from that muscle. Sampling of the muscle on the 2nd, 3rd, and 5th day shows that the glycogen content increased fourfold. In the opposite unexercised leg, there was no change in glycogen content. After the same animals were depleted of potassium, muscle glycogen content fell to extremely low values. In these depleted animals, electrical stimulation to the point of exhaustion was not followed by a measurable increase in muscle glycogen content. Thus, at least in dogs, potassium deficiency may impair the physiological process of "glycogen supercompensation." As an extension of this observation, it would appear that potassium deficiency may impair one of the most important biochemical adaptations to exercise training, namely glycogen synthesis. Simple endurance training leads to a substantial increase in muscle glycogen content and is a hallmark of the trained state. If potassium deficiency reduces muscle glycogen content in humans as it does in the dog, this could be partially responsible for the development of rhabdomyolysis with exercise, a process somewhat analogous to McArdle syndrome. Patients with McArdle's disease are unable to utilize their stores of muscle glycogen for energy production during exercise. If, in potassium-deficient humans, glycogen is absent, then there is no mechanism by which ATP can be generated under anaerobic conditions of intense exercise. Although the possibility that potassium deficiency impairs glycogen synthesis in humans has not been conclusively demonstrated, Bergstrom and Hultman (6) have shown a slight decline in muscle glycogen content in patients treated with thiazide diuretics for essential hypertension. There was no evidence that any of these patients became more potassium-deficient than the usual slight amount that occurs with such medication.

CLINICAL FEATURES OF HYPOKALEMIC MYOPATHY

The total content of potassium in the body of a 70-kg healthy man is about 50 mEq/kg or 3,500 mEq. To produce symptoms, a deficit of potassium in most cases must exceed 7% of total body stores, or about 250 mEq. The most common cause of potassium deficiency in industrialized nations is diuretic therapy. A large number of studies quantitating total body potassium before and after administration of diuretics usually show a deficit of about 200 or 300 mEq (29-31). The great majority of patients with such mild degrees of potassium deficiency are without symptoms. When they do occur, symptoms are vague and consist of weakness, muscular discomfort, easy fatiguability, lack of vigor, and, rarely, exercise-induced cramps. Some patients complain of fatigue-associated restlessness that is especially noticeable while sitting. This can be a very aggravating symptom which is relieved temporarily by sitting on one leg and then the other, crossing and uncrossing the legs, seeking different and variable positions of the legs, walking, or standing up and "stomping" the legs forcefully on the floor. Whether these particular symptoms derive from myopathy or neuropathy is difficult to ascertain. It somewhat resembles the "muscular impatience" described as akathisia in patients with a variety of neurological diseases or those with the "restless leg syndrome." These peculiar symptoms vanish following supplementation with potassium and correction of the mild hypokalemia usually associated with this disorder. In such instances, serum potassium concentration will generally range between 2.8 and 3.5 mEq/L. One can expect to find few, if any, physical abnormalities at this level.

Severe potassium deficiency, especially if it occurs rapidly, may result in florid weakness or frank paralysis. Although the progression of symptoms may resemble the Guillain-Barré syndrome, deep tendon reflexes may be retained despite paralysis. Muscle pain, tenderness, and weakness of such severity that the patient cannot lift the arms or stand usually indicate frank rhabdomyolysis. In the experimental animal with potassium deficiency, paralysis induced by insulin corresponds to provocation of hypokalemia of such severity that the sodium pump is depressed. This results in depolarization of the muscle and the inability to form action potentials (24). In clinical potassium deficiency, paralysis of muscles innervated by cranial nerves or those utilized for swallowing is unusual. The cause of death in patients paralyzed by hypokalemia is either arrhythmia or respiratory muscle paralysis with acute respiratory acidosis and hypoxia. In those with such severe potassium deficiency, the total deficit may exceed 25 or 30% of total body stores and serum values are almost invariably below 2.0 mEq/L. One should keep in mind that in any case of hypokalemia, symptoms will be proportionally worse in the presence of hypernatremia or hypercalcemia. Symptoms will also occur at higher relative levels of serum potassium concentration in the presence of hypernatremia or hypercalcemia. Symptoms will also be worse if hypokalemia occurs rapidly in contrast to those patients in whom severe hypokalemia develops over many weeks or months. In those patients who have developed frank rhabdomyolysis or paralysis, potassium deficiency is most often severe and has usually followed voluminous diarrhea, ingestion of two diuretics that act at different sites on the renal tubule, treatment for diabetic ketoacidosis, or in patients with distal or classic renal tubular acidosis. Rhabdomyolysis secondary to potassium deficiency may also occur in otherwise healthy men who have become potassium-depleted as a result of prolonged heat stress and then subject themselves to exhaustive, violent physical exercise (36).

In some respects, symptoms referable to skeletal muscle in patients with chronic longstanding potassium deficiency resemble those in patients with a number of so called "metabolic myopathies." Examples include vitamin D deficiency, chronic phosphorus depletion, or chronic alcoholic myopathy. In all, weakness is especially prominent in the legs and proximal muscle groups.

A number of investigators have made an association between potassium deficiency and myopathy in patients with chronic alcoholism who present with acute rhabdomyolysis (43,47). Studies from this hospital (3) have shown that although patients with alcoholic myopathy may sometimes be hypokalemic, analysis of muscle tissue shows that in about one-half of the cases hypokalemia is not associated with an abnormally low muscle potassium level. In such patients, hypokalemia is probably the result of respiratory alkalosis (11) or the hyperadrenergic state associated with alcoholic withdrawal (48). Unquestionably, patients with chronic alcoholism who have taken diuretics, or those who have experienced vomiting, diarrhea, or a low potassium intake, can become potassium-deficient. In such cases, it is my belief that muscle cells are probably injured in a subclinical manner by alcohol and the additional insult of potassium deficiency might be sufficient to trigger the myopathy into one that is clinically overt. A combination of noxious events is common in other instances of acute myopathy unrelated to either alcohol or potassium deficiency. A good example of such a relationship is the relative ease with which acute rhabdomyolysis may be induced in patients with certain hereditary metabolic abnormalities of skeletal muscle, such as McArdle syndrome or carnitine palmityl transferase deficiency. Both are conditions in which not only is metabolic production of energy impaired but also the demands for energy are markedly increased by exercise. In each situation, exhaustion of ATP stores and probable accumulation of hydrogen ions as the result of exercise result in cellular necrosis or rhabdomyolysis. Similarly, in most instances of major rhabdomyolysis that occur in potassium deficiency, some event has been superimposed upon muscle cells that precipitates the acute event.

LABORATORY FINDINGS IN PATIENTS WITH ACUTE RHABDOMYOLYSIS

Mild to moderate potassium deficiency does not necessarily cause hypokalemia, defined here as a serum potassium level below 3.5 mEq/L. If a patient's serum potassium level averaged 4.5 mEq/L before diuretic therapy, for example, a decline of 0.5 mEq/L could follow a 300-mEq depletion. Although the patient is potassium-deficient, he or she is not hypokalemic. When frank hypokalemia occurs, metabolic alkalosis is common, reflecting increased bicarbonate reabsorption as a result of volume contraction and also increased generation of bicarbonate because of potassium deficiency itself. When potassium deficiency becomes more severe, perhaps in excess of 350 mEq in a normal-sized individual, slight elevations of creatine kinase activity in serum might become detectable (31). Isoenzyme analysis of such samples will show a predominance of the MM fraction. More severe potassium deficiency, and especially that which produces frank rhabdomyolysis, will result in marked elevations of serum CK activity. In most cases in which CK activity approaches 100,000 IU/L, one can anticipate that a fraction of the total will be the MB isoenzyme. Up to 4% of skeletal muscle creatine kinase is of the MB moiety and therefore elevations of this fraction in patients with frank rhabdomyolysis do not necessarily infer the presence of myocardial infarction (22). In rhabdomyolysis, serum aldolase activity will also be elevated. Elevations of serum glutamic oxaloacetic transaminase SGOT and lactic dehydrogenase are commonly found but are not as specific as the elevations of CK.

A number of other laboratory abnormalities strongly suggest the presence of rhabdomyolysis (32). Hyperuricemia, sometimes to rather spectacular levels, reflects skeletal muscle injury with liberation of purine compounds into the circulation that are converted to urate in the liver (35). For example, patients have been observed shortly after the onset of massive rhabdomyolysis with a serum urea nitrogen concentration of 30 mg/dl, and a simultaneous value for serum urate as high as 60 mg/dl. Studies conducted on young men with mild degrees of exercise-induced rhabdomyolysis show that the hyperuricemia is the result of overproduction of urate, since total urinary excretion of uric acid was markedly increased (35). Some patients with substantial degrees of rhabdomyolysis show a disproportional elevation of serum creatinine concentration in relation to serum urea nitrogen at the time of onset. It is presumed that creatine is released from injured skeletal muscle, and then is spontaneously dehydrated to creatinine. The normal ratio of creatinine to serum urea nitrogen is about 0.1. Values for this ratio may become elevated to approximately 0.5 in patients with acute, severe rhabdomyolysis. If such patients are not in acute renal failure, this laboratory manifestation will usually disappear after the first 24 hr. Since muscle tissue contains a large quantity of phosphorus and potassium ions, frank muscle necrosis will commonly cause hyperphosphatemia and hyperkalemia. It is interesting that most patients with potassium deficiency retain the finding of hypokalemia despite severe muscle necrosis. Perhaps on the 2nd or 3rd hospital day, especially if the patients have developed acute renal failure as the result of rhabdomyolysis, hyperkalemia may then become a clinically important complication. Hyperphosphatemia, on the other hand, tends to occur early and will be especially exaggerated in patients with acute renal failure. An important finding in patients with massive rhabdomyolysis is severe hypoalbuminemia (26,32). Young men who had been in perfect health before the onset of rhabdomyolysis have shown serum albumin values as low as 1.5 g/dl. In such patients, there appears to be a high risk of the acute respiratory distress syndrome. It is my assumption that the hypoalbuminemia and the subsequent development of the acute respiratory stress syndrome reflect generalized capillary injury. It has been proposed that this complication results from liberation of proteolytic factors from lysosomal destruction in skeletal muscle cells (45). Severe hypocalcemia is an additional sign of severe rhabdomyolysis. It results from a combination of factors, including hypoalbuminemia, renal failure, and reduced vitamin D production and precipitation as calcium carbonate or calcium phosphate in injured skeletal muscle (33,41). Patients with rhabdomyolysis commonly pass urine that is stained dark brown or mahogany. Results of tests for heme pigment will be positive. Microscopic examination of urine sediment from such patients commonly shows pigmented casts that represent myoglobin. Since myoglobin is a relatively small molecule and is excreted rapidly in patients whose renal function remains normal, it is common to overlook or miss the urine samples that contain myoglobin. Negative results of urinary examination for the pigment do not exclude the diagnosis of rhabdomyolysis.

Electromyographic studies of patients with acute hypokalemic rhabdomyolysis characteristically show low-amplitude, short-duration, polyphasic motor units. Electrical hyperexcitability is suggested by the finding of sustained or profuse electrical activity in the form of runs of positive sharp waves and marked fibrillation potentials that clear with repletion of body potassium stores (47).

Microscopic examination of muscle tissue from patients with potassium deficiency has been reported to show vacuolar degeneration, loss of cross-striations of muscle fibers, fiber "dropout," cellular infiltration about decomposing fibers, and calcifications. Cellular infiltrates are composed of macrophages, large mononuclear cells, and lympocytes. Such findings do not specifically identify potassium deficiency but resemble the changes of acute rhabdomyolysis that may occur under a variety of circumstances.

REFERENCES

1. Akaike, N.: Contribution of an electrogenic sodium pump to membrane potential in mammalian skeletal muscle fibers. *J. Physiol.* 245:499–520, 1975.
2. Akaike, N.: Sodium pump in skeletal muscle: central nervous system-induced suppression by β-adrenoreceptors. *Science* 213:1252–1254, 1981.
3. Anderson, R., Cohen, M., Haller, R., Elms, J., Carter, N. W., and Knochel, J. P.: Skeletal muscle phosphorus and magnesium deficiency in alcoholic myopathy. *Mineral Electrolyte Metab.* 4:106–112, 1980.

4. Bartelheimer, H. K., Losert, W., Senft, G., and Sitt, R.: Storungen des Kohlenhydratstoffwechsels im Kaliummangel. *Naunyn Schmiedebergs Arch. Pharmacol.* 258:391-408, 1967.
5. Beck, F., Dorge, A., Mason, J., Rick, R., and Thurau, K.: Element concentrations of renal and hepatic cells under potassium depletion. *Kidney Int.* 22:250-256, 1982.
6. Bergstrom, J., and Hultman, E.: The effect of thiazides, chlorthalidone and furosemide on muscle electrolytes and muscle glycogen in normal subjects. *Acta Med. Scand.* 180:363-376, 1966.
7. Bergstrom, J., and Hultman, E.: Muscle glycogen synthesis after exercise: an enhancing factor localized to the muscle cells in man. *Nature* 210:309-310, 1966.
8. Bilbrey, G. L., Herbin, L., Carter, N. W., and Knochel, J. P.: Skeletal muscle resting membrane potential in potassium deficiency. *J. Clin. Invest.* 52:3011-3018, 1973.
9. Blachley, J., Long, J., and Knochel, J. P.: The effect of potassium deficiency on resting muscle glycogen content and its response to exercise. *Clin. Res.* 21:39, 1974.
10. Blaustein, M. P.: The interrelationship between sodium and calcium fluxes across cell membranes. *Rev. Physiol. Biochem. Pharmacol.* 70:33-82, 1974.
11. Burnell, J. M., Villamil, M. F., Uyeno, B. T., and Scribner, B. H.: Effect in humans of extracellular pH change on the relationship between serum potassium concentration and intracellular potassium. *J. Clin. Invest.* 35:935-939, 1956.
12. Burton, K. P., Hagler, H. K., Willerson, J. T., and Buja, L. M.: Abnormal lanthanum accumulation due to ischemia in isolated myocardium: effect of chlorpromazine. *Am. J. Physiol.* 241:H714-H723, 1981.
13. Dawes, G. S.: The vasodilator action of potassium. *J. Physiol. (Lond)* 99:224, 1941.
14. Gardner, L. I., Talbot, N. B., Cook, C. D., Berman, H., and Uribe, C.: The effect of potassium deficiency on carbohydrate metabolism. *J. Lab. Clin. Med.* 35:592-602, 1950.
15. Garrahan, P. J., and Glynn, I. M.: The stoichiometry of the sodium pump. *J. Physiol.* 192:217-235, 1967.
16. Gullner, H. G., Lake, C. R., Gill, J. R., Jr., and Lakatua, D. J.: Hypokalemia stimulates plasma epinephrine and norepinephrine in the rat. *Arch. Int. Pharmacodyn.* 260:78-82, 1982.
17. Hartsook, E. W., and Hershberger, T. V.: Tissue cation content of rats: effect of supplemental dietary amino acids in pyridoxine and potassium deficiencies. *J. Nutr.* 95:31-40, 1967.
18. Hastings, A. B.: Electrolytes of tissues and body fluids. *Harvey Lectures* 36:91-125, 1941.
19. Heppel, L. A.: The diffusion of radioactive sodium into the muscles of potassium-deprived rats. *Am. J. Physiol.* 128:449-454, 1940.
20. Hodgkin, A. L., and Katz, B.: The effect of sodium ions on the electrical activity of the giant axon of the squid. *J. Physiol. (London)* 108:37-77, 1949.
21. Irvine, R. O. H., and Dow, J. W.: Potassium depletion: effects on intracellular pH and electrolyte distribution in skeletal and cardiac muscle. *Aust. Annals Med.* 17: 206-213, 1968.
22. Jockers-Wretou, E., and Pfleiderer, G.: Quantitation of creatine kinase isoenzymes in human tissues and sera by an immunological method. *Clin. Chim. Acta* 58:223-232, 1975.
23. Kao, I., and Gordon, A. M.: Alteration of skeletal muscle cellular structures by potassium depletion. *Neurology* 27:855-860, 1977.
24. Kao, I., and Gordon, A. M.: Mechanism of insulin-induced paralysis of muscles from potassium-depleted rats. *Science* 188:740-741, 1975.
25. Kendig, J. J., and Bunker, J. P.: Extracellular space, electrolyte distribution, and resting potential in K depletion. *Am. J. Physiol.* 218:1737-1741, 1970.

26. Kendrick, W. C., Hull, A. R., and Knochel, J. P.: Rhabdomyolysis and shock after intravenous amphetamine administration. *Ann. Intern. Med.* 86:381–387, 1977.
27. Kernan, R. P.: Potassium ions in cell metabolism. *Cell Potassium,* New York, John Wiley & Sons, 1980, pp. 138–150.
28. Kjellmer, I.: Role of K ions in exercise hyperemia. *Med. Exp.* 5:50, 1961.
29. Knochel, J. P.: Diuretic-induced hypokalemia. *Am. J. Med.* 77(5A):18–27, 1984.
30. Knochel, J. P.: Neuromuscular manifestations of electrolyte disorders. *Am. J. Med.* 72:521, 1982.
31. Knochel, J. P.: Rhabdomyolysis and effects of potassium deficiency on muscle structure and function. *Cardiovasc. Med.* 3:247–261, 1978.
32. Knochel, J. P.: Rhabdomyolysis and myoglobinuria. *Annu. Rev. Med.* 33:435–443, 1982.
33. Knochel, J. P.: Serum clacium derangements in rhabdomyolysis and acute renal failure. Editorial. *N. Engl. J. Med.* 305(3):161–162, 1981.
34. Knochel, J. P., and Carter, N. W.: The role of muscle cell injury in pathogenesis of acute renal failure after exercise. *Kidney Int.* 10:S58–S64, 1976.
35. Knochel, J. P., Dotin, L. N., and Hamburger, R. J.: Heat stress, exercise, and muscle injury: effects of urate metabolism and renal function. *Ann. Intern. Med.* 81:321, 1974.
36. Knochel, J. P., Dotin, L. N., and Hamburger, R. J.: Pathophysiology of intense physical conditioning in a hot climate. I. Mechanisms of potassium depletion. *J. Clin. Invest.* 51:242–255, 1972.
37. Knochel, J. P., Foley, F. D., Jr., and Lipscomb, K.: High resting cardiac output with exercise-induced pulmonary edema in the conscious, potassium-deficient dog. *Mineral Electrolyte Metab.* 1:336–344, 1978.
38. Knochel, J. P., and Schlein, E. M.: On the mechanism of rhabdomyolysis in potassium depletion. *J. Clin. Invest.* 51:1750, 1972.
39. Knowles, H. C., Jr., and Guest, G. M.: Tissue electrolytes in alloxan-diabetic rats with ketoacidosis. *Proc. Soc. Exp. Biol. Med.* 79:552–554, 1952.
40. Leaf, A.: On the mechanism of fluid exchange of tissues in vitro. *Biochem. J.* 62: 241–246, 1956.
41. Llach, F., Felsenfeld, A. J., and Haussler, M. R.: Pathophysiology of altered calcium metabolism in rhabdomyolysis-induced acute renal failure. *N. Engl. J. Med.* 305(3): 117–122, 1981.
42. Losert, W.: Relationships between electrolyte balance and carbohydrate metabolism. *Dtsch. Med. Wochenschr.* 93:1723–1731, 1968.
43. Martin, J. B., Craig, J. W., Eckel, R. E., and Munger, J.: Hypokalemic myopathy in chronic alcoholism. *Neurology* 21:1160–1168, 1971.
44. Publicover, S. J., Duncan, C. J., and Smith, J. L.: The use of A23187 to demonstrate the role of intracellular calcium in causing ultrastructural damage in mammalian muscle. *J. Neuropathol. Exp. Neurol.* 37:5, 1978.
45. Reddy, M. K., Etlinger, J. D., Rabinowitz, M., Fischman, D. A., and Zak, R.: Removal of z-lines and α-actinin from isolated myofibrils by a calcium-activated neutral protease. *J. Biol. Chem.* 250:4278, 1975.
46. Riecker, G., Bolte, H. D., and Rohl, D.: Hypokaliamie und membranpotential. *Reanim Organes Artif* 1:41–50, 1964.
47. Rubenstein, A. E., and Wainapel, S. F.: Acute hypokalemic myopathy in alcoholism. *Arch. Neurol.* 34:553–555, 1977.
48. Sellers, E. M., Degani, N. C., Zilm, D. H., and MacLeod, S. M.: Propranolol-decreased noradrenaline excretion and alcohol withdrawal. *Lancet* 1:94–95, 1976.
49. Sen, A. K., and Post, R. L.: Stoichiometry and localization of adenosine triphosphate-dependent sodium and potassium transport in the erythrocyte. *J. Biol. Chem.* 239:345–352, 1964.

50. Skou, J. C.: Enzymatic basis for active transport of Na+ and K+ across cell membrane. *Physiol. Rev.* 45:596–617, 1965.
51. Thomas, R. C.: Membrane current and intracellular sodium changes in a snail neurone during extrusion of injected sodium. *J. Physiol. (London)* 201:495–514, 1969.
52. Torres, H. N., Birnbaumer, L., Garcia-Fernandez, M. D. C., Bernard, E., and Belocopitow, E.: Glycogen metabolism in muscle homogenates. I. The effect of potassium ions on glycogen synthesis. *Arch. Biochem. Biophys.* 116:59–68, 1966.
53. Vyskocil, F., Hnik, P., Rehfeldt, H., Vejsada, R., and Ujec, E.: The measurement of K^+ concentration changes in human muscles during volitional contractions. *Pflugers Arch.* 399:235–237, 1983.
54. Wei, J. W., and Sulakhe, P. V.: Sodium-calcium exchange carrier-supported calcium uptake in membrane vesicles isolated from brain, heart, skeletal muscle and liver. *Chin. J. Physiol.* 25:51–57, 1982.

8

Potassium Metabolism During Starvation and Hypocaloric States

DANIEL G. SAPIR
The Johns Hopkins University School of Medicine and Wyman-Park Health System Hospital, Baltimore, Maryland

To date, only a few published studies have examined potassium (K) loss during a period of total starvation in humans. This chapter will summarize these studies, outline K metabolism during a complete fast, discuss possible mechanisms of K wasting and K sparing during starvation, elucidate the relationship of K to nitrogen (N) wasting, and point out the possible dangers attendant on K loss during starvation. Finally, the discussion of K losses during fasting will be used as a background to discuss K depletion as a possible cause of death in persons who embark on weight loss programs by eating ill-devised hypocaloric diets. The chapter will focus on data from experiments performed in humans, but data from animal studies will be presented when they contribute to an understanding of K metabolism.

K METABOLISM DURING STARVATION

F.G. Benedict compiled his observations during the 31-day fast of one subject in his famous book entitled *A Study of Prolonged Fasting* (2). The pattern of urinary K loss observed by Benedict (the urine being the site of most of the K wastage that occurs during a total fast) has been confirmed in all subsequent studies. Table 1 shows the cumulative K excretion during successive 7-day periods in Benedict's report and two other studies performed in fasting humans. There was a higher rate of urinary K loss during the first week of fasting and progressively smaller losses over the next 3 weeks. Gamble et al. (12) reported their observations in four children who had grand mal epilepsy and who were fasted for 12 days. A lower rate of K excretion was seen in the children than during Benedict's study and the subsequent study, performed in adults (31).

Drenick and his colleagues (6) examined K metabolism during a prolonged fast in markedly overweight adults. During the first week of fasting, the mean cumulative urinary K loss was approximately 320 mEq, while the urinary loss during the first month in individual patients ranged between 485 and 819 mEq. We reported (31) similar values for cumulative urinary K loss during the first week of fasting, and similar rates of K excretion during an 18–28-day fast in grossly obese subjects. In our study, between-patient

Table 1 Weekly Total Urinary Potassium Excretion During Prolonged Fasting in Three Studies

	Study author		
	Benedict	Gamble	Sapir
1st Week	244	149[a]	309 ± 76[b]
2nd Week	141	78	187 ± 56
3rd Week	106	–	105 ± 20

[a]Observations over 6-day intervals.
[b]Mean ± SD.

variation of urine K loss was as great as that observed by Drenick et al. The latter also reported that administration of K supplements (134 mEq/day) during the period of starvation reduced K losses as did the ingestion of a hypocaloric (300 Kcal/day), low-K (30 mEq/day), diet prior to the initiation of fasting. In the fasting patients who ingested 134 mEq KCl/day, potassium balance was achieved on day 15 of the fast, and thereafter remained slightly positive for the remainder of the study, or the next 15 days. Administration of smaller quantities of KCl or $KHCO_3$ (0.5 mmol/kg per day after a period of total fasting lasting 18–28 days) induced a positive K balance also (31). In contrast, balance is never attained in individuals who are not taking K supplements during the fasting period. In both Drenick's study and ours, daily urinary K excretion was occasionally observed to fall to extremely low values, when K supplements were not given; at times these levels were less than 2 mEq/day during a fast lasting more than 1 month.

If K supplements are not given, serum K concentrations fall during a fast despite the presence of systemic acidemia. In general, the serum K concentration will not fall below 3.0 mEq/L even when supplemental K is not administered. However, we have observed occasional values as low as 2.5 mEq/L at the end of a 3-week period of starvation. Administration of 0.5 mmol K/kgBW per day after an 18–28-day total fast led to normalization of the serum K concentration (31). During Drenick's studies, serum K concentrations fell slowly during a prolonged fast, when K supplements were not given, so that by the 100th day of starvation, the serum K ranged between 2.8 and 3.2 mEq/L. Ingestion of 134 mEq KCL/day from the inception of the fast abolished any fall in serum K concentrations.

What fraction of total body K stores is lost during a fast? Is K lost selectively from different tissues during the course of fasting? What are the causes of K wastage and the pathologic changes that can be attributed to depletion of this cation?

Body K stores have been measured by determining exchangeable K after injection of the ^{42}K isotope, by counting the naturally occurring ^{40}K isotope, and by direct postmortem analysis of humans (11,26). By these methods of measurement, which are in relatively good agreement with each other, total body K is approximately 3,000 mEq in a 70-kg man, and when expressed on the basis of lean body or fat-free mass, K content is approximately 74 and 56 mEq/kg in men and women, respectively. Total body K is increased in markedly obese individuals, presumably because their lean body mass is greater than that of normal weight subjects (27). Fat itself has a very low K content (27). The distribution of K within the intracellular space, where 99% of body K is found, is not homogeneous, and thus the concentration of K varies within different tissues and organs (26). The skeletal muscle compartment contains the largest fraction of this cation (two-thirds).

The K loss in the subject studied by Benedict was approximately 640 mEq and this represented depletion of about 20% of the individual's total body potassium stores. Negative K balances of 900-1000 mEq observed after 4 weeks of fasting in some grossly obese subjects represent 25-30% of their total body K stores. In one study, measurements of total body K were made during a fast by measurement of the ^{40}K isotope (7). On this basis, Drenick et al. reported a loss of 13-36% of total body K during the course of 28-102 days of fasting in obese individuals.

Our knowledge of the contribution of various tissues to K loss during fasting is fragmentary. During the early phase of starvation, the liver may be a significant site of K loss. In the fed state, this organ contains a substantial quantity of glycogen and this complex sugar is deposited together with K in a relatively fixed ratio: 1 g glycogen/0.45 mEq K (3,10). Animal studies have shown that total depletion of glycogen occurs within a few hours after a fast is begun (10). It is unclear whether rapid hepatic glycogenolysis occurs during first hours or days of a fast in humans. Of course, one may question whether hepatic glycogenolysis leads to tissue K depletion anymore then does the loss of muscle K in the company of N. After the first days of a fast, muscle tissue, which contains the greatest quantity of potassium stored within the body, is probably the site from which most of the K is lost.

RELATIONSHIP OF K TO PROTEIN WASTAGE

Although substantial losses of K occur during fasting, one cannot simply equate the loss of this cation with tissue K depletion. The reason for this is the fixed relationship between K and protein (N) within lean tissue. Within this tissue compartment, the ratio K/N is approximately 3 mEqK/gN (8). Therefore, losses of K that occur together with N, at or below this ratio, may not represent true tissue K depletion. For example, the loss of a leg reduces both body K stores as well as total body N, but the remaining tissue is depleted neither of K nor N and certainly no one would claim that a now limbless person was necessarily K-depleted. During a fast, the loss of lean tissue measured as urinary N accounts for a substantial part of the K loss and only the remaining fraction of K lost in excess of the 3:1 ratio is thought to represent true tissue K depletion. In six fasting subjects previously studied in our laboratory (31), we observed that the mean ± SD cumulative K balance corrected for N losses was just −99.2 ± 59.3 mEq at the end of a 3-week period of fasting.

Although the K/N ratio of 3:1 is widely used in the interpretation of K balance data, its applicability in studies carried out in fasting humans may be limited for the following reasons. The 3:1 ratio applies to muscle tissue and the K/N ratio of other tissues may be considerably different; thus to the extent that K and N wastage arise from tissues other than muscle during starvation, use of a fixed ratio to evaluate K losses may be erroneous (22,26). In animals, partial repair of protein depletion may occur without K administration thereby demonstrating a dissociation of K and N balance (23). Such dissociation was also observed during our study (31) where approximately 50% of a K deficit arising during the course of a fast was repaired without provision of exogenous protein.

During fasting or hypocaloric states, the depletion of protein stores (lean body mass) is the main threat to continued survival. Not only is K present within muscle, where it is found in a fixed relationship with N, but also maintenance of the total body pool of this cation is essential for cellular metabolic processes (15). Without adequate K neither growth or maintenance of cells will occur and following K depletion, body cell mass will not be fully restored unless K is given in adequate quantities. The experiments performed

Table 2 Mean ± SEM Daily Excretion of NH_4^+, K^+, and Urine pH Before and After Administration of KCL or $KHCO_3$ (0.5 mmol/kg per day) During a Prolonged Fast

	KCL		$KHCO_3$	
	Control	Exp	Control	Exp
$U_{NH_4}V$ (mmol/day)	120.4 ± 21.5	83.4 ± 13.9[a]	128.9 ± 13.6	72.4 ± 12.8[a]
U_kV	12.2 ± 3.6	61.8 ± 6.0[a]	7.2 ± 3.5	45.2 ± 12.0[a]
UpH	6.00 ± 0.02	5.54 ± 0.06[a]	5.90 ± 0.11	5.59 ± 0.08[a]

[a] $p < 0.01$ from control value.

by Cannon et al. (4) clearly demonstrated diminution in growth rates of K-depleted rats, while Rudman and his co-workers (29) showed that patients' protein losses could not be repaired when intravenous alimentation solutions were administered without K. Potassium depletion produces histologic lesions that are the forerunner of cell death.

In view of the relationship between K and N, does provision of K during the course of a fast reduce N wastage? In humans, only three studies provide any answers to this question. Analysis of the data in Drenick's study (6) does not indicate that ingestion of a daily supplement of 134 mEq K reduced N wastage during a fast. A different conclusion can be reached when the data of Walker and his colleagues (37) are examined. These investigators demonstrated that provision of K as its gluconate salt reduced *total* N excretion in a group of fasting subjects below the levels of urea N excretion observed in another group of fasting subjects who were not taking any K supplements. Provision of small amounts of carbohydrate (CHO) calories, both as the gluconate salt of K and 15-30 g sucrose in the K solution, in those subjects whose total N excretion was lowered, opened their conclusion to question. Possibly their data remain valid because of the observation made during our studies that provision of CHO calories during a fast in quantities equal to the amount ingested by the subjects in Walker's study changed ammonium N (NH_4N), but not urea N excretion during a fast (33). Although the question of whether K supplements reduce urea N excretion during a fast remains open, the fact that K supplements produce an N-sparing effect during starvation has been established (31). The administration of 0.5 mmol/kg per day KCL or $KHCO_3$ during a prolonged fast reduced NH_4N excretion by approximately 40 mmol/day (Tables 2, 3). This occurred without a change in urine volume or organic acid excretion in the subjects who took $KHCO_3$ and with a fall in urine pH, the cause of which was a decline in buffer (ammonium) excretion. The data obtained in subjects who were given KCl supplements were similar to the experiments during which $KHCO_3$ was given, except that organic acid excretion fell in the subjects who took KCL supplements. Since glutamine is the major source material for synthesis of ammonium N (1), the provision of K may have decreased amino acid degradation or increased amino acid synthesis during the course of a fast. This effect was present as long as K supplements were given, but was reversed when K was no longer ingested. After 3 weeks of starvation, N excretion falls to very low levels, approximately 4-5 g/day, the major fraction of which is equally apportioned between urea and ammonium N (24). During our study, urinary ammonium N excretion fell by about one-third or 0.4 g/day following K supplementation. We did not observe a change in urinary urea N excretion when 0.5 mmol K/Kg per day was administered nor when larger quantities of $KHCO_3$ (1.5-2.0 mmol/kg per day) were ingested (31).

Table 3 Mean ± SEM Potassium Balance, Urine Urea Nitrogen Excretion, and Blood Glutamine Concentration Before and After Administration of KCL (0.5 mmol per day) During a Prolonged Fast

	Control	KCL
K balance (mEq/period)	−525 ± 71	+255 ± 35
UUN (g/day)	1.47 ± 0.2	1.49 ± 0.1
Blood glutamine (mmol)	387 ± 25	449 ± 35

PHYSIOLOGICAL DETERMINANTS OF K LOSS DURING FASTING

What are the physiological determinants of K loss during a fast and what mechanisms limit the wastage of this cation during starvation? Factors that alter the rate of K excretion include the rate of water and solute delivery to the distal nephron (17), the concentration of anions within the lumen of the distal tubule (21), circulating concentrations of mineralocorticoids (34), plasma acid-base balance (19), and the rate of renal ammoniagenesis (36). Increased rates of urine flow as well as sodium and solute delivery to the distal nephron heighten K excretion. Markedly obese individuals have elevated total body Na contents confirmed by the clinical presence of edema and early during the course of fasting may lose up to 6-7 L urine/day, resulting in total urinary Na loss of 6-800 mEq over the first 5 days of a fast (30). Despite these figures, we have not observed a correlation between the rate of urine flow and Na excretion and the rate of kaliuresis during fasting.

Within the distal nephron, K transfer into the tubular lumen may, in large part, be a passive process. This cation is excreted under the influence of an intraluminal negative electrical potential (20). Any physiological perturbations that increase this transluminal potential within the distal nephron will accelerate kaliuresis. One such manuever is infusion of Na_2SO_4 following which intraluminal concentration of the relatively poorly reabsorbed anion $SO_4^{=}$ increases (20). Stimulation of Na reabsorption will then increase further the potential difference and augment urinary K loss. During a fast, the urinary organic anion excretion of acetoacetate (AcAc) and B-hydroxybutyrate (B-OHB) will increase by several hundred times (32), reaching values as high as 300 mEq/day. We have shown that acetoacetate is almost completely reabsorbed and only a very small fraction of the quantity filtered appears in the urine. This contrasts with the urinary loss of B-OHB, whose fractional excretion rate is approximately one-third, and accordingly, this ketone body accounts for more than 80-90% of the total ketones appearing in the urine during a prolonged fast (32). Thus, during fasting, increased organic anion (ketone body) excretion may serve to increase urinary K loss. Moreover, urinary Na losses occurring early during a fast would increase plasma aldosterone concentration and heighten Na reabsorption, thereby creating an analogous situation to that observed following Na_2SO_4 infusions. But our data did not show any correlation between mean daily urinary K and ketone body excretion over 3 successive 7-day periods of starvation. The reason for this lack of correlation may be the increased renal ammonium excretion which almost completely matches the increased excretory rate of AcAc and B-OHB during a fast. To the extent that NH_4 excretion provides a cation to maintain urinary electroneutrality, the necessity to excrete K is diminished.

As mentioned previously, one other factor that could increase K wastage during fasting is an increase in plasma aldosterone concentrations. However, Cooke (unpublished observations) found that aldosterone secretory rates are elevated during starvation at a time when the rate of K excretion is minimal. On the 28th day of a fast, the mean ± SEM (n = 7) aldosterone secretory rate had risen to 597 ± 138 μg/day from a figure of 43 ± 13 μg/day one day before the start of starvation. The contribution of this hormonal alteration to K wastage is unknown, but clearly the influence is not significant, because high secretory rates of this hormone observed during the course of a fast occurred at a time when the rate of K excretion was minimal.

Previous studies have indicated that the lean body mass of grossly obese adults is increased. Total body K content is correlated with lean body mass, so that one of the physiological determinants of the quantity of K lost during a fast could be the initial lean body mass or K content of the individual and the subsequent rate of proteolysis during fasting. We demonstrated that the daily K excretory rate correlates with the initial body weight of obese subjects, but not with the daily excretion of either urea N or creatinine. Thus, it is possible that the rate of K excretion during fasting is a function of the initial K pool size.

An analysis of the pattern of urinary K loss at the beginning of a fast shows that K excretion occurs at the same rate as that observed in the fed state. Most grossly obese subjects on a self-selected diet excrete approximately 50-60 mEq K/day. Potassium excretion declines steadily, but somewhat erratically throughout fasting, reaching levels as low as 5-10 mEq/day during the 4th week of fasting. This suggests that any mechanism(s) that spares K during a fast is (are) slow in onset.

What then are the possible K-sparing mechanism(s) that limit excretion of this cation during a fast? Heightened renal ammonium excretion is one factor that limits K excretion and, although very effective, it is delayed in onset because the increase in daily urinary ammonium excretion is slow to reach maximal levels. Tannen has shown that renal K and ammonium metabolism are linked so that heightened renal ammoniagenesis and urinary ammonium excretion occur in the presence of hypokalemia and K depletion (36). Conversely hyperkalemia reduces renal ammoniagenesis and urinary ammonium excretion. Potassium is a controlling factor in the synthesis of ammonium at several enzymatic sites of the biochemical pathway in which the amide group of glutamine is removed and subsequently excreted as ammonium (36). During a prolonged fast, we observed that partial restoration of K balance and normalization of the serum K was associated with a significant increase in urinary K excretion and a decline in urinary ammonium output. The heightened output of ammonium during a fast provides a cation to be excreted in the company of the anionic urinary ketone bodies, thereby reducing the need for excretion of other cations including K (31).

Another factor limiting K output which is slow in onset is diminution of urine volume and urinary Na excretion during a fast. By the middle of the 2nd week of a total fast daily urinary Na excretion falls to less than 1 mEq/day and remains at that level for the duration of starvation. Urine volume diminishes consequent to low water intake in fasting subjects who have not been encouraged to drink and by the presence of low rates of solute excretion which, having progressively declined during a fast, attain minimal levels by the fourth week of starvation. The fall in urinary solute excretion is due primarily to reduction in urine urea nitrogen and urinary sodium output. We have observed urine volumes as low as 100 ml/day in several fasting subjects who did not have a change in measured renal function nor manifest renal or urinary tract stones. Similarly, low urine volumes as well as 24-hr periods of anuria were described by Runcie and Thomson (30) in a group of patients undergoing a total fast and by Drenick et al. (7). In the latter report, the authors describe one patient who had an average urine output of 120 ml/day over a 5-day period without change in renal function.

One of the major factors that enable humans to withstand the effects of total fasting is limitation of the rate of loss of protein stores (9). Factors involved in this process include the use of fat as the primary fuel during a fast (9), limitation of gluconeogenesis (9), utilization of ketone bodies rather than glucose as a fuel by the CNS (25), and increased renal ketone body reabsorption (32). Reduction of proteolysis minimizes K wastage by reducing the loss of body cell mass. By the 4th week of fasting, urinary N loss is reduced to 4-5 g/day from a value of 12-15 g/day during the first few days of a fast.

Potassium depletion may cause myocardial damage during a total fast. A number of experimental studies have demonstrated the presence of such damage in association with K depletion (5,16,28). Cardiac arrhythmias induced by K depletion could have caused the two sudden deaths that occurred during a total fast, reported by Spencer (35).

K LOSS DURING HYPOCALORIC STATES

Although total fasting has been used as a rapid method of losing weight throughout the United States, calorie-restricted diets are in much wider use than starvation. Some of the calorie-restricted diets are not only deficient in calories but also may lack the quantity and quality of protein necessary to maintain nitrogen balance. Potassium depletion may also be a feature of these diets because of deficient intake of this cation. To compound further the problem of K wastage, many dieters take diuretics in an attempt to hasten weight loss. Hypokalemia may cause further nitrogen depletion (36) and precipitate fatal cardiac arrhythmias (13).

The recent use of a diet based on a liquid protein supplement illustrates the possible hazards of nutritional deficiency. During a 6-month period beginning in July, 1977, at least 60 persons using a liquid protein diet supplement died (13). Observations made on 17 of 60 of these patients were reported by Isner et al. (14). Ten had episodes of ventricular tachycardia, nine prolongation of the QT interval, and nine had diminished amplitude of the QRS complex. Autopsy performed in 14 of these patients demonstrated attenuated myocardial fibers in 12 and increased myocardial lipofuchsin pigment in 11. Hypokalemia was a common finding in these patients, but its relationship to the cardiac arrhythmias and death was difficult to assess. Lantigua et al. (18) reported the occurrence of heart block, frequent premature ventricular contractions, and ventricular tachycardia in three of six patients on a diet that was based on a liquid protein supplement. Their patients sustained only a modest K deficit, in part because of the administration of a daily K supplement. This study demonstrated that arrhythmias occurred during the period of ingestion of this diet, and suggested that there is significant potential for the development of other cardiac arrhythmias when K supplementation was not added to the dietary regimen.

Bulimia, or self-induced postprandial vomiting is another dietary condition in which hypokalemia may contribute to morbidity and mortality.

CONCLUSIONS

1. Moderate potassium wasting occurs during fasting. There is a small loss of potassium in excess of that predicted from losses of nitrogen.
2. Moderate declines of serum potassium levels are present during a fast, but severe hypokalemia may occur in some patients. Cardiac arrythmias, one of the causes of death during a prolonged fast, may result from hypokalemia.
3. During a prolonged fast, potassium balance may affect nitrogen balance: Partial repletion of potassium stores produces a nitrogen-sparing effect during a fast by reducing renal ammonium excretion; during fasting, provision of potassium supplements improves potassium balance.
4. Potassium depletion may be a factor in the death of some persons on hypocaloric diets.

REFERENCES

1. Balagura-Baruch, S.: Renal metabolism and transfer of ammonia in the kidney, edited by Rouller, C., Muller, A. F., New York, London, Academic Press, Vol. 3, 1971.
2. Benedict, F. G.: *A Study of Prolonged Fasting*, Washington, Carnegie Institute of Washington, Publication No. 203, 1916.
3. Bergstrom, J., and Hultman, E.: Glycogen content of skeletal muscle in patients renal failure. *Acta Med. Scand.* 186:177-181, 1969.
4. Cannon, P. R., Frazier, L. E., and Hughes, R. H.: Influence of potassium on tissue protein synthesis. *Metabolism* 1:49-57, 1952.
5. Darrow, D. C., and Miller, H. C.: The production of cardiac lesions by repeated injections of desoxycorticosterone acetate. *J. Clin. Invest.* 21:601-611, 1942.
6. Drenick, E. J., Blahd, W. H., Singer, F. R., and Lederer, M.: Body potassium content in obese subjects and potassium depletion during prolonged fasting. *Am. J. Clin. Nutr.* 18:278-285, 1966.
7. Drenick, E. J., Swenseid, M. E., Blahd, W. H., and Tuttle, S. G.: Prolonged starvation as treatment for severe obesity. *JAMA* 187:100-105, 1964.
8. Elkinton, J. R., and Danowski, T. S.: *The Body Fluids.* Baltimore, Williams & Wilkins Co., 1955, p. 183.
9. Felig, P., Owen, O. E., Wahren, J., and Cahill, G. F. Jr.: Amino acid metabolism during prolonged starvation. *J. Clin. Invest.* 48:584-594, 1969.
10. Fenn, W. O.: The deposition of potassium and phosphate with glycogen in rat livers. *J. Biol. Chem.* 128:297-307, 1939.
11. Forbes, G. B., and Lewis, A. M.: Total sodium, potassium and chloride in adult man. *J. Clin. Invest.* 35:596-600, 1956.
12. Gamble, J. L., Ross, G. S., and Tisdall, F. F.: The metabolism of fixed base during fasting. *J. Biol. Chem.* 57:633-695, 1923.
13. Gregy, M. B. (Ed.): Deaths associated with liquid protein diets. *Morbid. Mortal. Weekly Rep.* 26:383, 1977.
14. Isner, J. M., Sours, H. E., Paris, A. L., Ferrans, V. J., and Roberts, W. C.: Sudden unexpected death in avid dieters using the liquid protein modified fast diet. *Circulation* 60:1401-1412, 1979.
15. Kernan, R. P.: *Cell K.* Washington, Butterworths, Molecular Biology and Medicine Series, 1965.
16. Keye, J. D.: Death in potassium deficiency. Report of a case including morphologic findings. *Circulation* 5:766-770, 1952.
17. Kunau, R. T., Webb, H. L., and Borman, S. C.: Characteristics of the relationship between flow rate of tubular fluid and potassium transport in the distal tubule. *J. Clin. Invest.* 54:1488-1495, 1974.
18. Lantigua, R. A., Amatruda, J. M., Biddle, T. L., Forbes, G. B., and Lockwood, D.: Cardiac arrhythmias associated with a liquid protein diet for the treatment of obesity. *N. Engl. J. Med.* 303:735-738, 1980.
19. Malnic, G., DeMello-Aires, M., and Giebisch, G.: Potassium transport across renal distal tubules during acid base disturbances. *Am. J. Physiol.* 221:1192-1208, 1971.
20. Malnic, G., Klose, R. M., and Giebisch, G.: Micropuncture study of distal tubular potassium and sodium transport in rat nephron. *Am. J. Physiol.* 211:529-547, 1966.
21. Malnic, G., Klose, R. M., and Giebisch, G.: Microperfusion study of distal, tubular potassium and sodium transfer in rat kidney. *Am. J. Physiol.* 211:548-599, 1966.
22. Mounib, M. S., and Evans, J. V.: The potassium and sodium contents of sheep tissues in relation to the potassium content of the erythrocytes and the age of the animal. *Biochem. J.* 75:77-82.

23. Muntwyler, E., and Griffin, G. E.: Tissue electrolyte content of potassium and protein deficient rats. *Proc. Soc. Exp. Biol. Med.* 89:349–352, 1955.
24. Owen, O. E., Felig, P., Morgan, A. P., Wahren, J., and Cahill, G. F. Jr.: Liver and kidney metabolism during prolonged starvation. *J. Clin. Invest.* 48:574–583, 1969.
25. Owen, O. E., Morgan, A. P., Kemp, H. G., Sullivan, K. M., Herrera, M. G., and Cahill, G. F. Jr.: Brain metabolism during fasting. *J. Clin. Invest.* 46:1589–1595, 1967.
26. Patrick, J.: Assessment of body potassium stores. *Kidney Int.* 11:476–490, 1977.
27. Pierson, R. N., Lin, D. H. Y., and Phillips, R. A.: Total body potassium in health: Effects of age, sex, height and fat. *Am. J. Physiol.* 226:206–212, 1974.
28. Rodriguez, C. E., Wolf, A. L., and Bergstrom, V. W.: Hypokalemic myocarditis. *Am. J. Clin. Pathol.* 20:1050–1055, 1950.
29. Rudman, D., Millikan, W. J., Richardson, R. J., Bixler, T. J., Stackhouse, W. J., and McGarrity, W. C.: Elemental balances during intravenous hyperalimentation of underweight adult subjects. *J. Clin. Invest.* 55:94–104, 1975.
30. Runcie, J., and Thomson, T. J.: Prolonged starvation—a dangerous procedure? *Br. Med. J.* 3:432–435, 1970.
31. Sapir, D. G., Chambers, N. E., and Ryan, J. W.: The role of potassium in the control of ammonium excretion during starvation. *Metabolism* 25:211–220, 1976.
32. Sapir, D. G., and Owen, O. E.: Renal conservation of ketone bodies during starvation. *Metabolism* 24:22–33, 1975.
33. Sapir, D. G., Owen, O. E., Cheng, J. T., Ginsberg, R., Boden, G., and Walker, W. G.: The effect of carbohydrates on ammonium and ketoacid excretion during starvation. *J. Clin. Invest.* 51:2093–2102, 1972.
34. Shambelan, M., Sebastian, A., and Hulter, H. N.: Mineralocorticoid excess and deficiency syndromes. In *Acid-Base and Potassium Homeostasis*, edited by B. M. Brenner and J. H. Stein, pp. 232–268.
35. Spencer, I. O. B.: Death during therapeutic starvation for obesity. *Lancet* 1:1288–1290, 1968.
36. Tannen, R. L.: Relationship of renal ammonia production and potassium homeostasis. *Kidney Int.* 11:453–465, 1977.
37. Walker, W. G., Sapir, D. G., Turin, M., and Cheng, J. T.: *Potassium Homeostasis and Diuretic Therapy. Modern Diuretic Therapy in the Treatment of Cardiovascular and Renal Disease.* Amsterdam, Excerpta Medica, 1972.

9

Potassium-Losing Tubulopathies: Bartter's Syndrome and Similar Disorders

JOHN R. GILL, JR.
National Heart, Lung and Blood Institute, National Institutes of Health, Bethesda, Maryland

In 1962 Bartter and associates described a syndrome of renal potassium loss, the essential features of which were hyperplasia of the juxtaglomerular apparatus with aldosteronism, hypokalemic alkalosis, normal blood pressure, decreased pressor responsiveness to angiotensin II, and growth retardation (2). Findings in the two reported patients were thought to represent a new syndrome caused by a primary resistance of the vasculature to angiotensin II. It is now clear that a number of disorders that cause potassium loss through the kidney or gastrointestinal tract can produce all of the above features initially attributed to Bartter's syndrome and may closely resemble one another (Table 1). For example, familial chloride diarrhea with loss of potassium chloride from the gastrointestinal tract may be associated with hyperplasia of the juxtaglomerular apparatus, hyperreninemia, aldosteronism, hypokalemic alkalosis, and decreased pressor resistance (30,32). Patients with potassium chloride loss, self-induced by laxative abuse or by covert vomiting, show similar clinical features (12,34,40). These disorders, similarly to Bartter's syndrome (17), show an overproduction of prostaglandins (PGs) which appear to mediate the pathophysiological changes of potassium depletion (14). Although the disorders listed in Table 1 have many clinical features in common, they also have differences which depend, in part, on the location of the potassium loss (whether through the kidney or gastrointestinal tract) and, in part, on the cause of that loss.

PATHOPHYSIOLOGY OF EXPERIMENTAL POTASSIUM DEPLETION

Potassium deficiency of approximately 8 mEq/kg was produced in dogs by hemodialysis and maintained for 21 days by feeding them a potassium-free diet (14). The hemodynamic consequences of prolonged potassium depletion were a decrease in peripheral vascular resistance, expansion of plasma volume, and an increase in cardiac output (Fig. 1). The hemodynamic changes were associated with an increase in renal PGE production, an increase in plasma renin activity, and decreased pressor responsiveness to angiotensin II (Fig. 2). Blood pressure was maintained because changes such as increases in cardiac

Table 1 Differential Diagnosis of Bartter's Syndrome

Bartter's syndrome
Covert diuretic abuse
Magnesium-losing tubulopathy
Calcium-losing tubulopathy
Chronic renal disease
Cystinosis
Nephritis
Gastrointestinal disorders
Covert vomiting
Covert laxative abuse
Familial chloride diarrhea

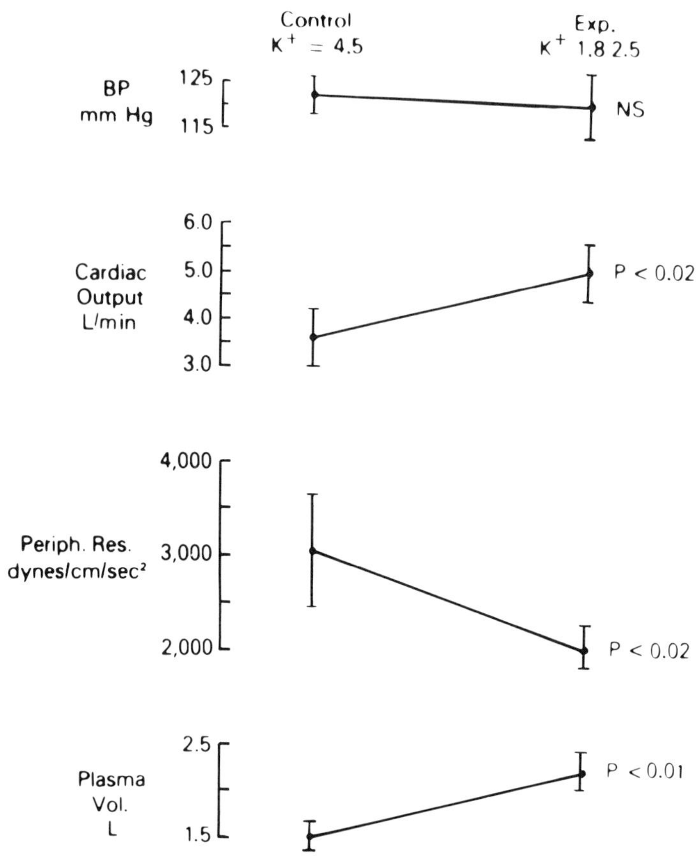

Figure 1 The changes in blood pressure (BP), cardiac output, peripheral resistance (Periph. Res.), and plasma volume (Vol) produced by prolonged potassium (K^+) depletion in the dog. (Data from Ref. 14.)

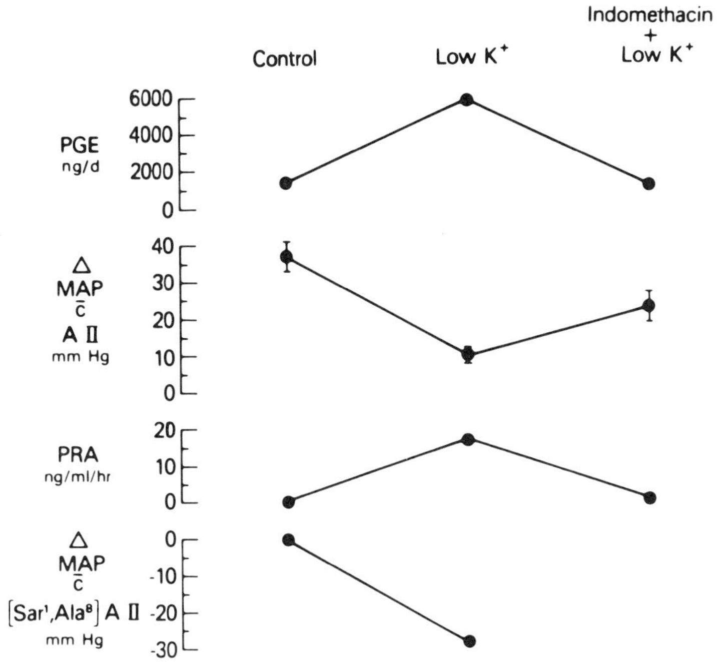

Figure 2 Changes in urinary prostaglandin E (PGE), response of mean arterial pressure (MAP) to infusion of angiotensin (A) II (10 ng/kg per min), changes in plasma renin activity (PRA), and response of MAP to infusion of [Sar^1, Ala^8] AII (10 μg/kg per min) produced by prolonged potassium (K^+) depletion and by superimposition of indomethacin (150 mg/day). (Data from Ref. 14.)

output and plasma renin activity compensated for the decreases in peripheral resistance and in vascular responsiveness to angiotensin II. The importance of hyperreninemia as a compensatory mechanism was indicated by the large fall in mean arterial pressure produced by a dose of an angiotensin II antagonist ([Sar^1,Ala^8] angiotensin II) that had no effect on blood pressure before potassium depletion was induced (Fig. 2). An increase in plasma epinephrine and norepinephrine in rats fed a potassium-deficient diet suggests that an increase in sympathoadrenal activity may also contribute to the maintenance of blood pressure during potassium depletion (21).

Potassium depletion stimulated renal synthesis and excretion of PGE and there are reasons to believe that it may have stimulated PG synthesis by vascular tissue to produce vasodilatation (14). First, prostacyclin is probably the major prostanoid synthesized by vascular tissue and release of this vasodilator PG from aortic strips was stimulated when they were incubated in media with a low potassium concentration (9). Second, a metabolite of prostacyclin, 6-keto $PGF_{1\alpha}$ increased to the same degree as PGE_2 in the urine of rats fed a potassium-deficient diet (20). Third, treatment of potassium-deficient dogs with indomethacin inhibited renal and probably vascular synthesis of PGs, and corrected the hyperreninemia and the vascular resistance to angiotensin II, presumably by correcting vascular vasodilatation (Fig. 2).

PATHOPHYSIOLOGY OF BARTTER'S SYNDROME

PGE_2 and 6-keto $PGF_{1\alpha}$ are increased in the urine of patients with Bartter's syndrome and indicate that the synthesis of PGE_2 and prostacyclin is increased (17,18). Although there are no estimates of peripheral vascular resistance in Bartter's syndrome, a number of observations suggest that vascular vasodilatation may be present in these patients and that it is prostaglandin dependent.

1. An angiotensin II antagonist, (Sar^1-Ile^8) angiotensin II, produced large falls in blood pressure in patients with Bartter's syndrome despite a further increase in plasma renin activity; when PG synthesis was inhibited by indomethacin, plasma renin activity fell to normal and the same dosage of (Sar^1-Ile^8) angiotensin II produced a rise in blood pressure (24,38). [(Sar^1-Ile^8) angiotensin II is both an antagonist and a weak agonist; when blood pressure is not dependent on angiotensin II and plasma renin activity is normal or low, its agonistic action may predominate.]
2. Large falls in blood pressure were also observed in patients with Bartter's syndrome when plasma angiotensin II was lowered to normal by administration of a converting enzyme inhibitor, captopril (1,13).
3. Sympathoadrenal activity was increased in patients with Bartter's syndrome and, since it was corrected by indomethacin, it, like the hyperreninemia, was presumably a compensatory response to prostaglandin-mediated vasodilatation (19).
4. Plasma bradykinin, a vasodilator, was supranormal in patients with Bartter's syndrome (41). Treatment with aprotinin, which inhibits the formation of bradykinin by kallikrein, partially corrected the vascular resistance to angiotensin II (35). Although the increase in plasma bradykinin was associated with increased PG synthesis and was corrected when the overproduction of PGs was corrected by treatment with indomethacin, the precise mechanism of the increase in bradykinin is unknown (41).
5. Treatment with indomethacin corrected the hyperreninemia and increase in sympathetic activity in Bartter's syndrome and restored sensitivity of the vascular system to the pressor effects of angiotensin II and norepinephrine to normal (19,33).

Although these observations suggest that increases in vascular vasodilator PGs and in plasma bradykinin were initially and principally responsible for the decrease in pressor responsiveness, down-regulation of angiotensin II receptors occurring in response to hyperreninemia may also have contributed to the pressor resistance to angiotensin II (22). Treatment with an inhibitor of angiotensin-converting enzyme lowered plasma angiotensin II to normal and partially corrected the pressor resistance to angiotensin II (13). The foregoing pathophysiological features of Bartter's syndrome and proposed schema for their interrelationship are presented in Figure 3. This schema is also applicable to the disorders listed in Table 1 and to experimental potassium depletion; these conditions all show pathophysiological changes similar to those of Bartter's syndrome.

Potassium depletion in Bartter's syndrome results from excessive renal excretion of potassium that persists during correction of PG overproduction, albeit at a somewhat reduced rate because of renal hemodynamic changes associated with inhibition of PG synthesis (3,17). Some patients with Bartter's syndrome have also shown excessive renal excretion of magnesium with hypomagnesemia. These patients with magnesium depletion also show an abnormally low urinary calcium level (36), presumably, because serum ionized calcium levels and the filtered load of calcium tend to be lower as a result of impaired release of parathyroid hormone and/or increased resistance to its calcium-mobilizing action.

Maximal urinary concentrating ability (6) and maximal urinary diluting ability (16) were both impaired and were not improved by treatment with indomethacin. These

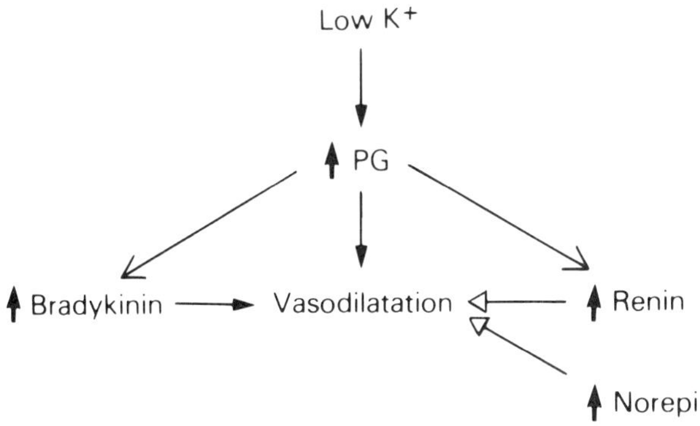

Figure 3 Proposed schema for the pathogenesis of Bartter's syndrome. Solid arrows indicate stimulation; open arrows indicate inhibition. (From Ref. 14.)

abnormalities in urinary concentration and dilution may be a result of the subnormal distal fractional chloride reabsorption in Bartter's syndrome (16). Since estimates of distal fractional chloride reabsorption during water diuresis provides an indirect assessment of chloride transport by the thick ascending limb of Henle's loop (7), this suggests that the location of the impaired distal chloride transport in Bartter's syndrome is the thick ascending limb. Not only does active transport of chloride with passive sodium reabsorption in this segment of the nephron generate most of the solute-free water excreted during a water diuresis, but it also supplies solute to the interstitium to maintain hypertonicity essential for concentration of tubular fluid (5). Impaired chloride reabsorption by the thick ascending limb, in addition to causing abnormalities in urinary concentration and dilution, may also cause potassium loss by decreasing potassium reabsorption in the thick ascending limb and by increasing delivery of tubular fluid to more distal nephron segments where potassium secretion is flow dependent (42).

Inhibition of prostaglandin synthesis did not improve either concentrating or diluting ability and only transiently decreased potassium loss; this suggests that a prostaglandin-independent impairment in chloride reabsorption by the thick ascending limb represents the most proximate cause of Bartter's syndrome yet identified. This proposed defect in chloride absorption, if it involved the macula densa, could also account for the especially prominent juxtaglomerular hyperplasia in Bartter's syndrome. Except in gastrointestinal disorders or furosemide abuse, in which the absorption of chloride by the macula densa may be limited by severe chloride deficiency or inhibited transport, the changes in the juxtaglomerular apparatus in other disorders of potassium depletion tend to be less marked than those in Bartter's syndrome.

Bartter's syndrome can be differentiated from gastrointestinal disorders with potassium depletion because losses of sodium and chloride from the gastrointestinal tract decrease their excretion in the urine (15). Differentiating Bartter's syndrome from other disorders that produce urinary potassium loss is more difficult, although chronic renal diseases that produce potassium loss are usually recognizable and covert diuretic abuse can usually be diagnosed by a diuretic screen of urine (23,29). Magnesium-losing and calcium-losing tubulopathies are frequently diagnosed as Bartter's syndrome because all three disorders closely resemble one another and correct identification may not be possible without detailed studies of renal function and histological characteristics. Although the molecular basis for none of these three tubulopathies is known, the disorders do appear to be separate entities that can be identified by detailed studies of renal function and histological findings.

MAGNESIUM-LOSING TUBULOPATHY

Numerous observations indicate that magnesium depletion may lead to hypokalemia, although the mechanism by which this occurs is poorly understood (Chap. 2). The hypomagnesemia and hypokalemia, in turn, stimulate renin release and the aldosteronism that ensues may further aggravate potassium and magnesium loss.

The clinical features of magnesium-losing tubulopathy are shown in Table 2. The disorder may be familial or acquired, and, when it has occurred in childhood, growth and development are normal (26,31). In most patients tetany was the major complaint and, in some patients, was not manifest except during illness or pregnancy. Hypocalcemia was present in some patients and appeared to be best explained as an inhibitory effect of magnesium depletion on action and/or release of parathyroid hormone (10,37). Magnesium supplementation with only partial correction of hypomagnesemia restored serum calcium levels to normal (10,37).

Renal histologic findings have usually been normal and the juxtaglomerular apparatus was not hyperplastic even though plasma renin activity was increased (10,26,31). Occasionally, patchy interstitial fibrosis and deposition of immunoglobulins in glomeruli and along the tubular basement membrane have been observed and suggest that the magnesium loss may have been acquired (10,37). The patterns of serum concentration and urinary excretion of cations indicate that urinary excretion of potassium and magnesium are inappropriately high for the serum concentrations of these cations (Table 3). The low urinary calcium reflects the low serum calcium concentration. Maximal urinary osmolality has shown little impairment despite the presence of hypokalemia (10,26,31). This finding is in accord with the observation that in experimental magnesium depletion concentrating ability was not impaired by the hypokalemia that developed (39). During water loading, minimal urinary osmolality was normal as was distal fractional chloride reabsorption (Gill, Jr., J.R., unpublished observations). Thus, although patients with magnesium-losing tubulopathy and those with Bartter's syndrome may have hypokalemia, alkalosis, hypomagnesemia, hyperreninemia, and aldosteronism, these conditions can usually be differentiated based on renal histological findings and results of tests of renal diluting and concentrating ability. This assumes that the diagnosis of Bartter's syndrome

Table 2 Clinical Findings in Magnesium-Losing Tubulopathy

Normal growth and development
Normal blood pressure
Tetany
Hypokalemic alkalosis
Hypomagnesemia
Hypocalcemia
Hyperreninemia with aldosteronism
Renal histological findings
Normal
Deposits of immune complexes

Table 3 Serum and Urine Cations and Renal Function in Magnesium-Losing Tubulopathy

Serum	Urine
Low K^+	High K^+
Low Mg^{++}	High Mg^{++}
Low Ca^{++}	Low Ca^{++}
	Normal Max osmolality
	Normal dilution

is reserved for patients with juxtaglomerular hyperplasia and subnormal distal fractional chloride reabsorption with an inability to dilute and concentrate urine normally.

CALCIUM-LOSING TUBULOPATHY

In some patients, calcium-losing tubulopathy may be associated with hypokalemic alkalosis, hyperreninemia, and aldosteronism (4,8,11,27,28). The clinical features of this disorder are presented in Table 4. The disorder may be sporadic or familial and children born with this tubulopathy have been frequently delivered prematurely after pregnancies complicated by polyhydramnios; subsequent growth and development were usually delayed. The cause of the impaired tubular reabsorption of calcium is unknown. Why the disorder should be associated with hyperreninemia, aldosteronism, and hypokalemia is also unclear but the inverse relationship between calcium concentration in the juxtaglomerular apparatus and renin secretion suggests that disordered renin secretion may be caused by abnormal calcium transport. Aldosteronism, stimulated by hyperreninemia, would lead, in turn, to increased renal potassium loss with hypokalemia. This hypothesis is supported by the observation that treatment with an inhibitor of prostaglandin synthesis which corrected the hyperreninemia also corrected the aldosteronism and hypokalemia (4,8).

Polyuria and polydipsia, reflecting the pronounced impairment in urinary concentrating ability, may be especially prominent in children. Nephrocalcinosis has been invariably present and the juxtaglomerular apparatus usually showed hyperplasia. The patterns of serum concentration and urinary excretion of cations indicate that serum calcium levels remain normal despite a high urinary calcium level whereas a low serum potassium level is associated with an inappropriately high urinary potassium level (Table 5). Serum and urinary magnesium levels are usually normal. Although maximal urinary osmolality has

Table 4 Clinical Features of Calcium-Losing Tubulopathy

Impaired growth and development
Normal or high blood pressure
Polyuria, polydipsia
Hypokalemic alkalosis
Hyperreninemia with aldosteronism
Renal histological findings
Nephrocalcinosis
Normal or hyperplastic juxtaglomerular apparatus

Table 5 Serum and Urine Cations and Renal Function in Calcium-Losing Tubulopathy

Serum	Urine
Low K^+	High K^+
Normal Mg^{++}	Normal Mg^{++}
Normal Ca^{++}	High Ca^{++}
	Low Max osmolality
	Normal dilution

been markedly impaired (4,8,11,27), presumably caused, at least in part, by hypercalciuria, diluting capacity has remained intact (25). Thus, patients with calcium-losing tubulopathy can be readily differentiated from patients with Bartter's syndrome by high urinary calcium levels, normal diluting ability and, occasionally, a normal juxtaglomerular apparatus.

In summary, Bartter's syndrome, magnesium-losing tubulopathy, and calcium-losing tubulopathy are different despite their many similarities. Renal histological findings, diluting ability, concentrating ability, and excretion of magnesium and calcium in the three tubulopathies are contrasted in Figure 4. As the results indicate, each tubulopathy differs from the other two in two or more respects. This suggests that one may correctly diagnose these tubulopathies using a systematic evaluation of renal function as outlined in Figure 4.

	Bartter's Syndrome	Magnesium-Losing Tubulopathy	Calcium-Losing Tubulopathy
Urinary Calcium	↓	↓	↑
Urinary Magnesium	↑	↑	Normal
Urinary Concentration	↓	Normal	↓
Urinary Dilution	↓	Normal	Normal
Juxtaglomerular Apparatus	Hyperplastic	Normal	Normal or Hyperplastic

Figure 4 Changes in urinary calcium, urinary magnesium, urinary concentration, urinary dilution, and juxtaglomerular apparatus in Bartter's syndrome, magnesium-losing tubulopathy, and calcium-losing tubulopathy.

REFERENCES

1. Aurell, M., and Rudin, A.: Effect of captopril on blood pressure, renal function, the electrolyte balance and the renin-angiotensin system in Bartter's syndrome. *Nephron* 33:274–278, 1983.
2. Bartter, F. C., Pronove, P., Gill, J. R. Jr., and MacCardle, R. C.: Hyperplasia of the juxtaglomerular complex with hyperaldosteronism and hypokalemic alkalosis. *Am. J. Med.* 33:811–828, 1962.
3. Bowden, R. E., Gill, J. R., Jr., Radfar, N., Taylor, A. A., and Keiser, H. R.: Prostaglandin synthetase inhibitors in Bartter's syndrome. *JAMA* 239:117–121, 1978.
4. Betend, B., David, L., Vincent, M., Hermier, M., and Francois, R.: Successful indomethacin treatment of two paediatric patients with severe tubulopathies. *Helv. Paediatr. Acta* 34:339–344, 1979.
5. Burg, M., and Good, D.: Sodium chloride coupled transport in mammalian nephrons. *Annu. Rev. Physiol.* 45:533–547, 1983.
6. Chan, J. C. M., Gill, J. R., Jr., and Bartter, F. C.: Lack of evidence for a role for prostaglandins in the mediation of impaired urinary concentrating ability in Bartter's syndrome. *Nephron* 35:116–119, 1983.
7. Danovitch, G. M., and Bricker, N. S.: Influence of volume expansion on NaCl reabsorption in the diluting segments of the nephron. A study using clearance methods. *Kidney Int.* 10:229–238, 1976.
8. Dillon, M. J., Shah, V., and Mitchell, M. D.: Bartter's syndrome: 10 cases in childhood. *Q. J. Med.* 48:429–446, 1979.
9. Düsing, R., Scherhag, R., Tippelmann, R., Budde, U., Glanzer, K., and Kramer, H. J.: Arachidonic acid metabolism in isolated rat aorta: dependence of prostacyclin biosynthesis on extracellular potassium concentration. *J. Biol. Chem.* 257:1993–2001, 1982.
10. Evans, R. A., Carter, J. N., Georg, C. R. P., Walls, R. S., Newland, R. C., McDonnell, G. D., and Lawrence, J. R.: The congenital magnesium-losing kidney. *Q. J. Med.* 197:39–52, 1981.
11. Fanconi, A., Schachenmann, G., Nussli, R., and Prader, A.: Chronic hypokalemia with growth retardation, normotensive hyperrenin-hyperaldosteronism ("Bartter's syndrome"), and hypercalciuria. *Helv. Paediatr. Acta* 26:144–163, 1971.
12. Fleischer, N., Brown, H., Graham, D. Y., and Delena, S.: Chronic laxative-induced hyperaldosteronism and hypokalemia simulating Bartter's syndrome. *Ann. Intern. Med.* 70:791–798, 1969.
13. Fujita, T., Ando, K., Sato, Y., Yamashita, K., Nomura, M., and Fukui, T.: Independent roles of prostaglandins and the renin-angiotensin system in abnormal vascular reactivity in Bartter's syndrome. *Am. J. Med.* 73:71–76, 1982.
14. Galvez, O. G., Bay, W. H., Roberts, B. W., and Ferris, T. F.: The hemodynamic effects of potassium deficiency in the dog. *Circ. Res.* 40:Suppl I:I-11–I-16, 1977.
15. Gill, J. R., Jr.: Prostaglandins in Bartter's syndrome and in potassium-deficient disorders that mimic it. *Mineral Electrolyte Metab.* 6:76–81, 1981.
16. Gill, J. R., Jr., and Bartter, F. C.: Evidence for a prostaglandin-independent defect in chloride reabsorption in the loop of Henle as a proximal cause of Bartter's syndrome. *Am. J. Med.* 65:766–772, 1978.
17. Gill, J. R., Jr., Frölich, J. C., Bowden, R. E., Taylor, A. A., Keiser, H. R., Seyberth, H. W., Oates, J. A., and Bartter, F. C.: Bartter's syndrome: a disorder characterized by high urinary prostaglandins and a dependence of hyperreninemia on prostaglandin synthesis. *Am. J. Med.* 61:43–51, 1976.
18. Güllner, H.-G., Bartter, F. C., Cerletti, C., Smith, J. B., and Gill, J. R.: Prostacyclin overproduction in Bartter's syndrome. *Lancet* 2:767–770, 1979.

19. Güllner, H.-G., Gill, J. R., Jr., Bartter, F. C., Lake, C. R., and Lakatua, D. J.: Correction of increased sympathoadrenal activity in Bartter's syndrome by inhibition of prostaglandin synthesis. *J. Clin. Endocrinol. Metab.* 50:857–861, 1980.
20. Güllner, H.-G., Graf, A. K., Gill, J. R., Jr., and Mitchell, M. D.: Hypokalemia stimulates prostacyclin synthesis in the rat. *Clin. Sci.* 65:43–46, 1983.
21. Güllner, H.-G., Lake, C. R., Gill, J. R., Jr., and Lakatua, D. J.: Hypokalemia stimulates plasma epinephrine and norepinephrine in the rat. *Arch. Int. Pharmacodyn Ther* 260:78–82, 1982.
22. Gunther, S., Gimbrone, M. A., Jr., and Alexander, R. W.: Regulation by angiotensin II of its receptors in resistance blood vessels. *Nature* 287:230–232, 1980.
23. Jamison, R. L., Ross, J. C., Kempson, R. L., Sufit, C. R., and Parker, T. E.: Surreptitious diuretic ingestion and pseudo-Bartter's syndrome. *Am. J. Med.* 73:142–147, 1982.
24. Kono, T., Oseko, F., Shimbo, S., Nanno, M., Ikeda, F., and Endo, J.: Blood pressure fall by angiotensin II antagonist in patients with Bartter's syndrome. *J. Clin. Endocrinol.* 43:692–695, 1976.
25. Kurtz, I., Maher, T., Jones, J. W., Sutton, J. M., Schambelan, M., Holter, H. N., Rector, R. C., Jr., Morris, R. C., Jr., and Sebastian, A.: Familial chloride-resistant renal alkalosis and hypokalemia with fasting hypercalciuria and medullary nephrocalcinosis: a unique variant of Bartter's syndrome without impaired renal diluting ability. *Clin. Res.* 29:555A, 1981.
26. McCredie, D. A., Blair-West, J. R., Scoggins, B. A., and Shipman, R.: Potassium-losing nephropathy of childhood. *Med. J. Aust.* 1:129–135, 1971.
27. McCredie, D. A., Rotenberg, E., and Williams, A. C.: Hypercalciuria in potassium-losing nephropathy: a variant of Bartter's syndrome. *Aust. Paediatr. J.* 10:286–295, 1974.
28. Meyer, W. J. III, Middler, S. A., Delea, C. S., and Bartter, F. C.: Hypercalciuria and increased plasma renin activity. In *Control of Renin Secretion,* edited by Assaykeen, A., New York, Plenum Press, 1972, pp. 246–262.
29. Nielsen, I., Hesse, B., and Christensen, P.: On the pathogenetic role of prostaglandins in Bartter's syndrome. *Acta Med. Scand.* 625(Suppl):135–140, 1979.
30. Pasternack, A., Perheentupa, J., Launiala, K., and Hallman, N.: Kidney biopsy findings in familial chloride diarrhoea. *Acta Endocrinol.* 55:1–9, 1967.
31. Paunier, L., and Sizonenko, P. C.: Asymptomatic chronic hypomagnesemia and hypokalemia in a child: cell membrane disease. *J. Pediatr.* 88:51–55, 1976.
32. Pearson, A. J. G., Sladen, G. E., Edmonds, C. J., Tavill, A. S., Wills, M. R., and McIntyre, N.: The pathophysiology of congenital chloridorrhoea. *Q. J. Med.* 167: 453–466, 1973.
33. Radfar, N., Gill, J. R., Jr., Bartter, F. C., Bravo, E., Taylor, A. A., and Bowden, R. E.: Hypokalemia, in Bartter's syndrome and other disorders, produces resistance to vasopressors via prostaglandin overproduction. *Proc. Soc. Exp. Biol. Med.* 158: 502–507, 1978.
34. Ramos, E., Hall-Craggs, M., and Demers, L. M.: Surreptitious habitual vomiting simulating Bartter's syndrome. *JAMA* 43:1070–1072, 1980.
35. Rodriguez, J. A., Lopez, J. M., and Mahana, D.: Inhibition of the kallikrein-kinin system and vascular reactivity in Bartter's syndrome. *Abstracts 7th International Congress of Endocrinology*, Excerpta Medica, Amsterdam, Elsevier, p. 1259, 1984.
36. Rudin, A., Sjogren, B., and Aurrell, M.: Low urinary calcium in Bartter's syndrome. *N. Engl. J. Med.* 310:1190, 1984.
37. Runeberg, L., Collan, Y., Jokinen, E. J., Lahdevirta, J., and Aro, A.: Hypomagnesemia due to renal disease of unknown etiology. *Am. J. Med.* 59:873–881, 1975.

38. Sasaki, H., Okumura, M., Asano, T., Arakawa, K., and Kawasaki, T.: Responses to angiotensin II antagonist before and after treatment with indomethacin in Bartter's syndrome. *Br. Med. J.* 2:975–1038, 1977.
39. Suh, S. M., and Firek, A. F.: The effect of hypomagnesemia with or without associated hypercalcemia on renal concentrating ability in rats. *J. Am. Coll. Nutr.* 4: 355–360, 1983.
40. Veldhuis, J. D., Bardin, C. W., and Demers, L. M.: Metabolic mimicry of Bartter's syndrome by covert vomiting. *Am. J. Med.* 66:361–363, 1979.
41. Vinci, J. M., Gill, J. R., Jr., Bowden, R. E., Pisano, J. J., Izzo, J. L., Jr., Radfar, N., Taylor, A. A., Zusman, R. M., Bartter, F. C., and Keiser, H. R.: The kallikrein-kinin system in Bartter's syndrome and its response to prostaglandin synthetase inhibition. *J. Clin. Invest.* 61:1671–1682, 1978.
42. Wright, F. S., and Giebisch, G.: Renal potassium transport: contributions of individual nephron segments and populations. *Am. J. Physiol.* 235:F515–F527, 1978.

10
Family Periodic Paralyses

KENNETH ZIERLER
The Johns Hopkins University School of Medicine, Baltimore, Maryland

DEFINITION

Let us begin by agreeing on the name of the disease. In 1885 Westphal described periodic paralysis (12). The report was in German. Westphal's description was "an arcane case of periodic paralysis of all four extremities." When the French published case reports of the disease they called it *familiale*. Germans called it *familiäre*.

The first reports in English referred to the disease as *family* periodic paralysis, and so it was known in English from 1902 until 1934. When Biemond and Daniels (2) reported that serum K^+ concentration is decreased during attacks, they seem to have also changed the English name to *familial* periodic paralysis. During the next few years both versions of the name appeared, but *familial* soon became more familiar, and *family* all but disappeared from use. In 1956, Andres and I (13) resurrected the original term, but our finger was too small for the hole in the dike. Nevertheless, as one who clings to such notions that *data* is plural and that *hemorrhage* is not a verb, I shall be discussing hypokalemic *family* paralysis.

CHARACTERISTICS

There are three kinds of periodic paralysis related to serum K^+ concentration: hyperkalemic, normokalemic, and hypokalemic. All three types appear to be inherited as an autosomal dominant, but, although the distribution is about 50:50 between males and females in normo- and hyperkalemic periodic paralysis, at least twice as many males as females experience hypokalemic periodic paralysis. There are differences in usual age of onset; the hyperkalemic form occurs earlier. Patients with hypokalemic periodic paralysis often have a sense or aura of impending paralysis, and they find they can avert paralysis by mild exercise. We know that exercise causes net K^+ loss from exercising muscles into the circulation, thus raising serum K^+ concentration. Attacks are brought on, usually, by rest after heavy exercise, or some hours after a large meal. We know that during rest, K^+ can move in the net from serum back into muscle, and is most likely to happen during

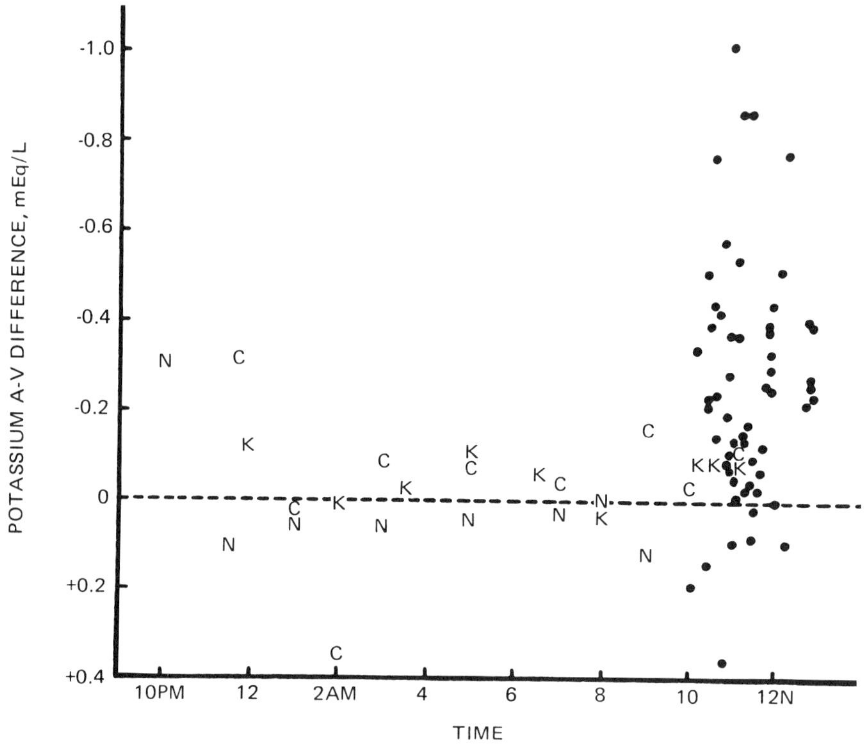

Figure 1 Time course of arteriovenous difference in plasma potassium concentration. C, K, and N refer to normal subjects followed during the night. Black dots represent all AV differences obtained in 19 additional subjects studied only between 10 a.m. and 1 p.m. (From Ref. 1.)

the night. Attacks of hypokalemic paralysis are most likely to begin during the night; those of hyperkalemia during active periods in daytime. But these generalities are unreliable in individual cases, and diagnosis must rest on measurement of serum K^+ concentration.

In studies of metabolism of muscles of the forearm in normal young adults, with the subject at rest, at about 9 a.m., about 14 or 15 hr after the last meal, there is a net loss of K^+ from forearm muscles into blood (1). However, this loss of K^+ is reversed after meals. In the studies shown in Figure 1, net K^+ movement between forearm muscles and blood was zero or slightly positive (net K^+ uptake by muscles) some 4-6 hr after supper, and continued that way throughout the night. From 7 or 8 until 10 a.m. in subjects still without food since supper the previous evening, increasing net K^+ was lost from muscle. This sets the stage for our understanding, at one level, what happens in family periodic paralysis.

Before we go further with discussing hypokalemic family periodic paralysis, we must be clear that we are discussing this condition specifically and not hypokalemic paralyses in general. Hypokalemia from any cause, some of which are listed in Table 1, can lead to paralysis. The mechanism of production of paralysis in hypokalemia from these other causes may be different from the mechanisms in family periodic paralysis. The hypo-

Table 1 Types of Hypokalemic Paralysis

Episodic (any cause of hypokalemia)
Hyperaldosteronism (Conn's syndrome)
K^+-wasting diuretics
Renal tubular acidosis
Bartter's syndrome
Diarrheal disease
Corticosteroids, licorice
Paraaminosalicylic acid
Diabetes mellitus
Alcoholism
Periodic
Hyperthyroidism
Nonhereditary
Family

kalemic periodic paralyses are of three sorts. First, there is the remarkable group associated with thyrotoxicosis, which is seldom seen in the United States but quite common in Japan. Paralytic attacks cease upon satisfactory treatment of the hyperthyroidism. Second, there are some occasional examples of spontaneous periodic paralysis, apparently not hereditary, but one wonders if the family history is simply incomplete. Finally, there is our subject, family periodic paralysis.

Hypokalemic family periodic paralysis is a flaccid paralysis, beginning in the extremities. One of its major serious aspects is that it can involve respiratory muscles.

POTASSIUM DISTRIBUTION DURING ATTACKS

During attacks, serum K^+ concentration decreases (2). This decrease is not due to hemodilution. There is a true loss of serum, and extracellular K^+, not due to urinary excretion. Urine K^+ content actually decreases (4). Where does the K^+ go?

Most of it goes into skeletal muscle (3). The time course of arterial and forearm venous K^+ concentrations before, during, and after an attack of paralysis appears in Figure 2. The attack occurred in a young man given a high-carbohydrate meal at 5:30 p.m. By midnight, there was already a marked fall in his arterial K^+, from the normal of 3.5 to 4, down to 2.5 mEq/L. K^+ in venous blood draining forearm muscles was only 1.7 mEq/L. That is, K^+ was already moving in the net out of blood into muscle. Weakness did not appear until an hour later, at 1 a.m., and there was quadriplegia at 3 a.m.

Note in Figure 2 that at the time indicated by each arrow the subject swallowed 5 g KCl, beginning at 4:10 a.m. Although arterial K^+ concentration rose, it remained less than normal for the next 2 hr and during all that time muscle continued to remove K^+ from blood; venous K^+ remained less than arterial. The tide did not reverse until 7 a.m.; venous K^+ concentration exceeded arterial; K^+ moved out of muscle into blood; there was a rapid rise in plasma K^+ concentration, actually to hyperkalemic levels. In fact, the reverse movement, loss of K^+ from muscle to blood, was greater than expected in normal subjects.

This point is emphasized by a study of another patient with family periodic paralysis. Patient H had a spontaneous paralytic attack during the night, which caught us unprepared to carry out our studies. By the time we were able to begin our studies, he had

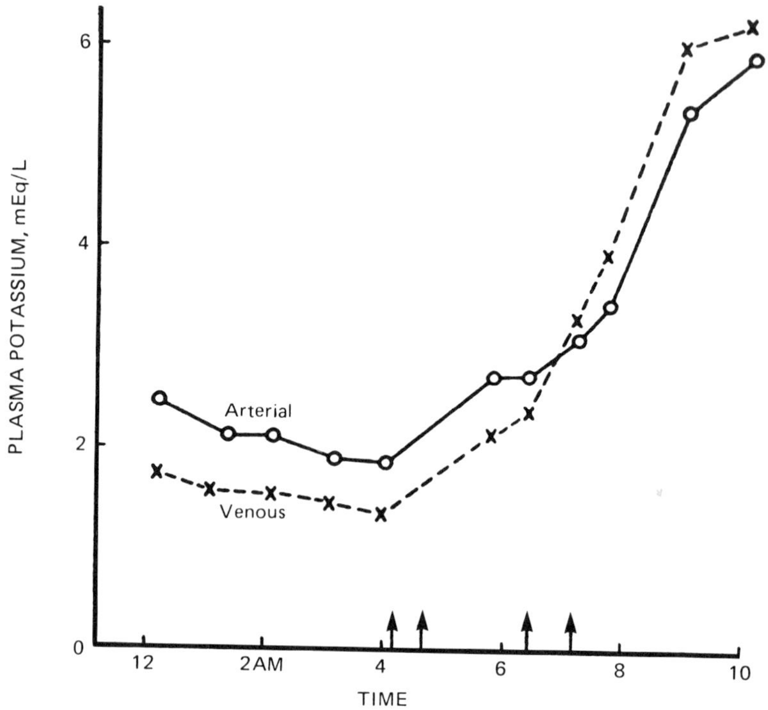

Figure 2 Arterial and venous plasma potassium concentrations during attack and recovery in a patient. At each time indicated by arrows, 5 g KCl was given orally. (From Ref. 13.)

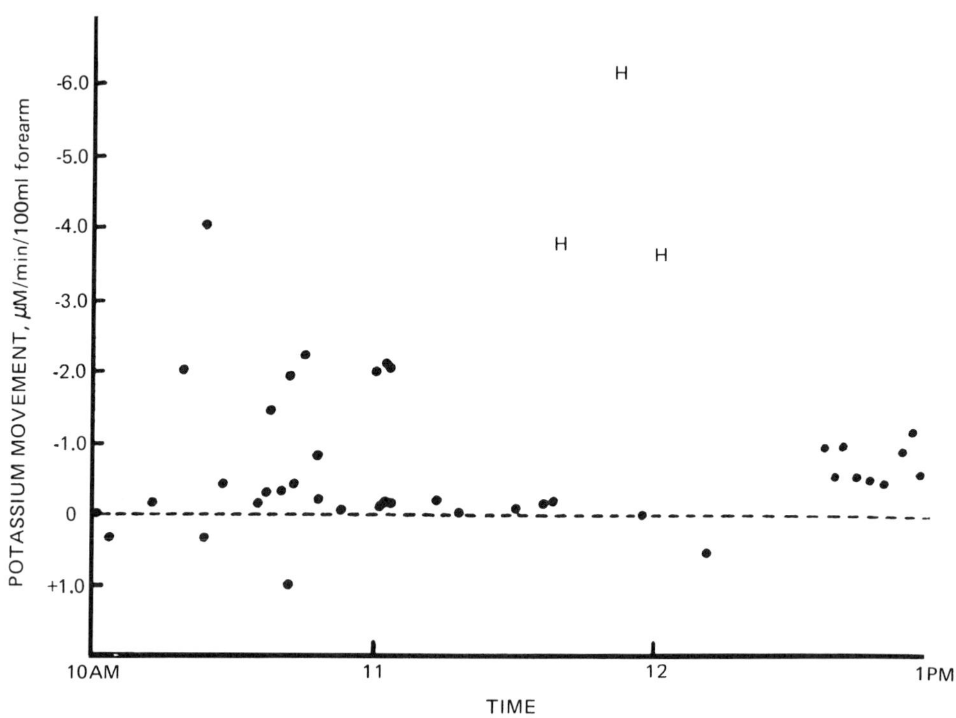

Figure 3 Potassium output from muscle to plasma during spontaneous recovery from a spontaneous attack of paralysis in subject M.H. ●, data from normal subjects in the basal state. (From Ref. 13.)

already recovered spontaneously, almost completely. During this spontaneous recovery period, at about 10 a.m. to 12 noon, his forearm muscles discharged K^+ into blood at rates many times greater than normal (Figure 3).

We suspect from these observations that, in patients with family periodic paralysis, muscles have an exaggerated response to normal stimuli to K^+ movement in both directions. Stimuli that evoke net K^+ uptake into muscle evoke greater uptake; stimuli that evoke net K^+ loss from muscle evoke greater K^+ loss in periodic paralysis.

CAUSE OF PARALYSIS

What is the cause of the paralysis? There is no disturbance of nerve conduction and no disturbance of myoneural transmission. The defect is, therefore, intrinsic in muscle. (See Reference 5 for citations of earlier studies of neurological deficit in family periodic paralysis. Westphal [12] reported in 1885 that muscle could not be stimulated during periodic paralysis.)

Long ago, before any measurements were made of electrical potential differences across muscle membranes in periodic paralysis, some of us guessed, incorrectly, that muscles would be hyperpolarized when serum K^+ concentration fell. A modified form of the classic Goldman-Hodgkin-Katz equation, applicable to skeletal muscle is:

$$\psi_m = -\frac{RT}{F} \ln \frac{P_K[K^+]_i + P_{Na}[Na^+]_i}{P_K[K^+]_o + P_{Na}[Na^+]_o}, \tag{1}$$

where ψ_m is a steady-state electrical potential difference between the inside and outside of a muscle fiber, R is the gas constant, T the absolute temperature, F is Faraday's constant (and RT/F is, therefore, a constant at a given temperature), *ln* denotes that what follows is the natural logarithm (log to base e), P_K and P_{Na} are permeability coefficients of the membrane to K^+ and Na^+, respectively (dimensions are those of velocity, cm/sec), and $[K^+]_i$ and $[Na^+]_i$, and $[K^+]_o$ and $[Na^+]_o$ are, respectively, intracellular and extracellular concentrations of K^+ and Na^+.

In mammalian skeletal muscle P_{Na} is not negligible. If P_{Na} were zero, the membrane potential would be the same as the K^+ equilibrium potential. But it is not: it is about 1-3% P_K. However, normal $[K^+]_o$ is only a little more than 3% $[Na^+]_o$. Therefore, the two terms in the denominator of the logarithmic factor have about equal weight at normal $[K^+]_o$. As $[K^+]_o$ decreases, the weight of the $P_{Na}[Na^+]_o$ term becomes greater, and, even if the permeability coefficients P_K and P_{Na} were not affected by reduced $[K^+]_o$, the membrane potential, although hyperpolarizing, would depart even further from the K^+ equilibrium potential.

As serum K^+ concentration falls, indicated here by $[K^+]_o$, the logarithmic factor in equation (1) gets larger; that is, the membrane hyperpolarizes. A hyperpolarized membrane requires a greater amount of depolarization to initiate or propagate an action potential. Without an action potential, there is no muscle contraction. This apparently reasonable sequence may indeed describe the way things work in some, but not all, of the hypokalemic paralysis secondary to hypokalemia from a variety of causes.

Only a few electrical studies have been made, and in only a few patients with family periodic paralysis (3,11). The resting membrane potential, instead of being hyperpolarized, is either essentially unchanged or slightly depolarized during an attack. It may even be slightly depolarized between attacks, when strength seems about normal. How do we explain this? The explanation lies in an examination of equation (1).

In the previous discussion of that equation we assumed that the permeability coefficients were constant, independent of the decrease in $[K^+]_o$. But, in fact, the permeability coefficient, P_K, is dependent upon $[K^+]_o$. The permeability coefficient tells us essentially the same thing about the membrane as the electrical conductance. The current through the membrane carried by net movement of K^+ is permitted to pass through some membrane machinery designated as the electrical conductance to K, g_K, the reciprocal of membrane resistance to passage of electrical current carried by translocation of K^+. Both Na^+ and K^+ conductance are voltage-sensitive. As hyperpolarization occurs, g_K decreases.

Ohm's Law tells us that current (i) equals conductance (g) times voltage (V) with conductance being constant. When we plot current (i) as a function of voltage (V) we get a straight line, with constant slope g. But in nerve and muscle, a plot of i against V is not a straight line. Conductance (g) is not constant. If we approach a given voltage from a hyperpolarized state the slope (= conductance) is different than when we approach that voltage from the depolarized state. This phenomenon is called rectification. (Inward rectification, as used here, refers to a voltage- or K-dependent change in conductance in which the ratio P_{Na}/P_K increases as external K concentration falls below normal.)

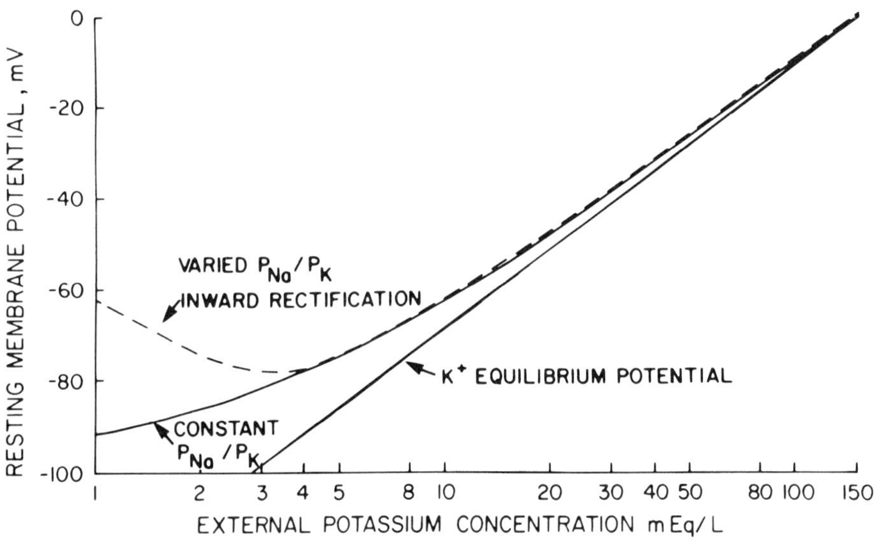

Figure 4 Steady-state electrical potential difference between the inside and outside of a mammalian skeletal muscle as a function of extracellular K^+ concentration. Two theoretical curves are shown, both constructed according to the modified Goldman-Hodgkin-Katz equation (equation 1). In one (heavy solid line), the ratio of permeabilities, P_{Na}/P_K, is constant at 0.02. In the other (broken line), the permeability ratio is constant for all $[K^+]_o \geqslant 4$ mEq/L, but increases progressively for all $[K^+]_o < 4$ mEq/L; that is, there is inward rectification, with progressive depolarization as $[K^+]_o$ decreases. The K^+ equilibrium potential, E_K, (i.e., the potential that would be measured if K^+ were the only permeant ion) is shown (light solid line) to emphasize that in resting mammalian muscle the observed electrical potential is less negative than E_K at all values of $[K^+]_o$ compatible with life, and the difference is exaggerated increasingly as $[K^+]_o$ decreases. The slope of the membrane potential curve is less than 59 mV for a 10-fold change in $[K^+]_o$, which is the expected slope of the E_K when all extracellular Na^+ is replaced by K^+. At that point, because there is no $[Na^+]_o$, the membrane potential is E_K.

A plot of membrane potential against logarithm of K^+ concentration in the bathing solution might look like either of the curves shown in Figure 4. In the presence of marked inward rectification, there might actually be depolarization as external K^+ concentration falls sufficiently far. Indeed, this is what Otsuka and Ohtsuki reported in diaphragms from rats fed a K-deficient diet (8).

A few other observations have been made on electrical properties of muscle during paralysis with hypokalemic periodic paralysis. Electrical stimuli, adequate to make a muscle contract during the normokalemic interval between attacks, failed to induce contraction or propagated action potentials (5,11) during hypokalemic paralysis. There are several situations in which muscle can be made inexcitable. In the laboratory this is most commonly done by blocking the voltage-dependent, fast-Na^+ channel, usually with drugs such as tetrodotoxin or scorpion venom.

These electrical studies are difficult to carry out in patients. What is needed is a laboratory model. Researchers have turned, therefore, to studies in K^+-depleted rats.

THE POTASSIUM-DEPLETED RAT

Muscle from K^+-depleted rats shows vacuolization similar to that seen in family periodic paralysis. Mechanical responses are abnormal. Most of the abnormality can be explained by an increase in a series elastic component, such as could be provided by incompetent diseased sarcomeres in series with normal sarcomeres strung along a muscle fiber.

Electrical responses are only partly reminiscent of what occurs in family periodic paralysis. The resting membrane potential is slightly depolarized (6), but not nearly enough to account for paralysis on the basis of a depolarization block. K^+ conductance is probably decreased (6), but that is to be expected in view of the pathological changes. Na^+ conductance has not been measured sufficiently unambiguously, but one can interpret the data as consistent with increased resting Na^+ conductance. There are abnormalities in the action potential and, as occurs in family periodic paralysis, an action potential cannot be generated during paralysis.

There are also similarities between the human disease and the K-deficient rat with respect to pathological muscle changes.

Figure 5 shows a longitudinal section through a muscle fiber. At the surface of every sarcomere, at intervals of one sarcomere length, is a ring of small openings, about 150-200 Å in diameter. These are the surface openings of transverse, or T, tubules, which run like spokes of a wheel to the center of the fiber. Running longitudinally in the fiber are a large number of tubes, also about 150-200 Å in diameter for most of their length, extending from T-tubule at one end of a sarcomere to T-tubule at the other. This is the sarcoplasmic reticulum (SR). Each tube ends in a large flattened globular dilatation, much larger than shown here, actually in close contact with about one-third of the length of the T-tubules. These dilatations are the terminal cisternae. The combined surface area of SR is many times greater than the surface area of T-tubules, and the combined surface area of T-tubules is about an order of magnitude greater than that of plasma membrane, the sarcolemma.

It is likely that the vacuoles seen in family periodic paralysis and in K^+-depleted rat muscle are dilated T-tubules and SR. When water moves between interstitial fluid and sarcoplasm, it is much more likely to take the path from sarcoplasm to the outside by way of the SR surface than by way of sarcolemma, because the former surface is about

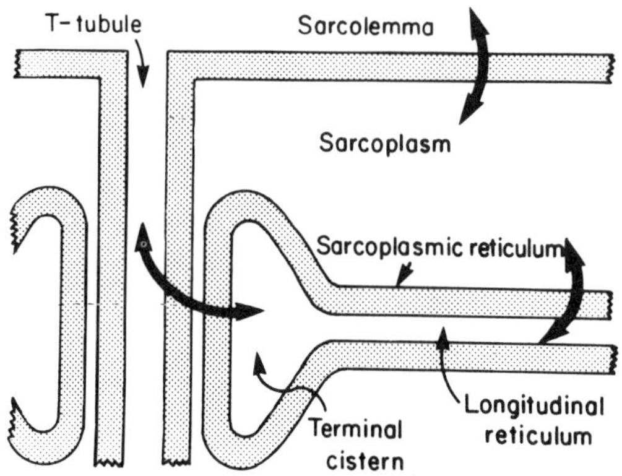

Figure 5 Paths water and small ions may take between interior and exterior of skeletal muscle (heavy double arrows). In each muscle sarcomere are many units of sarcoplasmic reticulum terminating at each end in bulbous terminal cisterns. The compound membrane (T-tubule membrane plus terminal cistern membrane) is more permeable to small molecules than is sarcolemma. Water, moving from sarcoplasm to outside, is more likely to take the path across SR than across sarcolemma because the former surface is at least 100 times greater. The bottle neck is the narrow T-tubule. Under certain conditions, in which there is massive water movement out of sarcoplasm, SR may become engorged, particularly the terminal cisterns, causing the large vacuoles seen in several diseases of muscle, including the periodic paralyses.

100 times greater. The bottle neck is at the mouth of the T-tubule. Hence, the T-tubule SR system dilates.

There are several effects of this dilation. One is upon conductance. In skeletal muscle at rest, Cl^-conductance is about twice as great as K^+ conductance, which, in turn, is about 50 times greater than Na^+ conductance. But virtually all Cl^-conductance is across the plasma surface membrane, while only about one-third of the K^+ conductance is across that surface. Most of the K^+ conductance is across the subsurface membranes. It is generally believed that about two-thirds of the K^+ conductance is across walls of T-tubules, but some of us entertain the possibility that it might also lie in walls of SR. In either case, when the integrity of these internal membranes is violated, as it appears to be in K^+ deficiency and in periodic paralysis, one expects to find K^+ conductance decreased.

MORE RECENT METABOLIC STUDIES

Because paralytic attacks can be induced in patients with family periodic paralysis by feeding them high-carbohydrate meals, physicians turned naturally to look at effects of insulin, which is known to decrease serum K^+ concentration. When insulin is infused into a brachial artery and forearm glucose uptake and net K^+ movement are measured, one finds a prompt response for both, but the effect on K^+ uptake is markedly prolonged beyond the effect on glucose uptake (14). That is, it takes less insulin to cause net K^+ uptake into muscle than to cause glucose uptake.

Studies of insulin effect in family periodic paralysis are sporadic, involve only a small number of subjects, and their interpretation is complicated by uncertainty as to what additional or complicating abnormalities an individual patient may have.

For example, one study shows an apparently decreased affinity between insulin and its receptors, while another shows increased binding, without either having data to differentiate the role of number of receptors from that of affinity. One study found insulin secretion rate increased; another found it to be normal.

There has been a good deal of speculation that these patients might be abnormally sensitive to insulin. As indicated earlier, I believe they are with respect to K^+ uptake, because they seem to be more sensitive to various stimuli to K^+ movement, whether net uptake by muscle or net output from muscle.

Minaker and co-workers (7) have recently studied responses to insulin in a patient with hypokalemic periodic paralysis. I am indebted to Dr. Minaker for detailed information in advance of publication. The patient had family periodic paralysis, but it must be noted that he was enormous: 1.9m, 163 kg, 43 years old, with a 33-year history of periodic paralysis. At approximately the same serum insulin concentration as the normals, the patient's tissues took up less glucose than normal during a euglycemic insulin infusion. But this is quantitatively what we expect to find in an obese person (9), even in the absence of periodic paralysis.

What was different was that the patient lowered his plasma K^+ concentration substantially more than the normals, which is not what occurs in obese persons normally.

CONJECTURES

It is premature to put all this together; nothing seems yet sufficiently solid. But we can summarize some proposed mechanisms.

First, whatever the mechanisms, there appears to be an exaggerated response to stimuli altering K^+ movement. There is increased net K^+ uptake by muscle in response to insulin, and probably to some other stimuli to K^+ uptake. There is increased net K^+ output from muscle in response to exercise, and probably to some other stimuli.

Does the paralysis have anything to do with K^+, or are the paralysis and K^+ alterations simply parallel manifestations of some more fundamental disturbance? With respect to the paralysis, it has been suggested that there may be depolarization block, that is, that Na^+ channels may be inactivated by depolarization. But the degree of depolarization observed is too small for this effect, so that one must then make the additional conjecture that, in these patients, Na^+ channel inactivation occurs with less depolarization than in normals.

Kao and Gordon (6) suggested that paralysis may be due to exaggerated inward rectification. As the concentration of K^+ bathing a muscle falls, permeability to K^+, or K^+ conductance, decreases. Rectification is the state in which current flows more easily in one direction than in the other, and it is a normal property of muscle membrane. During the late phase of the action potential, inward rectification occurs normally. Its cause has been a subject of investigation for decades, and is still elusive, but one possibility is that it is related to temporary accumulation of K^+ in SR or T-tubules. During this time it may be impossible to generate another action potential.

Finally, there is a fascinating suggestion, by Schipperheyn and Buruma (10), that underlying family periodic paralysis may be production of an abnormal, and totally hypothetical, protein with properties resembling those of scorpion venom. This protein blocks the voltage-dependent fast Na^+ channels, preventing action potentials, in the manner of tetrodotoxin. But, unlike tetrodotoxin, scorpion toxin increases resting Na^+ conductance, and so depolarizes resting potential.

REFERENCES

1. Andres, R., Cader, G., Goldman, P., and Zierler, K. L.: Net potassium movement between resting muscle and plasma in man in the basal state and during the night. *J. Clin. Invest.* 36:723–729, 1957.
2. Biemond, A., and Daniels, P.: Familial periodic paralysis and its transition into spinal muscular atrophy. *Brain* 57:91–108, 1934.
3. Creutzfeldt, O. D., Abbott, B. C., Fowler, W. M., and Pearson, C. M.: Muscle membrane potentials in episodic adynamia. *Electroencephalogr. Clin. Neurophysiol.* 15:508–519, 1963.
4. Ferrebee, J. W., Atchley, D. W., and Loeb, R. F.: A study of the electrolyte physiology in a case of familial periodic paralysis. *J. Clin. Invest.* 17:504–505, 1938.
5. Gordon, A. M., Green, J. R., and Langunoff, D.: Studies on a patient with hypokalemic familial periodic paralysis. *Am. J. Med.* 48:185–195, 1970.
6. Kao, I., and Gordon, A. M.: Mechanism of insulin-induced paralysis of muscles from potassium-depleted rats. *Science* 188:740–741, 1975.
7. Minaker, K. L., and Rowe, J. W.: Familial hypokalemic paralysis: insulin-induced potassium disposal is increased despite severely reduced glucose uptake. *Clin. Res.* 32:454A, 1984.
8. Otsuka, M., and Ohtsuki, I.: Mechanism of muscular paralysis by insulin with particular reference to familial periodic paralysis. *Nature* 207:300–301, 1965.
9. Rabinowitz, D., and Zierler, K. L.: Forearm metabolism in obesity and its response to intraarterial insulin. Characterization of insulin resistance and evidence for adaptive hyperinsulinism. *J. Clin. Invest.* 41:2173–2181, 1962.
10. Schipperheyn, J. J., and Buruma, O. J. S.: Familial periodic paralysis: low muscle potassium permeability or high sodium permeability? *Ann. Neurol.* 13:686, 1983.
11. Shy, G. M., Wanko, T., Rowley, P. T., and Engel, A. G.: Studies in familial periodic paralysis. *Exp. Neurol.* 3:53–121, 1961.
12. Westphal, C.: Ueber einen merkwürdigen Fall von periodscher Lähmung aller vier Extermitäten mit gleichzetigem Erlöschen der elektrischen Erregbarkeit während der Lähmung. *Berlin. Klin. Wochenschr.* 31:491–494, 1885.
13. Zierler, K. L., and Andres, R.: Movement of potassium into skeletal muscle during spontaneous attack in family periodic paralysis. *J. Clin. Invest.* 36:730–737, 1957.
14. Zierler, K. L., and Rabinowitz, D.: Effect of very small concentrations of insulin on forearm metabolism. Persistence of its action on potassium and free fatty acids without its effect on glucose. *J. Clin. Invest.* 43:950–962, 1964.

11

Cardiorenal Pathology in Hypokalemic Patients

WOLFGANG JOHANNES MERGNER, NGA NGUYEN, and RAFFAELE G. DAVID*
University of Maryland School of Medicine, Baltimore, Maryland

VIABILITY AND THE INTERIOR MILIEU OF EXCITABLE CELLS AND TRANSPORTING EPITHELIA

Pathological changes are alterations of the structural and functional integrity of tissues and cells. Chronic and acute hypokalemia produces morphological lesions and alteration or loss of function in the kidney, heart, and skeletal muscle. Pathological lesions have been recognized and described in hypokalemia since the early days of cellular pathobiology. Follis et al. (23), McPherson (56), Selye and Bajuz (83), French (27), Bajuz (7), Lowenhaupt et al. (53), Welt et al. (100), Relman and Schwartz (71), and Toback et al. (93-96) described focal necrosis in the heart and alterations in the distal convoluted tubules and collecting ducts of the kidney. Low levels of extracellular potassium interfere with structural integrity and viability of cells in certain target tissues. What is the pathogenetic mechanism?

Trump et al. (97,99) and Jennings et al. (39) have defined a viable cell as one that is able to maintain volume and to control its interior milieu. Is cell volume control and control over the electrolyte content of the cellular space altered in either acute total hypokalemia or chronic nutritional hypokalemia?

Why is such control limited, and what are the consequences? A number of examples of modification of extracellular ions have suggested a direct effect on ion control by changes in the cell environment; Trump and Ginn (98) have shown that replacement of extracellular sodium with potassium chloride caused total collapse of cellular volume control. These investigators showed in the flounder that kidney tubular cells were injured, and the injury was mediated by an inactivation of the Na-K-ATPase. Bulger and Trump (14) demonstrated a differential effect when they acutely replaced extracellular calcium and/or potassium in the isolated flounder tubule system. When potassium was acutely omitted in the bathing medium, the basal regions of tubular cells showed swelling. In contrast, the apical region was structurally altered if calcium was omitted. Omission of either or both

Current affiliation: Central Emek Hospital, Afula, Israel

K or Ca caused the cells to cease functioning. For example, dye transport into the lumen could not be observed. Pathophysiologically it may make a considerable difference if such change in the exterior environment of cells occurs acutely or chronically. Acute changes can be enhanced by change in the perfusion medium of the isolated heart or kidney. Chronic changes in nutritional hypokalemia occur gradually over a prolonged period of time, and are not total.

Assessment of body potassium stores is described by Patrick (65). Since 95% of the body's potassium is intracellular cation, the body stores of potassium are difficult to assess. Potassium depletion may be (a) a lowering of potassium in the extracellular fluid and in the intracellular fluid; (b) lowering of intracellular potassium, not appropriately related to extracellular potassium; or (c) lowering of total body potassium without direct change in concentrations. In prolonged and metabolically complex potassium deficiencies, measurement of plasma potassium is very unreliable.

Clinically, hypokalemia is defined as a serum potassium level of less than 3 mEq/L. We recognize that low levels of extracellular potassium, called hypokalemia, have systemic pathological effects. At the same time certain target tissues are preferentially affected. Pathogenic mechanisms, possibly hormonal in nature, cause localized lesions: in the proximal convoluted tubule, distal convoluted tubules, and collecting duct epithelium in humans or the distal nephron in the rat, as well as scattered lesions in the rat heart. Research aims to explore both, the general aspects as well as the mechanisms that cause local manifestation of disease.

METABOLIC ROLE OF POTASSIUM

Cellular ion gradients are important for a number of integrated functions such as volume control, electrochemical gradients of excitable membranes, and bioenergetics. Maintenance of ion gradients requires also the expenditure of metabolic energy. Interference with cellular energy metabolism will cause cells to lower the gradient of potassium. Kline and Murad (49) have demonstrated the rapid efflux of cellular potassium in hypoxia. Plasma membrane Na-K-ATPase, and cellular carbohydrate metabolism all may be affected by hypokalemia (28). Potassium and acid-base balance are also known to be interrelated. Reduction in body potassium stores often induces sustained metabolic alkalosis (2). We would like to think that alterations in mitochondria may be significant changes experienced in hypokalemia (38). Gustafson et al. (33) documented depressed protein metabolism in kidney, liver, muscle, and heart in potassium-deficient rats. Lubin (54) has also shown that hypokalemia slows growth in *E. coli* and *B. subtilis* by limiting transfer of amino acids from amino acyl-RNA to polypeptide, thus limiting protein synthesis. Interference with cell maintenance may be a chronic effect of low environmental or intracellular potassium levels.

Hypokalemia is also interrelated with hormonal regulation. Güllner et al. (31) found that after 45 days of hypokalemia, norepinephrine levels in the serum increased by 80% and epinephrine levels increased by 270%. Hypokalemia stimulated prostacycline synthesis in the rat (30). Both changes may be interrelated. The implication of the hormonal changes are discussed elsewhere in this volume.

Control of Intracellular Potassium in the Kidney

Control of electrolytes involves control over inflow and outflow. Potassium is accumulated intracellularly as a consequence of energy-dependent sodium extrusion (55). Potassium apparently can leave the cell rapidly, the permeability of many membranes towards potassium being greater than to sodium. There is a structural polarity in K^+ permeability of cells, allowing great permeability of K^+ at the basilar membrane but not at the luminal membranes of proximal tubular cells. Thus, the columnar epithelial cellular membrane regulates potassium mainly at the basilar surface. This process involves an exchange of K^+ between extracellular fluid and cellular fluid. The Na-K-ATPase is not equally distributed over the cell surface. In epithelial cells the ouabain-inhibited ATPase is mainly on the basolateral border. Potassium accumulation in renal tissue is essentially dependent on sodium transport.

Wright (103) stresses that renal tubules are capable of transporting potassium in both reabsorptive and secretory directions. Reabsorption is the principal process in the proximal portion of the nephron, whereas in the more distal segments secretion into the tubules is the dominant activity. This means that most urinary potassium is derived not from filtered potassium but from secreted potassium. Khuri and co-workers (46) found that tubular fluid potassium levels declined between paraglomerular and later segments of the proximal tubules. The descending limb of the loop of Henle apparently secretes K actively into the tubules (i.e., towards the tip of the medulla), while the ascending limb again shows reabsorption. The distal convoluted tubule and collecting duct reveal both activities: secretion and reabsorption. Morel and colleagues (59) have observed that the distal convoluted tubules, at least the superficial segments consists of three segments: (a) a tortuous segment with a bright cytoplasmic appearance; (b) a segment with a large diameter and granular cellular appearance; and (c) a narrow segment with light appearance. It is thought that one segment or several segments of the last part of the distal convoluted tubule collects K^+. The intracellular potassium level in distal convoluted tubular cells is less well known, even less is known about the control of cellular K in the distal convoluted tubule. Potassium secretion is dependent on cellular potassium and aldosterone. The role of aldosterone is not clear. There is evidence of a luminal potassium pump in collecting tubules which is inhibited by luminal hydrogen ions. The anatomical arrangement and control of potassium vary between species. Renal ammonia production appears to be intimately related to potassium homeostasis (91). Chronic potassium depletion stimulates ammonia production; hyperkalemia inhibits it. With increased ammoniogenesis potassium excretion decreases. A link has also been postulated to hydrogen ion regulation.

Control of Intracellular Potassium in the Heart

The heart and Purkinje's fibers are examples of membranes that periodically change their transmembrane gradient. The reestablishment of this gradient is dependent on the Na-K pump and the Na/Ca exchange system. Potassium regulation is at least two-faced, being interlinked with sodium and calcium regulation. There are also close interrelationships with magnesium chloride, hydrogen ions, and phosphate.

Potassium efflux occurs through selective potassium channels which are responsible for maintaining a resting membrane potential and for repolarization of the membrane. Potassium uptake is maintained through the sodium pump, though some uptake can occur through a potassium-selective channel (68).

Mitochondria and Potassium

Jung et al. (40) described the energy-dependent exchange of K^+ in heart mitochondria. Extracellular potassium depletion produces a decrease in the mitochondrial content of potassium, magnesium, and sodium.

A number of studies have quite convincingly demonstrated that potassium is required for proper mitochondrial function. For example, Pressman and Lardy (70) and Gomez-Pyon et al. (29) have proposed that oxidative phosphorylation is dependent on the intramitochondrial levels of potassium. This applies to the overall function of oxidative phosphorylation and to partial functions. Kimmick and Rasmussen (47) have illustrated that respiration is decreased when potassium is reduced. Gomez-Pyon et al. (29) have shown that phosphorylation reactions and phosphate exchange are dependent on potassium. Harrison et al. (38) described the interrelationship and depression of mitochondrial function in potassium-depletion cardiomyopathy.

Based on the existing data, we propose that energy metabolism is the pivotal element in a patient's vulnerability to acute and chronic potassium depletion. Organ and cell functions that are highly dependent on oxidative phosphorylation show the most severe alterations.

CHRONIC EFFECTS OF HYPOKALEMIA

Balance Studies

Potassium Excretion and Balance

In humans the daily uptake of K^+ is 80 mEq; the daily excretion is 72 mEq in the urine and 8 mEq in the feces (17,48). Cohen (17), who reviews the role of the kidney in disorders of potassium balance, stresses the narrow limits within which potassium is maintained extracellularly at 4-5 mEq/L and intracellularly at 150 mEq/L based on the function of two hormones that regulate intake of potassium: insulin and aldosterone. In rats on a hypokalemic diet, the serum potassium level fell to 2.6 mEq/L (normal, 3.5-5.5 mEq/L but considerable variations could be seen). Urinary potassium levels fell to 1.5 mEq/L within 2 days (normal, 72-130 mEq/L) and potassium in the feces was reduced to 4nmol/kg dry weight (normal, 40 mmol/kg dry weight). This indicated an intense effort by the body to conserve K^+. In the overall balance, the calculated daily loss of potassium fell to 15 mEq/kg body weight.

Weight Gain and Organ Weights

Rats fed a hypokalemic diet (TEKLAD) for 35 days showed reduced growth compared to normokalemic controls. The average weight gain over 35 days was 110%, compared to 170% in controls. The organ weight of kidney was almost unchanged over controls. The weight of the liver, spleen, and heart was reduced (see Table 1).

Table 1 Organ Weights (g) in Rats Fed Hypokalemic Diet for 4 Weeks, Compared with Normal Controls

Organ	Hypokalemia (n = 20)	% Body weight	Control (n = 15)	% Body weight
Heart	0.85	0.26	1.188	0.27
Liver	10.15	3.00	16.7	3.00
Kidney	1.65	0.5	1.73	0.4
Spleen	0.56	0.17	0.87	0.18
Total body	323.19		433.25	

Electrolytes in Various Organs

Whole-body balance studies by Southon and Heaton (85) have shown that the cells in the different tissues differ in their susceptibility to potassium depletion. Significant potassium loss was observed in skeletal muscle, heart, and kidney, while brain and liver were relatively unaffected. Cellular sodium in the same tissues was increased but only the heart tissue revealed an increase in calcium. The situation is complicated since potassium and magnesium deficiency frequently occur together in nutritional hypokalemia (79,80).

Several studies during potassium depletion show that the kidney actively reduces potassium losses (8, Mergner et al., in progress). Another physiological change observed is impaired urinary concentrating ability. Polyuria is a consistent feature of nephropathy of potassium depletion (71). The cellular mechanism has been suggested to be twofold: an alteration of responsiveness of the cyclic AMP system in kidney cells (9) that alters the hormonal response; and polydipsia as a result of stimulation of the thirst mechanism (10). In our balance studies we saw a rapid onset of polydipsia, polyuria, and secretion of urine with low specific gravity and low K^+ content (Mergner et al., in preparation).

Studies on the Heart

Structure and Viability

Hypokalemic rat hearts had a significantly reduced mass. The hearts of the control rats showed an average weight of 1.5 g, the hypokalemic rats' hearts had an average weight of 0.85 g (Figure 1). On day 32 no heart failure could be seen but on day 42 the majority of hearts showed ventricular dilatation. Perkins et al. (66), Harrison et al. (37), and Abbrecht (1) reported congestive heart failure in chronic hypokalemia. Human cases showed histopathological evidence of loss of heart muscle striations, interstitial cellular infiltration, and varying degrees of cell necrosis and/or scarring (73). The clinical studies correlated well with studies on the isolated papillary muscle of the cat which showed, in chronic hypokalemia, depressed velocity of contraction, reduced extent of shortening, and reduced maximally-developed isometric tension (32). Harrison et al. (38) proposed that mitochondrial alteration occurs as the result of chronic hypokalemia.

Follis et al. (23) described the genesis of the lesions in the heart and kidney. The heart showed tiny, opaque grayish areas beginning at 15 days of potassium depletion. The lesion grew and could be seen in all animals at 6 weeks of hypokalemia. Lesions were numerous in the endocardium and epicardium. Loss of striation was another pathological observation. Our group was particularly interested in the effect of hypokalemia on the ultrastructure of the heart (21). We found scattered lesions of cell necrosis in the middle portions of the wall; these were particularly common in the endocardial region of the free wall and septum. The lesions characteristically provoked a mononuclear response by macrophages or nonspecific phagocytic cells. These cells are characterized by bland cytologic features and an abundance of ribosomes. Phagocytic cells entered the basement membrane, which reflected around the point of entry but remained intact (Figure 2). No polymorphonuclear leukocytes were seen. Cell injury was peculiar because it occurred as single cell necrosis. Dead cells were often found linked to adjacent intact cell. Cell necrosis and mononuclear infiltrate were also reported by Savoie (79) who found focal calcification as well. Selye and Bajusz (83) reported greater sensitivity of hypokalemic rats to stress, which introduced focal necrosis. Focal necrosis was also documented by Bajusz (7), Follis et al. (23), Molnar et al. (58), and Cowan et al. (18). X-ray microanalysis

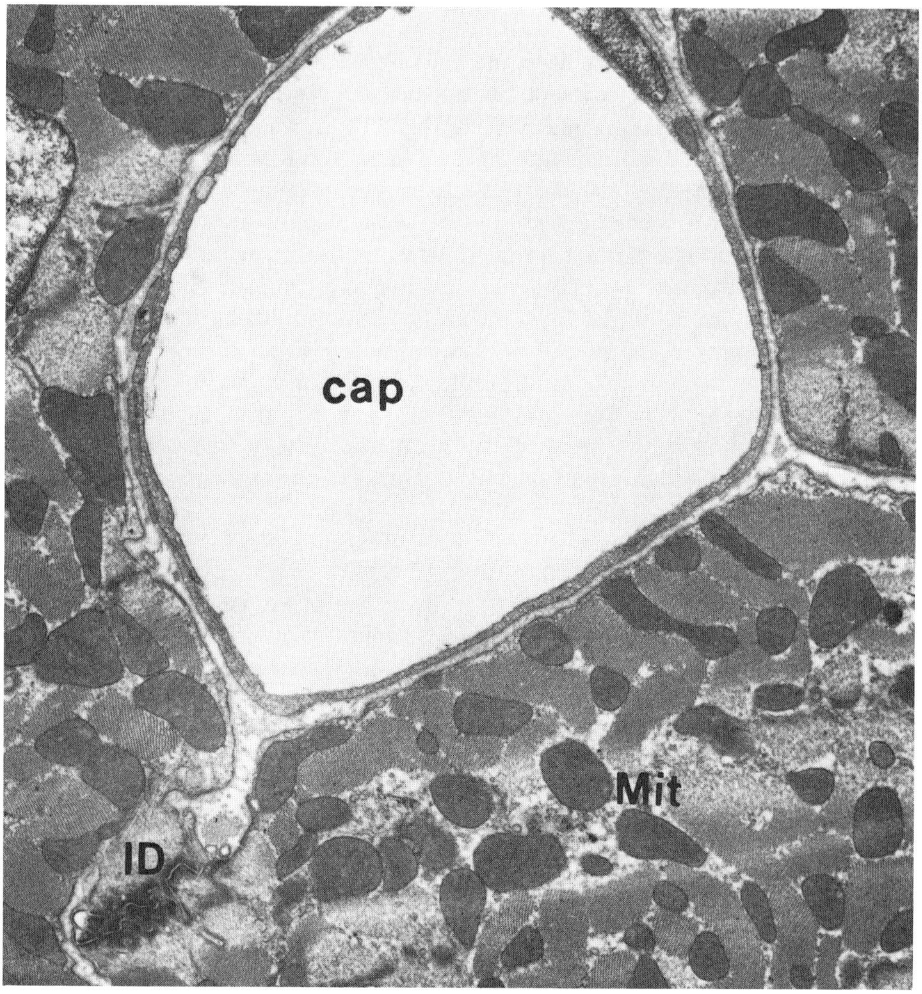

Figure 1 Myocardium after perfusion fixation. Since the lesions are focal one can find numerous cross sections with normal cardiac structures. ID, intercalated disk; cap, capillary; N, nucleus; Mit, mitochondria. Original magnification, 3,000.

of hypokalemic myocardium was performed by scanning microscopy of thick frozen and dehydrated sections according to the technique of Orsonio-Vargas et al. (64). The hypokalemic myocardium showed elevated levels of cellular sodium, chloride, and calcium, and depression of cellular potassium similar to the changes seen in ischemic cell injury. The cellular elevation of calcium, however, was not consistent and varied considerably between different scans. It was reported that necrosis occurred in the rat if the myocyte potassium level had decreased to 72 mEq/kg wet weight.

Vacuolization

Many heart cells developed huge vacuoles which ranged from 10 to 15 μm in diameter and were frequently adjacent to the cell surface or extended from the intercalated disk

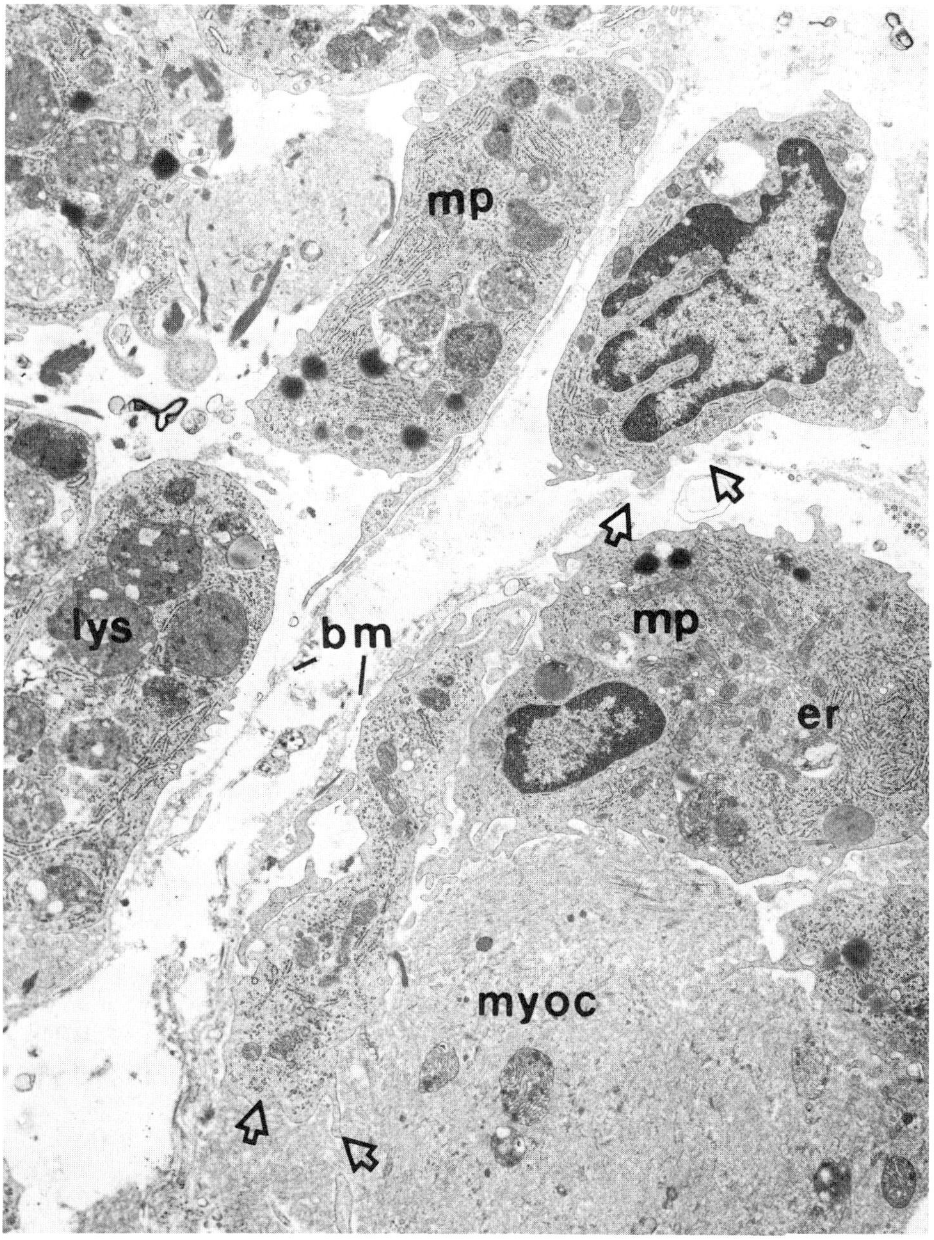

Figure 2 Necrotic myocyte (myoc) invaded by phagocytic cells (mp). Note the reflection of the basement membrane (bm) at the entry point (arrows). er, endoplasmic reticulum; lys, lysosomes. Original magnification, 5,000.

(Figure 3). We often observed a "neck" extending into the region of the intercalated disk. The vacuoles contained cell constituents including myofilaments and mitochondria. These mitochondria could be seen in different stages of alteration. Mitochondria in adjacent vacuoles often appeared in different stages of degeneration indicating, perhaps, different times of development. Adjacent cytoplasmic mitochondria commonly appeared to be normal. Other constituents of these vacuoles included cellular filaments which were in various stages of disarray and dissolution. The intercalated disks often appeared flattened (Figure 4), but just as frequently the disks were normal. Histochemical stain for phosphatases showed that the vacuoles contained little or no reaction product. It is our interpretation that these vacuoles represent invaginations of heart cells into adjacent heart cells. The observed degeneration may occur by lytic enzymes associated with cellular organelles. At a late stage, lysosomal enzymes may gain access to these vacuoles. The similarity of vacuole lesion to these produced by catecholamines is striking.

Phospholipids

Myocytes specially fixed with a mixture of 4% tannic acid and 2.5% glutaraldehyde, according to Kalina and Pease (41,42), Seagull and Heath (82), and Bonilla (12,13), showed an array of multilamellar bodies. These darkly staining structures surrounded single mitochondria. They were also frequently seen adjacent to the plasma membrane, between the intercalated disk, in the interstitium, and in the cytoplasm of endothelial cells (Figure 5).

Structural Changes of Mitochondria

Frequent alterations in myocardial mitochondria could be seen. Those changes occurred scattered in cells, with selected mitochondria often singled out (Figures 6 & 7). Normal mitochondria could be seen adjacent to abnormal ones in single heart cells. A few mitochondrial changes were more widely distributed, such as increased matrix granules (Figure 8), but even those were not seen in all myocytes and all animals. A number of structural changes in mitochondria were observed. First, there were mitochondrial changes of mitochondria secluded in vacuoles (Figure 1). These included mitochondrial degenerations, as are seen in other cell injuries such as ischemia, predominantly swelling and flocculent densities in the matrix space. Mitochondria in living myocytes also showed significant changes, including alteration of some and all of the cristae (Figure 6), increased granules in the matrix space (Figure 8), and large lytic vacuoles that occupied the matrix space (Figure 7). These vacuoles distorted the cristae. They contained some electron-dense precipitate and were seen frequently together with matrix flocculent densities.

Functional Changes of Mitochondria

Ledwoch et al. (51) investigated the influence of chronic potassium deficiency on energy production, calcium metabolism, and phospholipid composition of isolated heart mitochondria. After 28 days on a K-deficient diet rabbits showed potassium-deficient cardiomyopathy. Evidence for the severe hypokalemia was the depression of the potassium levels in serum and heart tissue. While sodium levels became elevated, Ca and Mg levels remained unchanged. Functionally, mitochondria showed increased state 4 respiration and increased calcium uptake in the presence of ATP, indicating that hypokalemic heart mitochondria take up more calcium and store it in mitochondria. Phosphatidylcholine levels were depressed in mitochondria and the linoleic acid content of mitochondrial cardiolipin was increased after chronic hypokalemia. All the above changes were considered

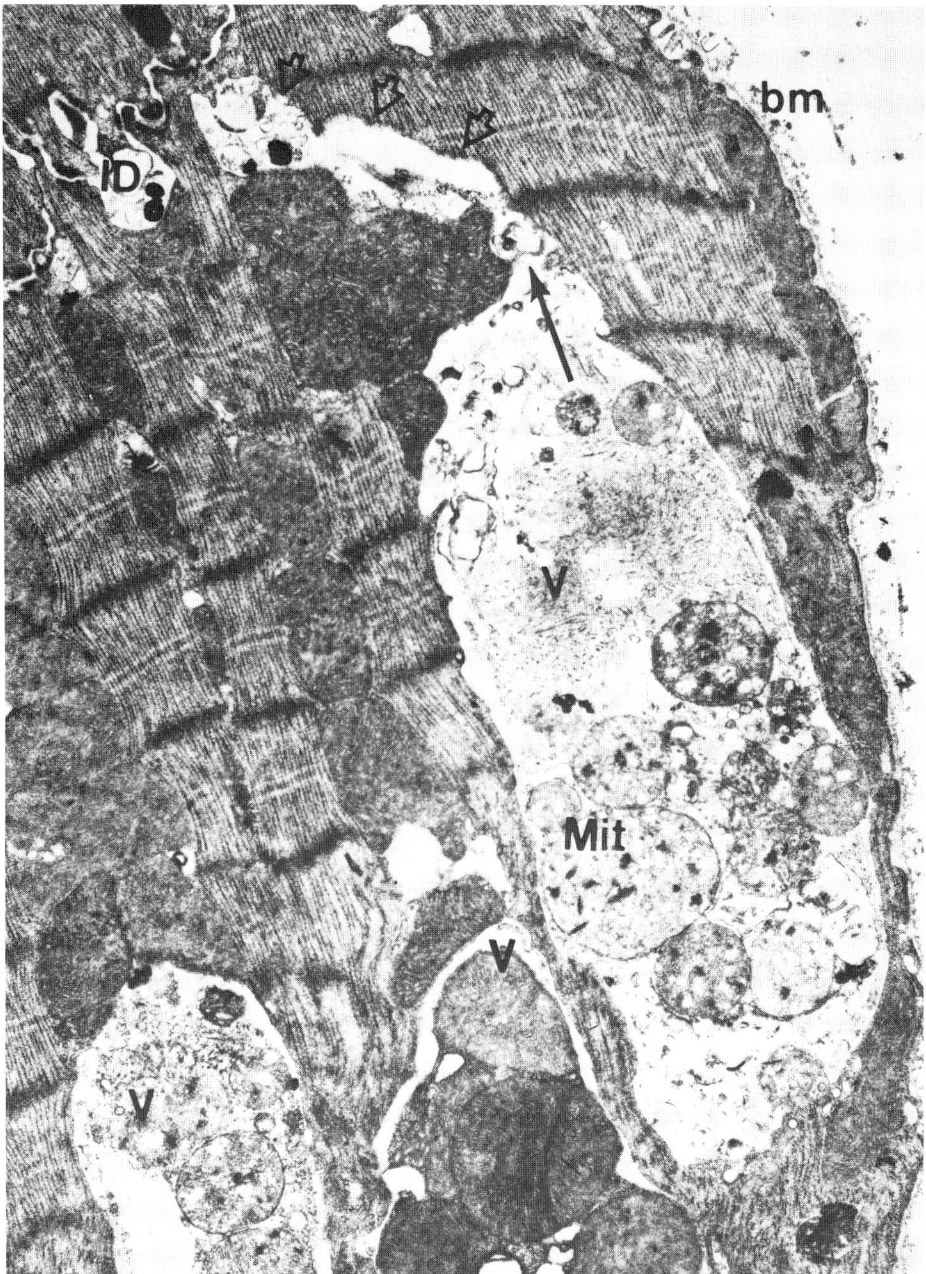

Figure 3 Two adjacent myocytes are seen. One contains three large vacuolar lesions containing altered organelles such as mitochondria (Mit) and filaments. Note the neck (arrow) connecting one vacuole to the intercalated disc (ID). V, vacuoles; bm, basement membrane. Original magnification, 3,500.

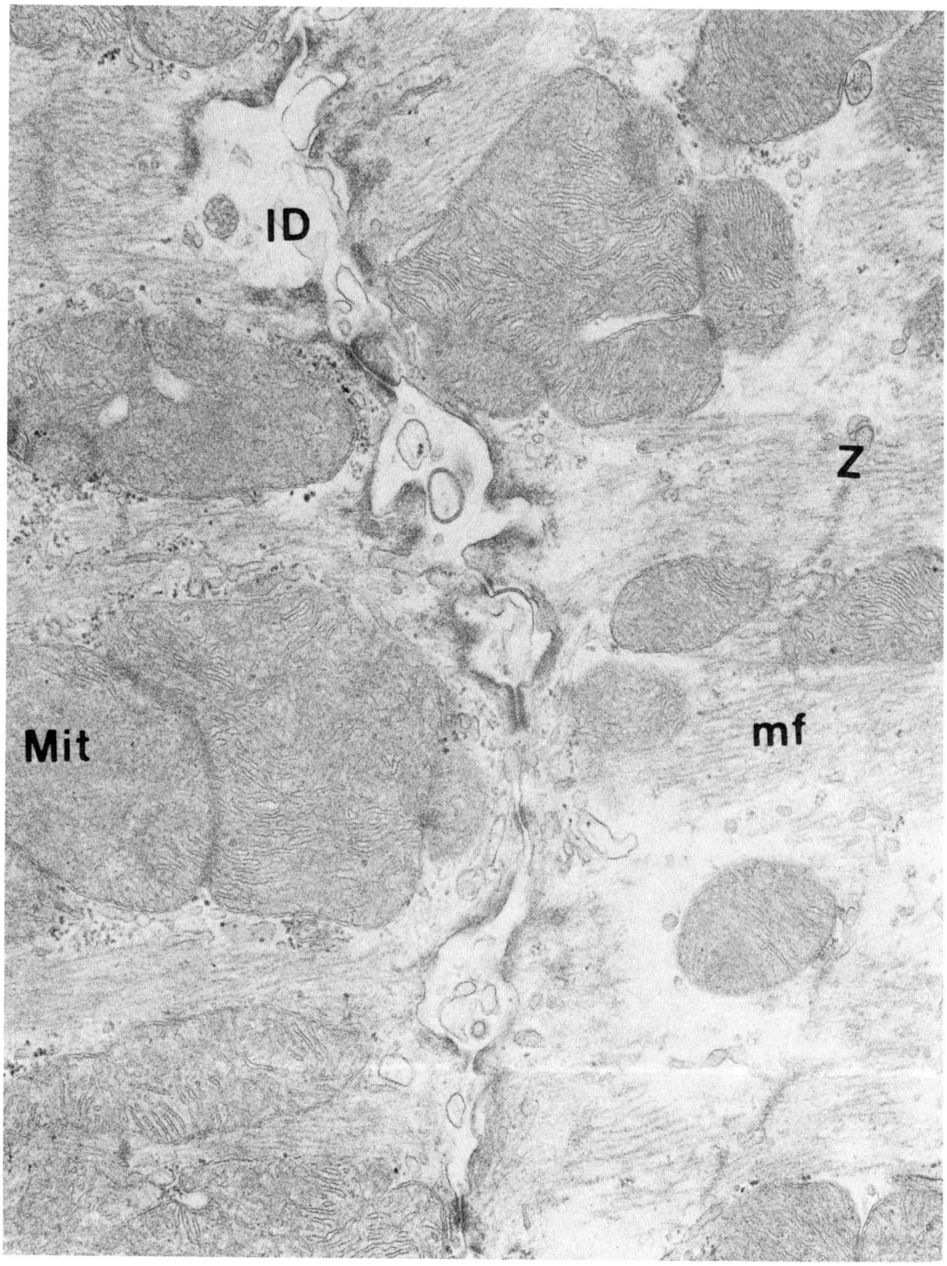

Figure 4 Intercalated disk (ID) separating two myocytes. Note the flattening of the disc, possibly a sign of cell swelling. Mit, mitochondria; mf, myofilaments; Z, z band.

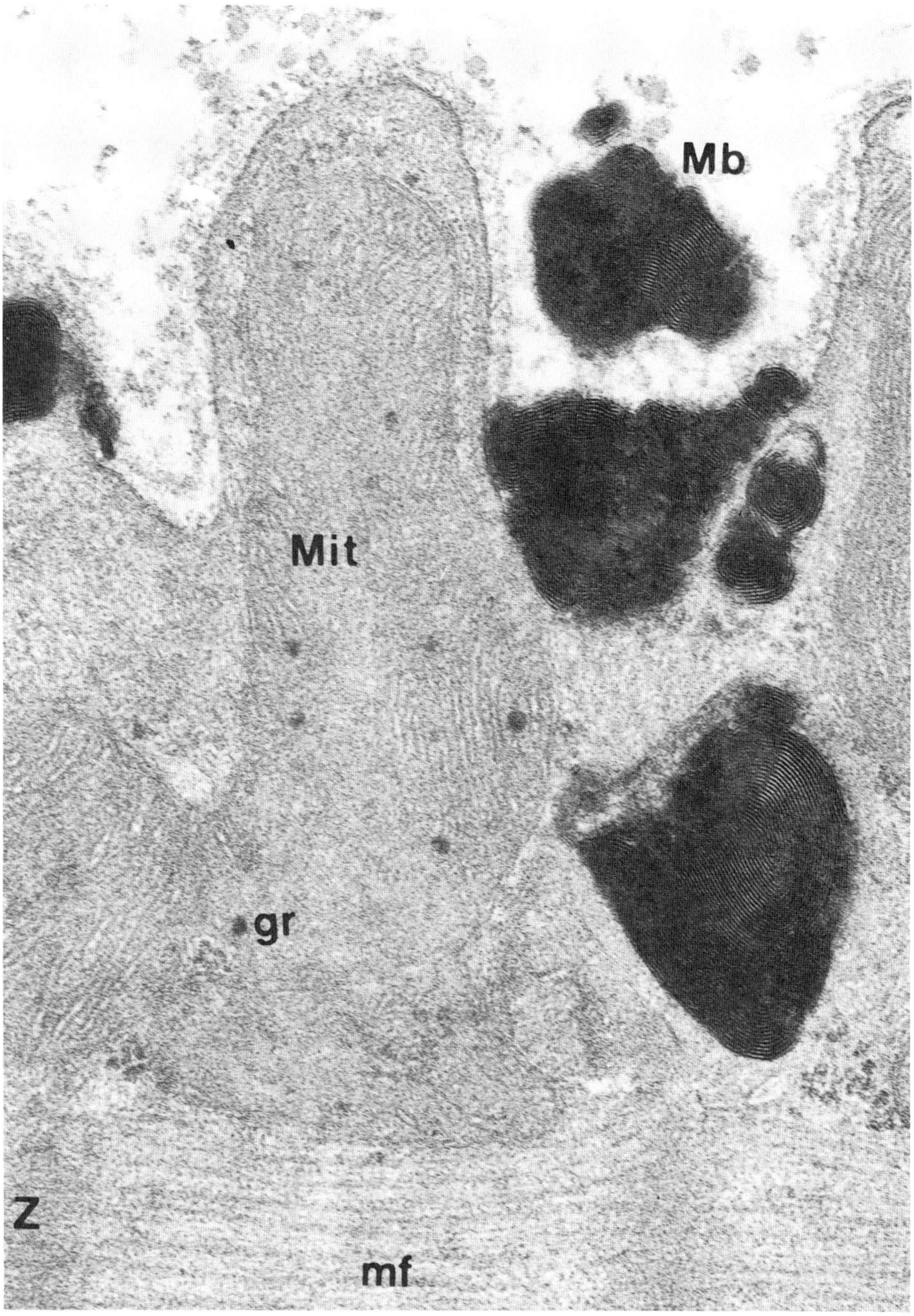

Figure 5 Lateral border of myocyte with "myelin bodies" (Mb) displaying fingerprint pattern. Fixed in glutaraldehyde 2.5% and tannic acid 3%. Mit, mitochondria; gr, granules; Z, z band; mf, myofilaments. Original magnification, 20,000.

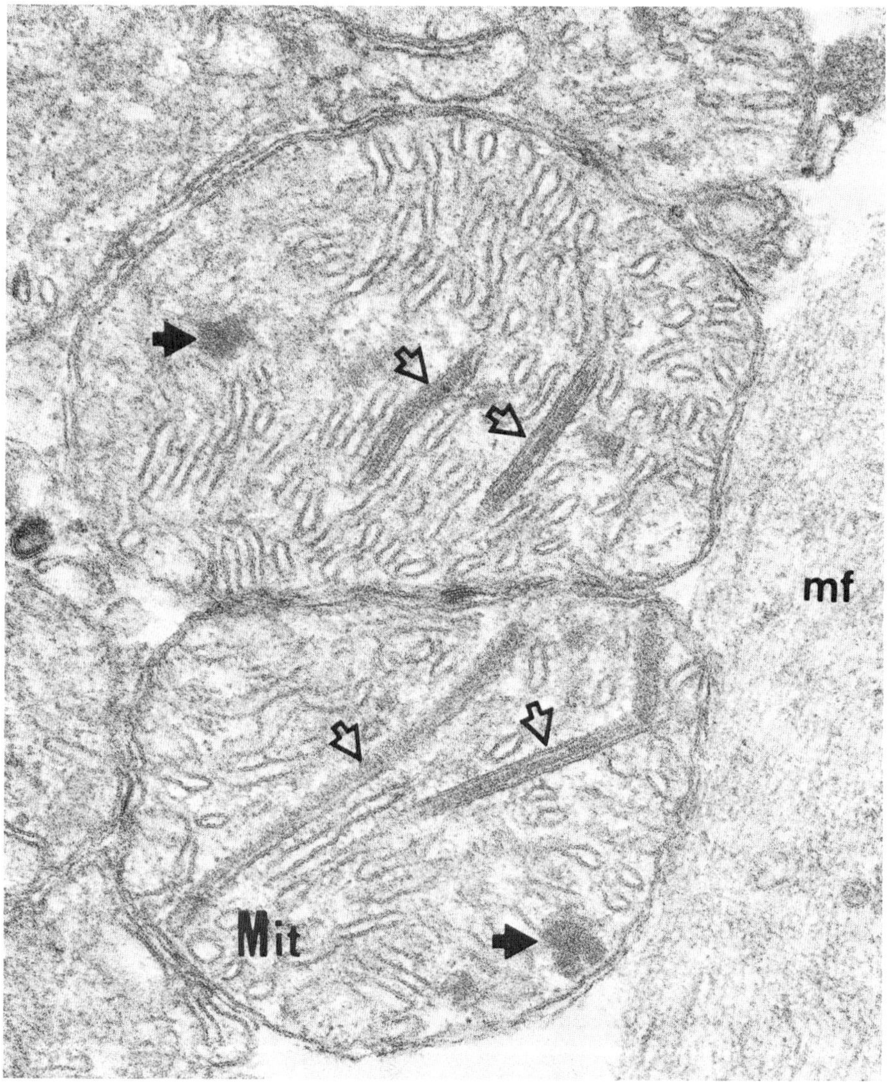

Figure 6 Histological section shows an altered myocyte with "flocculent densities" (solid arrow) and "zipperlike" fusion (open arrow) of cristae in mitochondria (Mit). mf, myofilaments. Original magnification, 20,000.

an adaptional change accompanied by a shift of calcium from sarcoplasmic reticulum to the mitochondria. Increased autophagocytosis was noted (Figure 9).

The Conduction System

Chah et al. (16) studied the effect of hypokalemia on the different parts of the conduction system following the acutely lowered serum K by dialysis. The AV conduction time was prolonged by 250% above control. His bundle and atrial conduction were less significantly affected than the remainder of the conduction tissue. Hypokalemic conduction tissue was more sensitive to lithium carbonate overdosage (34) as well as digitalis (36).

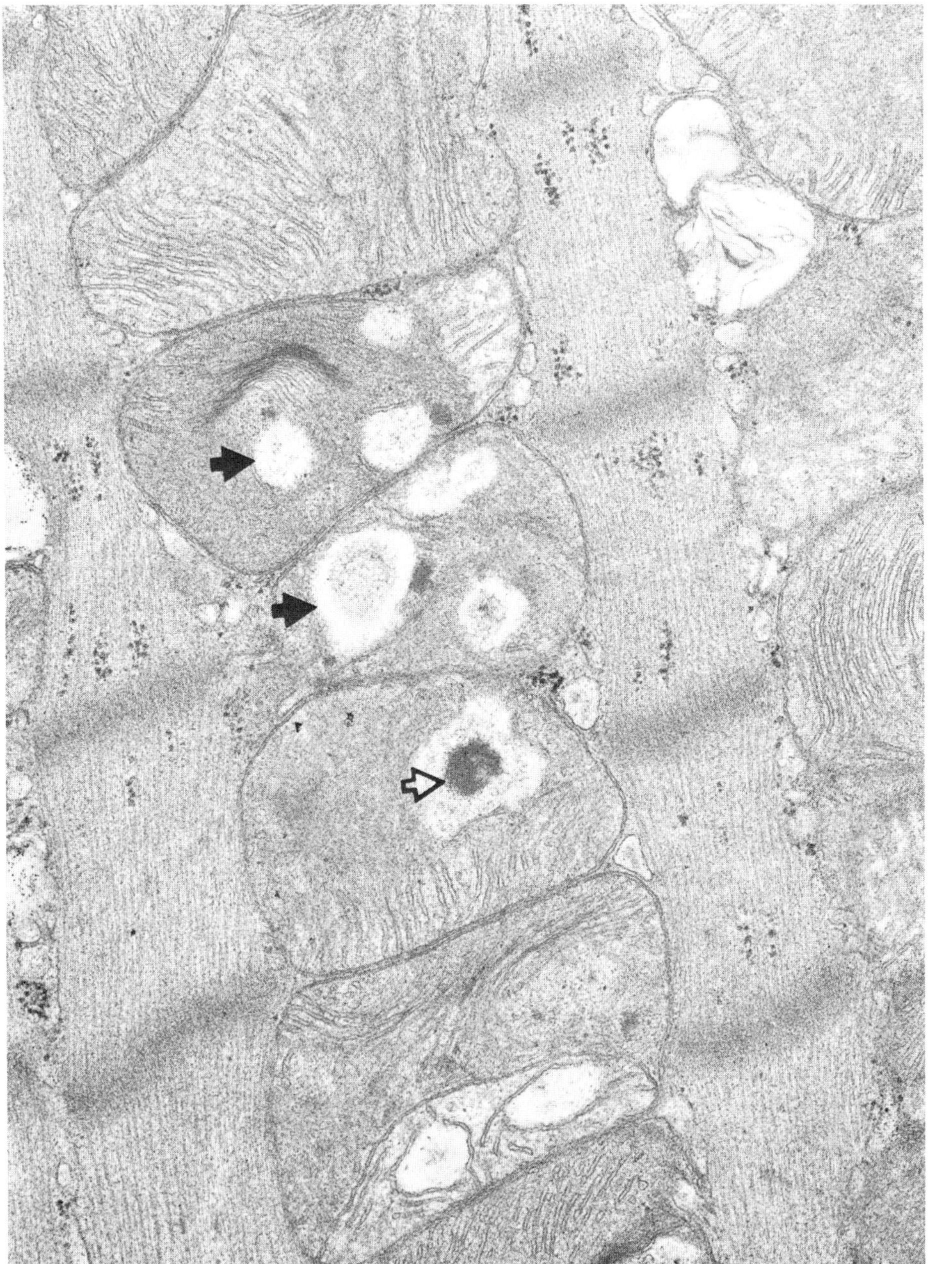

Figure 7 Mitochondria with large "flocculent densities" (open arrow) and "mitochondrial vacuoles" (solid arrows). The latter lesion was seen in viable and necrotic cells. Original magnification, 7,000.

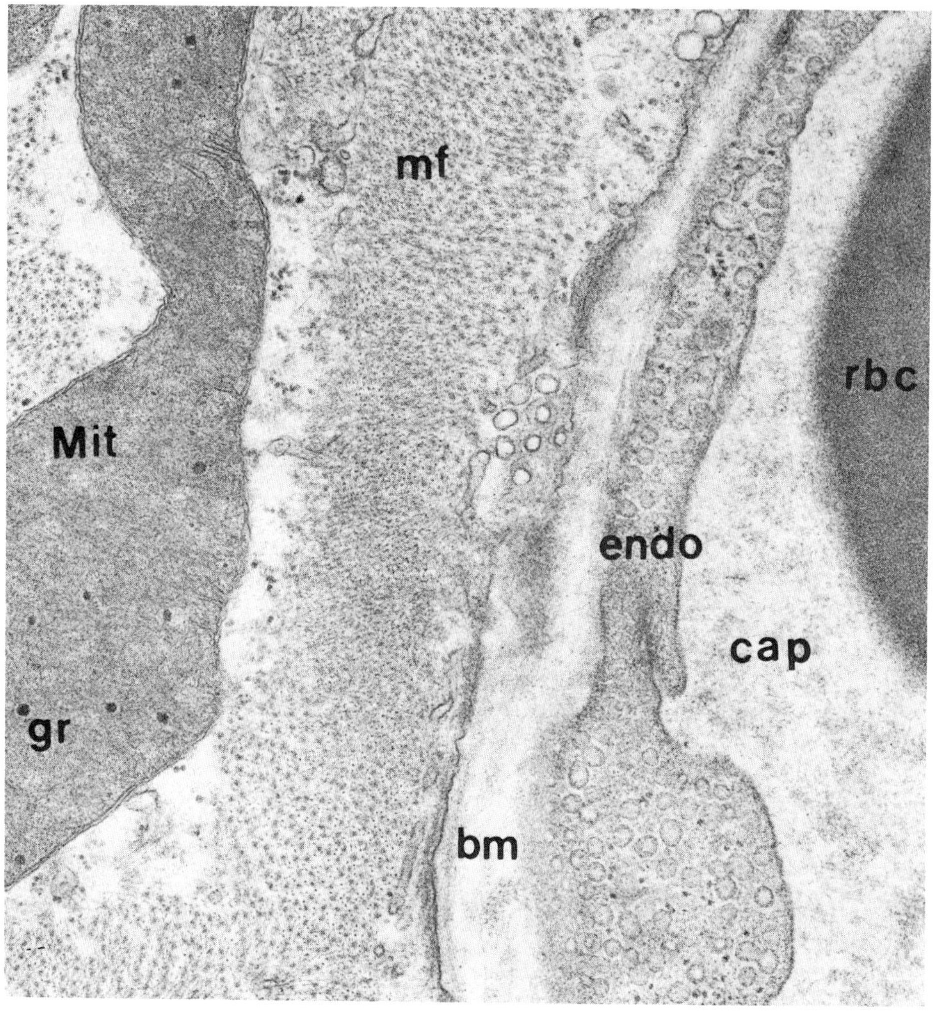

Figure 8 The section focuses on the capillary (cap) interface with a myocyte. Many mitochondria (Mit) were seen, with an apparently increased number of matrix granules (gr). mf, myofilaments; bm, basement membrane; endo, endothelium; rbc, red blood cells. Original magnification, 15,000.

Studies on the Kidney

Structural Alteration

The kidney shows marked zonal changes displaying different effects of potassium depletion on different cell types. Rapid growth has been reported by Oliver et al. (62) and by Toback et al. (93) in the kidney of rats fed a potassium-deficient diet. The most striking structural changes in rats take place in the collecting tubules of the inner strip which displays adenomatous hyperplasia. Functionally, the rat kidney subjected to potassium depletion shows a marked loss of the ability to concentrate urine and evidence shows that energy production in this zone is altered. Kannengiesser and Lee (43), Relman and

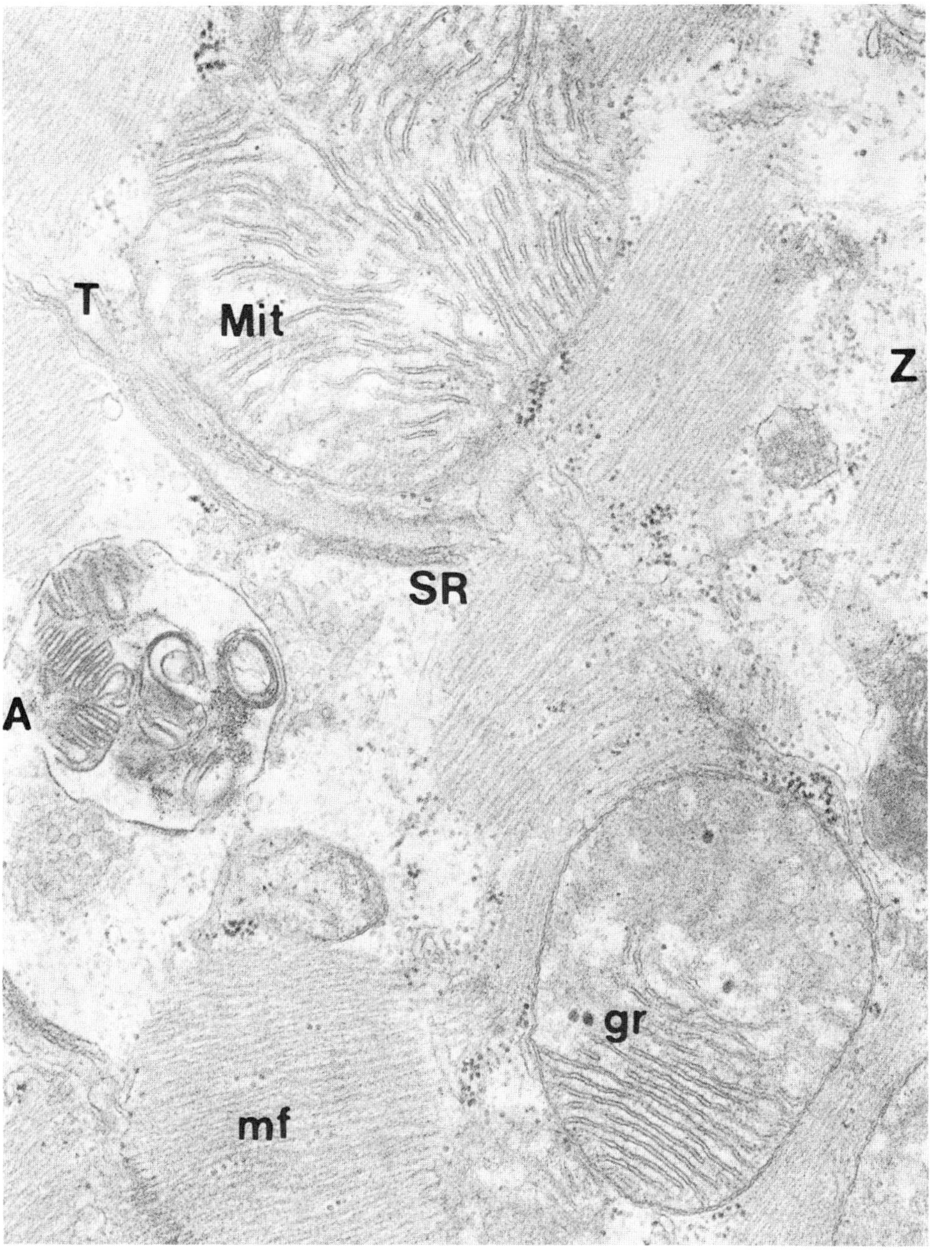

Figure 9 Autophagocytosis (A) of mitochondria (Mit). T, T-tubules; SR, sarcoplastic reticulum; Z, Z-band; mf, myofilaments; gr, granules. Original magnification, 20,000.

Schwartz (71), and Toback et al. (94) could show that during potassium depletion cell replication increased two to five times in the collecting tubules, thick limbs of Henle's loop, and interstitium. Potassium repletion halted cell proliferation and reduced the number of labled nuclei to control levels or below control levels. Papillary cells have been shown to become filled with lysosomes (5). In humans, hypokalemia causes different structural alterations. Relman and Schwartz (71,81), Bock et al. (11), Cremer and Bock (19), and Riemenschneider and Bohle (72) described the appearance of hypokalemia in renal biopsy specimens. There are dilated proximal tubules with swollen epithelial cells and cytoplasmic vacuoles. This is called foamy degeneration. Epithelial atrophy was seen. Spread of these lesions is not consistent and the distal convoluted tubules may be spared, as may be the collecting system. Humans do not show the proliferating distal tubular changes seen in rats. Long-standing human hypokalemia may be accompanied by scarring and interstitial nephritis. We do not know how much these lesions are able to regress (84). Osmophilic bodies were seen by electron microscopy, as was mitochondrial swelling. These changes correlate with an inability to concentrate, alteration in diluting capacity, and impaired tubular secretion (Figures 10 and 11).

Lysosomes

In potassium-depleted humans (24-26) and experimental rats (86), large droplets have been demonstrated in the cells of the inner medulla. Hydrolytic enzymes characteristic of lysosomes may also have increased. Labeling of proteins suggested an increased synthesis of lytic enzymes. In the same zone increased phospholipid synthesis was also demonstrated.

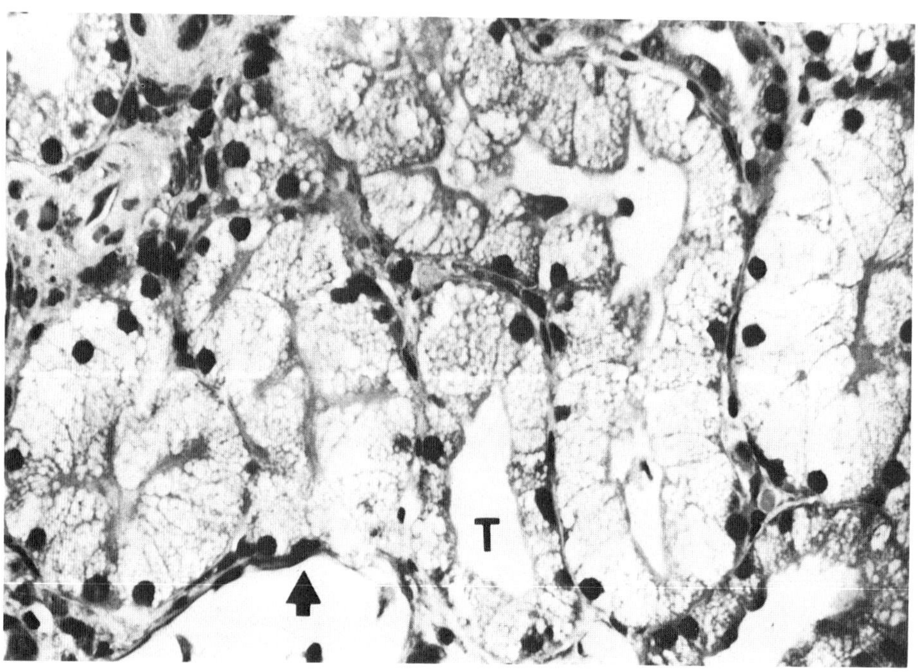

Figure 10 Light micrograph shows markedly foamy proximal tubular cells in this renal biopsy specimen. Original magnification, 400. (Courtesy of M. Hall-Craggs, University of Maryland, Baltimore, Maryland.)

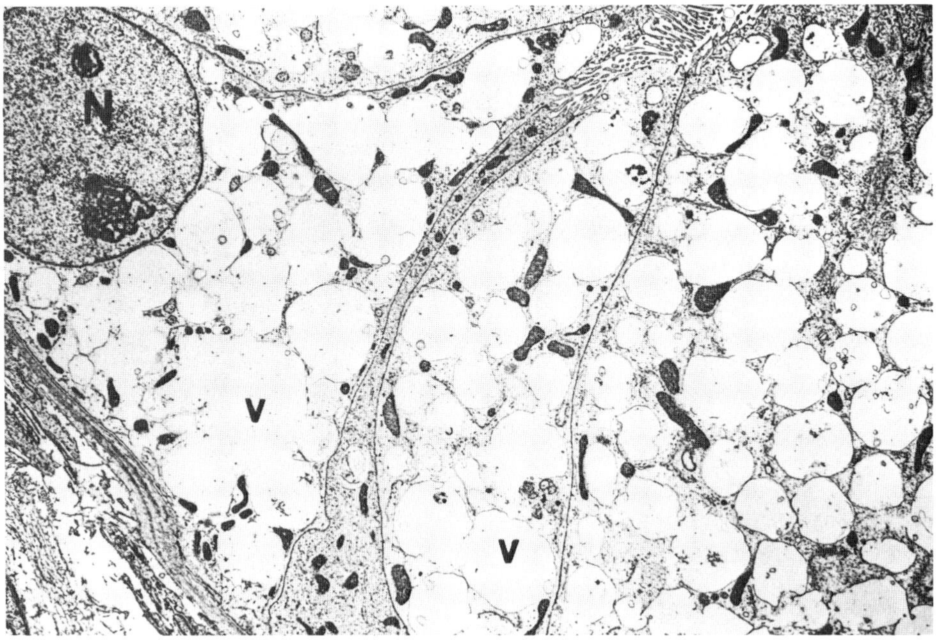

Figure 11 Electron micrograph of tubular cells shows abundant empty-appearing cytoplasmic vacuoles. (Courtesy of M. Hall-Craggs, University of Maryland, Baltimore, Maryland.)

Functional Alteration

Loss of urinary concentrating ability also occurs during potassium depletion. This change may be related to an aberration in renal energy metabolism (19). Bock et al. (11) describe chronic hypokalemic nephropathy in some patients.

Energy Metabolism

Aithal et al. (4) measured energy production in rat medulla after chronic nutritional potassium deficiency. Substrate oxidation decreased in mitochondria isolated from the inner strip for malate and pyruvate as well as succinate, as did phosphorylation of ADP. This selective defect was confined to the inner strip of the medulla that also showed adenomatous hyperplasia. Such hyperplasia is specific for the hypokalemic rat model. These mitochondria also showed potassium levels decreased by 36%. Upon reinfusion of potassium this localized defect returned to normal within less than 1 hr. This defect of bioenergetics in proliferating renal cells during potassium depletion was defined by Toback et al. (94), who studied DNA synthesis, anaerobic glycolysis, and oxidative phosphorylation. During potassium depletion, DNA labeling with thymidine was increased over the proliferating cells of collecting tubules, the thick limbs of Henle's loop, and the interstitial cells. It was also evident that the proliferating cells showed a shift towards anerobic glycolysis and decreased oxidative phosphorylation.

ACUTE EFFECT OF HYPOKALEMIA

Studies on the Heart

Adenosine Triphosphate, Inorganic Phosphate, and Creatine Phosphate

Acute hypokalemia was produced in the isolated perfused heart preparation in collaboration with the Department of Cardiology of Johns Hopkins University School of Medicine, in the laboratory of Drs. Jacobus, Hoerter, and Micelli (unpublished). When hearts were perfused with a solution in which potassium was omitted, cardiac activity ceased within 8.5 min. During the same time period inorganic phosphate increased significantly while adenosine triphosphate and creatine phosphate levels dropped rapidly.

pH in Acute Hypokalemia and in Chronic Hypokalemic Rats

Phosphate nuclear magnetic resonance permits us to estimate the intracellular pH in the isolated perfused rat heart. Test results showed a depression of intracellular pH when the perfusion medium was acutely switched to one that was potassium-free. This pH deflection, however, quickly returned to the original pH, even before the heart was returned to potassium-containing solutions.

Chronically potassium-deficient hearts also showed no consistent depression of pH, but reacted with a rapid upward deflection into alkalinity when the solution was changed from 2.8 mmol KCl to 5.9 mmol KCl and a downward deflection into acidity when switched again from a solution with 5.9 mmol KCl to one with 2.8 mmol KCl. In all these circumstances, the speed of correction was remarkable and suggests a buffering reaction between the intracellular space and the electrolytes and protons (2).

Recovery from Acute Hypokalemia

The heart recovered after acute hypokalemia, regained a regular beat, and systolic pressure returned to control level following reperfusion with potassium-containing solutions. There was, however, an elevation of end-diastolic pressure. Measurements of inorganic phosphate showed a decline of phosphate and a rise in creatine phosphate levels, while adenosine triphosphate did not reach control levels.

Hypothesis

It is our hypothesis that potassium deprivation in the perfusion medium has its primary effect on plasma membrane Na-K-ATPase. The ATPase is inhibited, allowing loss of cellular potassium and possible gain of cellular sodium and calcium. This leads to membrane alterations, because of the inability of mitochondria to regulate cellular calcium by a mechanism described by Alto and Dhalla (6) in calcium paradox and by Dhalla et al. (22) in acute hypokalemic perfusion. The alteration of the Na-K-ATPase has been elegantly shown by Cumberbatch and Morgan (20) and Rubython and Morgan (75) by testing erythrocytes' electrolyte control in hypokalemia. These investigators could show that hypokalemia caused a reduction in rate constant of the ouabain-sensitive ATPase. A compensatory increase in the number of pumps occurred in chronic hypokalemia.

RECOVERY FROM CHRONIC HYPOKALEMIA

Repairs of Myocardial Lesions of Chronic Hypokalemia

Abbrecht (1) studied in the dog the physiological effects of potassium depletion on arterial blood pressure, cardiac output, left ventricular stroke volume, renal blood flow, potassium balance, and plasma potassium concentration. During a 30-day depletion period he found progressive reduction in blood pressure, cardiac output, renal blood flow, stroke volume, and blood pressure. The values bounced back to normal during the repletion period (92). No strict relationship could be shown between hypokalemia and the severity of the myocardial lesions. Therefore, we suspect that hypokalemia involves both systemic effects on the myocardium and localized actions. It is, for example, documented that circulating epinephrine and norepinephrine are considerably increased during hypokalemia, possibly as a reactive adaption. These localized lesions, such as scattered myocardial necrosis, may be due to catecholamine action in the face of generalized metabolic stress as already described by Selye and Bajusz (7,83). Yet several aspects of extreme interest differentiate the recovery of myocardial lesions from hypokalemia: During hypokalemic injury and necrosis, the basement membrane remains intact, as do the vascular spaces (76,78, Mergner et al., in preparation). The lesions are devoid of typical inflammatory cells such as neutrophils, lymphocytes, or plasma cells; instead, the proliferating cells appear as mononuclear cells on light microscopy and as heavily phagocytic cells on electron microscopy. These phagocytic cells, however, differ from normal macrophages by characteristics of the cytosol which is studded with ribosomes (Figure 12) (21,58). It has been postulated that this process of phagocytosis and proliferation of phagocytic cells is different and the participating cells sufficiently specific to warrant special investigation (78). When the kaliopenic animals are resupplied with potassium the lesions were shown to regress and heal without scar formation (27,52,56, Mergner et al., in preparation). The repair process is quick: it is initiated in less than 24 hr and is completed in 3 days to 1 week. Several processes could be responsible for replacing the necrotic myocytes: the adjacent myocytes may hypertrophy and rearrange their alignment to fill the spaces left by necrotic cells; mature myocytes may divide and replace the necrotic cells (we have shown that this is not the case); Sarkas and Levine (78) proposed that the myocytes are replaced by proliferating nonspecialized interstitial cells which subsequently differentiate into mature myocytes. We tested the latter possibility and found, upon refeeding, proliferation of mononuclear cells that appeared with 1 day to 1 week following refeeding; these cells apparently dropped into the interstitial lattice during the recovery phase (52). Sarkas and Levine (78) observed that within a day or two of when the experimental animals' levels of serum potassium reached control values, the lesions showed early repletion by small myofibers with the early stages of myofilament precipitation, followed by an increasing parallel arrangement of the filaments and the appearance of Z-bands as well as intercellular attachments and intercalated disks. As soon as myofiber differentiation was apparent, the lysosomal bodies and any evidence of excessive phagocytosis disappeared.

Recovery in the Kidney

The recovery in the kidney is equally rapid, as described by Toback et al. (96) and Ordonez et al. (63) with a rapid reversal of the alteration of the pathophysiological metabolism as well as formation of abundant autophagosomes. Two patterns of involuntionary changes were seen in the collecting tubules upon repletion of potassium in the rat. A wave of autophagocytosis appeared within 3 hr in the hyperplastic cells typical of the rat renal reaction. Lysosomes showed rapid reduction. The process had recovered after 3 days. The rate of phosphotidylcholine breakdown increased and the rate of choline incorporation into phospholipids decreased. Phospholipase A activity, which was depressed during hypokalemia, increased during repletion within 12 hr. The increase in lysosomes was also seen in humans during hypokalemic nephropathy.

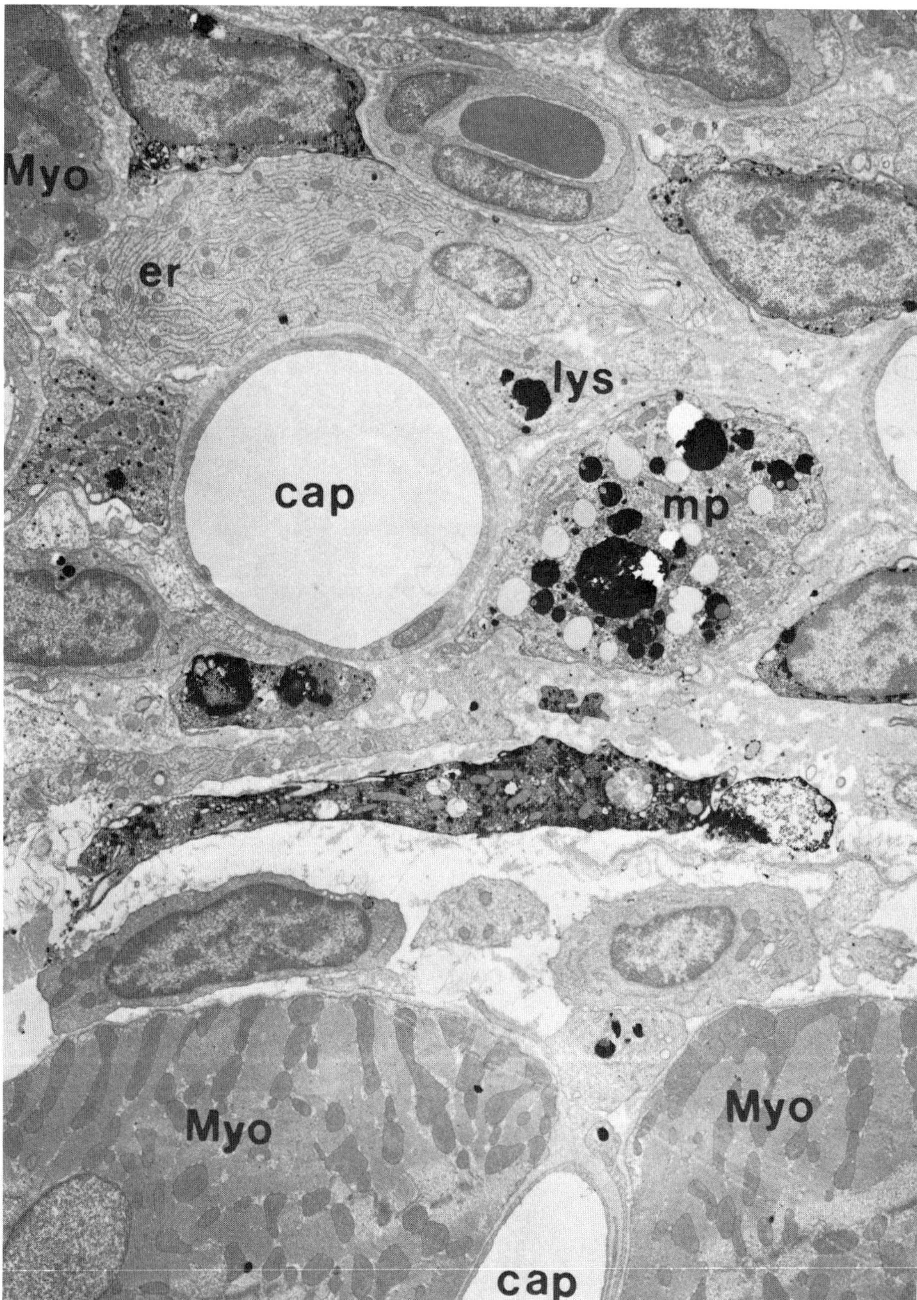

Figure 12 Histochemical stain for hydrolases shows the pericapillary proliferation of mononuclear cells. Myo, myocytes; er, endoplasmic reticulum; lys, lysosomes; cap, capillary. Original magnification, 3,000. (Courtesy of R. Broadwell, University of Maryland, Baltimore, Maryland.)

As seen in human biopsy specimens by Relman and Schwartz (71,81) recovery of hypokalemic nephropathy in humans is also rapid and usually complete.

SUMMARY

Hypokalemia causes pathological lesions in the heart and kidney of humans and animals. Two experimental conditions were utilized to uncover these effects: acute replacement of extracellular potassium in the perfusion medium and chronic nutritional potassium depletion. The two effects are: a systemic effect that may be mediated by depressed energy metabolism and/or disturbed plasma membrane electrolyte control, and a localizing effect that causes scattered cardiac cell necrosis and distal tubular epithelial lesions in the rat kidney or proximal and distal lesions in humans. These lesions may be the localizing effects of specific physiological reactions to the state of hypokalemia. We are impressed with the similarity of catecholamine-induced myocardial necrosis and hypokalemic lesions (74). The rapid recovery of all these lesions is a remarkable feature of the animal model. It is not known if this recovery is also as efficient in human cardiac or renal lesions.

ACKNOWLEDGMENT

This work was supported by grant RO1 HL 22281-03 and by the Universuty of Maryland Foundation.

REFERENCES

1. Abbrecht, P. H.: Cardiovascular effects of chronic potassium deficiency in the dog. *Am. J. Physiol.* 223:555–560, 1972.
2. Adler, S., and Fraley, D. S.: Potassium and intracellular pH. *Kidney Int.* 11:433–442, 1977.
3. Aithal, H. N., and Toback, F. G.: Defective mitochondrial energy production during potassium depletion nephropathy. *Lab. Invest.* 39:186–192, 1978.
4. Aithal, H. N., Toback, F. G., Ordonez, N. G., and Spargo, B. H.: Functional defects in mitochondria of renal inner red medulla during potassium depletion nephropathy. *Lab. Invest.* 37:423–429, 1977.
5. Aithal, H. N., Toback, F. G., Dube, S., Getz, G. S., and Spargo, B. H.: Formation of renal medullary lysosomes during potassium depletion nephropathy. *Lab. Invest.* 36:107–113, 1977.
6. Alto, L. E., and Dhalla, N. S.: Myocardial cation content during induction of calcium paradox. *Am. J. Physiol.* 237:713–719, 1979.
7. Bajusz, E.: The role of some essential nutrients in the pathogenesis of cardiac necrosis (studies on K-, Mg-, Na-, and Cl-deficiencies). *Rev. Can. Biol.* 20:713–721, 1961.
8. Bank, N., and Aynedjian, H. S.: Micropuncture study of potassium excretion by the remnant kidney. *J. Clin. Invest.* 52:1480–1486, 1973.
9. Beck, N., and Webster, S. K.: Impaired urinary concentrating ability and cyclic AMP in K depleted rat kidney. *Am. J. Physiol.* 231:1204–1208, 1976.
10. Berl, T., Linas, S. L., Aisenbrey, G. A., and Anderson, R. J.: On the mechanism of polyuria in potassium depletion: The role of polydipsia. *J. Clin. Invest.* 60:620–625, 1977.

11. Bock, K. D., Cremer, W., and Werner, U.: Chronic hypokalemic nephropathy: A clinical study. *Klin. Wochenschr.* 56:91–96, 1978.
12. Bonilla, E.: Staining of transverse tubular system of skeletal muscle by tannic acid-glutaraldehyde fixation. *J. Ultrastruct. Res.* 58:162–165, 1977.
13. Bonilla, E., Schotland, D. L., and Wakayama, Y.: Lamellar bodies at the cell periphery of human muscle fibers. *Eur. J. Cell Biol.* 20:159–167, 1979.
14. Bulger, R. E., and Trump, B. F.: Ca and K ion effects on ultrastructure of isolated flounder kidney tubules. *J. Ultrastruct. Res.* 28:301–319, 1969.
15. Buruma, O. J., Schipperheyn, J. J., and Bots, G. T.: Heart muscle disease in familial hypokalemic periodic paralysis. *Acta Neurol. Scand.* 64:12–21, 1981.
16. Chah, Q. T., Braly, G., Bokuzouita, K., and Faucon, G.: Effects of hypokalemia on the various parts of the conduction system of the dog heart in-situ. *Naunyn Schmiedebergs Arch. Pharmacol.* 319:178–183, 1982.
17. Cohen, J. J.: Disorders of potassium balance. *Hosp. Pract.* 14:119–128, 1979.
18. Cowan, M. J., Giddens, W. E., and Reichenbach, D. D.: Selective myocardial cell necrosis in non-human primates. *Arch. Pathol. Lab. Med.* 107:34–39, 1983.
19. Cremer, W., and Bock, K. D.: Symptoms and course of chronic hypokalemic nephropathy in man. *Clin. Nephrol.* 7:112–119, 1977.
20. Cumberbatch, M., and Morgan, D. B.: Erythrocytes sodium and potassium in patients with hypokalemia. *Clin. Sci.* 64:167–176, 1983.
21. David, R., Trifillis, A., and Mergner, W. J.: Tannic acid-glutaraldehyde fixation in the study of hypokalemic cardiomyopathy. *Fed. Proc.* 40:752, 1981.
22. Dhalla, N. S., Lee, S. L., Singal, P. K., Yates, T. C., and Ulrich, H. W.: Subcellular changes in rat hearts perfused with potassium free medium. *Am. J. Physiol.* 237: 61–69, 1979.
23. Follis, R. H., Orent-Keiles, E., and McCollum, E. V.: The production of cardiac and renal lesions in rats by a diet extremely deficient in potassium. *Am. J. Pathol.* 18: 29–39, 1942.
24. France, R.: Intracellular granules of renal medulla in potassium depletion. *Trans. Am. Clin. Climatol. Assoc.* 74:211–230, 1963.
25. France, R., Shelley, W. M., and Gray, M. E.: Abnormal intracellular granules of the renal papilla in a child with potassium depletion (Batter's syndrome) and renal tuberous sclerosis. *Johns Hopkins Med. J.* 135:274–285, 1974.
26. France, R., Gray, M. E., Stone, W. J., and Swift, L. L.: Intracellular granules of the renal medulla in a case of potassium depletion due to renal potassium wasting. Electron microscopic comparison with renal medullary granules in the potassium depleted rat. *Am. J. Pathol.* 91:299–312, 1978.
27. French, J. E.: A histological study of heart lesions in potassium deficient rats. *Arch Pathol.* 18:485–491, 1952.
28. Fuhrmann, G. F., Boehm, C., and Theuvenet, A. P. R.: Sugar transport, and potassium permeability in yeast plasma membrane vesicles. *Biochem. Biophys. Acta* 433: 583–596, 1976.
29. Gomez-Puyon, A., Sandoval, F., Chavez, E., and Thena, M.: On the role of potassium on oxidative phosphorylation. *J. Biol. Chem.* 215:5239–5247, 1970.
30. Güllner, H. G., Graf, A. K., Gill, J. R., and Mitchell, M. D.: Hypokalemia stimulates prostacyclin synthesis in the rat. *Clin. Sci. (London)* 65:43–46, 1983.
31. Güllner, H. G., Lake, C. R., Gill, J. R., and Lakata, D. J.: Hypokalemia stimulates plasma epinephrine and norepinephrine in the rat. *Arch. Int. Pharmacodyn. Ther.* 260:78–82, 1982.
32. Gunning, J. F., Harrison, C. E., and Coleman, H. N.: The effect of chronic potassium deficiency on myocardial contractility and oxygen consumption. *J. Mol. Cell Cardiol.* 4:139–153, 1972.

33. Gustafson, A. B., Shear, L., and Gabuszda, G. J.: Protein metabolism in-vivo in kidney, liver, muscle and heart of potassium-deficient rats. *J. Lab. Clin. Med.* 82: 287-296, 1973.
34. Habibzadeh, H. A., and Zeller, N. H.: Cardiac arrhythmia and hypopotassemia in association with lithium carbonate overdose. *South. Med. J.* 70:628-630, 1977.
35. Hadler, H. I., and Dimitriou, J. M.: The immediate uptake of potassium ion by mitochondria requiring gramicidin and 2,2-dimethyl succinic anhydride. *Eur. J. Biochem.* 69:315-30, 1976.
36. Hall, R. J., Gelbart, A., Billingham, H., Snidow, G., and Goldmand, R. H.: Effect of chronic potassium depletion on digitalis-induced inotropy and arrhythmias. *Cardiovasc. Res.* 15:98-107, 1981.
37. Harrison, T. R., Pitcher, C., and Ewing, G.: Studies on congestive heart failure. IV. Potassium content of skeletal and cardiac muscle. *J. Clin. Invest.* 8:325-235, 1930.
38. Harrison, C. E., Cooper, G., Zusko, K. J., and Coleman, H. N.: Myocardial and mitochondrial function in potassium depletion cardiomyopathy. *J. Mol. Cell. Cardiol.* 4:633-649, 1972.
39. Jennings, R. B., Baum, J. H., and Herdson, P. B.: Fine structural changes in myocardial ischemic injury. *Arch. Pathol.* 79:135-143, 1965.
40. Jung, D. W., Chavez, E., and Brierly, G. P.: Energy-dependent exchange of K in heart mitochondria. *Arch. Biochem. Biophys.* 183:452-459, 1977.
41. Kalina, M., and Pease, D.: The preservation of ultrastructure in saturated phosphatidyl cholines by tannic acid in model systems and type II pneumocytes. *J. Cell. Biol.* 74:726-741, 1977.
42. Kalina, M., and Pease, D. C.: The probable role of phosphatidyl cholines in the tannic acid enhancement of cytomembrane electron contrast. *J. Cell. Biol.* 74:742-746, 1977.
43. Kannengiesser, H., and Lee, J. B.: Role of outer renal medullary metabolism in the concentrating defect of K-depletion. *Am. J. Physiol.* 220:1701-1709, 1971.
44. Kashgarian, M., Hayslett, J. P., and Spargo, B. H.: Renal disease. *Am. J. Pathol.* 89:183-272, 1977.
45. Khuri, R. N., Agulian, S. K., and Kalloghlian, A.: Intracellular potassium in cells with distal tubule. *Pflugers Arch.* 335:297-308, 1972.
46. Khuri, R. N., Agulian, S. K., and Bogharian, K.: Electrochemical potentials of potassium in proximal renal tubule of rat. *Pflugers Arch.* 346:319-326, 1974.
47. Kimmick, G. A., and Rasmussen, H.: Inhibition of mitochondrial respiration by loss of mitochondrial K. *Biochem. Biophys. Acta* 131:413-420, 1967.
48. Kliger, A. S., and Hayslett, J. P.: Disorders of potassium balance. In *Acid-Base and Potassium Homeostasis*, Current Issues in Nephrology, Vol. 2, edited by Bremer, B. N., and Stein, W. H., New York, Churchill Livingstone, 1978.
49. Kline, R., and Murad, M.: Potassium efflux and accumulation in heart muscle. Evidence from K electrode experiments. *Biophys. J.* 16:367-372, 1978.
50. Koide, T., Ozeki, K., Kaihara, S., Kato, A., Hurao, S., and Kono, H.: Etiology of QT-prolongation and T wave changes in chronic alcoholism. *Jpn. Heart J.* 22:151-166, 1981.
51. Ledwoch, W., Greeff, K., Heinen, E., and Noak, E.: The influence of chronic potassium deficiency on energy production, calcium metabolism and phospholipid composition of isolated heart mitochondria. *J. Mol. Cell. Cardiol.* 11:77-89, 1979.
52. Levine, D. Z., Sarkas, K., Nash, L., and Rakusan, K.: The influence of potassium depletion on cardiac growth response to pressure overload. *Basic Res. Cardiol.* 78: 53-61, 1983.
53. Lowenhaupt, E., Schulman, M. P., and Greenberg, D. M.: Basic histologic lesions of magnesium deficiency in the rat. *Arch Pathol.* 49:427-433, 1950.

54. Lubin, M.: Intracellular potassium and control of protein synthesis. *Fed. Proc.* 23: 994–1007, 1964.
55. Macknight, A. D.: Epithelial transport of potassium. *Kidney Int.* 11:391–414, 1977.
56. McPherson, C. R.: Myocardial necrosis in the potassium depleted rat: A reassessment. *Br. J. Exp. Pathol.* 37:279–285, 1956.
57. Mergner, W. J., David, R., and Nguyen, N.: Ultrastructural physiological and biochemical changes in hypokalemic cardiomyopathy, in preparation.
58. Molnar, Z., Larsen, K., and Spargo, B.: Cardiac changes in the potassium-depleted rat. *Arch. Pathol.* 74:339–353, 1962.
59. Morel, F., Charbades, D., and Imbert, M.: Functional segmentation of rabbit distal tubule by microdetermination of hormone-dependent adenylate cyclase activity. *Kidney Int.* 9:264–277, 1976.
60. Muelrick, R. C., and Rosen, S.: Hypokalemic nephropathy in rat and man: A light and electron microscopic study. *Lab. Invest.* 13:1359–1365, 1964.
61. Nardone, D. A., McDonald, W. J., and Girard, D. E.: Mechanisms in hypokalemia: Clinical correlation. *Medicine (Baltimore)* 57:435–446, 1978.
62. Oliver, J., MacDowell, M., Welt, L. G., Holliday, M. A., Hollander, W. Jr., Winters, R. W., Williams, T. F., Segar, W. E.: The renal lesions of electrolyte imbalance. I. The structural alteration in potassium depleted rats. *J. Exp. Med.* 106:563–572, 1957.
63. Ordonez, N. G., Toback, F. G., Aithal, H. N., and Spargo, B. H.: Zonal changes in renal structure and phospholipid metabolism during reversal of potassium depletion nephropathy. *Lab. Invest.* 36:33–47, 1977.
64. Orsonio-Vargas, A. R., Berezesky, I. K., and Trump, B. F.: Procession of ion movement during acute myocardial infarction in the rat. An x-ray microanalysis study. *Scan Electronmicros.* 2:463–471, 1981.
65. Patrick, J.: Assessment of body potassium stores. *Kidney Int.* 11:476–490, 1977.
66. Perkins, J. G., Petersen, A. B., and Riby, J. A.: Renal and cardiac lesions in potassium deficiency due to chronic diarrhea. *Am. J. Med.* 8:115–119, 1950.
67. Pettit, G. W., Vick, R. L., and Kasello, M. D.: The contribution of renal and extrarenal mechanism to hypokalemia induced by glucagon. *Eur. J. Pharmacol.* 41: 437–441, 1977.
68. Pitts, B. J., and Entman, M. L.: The heart and cellular potassium fluxes. In *Potassium, Its Biological Significance*, edited by Whang, R., Boca Raton, CRC Press, Inc., 1983, pp. 110–118.
69. Potts, J. L., Dalakos, T. G., Streeten, D. H., and Jones, D.: Cardiomyopathy in an adult with Barter's syndrome and hypokalemia. Hemodynamic, angiographic and metabolic studies. *Am. J. Cardiol.* 40:995–999, 1977.
70. Pressman, B. C., and Lardy, H. A.: Further studies on the potassium requirements of mitochondria. *Biochem. Biophys. Acta* 18:682–687, 1955.
71. Relman, A. S., and Schwartz, W. B.: The nephropathy of potassium depletion: A clinical and pathological entity. *N. Engl. J. Med.* 255:195–203, 1956.
72. Riemenschneider, T., and Bohle, A.: Morphologic aspects of low-potassium and low-sodium nephropathy. *Clin. Nephrol.* 19:271–279, 1983.
73. Rodriguez, C. E., Wolfe, A. E., and Bergstrom, V. W.: Hypokalemic myocarditis: Report of two cases. *Am. J. Clin. Pathol.* 20:1050–1056, 1950.
74. Rona, G., Chappel, C. I., and Balazs, T.: An infarct-like myocardial lesion and other toxic manigestations produced by isoproterenol in the rat. *Arch. Pathol. Lab. Med.* 67:443–455, 1959.
75. Rubython, E., and Morgan, D. B.: Effect of hypokalemia on the ouabain-sensitive sodium transport and the ouabain-binding capacity in human erythrocytes. *Clin. Sci.* 64:177–182, 1983.

76. Rumanyantsev, P. P.: Interrelations of the proliferation and differentiation process during cardiac myogenesis and regeneration. *Int. Rev. Cytol.* 51:186–273, 1977.
77. Sack, D. W., Kim, N. D., and Harrison, C. E.: Contractility and subcellular calcium metabolism in chronic potassium deficiency. *Am. J. Physiol.* 226:756–763, 1974.
78. Sarkas, K., and Levine, D. Z.: Repair of myocardial lesions during potassium repletion of kaliopenic rats: An ultrastructural study. *J. Mol. Cell. Cardiol.* 11:1165–1172, 1979.
79. Savoie, L.: Effet d'antikaliuretiques dans le development des lesions cardiaques chez le rat deficient en potassium ou en magnesium. *Can. J. Biol.* 30:287–296, 1971.
80. Schrader, G. A., Prickett, C. O., and Salmon, W. D.: Symptomatology and pathology of potassium and magnesium deficiencies in the rat. *J. Nutr.* 14:15–21, 1937.
81. Schwartz, W. B., and Relman, A. S.: Effect of electrolyte disorders on renal structure and function. *New Engl. J. Med.* 276:452–458, 1967.
82. Seagull, R. W., and Heath, I. B.: The effect of tannic acid on the in-vivo preservation of microfilaments. *Eur. J. Cell. Biol.* 20:184–188, 1979.
83. Selye, H., and Bajusz, E.: Sensitization by potassium deficiency for the production of myocardial necrosis by stress. *Am. J. Pathol.* 35:525–550, 1959.
84. Solez, K.: Sundry conditions affecting the renal tubules. In *Renal Pathology* Vol. 2, edited by Heptinstall, R. H., Boston, Little, Brown, 1980, pp. 1557–1565.
85. Southon, S., and Heaton, F. W.: Changes in cellular and subcellular composition during potassium deficiency. *Comp. Biochem. Physiol.* 72:415–419, 1982.
86. Spargo, B. H.: Kidney changes in hypokalemic alkalosis in the rat. *J. Lab. Clin. Med.* 43:802–812, 1954.
87. Spargo, B. H.: Pathologic lesions producing nephrotic syndrome. *Monogr. Pathol.* 20:56–75, 1979.
88. Stanton, B. A., and Giebisch, G. H.: Potassium transport by the renal distal tubule. *Am. J. Physiol.* 243:F487–F493, 1982.
89. Stockigt, J. R.: Potassium metabolism. *Anesth Intensive Care* 5:317–325, 1977.
90. Struthers, A. D., Reid, J. L., Whitesmith, R., and Rodgers, J. C.: The effects of cardio-selective and non-selective beta-adrenoreceptor blockade on the hypokalemic and cardiovascular responses to adrenomedullary hormones. *Clin. Sci. (London)* 65:143–148, 1983.
91. Tannen, R.: Relationship of renal ammonia production and potassium homeostasis. *Kidney Int.* 11:453–465, 1977.
92. Tate, C. L., Bagdon, W. J., and Bokelman, D. L.: Morphologic abnormalities in potassium deficient dogs. *Am. J. Pathol.* 93:103–116, 1978.
93. Toback, F. G., Ordonez, N. G., Bortz, S. L., and Spargo, B. H.: Zonal change in renal structure and phospholipid metabolism in potassium deficient rats. *Lab. Invest.* 34:115–121, 1976.
94. Toback, F. G., Aithal, H. N., Ordinez, N. G., and Spargo, B. H.: Altered bioeñergetics in proliferating renal cells during potassium depletion. *Lab. Invest.* 41:265–267, 1979.
95. Toback, F. G., Havener, L. J., and Spargo, B. H.: Stimulation of renal phospholipid formation during potassium depletion. *Am. J. Physiol.* 233:E212–E216, 1977.
96. Toback, F. G., Havener, L. J., Dodd, R. C., and Spargo, B. H.: Phospholipid metabolism during renal regeneration after acute tubular necrosis. *Am. J. Physiol.* 232:216–222, 1977.
97. Trump, B. F.: Ion movement in cell injury. Proceedings, 4th International Congress on Nephrology, Stockholm, Vol. 1, Basel, Karger, 1970, pp. 88–101.
98. Trump, B. F., and Ginn, F. L.: Studies of cellular injury in isolated flounder tubules. II. Cellular swelling in high potassium media. *Lab. Invest.* 18:341–51, 1968.
99. Trump, B. F., Strum, J. M., and Bulger, R. E.: Studies on the pathogenesis of

ischemic cell injury. I. Relation between ion and water shifts and ultraastructure in rat kidney slices during swelling at 0–4 degrees C. *Virchows Arch.* [*Cell Pathol*] 16:1–34, 1974.

100. Welt, L. G., Hollander, W., and Blythe, W. B.: The consequences of potassium depletion. *J. Chron. Dis.* 11:213–254, 1960.
101. Wener, J., Pietruschkar, F., and Simon, M. A.: The effect of prolonged hypomagnesia on the cardiovascular system of young dogs. *Am. Heart J.* 67:221–229, 1964.
102. Whang, R.: *Potassium: Its Biological Significance*, Boca Raton, CRC Press, Inc., 1983.
103. Wright, F. S.: Sites and mechanism of potassium transport along the renal tubule. *Kidney Int.* 11:415–432, 1977.
104. Zeluff, G. W., Suki, W. N., and Jackson, D.: Depletion of body phosphate—ubiquitous, subtle, dangerous (Clinical Conference). *Heart Lung* 6:519–522, 1977.

HYPOKALEMIA AND CARDIAC ARRHYTHMIAS DURING ACUTE MYOCARDIAL INFARCTION

12

Relationship Between Initial Serum Potassium Values and Cardiac Arrhythmias in Patients with Acute Myocardial Infarction

WARREN D. COOPER and MALCOLM J. VANDENBURG*
Merck Sharp & Dohme, Ltd., Hoddesdon, Hertfordshire, England

The possibility that an easily measurable biochemical marker could predict the subsequent development of a life-threatening cardiac arrhythmia, in patients with acute myocardial infarction, merits the attention of practicing physicians. The recent appearance in the literature of several reports (1,4-7,10,11,15) concerning the significant relationship between the serum potassium level at admission and the occurrence of cardiac arrhythmias after myocardial infarction would appear to represent just such a situation. There has also been a suggestion that low potassium may be related to early mortality (6,12) though this is far from being confirmed.

The link between potassium and arrhythmias is theoretically predictable from basic electrophysiological considerations. The serum potassium level, however, is not a static variable but one that is known to change rapidly in acute illness (9) and that can also be modified by exogenous factors such as diet or drugs, particularly diuretics (8). The occurrence of cardiac arrhythmias as a consequence of the serum potassium level in patients with acute myocardial infarction may be complicated by factors other than these two primary variables. This report reviews the possible association between potassium and arrhythmias in the context of other potentially relevant factors.

PATIENTS AND METHODS

The case records of 1,395 consecutive patients admitted to the coronary care units of two large district general hospitals have been retrospectively reviewed. Five hundred and eighty-six patient records were drawn from East Birmingham Hospital and 809 from the Royal United Hospital in Bath. Patients considered in this review had a confirmed acute myocardial infarction (AMI) diagnosed on the basis of a history of chest pain, sequential ST and T wave changes on the electrocardiogram, and an associated rise in the level of serum glutamic oxalacetic transaminase (SGOT). The development of pathological Q

**Current affiliation*: Oldchurch and Rush Green Hospitals, Romford, Essex, England waves was not mandatory for the diagnosis of AMI. These patients also had blood taken for estimation of serum electrolytes on admission. All data reported here relate to blood samples obtained prior to any acute drug use in the coronary care unit, other than analgesics.

All patients had precordial electrocardiographic monitoring for a minimum of 24 hr. Tape recording facilities for storage of cardiac rhythm data were not available in these centers. All arrhythmias observed by nursing or medical staff were noted and samples of the rhythm disturbance were stored in the case notes when feasible.

The data from each of the two centers showed a relationship between potassium and arrhythmias (5,15) and, because of the complex interactions found, it was considered appropriate to combine the information to create a larger data base. Other factors found to be potentially relevant and available have now been examined and include age, sex, and history of diuretic therapy prior to admission. Neither the effects of the time delay from onset of symptoms to hospital admission, nor the type, dosage, and length of therapy with previously prescribed diuretics, nor the reason for which they had originally been prescribed have been evaluated. Insufficient results of cardiac enzyme assays precluded attempts to correlate our arrhythmia and potassium findings with "infarct size."

DATA ANALYSIS

We report here the combined results from two district hospitals after the information from each data set was analyzed separately (5,15). Both data sets were comparable in the distribution of patients' age, sex, diuretic use, potassium values, and incidence of arrhythmias. The primary method by which these data were analyzed has been fully reported (5).

Following this analysis of the relationship between arrhythmias and potassium, the influence of age, sex, and prior use of diuretics was examined with regard to the distribution of potassium values and the occurrence of arrhythmias. After we examined each of the possible combinations of any two of these five variables, a multivariate analysis was performed using a logistic regression method.

RESULTS

The 1,395 patient case records contained 1,103 men (79.1%) with a mean age of 62.1 years and 277 women (19.9%) with a mean age of 57.6 years. Matched age and sex data were missing for 15 individuals (1%).

Potassium and Arrhythmias

In the entire study population of 1,395 cases, the initial potassium values were normally distributed (Figure 1). When the findings are divided according to whether or not an arrhythmia occurred, the two distributions of potassium values were different and neither was normal. The distribution of potassium values in those patients who had an arrhythmia was skewed to the right (Figure 2) whereas those with no subsequent arrhythmia had a pattern of values skewed to the left (Figure 3). For this reason simple statistical comparisons between the two groups with regard to potassium may be misleading without prior data transformation. This is further confirmed by the effect of this transformation on the statistical significance of the comparison of the mean potassium values for the arrhythmia

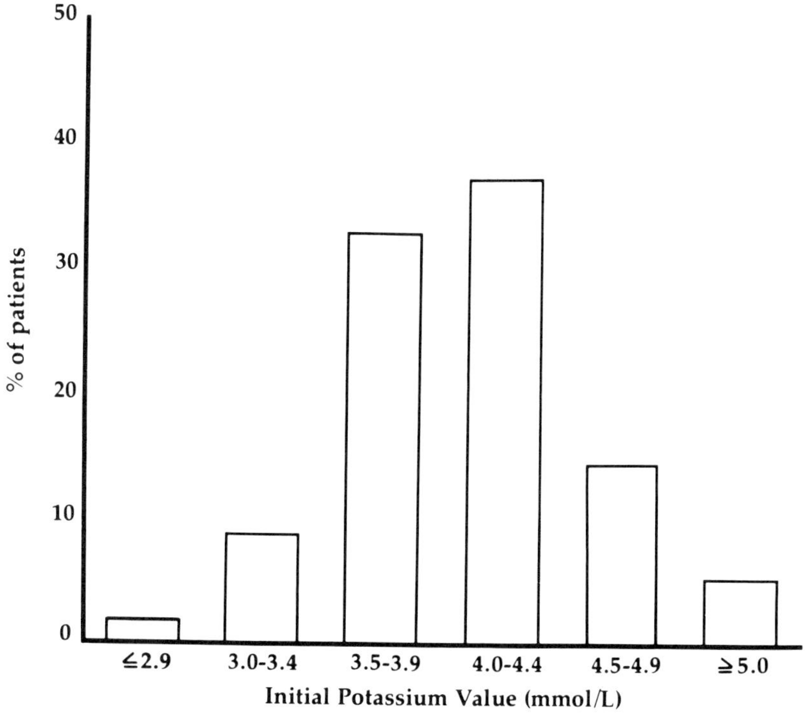

Figure 1 Distribution of initial serum potassium values for all patients.

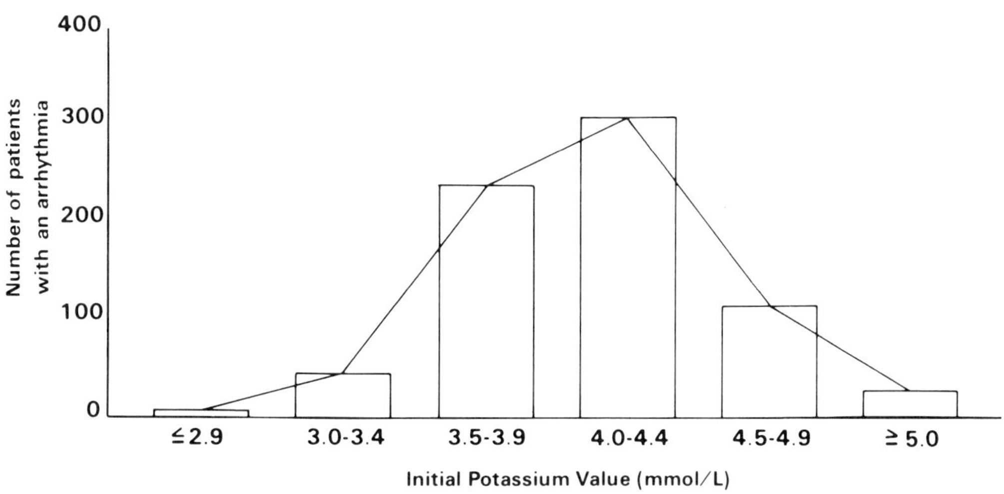

Figure 2 Distribution curve of initial serum potassium values for patients with an arrhythmia.

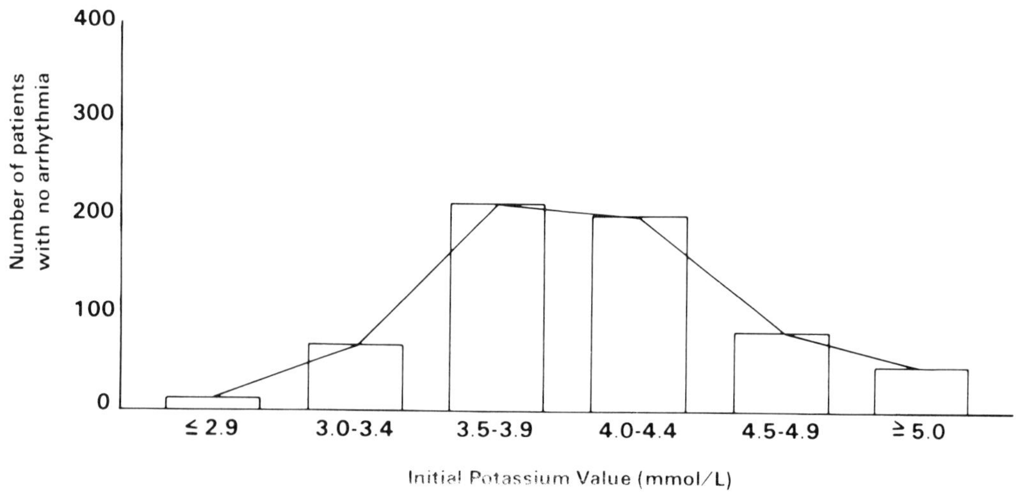

Figure 3 Distribution curve of initial serum potassium values for patients with no arrhythmia.

and nonarrhythmia groups. When nontransformed data were used, the mean potassium values of the arrhythmic group (4.09 ± 0.48 mmol/L) and the nonarrhythmic group (4.05 ± 0.62 mmol/L) were not significantly different from each other. However, after logarithmic transformation, the mean log serum potassiums were significantly different ($p<0.005$).

The distribution of patients with any arrhythmia compared to those with no arrhythmia was significantly different across the range of initial potassium values ($X^2 = 35.88$, $p<0.001$). This is represented in Figure 4; partitioned analysis revealed that the incidence of arrhythmias was significantly greater at potassium levels of <3.9 and >5.0 mmol/L when compared to the incidence in the 4.0–4.9 mmol/L range.

Figure 5 again shows the potential error of comparing mean potassium values between groups of patients. The U-shaped nature of the distribution of patients with an arrhythmia yielded a mean potassium value very similar to that of the nonarrhythmia group, despite their different and reciprocal-shaped curves.

Examination of the incidence of specific arrhythmias with respect to potassium showed that the strongest association occurred for ventricular fibrillation, ($X^2 = 81.42$, $p<0.001$). The incidence of ventricular fibrillation was significantly increased in potassium ranges <3.9 mmol/L and >5.0 mmol/L compared to the range 4.0–4.9 mmol/L (Figure 6).

The incidence of premature ventricular beats was also significantly increased when the potassium level was <3.9 mmol/L ($X^2 = 25.17$, $p<0.001$) (Figure 7). The incidence of complete heart block was increased the higher the potassium value ($X^2 = 45.43$, $p<0.001$) (Figure 8). No other specific arrhythmia bore a significant relationship to potassium, as determined by this method of analysis.

Age and Arrhythmias

The incidence of arrhythmias, considered in total, increased with age as shown in Figure 9 ($X^2 = 27.36$, $p<0.001$). The relationship was mainly a result of a significantly higher

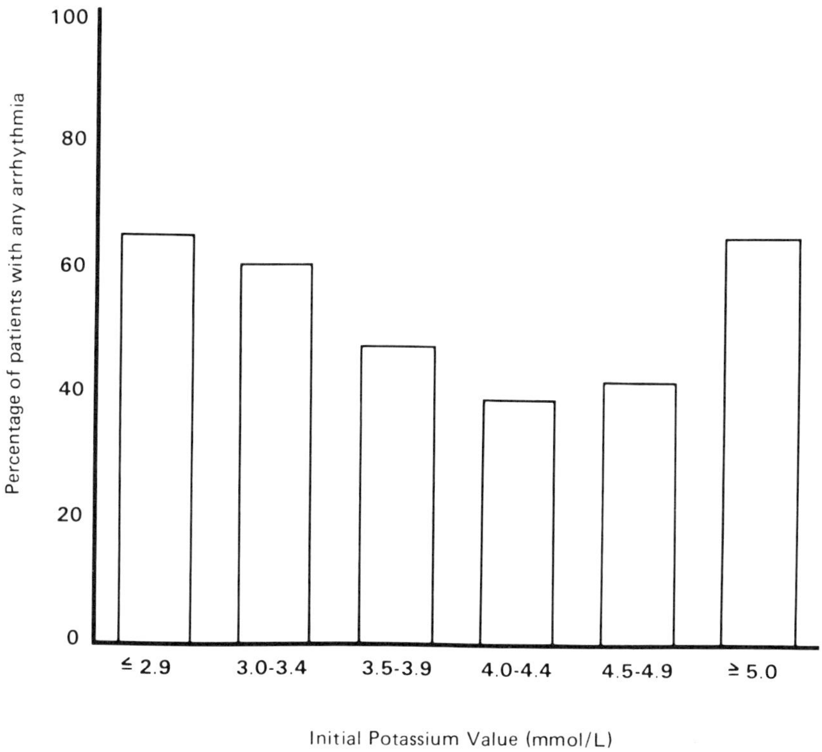

Figure 4 Incidence of arrhythmias relative to initial serum potassium value.

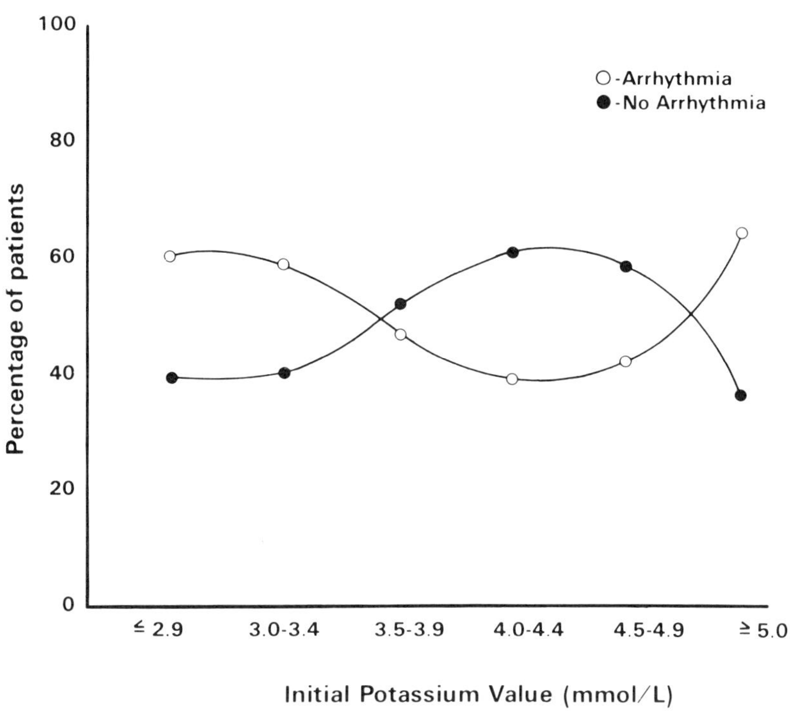

Figure 5 Comparative incidence of patients with or without an arrhythmia relative to initial serum potassium value.

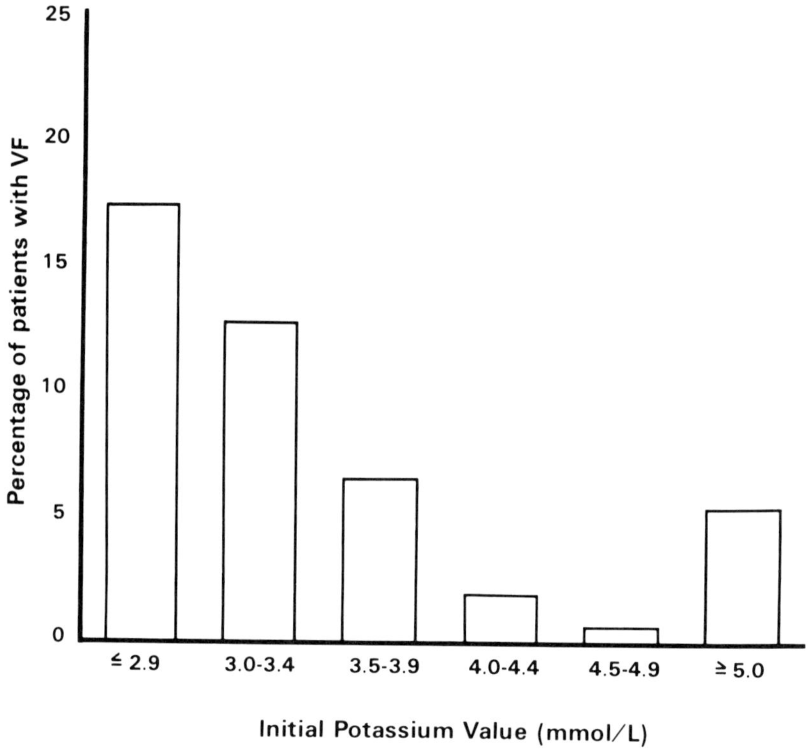

Figure 6 Incidence of ventricular fibrillation relative to initial serum potassium value.

incidence of arrhythmias in patients over 70 years of age. In particular, complete heart block (7.5% in the elderly vs. 2.3 in those under 70), interventricular conduction defects (6.3% vs. 2.9%), and atrial fibrillation (10.9% vs. 3.7%) were significantly more common in patients over 70.

Age and Potassium

The mean potassium value was not significantly different across each decile of the age range in this study. It varied only from 4.02 ± 0.48 mmol/L in the patients aged 30-39 years to 4.10 ± 0.64 mmol/L in those aged 70-79 years. Despite this, analysis of the categorical data for age and potassium showed a significant but complex relationship.

Age and Diuretics

The frequency of a positive history of preadmission diuretic use increased with age (X^2 = 21.55, $p<0.001$) being found in 0.02% of those less than 40 years old and 17.2% in those over 70 (Figure 10).

Sex and Potassium

Figure 11 shows a cumulative distribution curve for initial potassium values for men and women. These curves were significantly different from one another ($p<0.001$), showing

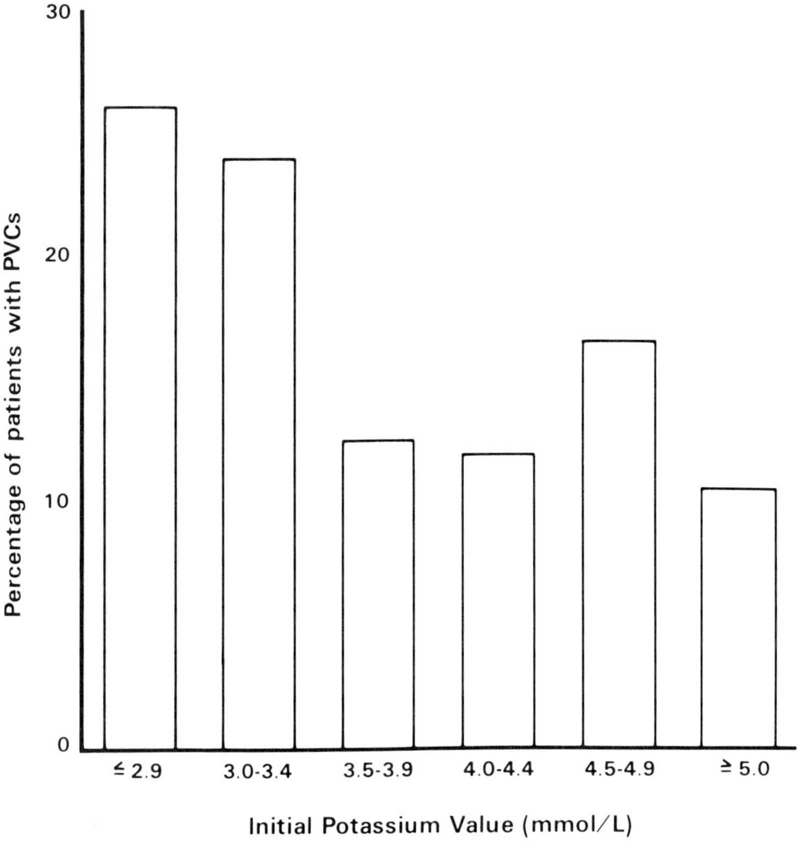

Figure 7 Incidence of premature ventricular beats relative to initial serum potassium value.

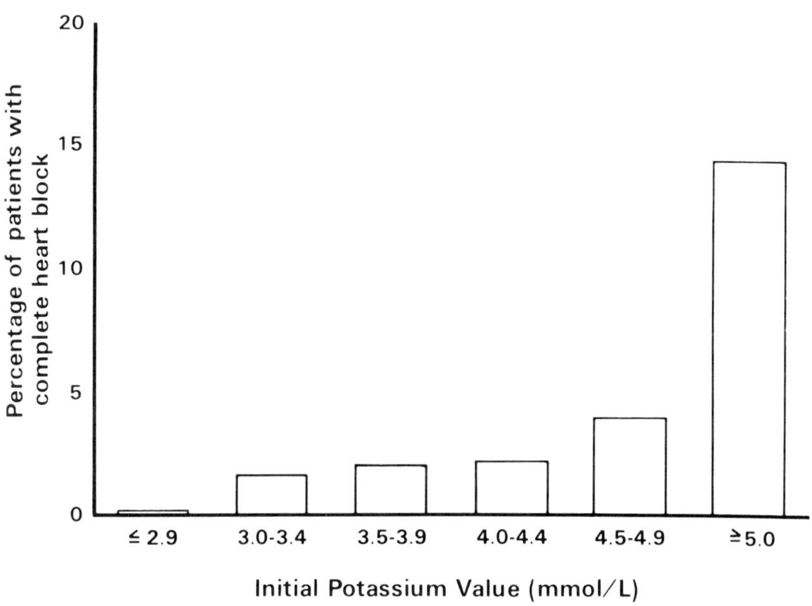

Figure 8 Incidence of complete heart block relative to initial serum potassium value.

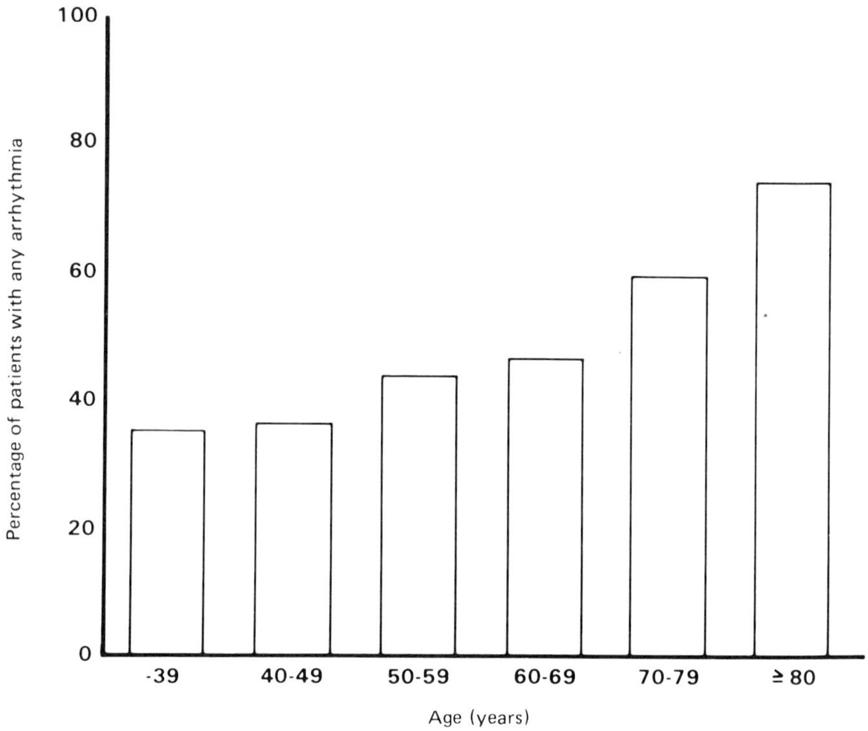

Figure 9 Incidence of arrhythmias relative to age.

that women tended to have lower serum potassium values. The mean potassium value in women was 3.98 ± 0.56 mmol/L, which was significantly lower than that for men: 4.09 ± 0.53 mmol/L ($p<0.001$).

Sex and Diuretics

The level of diuretic use determined in this study was low; 10.5% of all patients overall. However, proportionally more women (17.7%) than men (8.9%) were taking a diuretic prior to admission and this difference was highly significant ($X^2 = 18.03$, $p<0.001$).

Sex and Arrhythmias

More women (50.2%) had an arrhythmia than did men (44.8%), but this difference did not reach statistical significance.

Potassium and Diuretics

Figure 12 shows the distribution curves of potassium values for those patients taking a diuretic prior to admission compared to those with no history of diuretic use. The curve is shifted significantly to the left for those taking a diuretic. The incidence of hypokalemia, defined as a potassium value of less than 3.5 mmol/L, was 8.8% in those not taking a diuretic and 20.4% in those taking a diuretic ($X^2 = 19.58$, $p<0.001$).

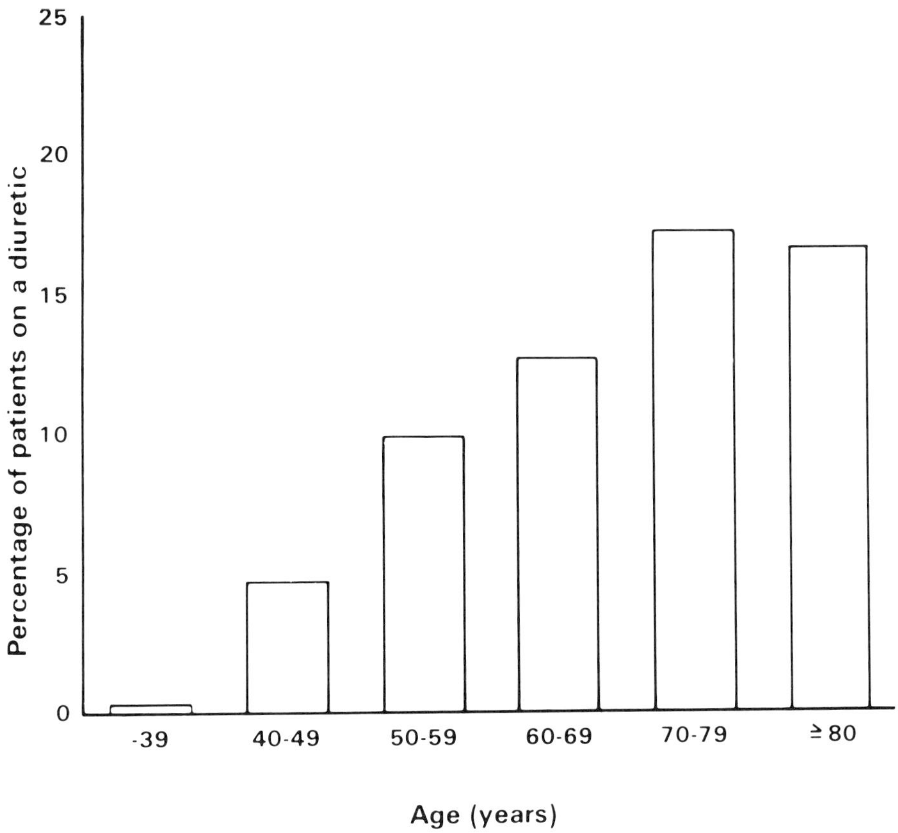

Figure 10 Prevalence of diuretic usage relative to age.

Diuretics and Arrhythmias

More patients previously taking a diuretic exhibited an arrhythmia during the first 24 hr after hospital admission. Of those with a history of diuretic use 59.1% had an arrhythmia, compared to an incidence of 44.1% of those with no such history ($X^2 = 12.11$, $p<0.001$). Furthermore, the highest incidence of arrhythmias (70%) occurred in those taking a diuretic who also had a potassium value below 3.5 mmol/L.

Overall Analysis

The above results in which pairs of variables were compared demonstrated several significant associations, thus making a more complex multivariate analysis not only appropriate but highly necessary. (The complex interrelationship of these major variables is summarized in Table 1.)

A logistic regression analysis was performed considering age, sex, potassium value, diuretic history, and occurrence of arrhythmia. For the reasons given above concerning the failure of the curve of potassium values to be normally distributed, logarithmically transformed potassium values were used in the multivariate analysis in addition to the categorical values: <2.9, 3.0–3.4, etc.

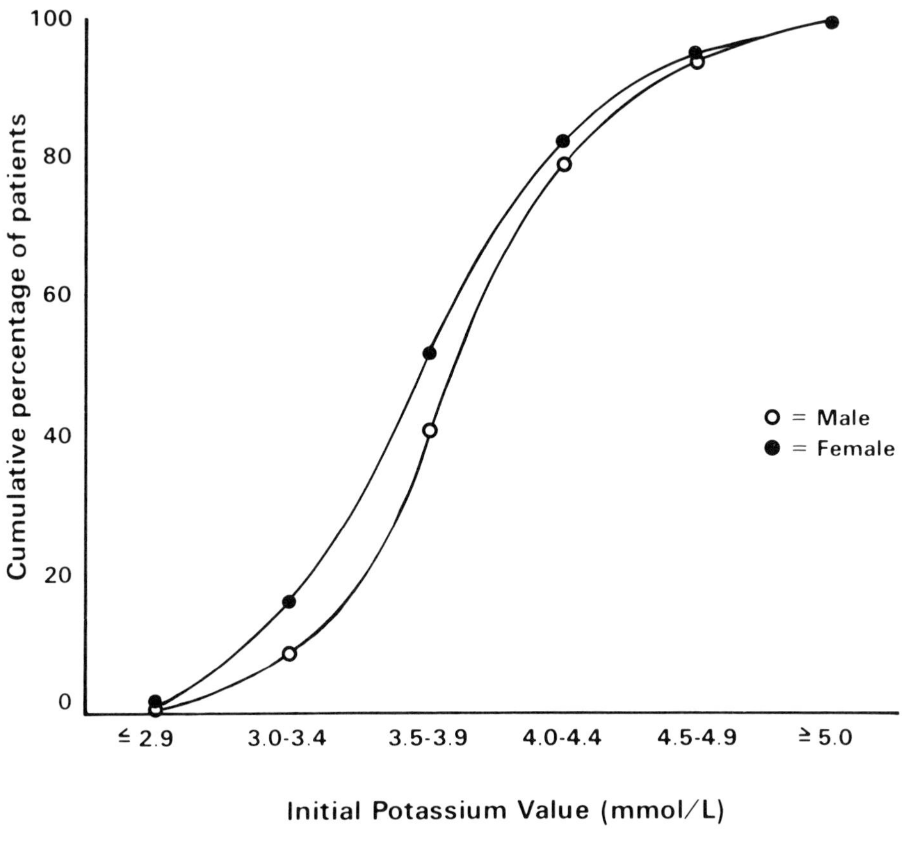

Figure 11 Distribution curve of initial serum potassium values relative to sex.

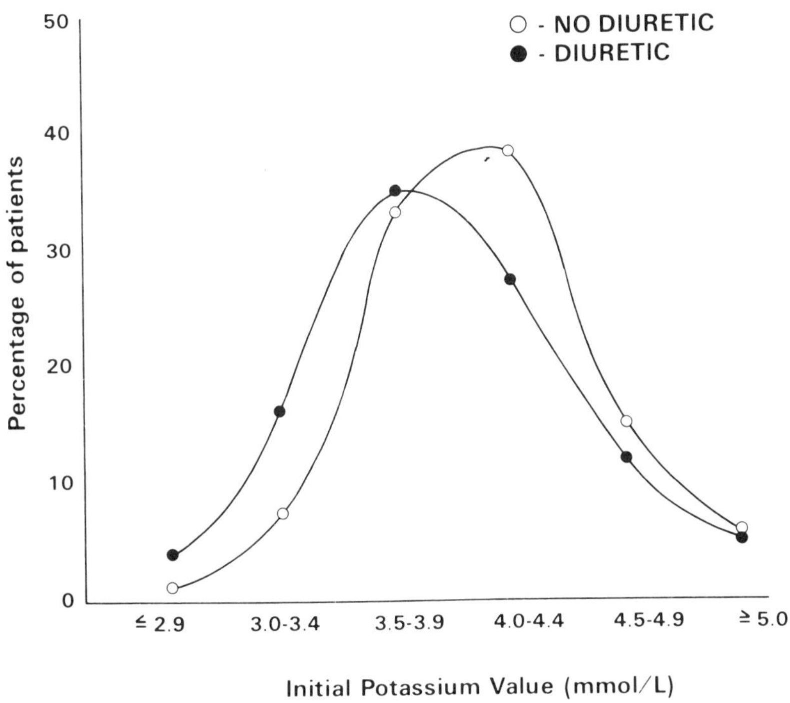

Figure 12 Distribution curves of initial serum potassium values relative to diuretic use.

Table 1 Interrelationships Among Major Study Variables

	Age	Sex	Potassium	Diuretics	Arrhythmias
Age	–	Women were older[a]	Complex[a]	Increased use with age[a]	More common in old[a]
Sex		–	Women had lower K levels[a]	More women were taking diuretics[a]	More common in women
Potassium			–	K level lower in patients taking diuretics[a]	More common with low K level[a]
Diuretics				–	More common in patients taking diuretics[a]
Arrhythmias					–

[a]Significant interaction

The results of this analysis showed that three variables were independently and significantly associated with the occurrence of arrhythmias: age ($p<0.0125$), serum potassium level ($p<0.0001$), and diuretic use ($p<0.0125$). The significance of the potassium association occurred irrespective of whether logarithmic potassium or categorical potassium values were used.

DISCUSSION

The various analytical methods we have used to examine these data confirm the previously described relationship between the initial serum potassium level and the subsequent occurrence of early cardiac arrhythmias after patients are admitted to hospital for acute myocardial infarction. This relationship is far more complex than has previously been recognized, or reported, and may reflect a failure to appreciate the possible interaction of other major variables.

We believe that the relationship between potassium and arrhythmias in this clinical setting is complex because the potassium values in those who had an arrhythmia, as well as in the group who had no arrhythmias, were not normally distributed. This makes it inappropriate to compare the group mean potassium values without prior transformation of the data. Using mean potassium is again inappropriate because the highest incidences of arrhythmias occurred at the two extremes of the potassium distribution curve, resulting in a U-shaped curve. Analytical handling of such a distribution is complex.

Within this U-shaped distribution are likely to be different causative factors influencing the relationship between potassium and arrhythmias, as evidenced by the equally significant but different patterns of the incidence of ventricular fibrillation and complete heart block with respect to potassium. It is difficult to group together all cases of ventricular fibrillation as having a common link to potassium, since the incidence of this arrhythmia is increased at the two extremes of the potassium range. Although our cases of ventricular fibrillation (VF) cannot at this stage be divided into primary or secondary forms, differences in the relationship to potassium of these forms of VF with different causes have previously been reported (3).

We have shown that age is a strong, independent variable that influences the occurrence of cardiac arrhythmias irrespective of the potassium value. Wilcox and Hampton (16) have reported that age is an important predictor of early mortality after hospital admission for definite or probable myocardial infarction. However, the extent of the interaction between age and the other major variables is difficult to ascertain from our data. Furthermore, it is possible that bias in admission policy may have influenced our results with regard to the extent of the effect of age. Some very elderly patients may not have been admitted to the hospital but have been cared for at home or within geriatric institutions. If admitted to hospital, they may not have been referred for coronary care unless an arrhythmia or other complication had occurred while they were in a general ward. Nevertheless, so strong was the influence of age on arrhythmias in our analysis that we believe this correlation to be a real finding.

Similarly, the history of prior diuretic therapy significantly influenced the occurrence of arrhythmias, independent of the admission potassium value. The question is immediately raised as to whether this is only because diuretics lower the serum potassium value or because of some other inherent metabolic property. The significant degree to which the distribution curve of potassium values was shifted to the left in the diuretic-treated group would tend to support the former view. Diuretic use may also be a reflection of the underlying disease for which the drug was initially prescribed, for example hypertension or cardiac failure, and such disease states could themselves influence the occurrence of arrhythmias. However, Nesje (10) has reported that the incidence of early postinfarction arrhythmias was the same in hypertensive patients and those with heart failure, not treated with diuretics, compared to those with no such previous disease. He also reported that the incidence of arrhythmias was higher in those patients with hypertension or heart failure who had received diuretics. To answer properly this question of how diuretics are influencing the occurrence of arrhythmias, one has to consider not only the absolute serum potassium level but also the change in the potassium level from before the onset of infarction and also from that level before diuretic therapy. These requirements obviously have practical limitations. However, based on electrophysiological considerations relating the ratio of the serum potassium value to the level within the myocardium, a large change in the former, from 5.0 to 4.0 mmol/L, while staying within the "normal range,"could influence membrane potential to as great an extent as a change of similar magnitude from the "normal" to the "abnormal" range, for example, 4.0 to 3.0 mmol/L.

Increased levels of circulating catecholamines, which are known to occur at the time of acute infarction, in some direct proportion to infarct extent, have a rapid potassium-lowering effect (3,16). This is likely to be of considerable relevance to this subject particularly since the hypokalemic tendencies of catecholamines and diuretics appear to be additive (13).

Perhaps the most important findings from our study are methodological and analytical. We believe that our initial approach, similarly to that used in the previously published relevant literature, failed to appreciate the complexity of interactions of other variables. We would urge other workers in this field to use a multivariate analytical approach to their data on the grounds that this is more realistic.

Our work supports a link between a lowered potassium level and arrhythmias following myocardial infarction and demonstrates that other factors, such as age and diuretics, may also be influential.

ACKNOWLEDGMENTS

We wish to thank Dr. R. D. Thomas of the Royal United Hospital, Bath, and Dr. S. R. Reuben, formerly of the East Birmingham Hospital, for allowing us to use data from their patients.

REFERENCES

1. Beck, O. A., and Hochrein, H.: Serum potassium levels and cardiac arrhythmias in acute myocardial infarction. *Z. Kardiol* 66:187–190, 1977.
2. Brown, M. J., Brown, D. C., and Murphy, D.: Adrenaline associated hypokalemia and tachycardia are selectively antagonised by β-2 receptor blockade in man. *Clin. Sci.* 64:71P, 1981.
3. Campbell, R. W. F.: Plasma potassium levels and ventricular fibrillation in acute myocardial infarction. *Int. Med.* Suppl. 4:10–11, 1983.
4. Cole, A. G., Arkin, D., and Solomon, R.: Arrhythmias and myocardial infarction: The role of potassium. In *Arrhythmias and Myocardial Infarction: The Role of Potassium*, edited by Wood, C., and Somerville, W., Royal Society of Medicine International Congress and Symposium Series No. 44:47–53, 1981.
5. Cooper, W. D., Kuan, P., Reuben, S. R., and VandenBurg, M. J.: Cardiac arrhythmias

following acute myocardial infarction: associations with the serum potassium level and prior diuretic therapy. *Eur. Heart J.* 5:464–469, 1984.

6. Dyckner, T., Helmers, C., Ludman, T., and Wester, P. O.: Initial serum potassium level in relation to early complications and prognosis in patients with acute myocardial infarction. *Acta Med. Scand.* 197:207–210, 1975.
7. Hulting, J.: In-hospital ventricular fibrillation and its relation to serum potassium. *Acta Med. Scand.* Suppl. 647:109–116, 1981.
8. Morgan, D. B., and Davidson, C.: Hypokalaemia and diuretics: an analysis of publications. *Br. Med. J.* 280:905–908, 1980.
9. Morgan, D. B., and Young, R. M.: Acute transient hypokalaemia: new interpretation of a common event. *Lancet* 2:751–752, 1982.
10. Nesje, O. A.: Hypokalaemia and arrhythmias after myocardial infarction in patients receiving prolonged treatment with diuretics. *Tidsskr. Nor. Laegeforen.* 24:1257–1259, 1976.
11. Nordrehaug, J. E.: Serum potassium and arrhythmias in acute myocardial infarction: a preliminary report. In *Arrhythmias and Myocardial Infarction: The Role of Potassium*, edited by Wood, C., and Somerville, W., Royal Society of Medicine International Congress and Symposium Series No. 44:83–86, 1981.
12. Rao, S. K.: The arrhythmic danger of hypokalaemia. *Curr. Med. Res. Opin.* (Supp. 1):83–86, 1982.
13. Struthers, A. D., Reid, J. L., Whitesmith, R., and Rodger, J. C.: The effect of intravenous adrenaline on the blood pressure, electrocardiogram and serum electrolytes. *Br. Heart J.* 49:90–93, 1983.
14. Struthers, A. D., Whitesmith, R., and Reid, J. L.: Prior thiazide diuretic treatment increases adrenaline-induced hypokalaemia. *Lancet* 1:1358–1361, 1983.
15. Thomas, R., and Hicks, S.: Myocardial infarction: ventricular arrhythmias associated with hypokalaemia. *Clin. Sci.* 60:32P, 1981.
16. Wilcox, R. G., and Hampton, J. R.: Importance of age in prehospital and hospital mortality of heart attacks. *Br. Heart J.* 44:503–507, 1980.

13

Importance of Potassium in the Development of Arrhythmias During Acute Myocardial Infarction

RICHARD J. SOLOMON
Brown University Program in Medicine, Roger Williams General Hospital, and Veterans Administration Medical Center, Providence, Rhode Island

There is little controversy concerning the ability of several electrolyte disturbances to promote cardiac arrhythmias. The central issue is to determine whether the frequently occurring electrolyte disturbances produce clinically significant rhythm disturbances. Patients with coronary heart disease are a group frequently focused upon in investigations of this effect. These are the patients who are most at risk for the development of clinically serious arrhythmias. For example, 80% of sudden death victims (presumably resulting from ventricular fibrillation) have evidence of significant coronary heart disease (1). The large numbers of these patients not only make clinical studies of the relationship between arrhythmias and electrolyte disturbances feasible but also highlight the potential importance of this information. Nearly 360,000 deaths each year are attributable to the sudden death syndrome and sudden death continues to be the leading cause of mortality in men over the age of 20 years (4). Because of the often catastrophic nature of these sudden arrhythmias, efforts to identify modifiable risk factors are clearly necessary for the development of preventive strategies. Electrolyte disturbances might be particularly good targets for such preventive efforts because they are easily and inexpensively identified and treated.

While the focus of this chapter is on patients with acute myocardial infarctions, the results can likely be extrapolated to others with less severe ischemic heart disease. This derives from the fact that the infarcted tissue is electrically inert and does not directly contribute to the pathogenesis of the arrhythmias. Arrhythmias probably have their origin in the areas of electrically viable but ischemic tissue.

METHODS

We examined retrospectively the hospital records of 153 patients consecutively treated between 1976 and 1978 for acute myocardial infarction at the Roger Williams General Hospital and the Veterans Administration Medical Center, Providence, Rhode Island. Myocardial infarction was documented by appropriate serum enzyme elevations and serial electrocardiographic abnormalities. The muscle-brain fraction of creatine phosphokinase was present in serum of all patients studied. Patients were initially admitted to the coronary care or the intensive care units and underwent constant electrocardiographic monitoring for the first 3 hospital days. All arrhythmias were documented by evaluation of an oscilloscope representation and/or automatically recorded rhythm strips.

The following information was extracted from the hospital charts: the nature and frequency of all ventricular arrhythmias, the level of serum potassium at admission, and the serum potassium level at the time of any arrhythmia. Serum potassium was determined within 12 hr of the ventricular arrhythmia in most cases. When this level was not available, the level closest in time to the occurrence of the arrhythmia was recorded. In addition, the use of potassium-wasting diuretics and cardiac glycosides either prior to admission or within the first 3 hospital days was noted. Serum potassium levels were measured by flame photometry. Patients were considered hypokalemic when serum potassium was 3.5 mmol/L or less.

Arrhythmias included in the study were as follows:

1. Ventricular tachycardia (three or more beats of ventricular origin at a rate greater than 150 bpm) or fibrillation occurring at any time during the hospital course, or
2. VPBs occurring more frequently than three/min during the first 3 days of hospitalization

VPBs occurring after the first 72 hr were excluded, because constant electrocardiographic monitoring of all patients was not performed after the 3rd hospital day. Two records were omitted from the study because the patients died of cardiogenic shock on the day of hospitalization. Statistical analysis was performed by the X^2 technique, using the Yates correction factor.

RESULTS

Twenty-one of the 151 patients studied (14%) had a serum potassium level of 3.5 mmol/L or less. The mean age of the hypokalemic patients was not different from that of the normokalemic patients (60 vs. 64 years, respectively). A similar distribution of male and female patients was also seen in the two groups (Table 1).

There were 64 patients taking diuretics of whom 15 (23%) were hypokalemic. In contrast, there were only 6 hypokalemic patients among 87 (7%) patients not receiving

Table 1 Incidence of Ventricular Arrhythmias in Patients with Acute Myocardial Infarction

	Normokalemic (N=130)	Hypokalemic (N=21)
Age (years)	64	60
Male (%)	81	86
Arrhythmia (%)		
VPB[a]	35	36
VT/VF[b]	21	48[c]

[a]VPB, ventricular premature beats without VT/VF.
[b]VT/VF, ventricular tachycardia and/or ventricular fibrillation.
[c]$p < 0.01$ by χ^2 test with Yates correction.

diuretics ($p < 0.01$). Thus, a history of diuretic use was associated with a threefold increase in the incidence of hypokalemia.

A total of 37 patients (25%) experienced ventricular tachycardia or fibrillation. Ten of 21 hypokalemic patients (48%), compared to 27 of 130 normokalemic patients (21%), had ventricular tachycardia or fibrillation ($p < 0.01$). Thus, malignant ventricular arrhythmias occurred 2.3 times more often in the hypokalemic patients than in normokalemic patients (Table 1). The likelihood of ventricular arrhythmia was inversely related to the level of serum potassium. As shown in Figure 1, the highest frequency of ventricular arrhythmia was found among those patients with the lowest serum potassium levels. Among those with serum potassium levels $\leqslant 3.0$ mmol/L, 67% experienced ventricular tachycardia or fibrillation, compared to 40% of those with serum potassium levels between 3.1 and 3.5 mmol/L and 20% of normokalemic patients. An increase in ventricular tachycardia and fibrillation was also noted among those patients with a serum potassium level > 5 mmol/L, although to a lesser extent than that found in the hypokalemic group. However, two patients had serum potassium levels > 6.5 mmol/L and did not experience arrhythmias.

Hypokalemia was not associated with an increased incidence of VPBs. Among those without either ventricular tachycardia or ventricular fibrillation, 36 of 103 normokalemic patients (35%) had VPBs, compared to 4 of 11 hypokalemic patients (36%) (Table 1).

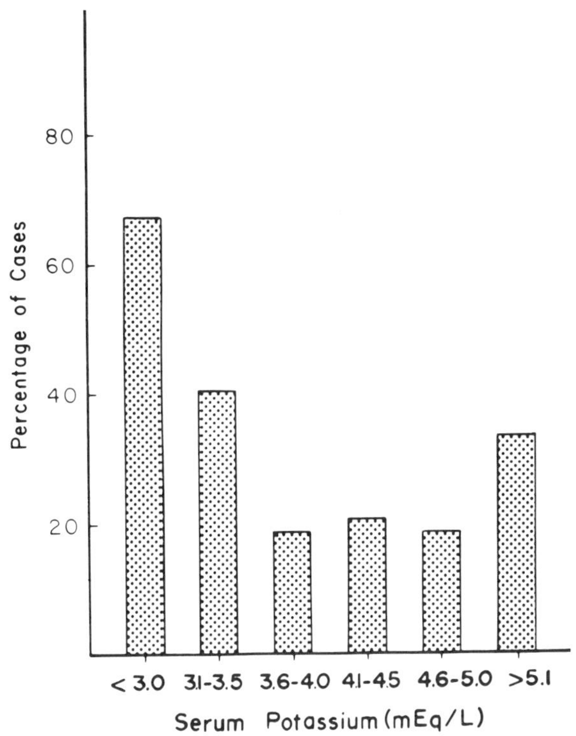

Figure 1 The relationship between the level of serum potassium (mmol/L) and the incidence of ventricular tachycardia and/or ventricular fibrillation in 151 patients with acute myocardial infarction.

Table 2 Ventricular Tachycardia and Fibrillation: Role of Diuretic Treatment

	Using diuretics	Not using diuretics
Mean serum potassium level (mmol/L)	4.29	4.27
Frequency of VT/VF (%)	19	23

These results suggest a relationship between hypokalemia and serious ventricular arrhythmias. However, since 71% of the hypokalemic patients had received diuretics, in contrast to only 40% of the normokalemic patients, a possible adverse effect of diuretics unrelated to potassium was considered. For example, patients receiving diuretic treatment may have a more severe or complicated cardiac condition which might increase the likelihood of severe ventricular arrhythmias independently of electrolyte disturbances. To address this possible complicating effect, we looked at the relationship between diuretic usage and arrhythmias when hypokalemia was not present.

In this group, 12 of 52 patients (23%) taking diuretics experienced arrhythmias compared to 15 of 78 patients (19%) not taking diuretics (Table 2). While the numbers are admittedly small, they do not suggest an association between diuretic use and ventricular arrhythmias which is related to the underlying cardiac condition for which diuretics were prescribed. That the hypokalemia itself is the key factor is demonstrated by the finding of a similar incidence of severe arrhythmia in hypokalemic patients not taking diuretics as in those receiving diuretic treatment.

The possible influence of concomitant therapy with cardiac glycosides on this relationship between ventricular arrhythmias and serum potassium was also considered. Patients receiving digitalis may be at increased risk for the development of arrhythmias in the presence of hypokalemia. Forty-two percent of the patients took cardiac glycosides during the study. Ventricular tachycardia and ventricular fibrillation occurred with equal frequency in the presence and absence of concomitant digitalis administration (Table 3). An increase in serious arrhythmias was noted in the hypokalemic patients not taking digitalis. Such arrhythmias accounted for the majority seen in this study. In patients who were receiving digitalis, hypokalemia was not associated with an increased incidence of ventricular tachyarrhythmias. A particularly high incidence of arrhythmias was noted in this group, however, which may have obscured any effect of hypokalemia. This may have resulted from a more severe underlying cardiac status (necessitating digitalis treatment) or a pharmacological effect of digitalis itself. Whatever the explanation of this observation, the important point is that patients not taking digitalis are at risk for the development of serious arrhythmias when hypokalemia is present.

Table 3 Ventricular Tachycardia and Fibrillation: Role of Digitalis

	Frequency of VT/VF (%)	
	Patients using digitalis	Patients not using digitalis
Normokalemic	30	14
Hypokalemic	20	38[a]

[a]$p < 0.05$ compared to normokalemic group.

DISCUSSION

A number of similar studies have now been reported encompassing a total of nearly 4,000 patients (2,3,6-9,11) (Table 4). In all these studies, an increase in the incidence of serious ventricular arrhythmias has been noted in hypokalemic patients. Such data do not necessarily mean that hypokalemia caused the arrhythmias, however. For example, hypokalemia may simply be a marker of catecholamine secretion. Since beta agonists facilitate potassium movement into cells, the lowest serum potassium levels might be associated with the highest levels of serum catecholamines (10). The high serum catecholamine levels may be the primary arrhythmogenic factor rather than the low potassium. Arguing against this interpretation is the considerable data in animals and humans that hypokalemia per se is capable of increasing myocardial irritability. Until further observations on the relationship between serum catecholamines and serum potassium are available in patients with ischemic heart disease, hypokalemia must be considered to have primary arrhythmogenic potential.

If hypokalemia is indeed a factor contributing to the development of serious arrhythmias in patients with acute myocardial infarctions, what implications does this have for patients with less severe forms of ischemic heart disease? In one large study, Hulting found a similar inverse relationship between the serum potassium level and the incidence of ventricular fibrillation in patients admitted with angina but without evidence of acute infarction (3). This suggests that the arrhythmia risks related to hypokalemia extend to patients with lesser degrees of ischemic heart disease.

Still, the clinical importance of potassium disturbances as a risk factor for serious ventricular arrhythmias cannot as yet be precisely determined. First, it must be determined whether the serum potassium level per se or the change in serum potassium induced by diuretics or catecholamines is most important. This has obvious implications for therapeutic decisions. For example, not all interventions designed to prevent potassium loss resulting from diuretics will also prevent catecholamine-induced transcellular shifts of potassium. In addition, the prevalence of either of these electrolyte disturbances in patients with serious arrhythmias needs to be determined. Few data exist on this point. In a small series, Lown found that 24% of patients with sudden death were hypokalemic (5). Based upon the studies in patients with acute infarction cited above, 26% of all the episodes of in hospital ventricular fibrillation occurred in hypokalemic patients. It should be appreciated that the majority of deaths in patients with infarction

Table 4 Relationship of Ventricular Arrhythmias and Hypokalemia in Various Studies

Study	No patients	Interval K-VT/VF (hr)	VT/VF[a] K < 3.5 vs. K > 3.5 (%)
Dyckner, 1975	444	up to 24	48 vs. 43
Solomon, 1980	151	up to 12	48 vs. 21
Nordehaug, 1981	1035	2-9	26 bs. 16
Hulting, 1980	537	up to 24	10 vs. 4[a]
Thomas, 1982	809	up to 48	4.2 vs. 1.8[a]
Reuben, 1982	405[b]	up to 24	6.9 vs. 0.4[a]
Reuben, 1984	586	up to 24	21 vs. 5

[a]Ventricular fibrillation only.
[b]Aged 65 years and older.

occur outside the hospital. The importance of potassium disturbances in these patients cannot be determined. However, the observation of Cobb et al. that patients resuscitated from out-of-the-hospital ventricular fibrillation had lower serum potassium levels than patients resuscitated from acute infarctions adds further to the clinical importance of potassium disturbances (12). Finally, the prevention of either of these electrolyte disturbances must be shown in prospective studies to diminish the incidence of serious arrhythmias. Such studies are underway and we anxiously await the results.

REFERENCES

1. Cobb, L. A., Werner, J. A., and Trobough, G. B.: Sudden cardiac death. I. A decade's experience with out-of-hospital resuscitation. *Mod. Concepts Cardiovas. Dis.* 49:31–36, 1980.
2. Dyckner, T., Helmers, C., Lundman, T., and Wester, P. O.: Initial serum potassium level in relation to early complications and prognosis in patients with acute myocardial infarction. *Acta Med. Scand.* 197:207–210, 1975.
3. Hulting, J.: In-hospital ventricular fibrillation and its relation to serum potassium. *Acta Med. Scand.* (Suppl.) 647:190–116, 1981.
4. Lown, B.: Sudden cardiac death: the major challenge confronting contemporary cardiology. *Am. J. Cardiol.* 43:313–328, 1979.
5. Lown, B., Calvert, A. F., Armington, R., and Ryan, M.: Monitoring for serious arrhythmias: monitoring for serious arrhythmias and high risk of sudden death. *Circulation* 51, 52 (Suppl.):189–197, 1975.
6. Nordrehaug, J. E.: Malignant arrhythmias in relation to serum potassium values in patients with an acute myocardial infarction. *Acta Med. Scand.* (Suppl.) 647:101–107, 1981.
7. Reuben, S. R., and Kuan, M. A.: The role of potassium in arrhythmias after myocardial infarction. *Int. Med.* Suppl. 5:9–11, 1983.
8. Reuben, S. R., and Thomas, R. D.: The relationship between serum potassium and cardiac arrhythmias following cardiac infarction in patients aged over 65 years. *Curr. Med. Res. Opin.* 7 (Suppl. 1):79–82, 1982.
9. Solomon, R. J., and Cole, A. G.: Importance of potassium in patients with acute myocardial infarction. *Acta Med. Scand.* (Suppl.) 647:87–93, 1981.
10. Struthers, A. D., Reid, J. I., Whitesmith, M. B., and Rodger, J. C.: The effect of cardioselective and nonselective beta-adrenoceptor blockade on the hypokalemic and cardiovascular responses to adrenomedullary hormones in man. *Clin. Sci.* 65:143–147, 1983.
11. Thomas, R. D.: Ventricular fibrillation in myocardial infarction: the role of potassium. *Int. Med.* (Suppl.) 4:7–9, 1983.
12. Thompson, R. G., and Cobb, L. A.: Hypokalemia after resuscitation from out-of-hospital ventricular fibrillation. *JAMA* 248:2860–2863, 1982.

14

Association Between Hypokalemia and Cardiac Arrhythmias in Patients with Acute Myocardial Infarction

JAN ERIK NORDREHAUG*
Diakonissehjemmet Hospital, Bergen, Norway

Arrhythmias in acute myocardial infarction may be caused by a variety of electrophysiological and pathological mechanisms. Infarct size is without doubt one of the important determinants of the type and severity of arrhythmias (2) and of their mortality. The concept of electrical instability (17) has been derived from the observation that ventricular arrhythmias also occur independent of infarct size. The relative importance of electrical instability and infarct size for prognosis is demonstrated by the differentiation between primary and secondary (complicated) ventricular fibrillation (16) occurring in patients, respectively, without or with heart failure and hypotension. In primary ventricular fibrillation, the rate of successful resuscitation is high in contrast to a high mortality in patients with secondary ventricular fibrillation (16) in whom the bad outcome is likely to be a result of their large infarctions.

Several reports (1,4-6,13,18,22) have shown an association between low extracellular potassium concentrations and increased occurrence of arrhythmias in acute myocardial infarction. In these reports hypokalemia was defined as a serum potassium level <3.5 mmol/L or <3.6 mmol/L, thus including patients with mild hypokalemia. Hypokalemia has also been associated with increased mortality in acute myocardial infarction (4).

Electrical instability may result from the electrophysiological consequences of a low serum potassium level (8) which could be the cause of the increased arrhythmic occurrence in hypokalemic patients with acute myocardial infarction. On the other hand, hypokalemia may be only a passive marker of other arrhythmogenic events. Thus, hypokalemia may result from diuretic treatment after hospital admission of patients with large infarctions and, therefore, a high risk of arrhythmias. Furthermore, high catecholamine levels are arrhythmogenic, but can also cause hypokalemia via $beta_2$-adrenoreceptor stimulation (24). With high catecholamine levels, hypokalemia may only be a passive marker of catecholamine levels, or may have additive arrhythmogenic potential.

**Current affiliation*: Haukeland Hospital and University of Bergen, Bergen, Norway

This chapter assesses the importance of hypokalemia in patients with arrhythmias and acute myocardial infarction based on experimental and clinical data.

EXPERIMENTAL STUDIES

Although potassium is mainly an intracellular ion, extracellular potassium is important for the cardiac resting cell membrane potential (8,30). A lowering of the extracellular potassium concentration makes the cell membrane potential more negative. Thus, the speed of conduction during upstroke of the action potential is increased, as is the rate of spontaneous depolarization, and the repolarization phase is prolonged (8,25). A prolonged repolarization phase predisposes to arrhythmias (25), and an increased rate of depolarization may induce automaticity in latent automatic fibers (8). Hypokalemia may induce atrioventricular conduction blocks in experimental animal hearts, but conduction blocks grade 2 and 3 are generally only observed at serum potassium levels <2.0 mmol/L (21).

The influence of hypokalemia on arrhythmias during acute cardiac ischemia in the experimental animal has not been elucidated and therefore remains subject to speculation. Profound hyperkalemia occurs in the ischemic area within a few minutes of coronary ligation in animals (3,11), and may cause ventricular fibrillation (9). However, ventricular fibrillation may also be initiated by currents in normal Purkinje's fibers located at the normal side of the ischemic border (14), that is, in areas that may have extracellular potassium concentrations reflecting those of the general circulation, and where low extracellular potassium can induce ectopic currents. Furthermore, variability of the extracellular potassium level within the myocardium creates inhomogeneity of the action potentials and enhances the risk of arrhythmias.

Chronic hypokalemia can cause a reversible nephropathy, thus the possibility remains that chronic hypokalemia resulting from diuretic therapy may cause structural changes in the myocardium. This possibility of myocardial damage and thereby arrhythmic potential has not been extensively investigated.

CLINICAL STUDIES

General Problems

An association between hypokalemia and increased occurrence of arrhythmias in acute myocardial infarction is evident from clinical studies (1,4-6,13,18,22,26). However, these studies do not give conclusive evidence of hypokalemia as an independent risk factor for arrhythmias. Such evidence would have to come from studies with a different design. For example, the prevention of arrhythmias by potassium correction, which was not attempted in any of the studies, would provide more direct evidence.

The classification of patients into groups based on potassium values has been done in different ways. Some studies have grouped patients based on the potassium value obtained nearest in time to the particular arrhythmia under review. In this instance, patients without arrhythmias are classified according to serum potassium concentration on admission to hospital. This ensures a better temporal relationship between the serum potassium measurement and the arrhythmia but has three major drawbacks as well. First, a fall in potassium concentration resulting from in-hospital diuretic treatment only will be observed in some patients with arrhythmias, resulting in a falsely high incidence of hypokalemia in such patients. Second, patients in need of diuretic treatment with poor left ventricular function, and therefore a high risk of arrhythmias, tend to be clustered in the hypokalemia group, resulting in a high rate of mortality and arrhythmias in this group, and making the comparison of rates of arrhythmias with the normokalemic group difficult. Third, classification into groups based on serum potassium obtained after ventricular fibrillation and resuscitation may not be indicative of the potassium concentration before the onset of ventricular fibrillation, since increased catecholamine levels and infusion of glucose and sodium bicarbonate during resuscitation may influence the level of serum potassium.

To avoid these problems, another approach has been to base the groups on potassium concentration obtained at hospital admission for all patients. This may result in a loss of temporal relationship between potassium measurement and arrhythmias, but has a better chance of documenting potassium measurements at the same time of infarct evolution in the two potassium groups (18).

A closer temporal relationship between initial serum potassium concentration and arrhythmias can be reached by detecting arrhythmia for only a short interval (1). Again, this has several drawbacks. First, the period of arrhythmia monitoring has to be short because hypokalemia due to rapidly changing epinephrine levels early in acute myocardial infarction (15) may be transient in nature. Such short-term arrhythmia monitoring may be inadequate for comparison of hypo- and normokalemic groups because of the chance of spontaneous variation in the occurrence of arrhythmias (29). Second, clinical studies generally consist of a small hypokalemic and a large normokalemic group, which may lead to a greater risk of detecting arrhythmias at different stages of ischemia and infarct evolution in the two potassium groups.

Digitalis therapy may have different actions according to extracellular potassium concentrations. In the presence of normokalemia, digitalis may prevent arrhythmias, especially supraventricular arrhythmias. In contrast, hypokalemia may induce increased sensitivity to digitalis (23), which may provoke arrhythmias (7). In this way, digitalis therapy in clinical studies may preclude some comparisons of arrhythmia between patients classified into different potassium groups.

Some studies have reported on ventricular arrhythmias based on conventional detection of arrhythmia. This method has been clearly shown to underestimate the frequency of arrhythmias, especially premature ventricular contractions and ventricular tachycardia, as compared with detection by arrhythmia computer (28) or continuous electrocardiographic recording analyzed beat-by-beat (12).

Hypokalemia is associated with diuretic treatment in the studies of acute myocardial infarction. A proportion of the patients with hypokalemia have not been treated with diuretics, however, and there is generally little information in the reports about the cause of hypokalemia in these patients. Of greatest interest would be information about factors that can cause hypokalemia and at the same time influence the heart independently of hypokalemia, such as epinephrine, which have not been measured in the clinical studies. Another factor is alcohol consumption, which may be difficult to assess exactly. A high level of alcohol consumption can cause hypokalemia and also a cardiomyopathy which in itself may have an arrhythmogenic potential.

Atrioventricular Conduction Blocks

Complete and second-degree heart block have not been shown to occur more frequently in patients with hypokalemia than with normokalemia in acute myocardial infarction (1,6,19). Hypokalemia does cause conduction blocks in experimental animals, and the discrepancy between clinical and animal studies may be related to the degree of hypokalemia. While complete and second-degree heart block can be most easily induced at a serum potassium level <2.0 mmol/L (21) in animal heart experiments, such potassium values probably rarely occur in patients with acute myocardial infarction. In one study of more than 1,000 patients the lowest serum potassium value observed was 2.3 mmol/L (18).

Supraventricular Arrhythmias

Atrial fibrillation and flutter are prognostically important during acute myocardial infarction (27). Dyckner et al. (6) showed a significantly higher incidence of these arrhythmias in hypokalemic as compared to normokalemic patients. Other supraventricular arrhythmias were not different between the hypo- and normokalemic groups. The percentage of digitalis treatment was 35 and 31%, respectively.

A first incident of atrial fibrillation or flutter lasting more than 2 min during the acute phase of infarction was one of the criteria for classifying patients in a special high-risk group in the Norwegian multicenter study on use of timolol after acute myocardial infarction (20). In a cohort of 1,033 of the 1,884 patients later included in the timolol study (20), there were significantly ($p < 0.01$) more hypokalemic [23 of 96 patients (24%)] than normokalemic [102 of 937 patients (11%)] patients with atrial fibrillation, atrial flutter, or both arrhythmias.

Ventricular Arrhythmias

Premature ventricular contractions have been classified in several ways, for instance, according to number per minute or hour, as "warning arrhythmias," or in other ways. Regardless of the classification and monitoring method used, clinical studies have not shown significant differences between hypokalemic and normokalemic patients. When potassium subgroups and subclasses of premature ventricular contractions between the hypo- and normokalemic groups were analyzed, some significant differences have been reported (1, 13). However, subgrouping and subclassing often produce so many variables to compare that significance levels may be reached more easily by chance.

Several studies (1,13,18,22) of patients with acute myocardial infarction have shown an association between hypokalemia and an increased incidence of ventricular tachycardia and/or ventricular fibrillation. One report found an increased occurrence of ventricular fibrillation in patients with a serum potassium level <4.0 mmol/L than in those with a level ⩾4.0 mmol/L (26). Some workers have compared the number of patients with ventricular tachycardia or ventricular fibrillation or both arrhythmias in group with low and normal potassium levels (1,22), and have found significantly more patients with these arrhythmias in the hypokalemic group. Since differentiating between these arrhythmias may be difficult in clinical studies, grouping them together may be advocated. However, when differentiation has been attempted (1,13), the increased rate of arrhythmia in patients with hypokalemia seems to be due to ventricular fibrillation only (Figure 1).

Hypokalemia, Ventricular Fibrillation, and Comparability of Potassium Groups

In a study of 1,074 patients, including both those studies later included in and excluded from the Norwegian multicenter study on timolol after acute myocardial infarction (20)

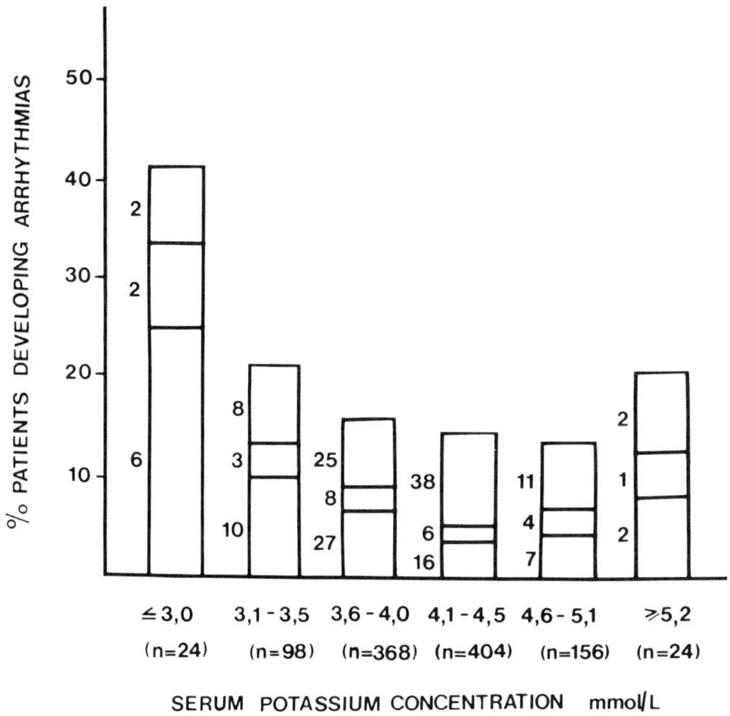

Figure 1 Number and percentage of patients developing ventricular fibrillation (lower part of columns) (18), ventricular tachycardia (upper part), or both arrhythmias (middle) (18) in relation to serum potassium concentration. Of the 122 patients with hypokalemia 25.4% developed these arrhythmias, compared with a rate of 15.4% in the remaining patients ($p < 0.01$).

in 5 of the 20 participating hospitals, hypokalemia on admission to hospital predicted an increased likelihood and early occurrence of ventricular fibrillation (18). The number of patients with ventricular tachycardia, ventricular fibrillation, or both arrhythmias during their stay in hospital is shown in Figure 1. The patients classified as having ventricular fibrillation all had clinical signs of this arrhythmia with circulatory standstill, and an attempt at resuscitation was made in all. The difference in occurrence of ventricular fibrillation between the potassium groups was still significant even after one excludes the small number of patients (18) who had ventricular fibrillation at the time of their admission to hospital and thus had their study serum potassium measured after the onset of the arrhythmia. The number of patients with ventricular tachycardia was not significantly different in the groups with low and normal serum potassium levels.

The lowest incidence of ventricular fibrillation was seen in patients whose serum potassium level was between 4.1 and 5.1 mmol/L. At levels below this there was an inverse relationship between potassium concentration and the frequency of ventricular fibrillation, and at potassium values of ≤ 3.0 mmol/L, 33% of the hypokalemic patients developed ventricular fibrillation. Hypokalemia was significantly more common in women, as was diuretic therapy. The frequency of ventricular fibrillation was about the same in the hypo- and normokalemic groups of women and men and thus the occurrence

Table 1 Number and Percentage Distribution of Patients According to Potassium Group and Time from Hospital Admission to the Occurrence of Ventricular Fibrillation

	Serum potassium ⩽ 3.5 mmol/L		Serum potassium ⩾ 3.6 mmol/L	
Number of patients with ventricular fibrillation	21		71	
0–2 hours (%)	16	(76)	28	(39)
2–12 hours (%)	3	(14)	13	(18)
After 12 hours (%)	2	(10)	30	(42)
Time from hospital admission to onset of ventricular fibrillation (median hr)	0.3[a]		7	
Time from onset of symptoms to hospital admission (hr)				
Mean	3		3.8	
Median	1		1	

[a] $p < 0.01$
Source: Ref. 18.

of ventricular fibrillation depended on the number of patients with hypokalemia but not on the distribution of women or men in the potassium groups.

The mean time from onset of symptoms of acute myocardial infarction to hospital admission was approximately the same in the two potassium groups (Table 1), consequently the potassium measurements on admission to hospital were done at comparable mean times of infarct evolution in all the groups. This minimizes the chance of inhomogeneity between the groups in having observed arrhythmias at different phases of ischemia according to the Harris model (10). When the patients were subgrouped according to time between hospital admission and the onset of ventricular fibrillation (Table 1), patients with hypokalemia had ventricular fibrillation significantly earlier than the normokalemic group. Since 76% of the patients with hypokalemia and ventricular fibrillation experienced this arrhythmia within the first 2 hr after hospital admission, there was an impressive temporal relationship between the potassium estimations and ventricular fibrillation in that group.

The hypo- and normokalemic groups of patients with ventricular fibrillation have been compared for a substantial number of demographic and clinical variables (18). There were fewer patients with signs of heart failure among those with ventricular fibrillation and hypokalemia as compared to normokalemia, but no other significant differences were found. More patients with hypokalemia and ventricular fibrillation had been treated with diuretics prior to hospital admission, but this difference did not reach significance, possibly because of the small number of patients involved.

Among the hypokalemic and normokalemic patients with ventricular fibrillation, 33 and 44%, respectively, died within the first 3 months. Corresponding figures for the patients who had ventricular fibrillation within the first 2 hr of hospital admission (Table 1) were 19 and 29%. No intravenous potassium correction was used. The lower percentage of deaths among the patients with early ventricular fibrillation suggests that most such subjects had primary ventricular fibrillation. An early occurrence of primary ventricular fibrillation is also in accordance with other studies (16). Patients who had ventricular fibrillation more than 2 hr after hospital admission had a higher death rate, and the occurrence of ventricular fibrillation was not significantly different between the hypo- and normokalemic groups.

The mortality at 3 months was not different between the total number of patients with hypokalemia (16%) and normokalemia (16%) despite the association of hypokalemia with ventricular fibrillation. This may have been a consequence of both the relatively small subgroup of patients in which the occurrence of ventricular fibrillation showed the largest difference between the two potassium groups, and the relatively good prognosis of these particular patients when resuscitated.

In conclusion, there is supportive evidence for the concept that hypokalemia is a risk factor for early ventricular fibrillation in acute myocardial infarction. The risk conferred by hypokalemia is independent of infarct size and left ventricular function.

IMPLICATIONS FOR TREATMENT

At present, the management of patients with hypokalemia and acute myocardial infarction must be viewed from the perspective that no prospective, randomized, placebo-controlled studies of potassium correction for the prevention of arrhythmias have been done. Consequently, neither the effects of treatment nor the rate of complications of such treatment is known. The management is further complicated by the early occurrence of ventricular fibrillation. Since the prognosis during the first 3 months is about the same for patients with hypokalemia and normokalemia who experience ventricular fibrillation during an acute myocardial infarction (18) without the early use of intravenous potassium correction, this arrhythmia seems to be well handled without such prophylaxis, which in itself may provoke arrhythmias in some patients (30).

The evidence of an association between hypokalemia and other arrhythmias in patients with acute myocardial infarction who are not taking digitalis is scarce, and further studies must be awaited.

The early occurrence of ventricular fibrillation in patients with hypokalemia may have important implications for the prehospital phase of the infarction and the many deaths known to occur from ventricular fibrillation outside the hospital. The first logical step seems to be prevention of hypokalemia, especially in diuretic-treated patients, before they experience acute myocardial infarction.

REFERENCES

1. Beck, O. A., and Hochrein, H.: Initial serum potassium level in relation to cardiac arrhythmias in acute myocardial infarction. *Z. Kardiol.* 66:187–190, 1977.
2. Bigger, J. T., Jr, Dresdale, R. J., Heissenbuttel, R. H., Weld, F. M., and Wit, A. L.: Ventricular arrhythmias in ischemic heart disease: mechanism, prevalence, significance, and management. *Prog. Cardiovasc. Dis.* 19:255, 1977.
3. Case, R. B., Nasser, M. G., and Crampton, R. S.: Biochemical aspects of early myocardial ischemia. *Am. J. Cardiol.* 24:766, 1969.
4. Donelly, T., Gray, H., Simpson, E., and Rodger, J. C.: Serum potassium in acute myocardial infarction. *Scott. Med. J.* 25:176, 1980.
5. Duke, M.: Thiazide-induced hypokalemia. Association with acute myocardial infarction and ventricular fibrillation. *JAMA* 239:43–45, 1978.
6. Dyckner, T., Helmers, C., Lundman, T., and Wester, P. O.: Initial serum potassium

level in relation to early complications and prognosis in patients with acute myocardiol infarction. *Acta Med. Scand.* 197:207–210, 1975.

7. Evered, D. C., and Chapman, C.: Plasma digoxin concentrations and digoxin toxicity in hospital patients. *Br. Heart J.* 33:540–545, 1971.
8. Fisch, C.: Relation of electrolyte disturbances to cardiac arrhythmias. *Circulation* 47:408–419, 1973.
9. Harris, A. S., Bisteni, A., Russel, R. A., Brigham, J. C., and Firestone, J. E.: Excitatory factors in ventricular tachycardia resulting from myocardial ischemia: potassium a major excitant. *Science* 119:200, 1954.
10. Harris, A. S.: Delayed development of ventricular ectopic rhythms following experimental coronary occlusion. *Circulation* 1:1318–1329, 1950.
11. Hill, J. L., and Gettes, L. S.: Effect of acute coronary occlusion on local myocardial extracellular K^+ activity in swine. *Circulation* 61:768–778, 1980.
12. Holmberg, S., Rydén, L., and Waldenström, A.: Efficiency of arrhythmia detection by nurses in a coronary care unit using a decentralised monitoring system. *Br. Heart J.* 39:1019–1025, 1977.
13. Hulting, J.: In-hospital ventricular fibrillation and its relation to serum potassium. *Acta Med. Scand.* Suppl. 647:109–116, 1981.
14. Janse, M. J., van Capelle, F. J. L., Morsink, H., Kleber, A. G., Wilms-Schopman, F., Cardinal, R., D'Alnoncourt, C. N., and Durrer, D.: Flow of "injury" current and patterns of excitation during early ventricular arrhythmias in acute regional myocardial ischemia in isolated porsine and canine hearts. *Circ. Res.* 47:151–165, 1980.
15. Karlsberg, R. P., Cryer, P. E., and Roberts, R.: Serial plasma catecholamine response early in the course of clinical acute myocardial infarction: relationship to infarct extent and mortality. *Am. Heart J.* 102:24–29, 1981.
16. Lawrie, D. M., Higgins, M. R., Godman, M. J., Oliver, M. F., Julian, D. G., and Donald, K. W.: Ventricular fibrillation complicating acute myocardial infarction. *Lancet* 2:523–8, 1968.
17. Lesch, M.: VPB's—the benign and the malignant. *N. Engl. J. Med.* 297:782–783, 1977.
18. Nordrehaug, J. E., and von der Lippe, G.: Hypokalaemia and ventricular fibrillation in acute myocardial infarction. *Br. Heart J.* 50:525–529, 1983.
19. Nordrehaug, J. E.: Serum potassium and arrhythmias in acute myocardial infarction: a preliminary report. *Int. Congress Sympos. Series* 44:83–86, 1981.
20. Norwegian Multicenter Study Group: Timolol-induced reduction in mortality and reinfarction in patients surviving acute myocardial infarction. *N. Engl. J. Med.* 304: 801–807, 1981.
21. Paes de Carvalho, A., and Langhan, W. B.: Influence of extracellular potassium levels on atrioventricular transmission. *Am. J. Physiol.* 205:375–381, 1963.
22. Solomon, R. J., and Cole, A. G.: Importance of potassium in patients with acute myocardial infarction. *Acta Med. Scand.* Suppl. 647:87–93, 1981.
23. Steiness, E., and Olesen, K. H.: Cardiac arrhythmias induced by hypokalemia and potassium loss during maintenance digoxin therapy. *Br. Heart J.* 38:167–172, 1976.
24. Struthers, A. D., Reid, J. L., Whitesmith, R., and Rodger, J. C.: Effect of intravenous adrenaline on electrocardiogram, blood pressure, and serum potassium. *Br. Heart J.* 49:90–93, 1983.
25. Surawicz, B.: Role of electrolytes in etiology and management of cardiac arrhythmias. *Prog. Cardiovasc. Dis.* 8:364–386, 1966.
26. Thomas, R. D.: Ventricular fibrillation and initial plasma potassium in acute myocardial infarction. *Postgrad. Med. J.* 59:354–356, 1983.
27. Vedin, A., Wilhelmsen, L., Wedel, H., Pettersson, B., Wilhelmsson, C., Elmfeldt, D.,

and Tibblin, G.: Prediction of cardiovascular deaths and non-fatal reinfarctions after myocardial infarction. *Acta Med. Scand.* 201:309–316, 1977.

28. Vetter, N. J., and Julian, D. G.: Comparison of arrhythmia computer and conventional monitoring in coronary-care unit. *Lancet* 1:1151–1154, 1975.
29. Winkle, R. A.: Antiarrhythmic drug effect mimicked by spontaneous variability of ventricular ectopy. *Circulation* 57:1116–1121, 1978.
30. Zipes, D. P.: Electrolyte derangements in the genesis of arrhythmias. In *Cardiac Arrhythmias*, edited by Dreyfus and Likoff, 1973, pp. 55–69.

15

Catecholamines and Hypokalemia During and After Myocardial Infarction

JOHN L. REID
University of Glasgow and Stobhill General Hospital, Glasgow, Scotland

BACKGROUND

Hypokalemia has been observed relatively frequently in patients presenting within hours after acute myocardial infarction (11,13,30,39). In the majority of these patients there are no obvious explanations such as diuretic therapy, diarrhea, vomiting, or dietary fads. Several retrospective series have suggested that low serum potassium levels on presentation indicate a poor prognosis (11,13,30). Hypokalemic patients were reported to have a higher frequency of serious arrhythmias including ventricular fibrillation and a greater early mortality rate (11,13,30). It is tempting to conclude that hypokalemia contributed to increased fatal arrhythmias and directly to death. An alternative view is that hypokalemia may be associated with larger more extensive infarcts and that these patients had a worse prognosis for other reasons unrelated to serum potassium levels. Although the second possibility cannot be excluded, particularly in some of the earlier retrospective surveys, it is unlikely that hypokalemia was an incidental unrelated confounding factor in patients who had the most severe infarctions.

Hypokalemia has been observed in a review of acute medical admissions to hospital (25). In the majority of cases previous diuretic therapy could not be implicated and other clinical explanations for hypokalemia were not obvious from the history or the patients' case records. Serum potassium levels recovered spontaneously in these patients over a few days. There was no evidence that oral or intravenous potassium supplementation substantially influenced the recovery of serum levels. In our clinical practice we have also observed occasional patients with unexplained hypokalemia which recovered spontaneously. We became interested in the possible mechanisms of hypokalemia of acute illness, including myocardial infarction and its link to the genesis of cardiac arrhythmias. Our studies over the last 3 years lead us to believe that serum potassium levels can be profoundly influenced by changes in plasma catecholamines particularly epinephrine (35,37, 38). Epinephrine-induced hypokalemia causes changes in the electrocardiogram similar to those seen with hypokalemia of other causes (37). We conclude that stress-related epinephrine release from the adrenal medulla could be an important mechanism causing hypokalemia in acute myocardial infarction and an additional factor in predisposing to arrhythmias (34).

MECHANISM OF EPINEPHRINE-INDUCED HYPOKALEMIA

Circulating epinephrine is principally a bloodborne hormone which achieves its activity by stimulating catecholamine receptors accessible to the intravascular compartment (8). Epinephrine is released from the adrenal medulla following a range of stimuli as part of a series of differentiated sympathoadrenal and sympathoneural responses under central nervous control (8). Norepinephrine is only released in small amounts from the adrenal medulla but is the neurotransmitter released from sympathetic nerves to act on local intrasynaptic catecholamine receptors. Plasma levels of norepinephrine are thus less important determinants of response to this amine than intrasynaptic levels. In contrast, plasma levels of epinephrine determine the response observed and most changes in plasma epinephrine will influence a range of metabolic functions. We have observed in humans that changes in plasma epinephrine within the range observed in pathological and pathophysiological states of stress (3-5 nm), such as insulin-induced hypokalemia, can lower serum potassium by up to 1 mmol/L (37). These observations confirm many previous reports from animal studies (12,42) and with higher dosages of catecholamine agonists in humans (4,44). The role of catecholamines in the regulation of serum potassium has been recently reviewed (1,3,14,34).

The model we have used to study metabolic and hemodynamic effects of epinephrine is shown in Figure 1. In healthy young subjects 5% dextrose vehicle was infused intra-

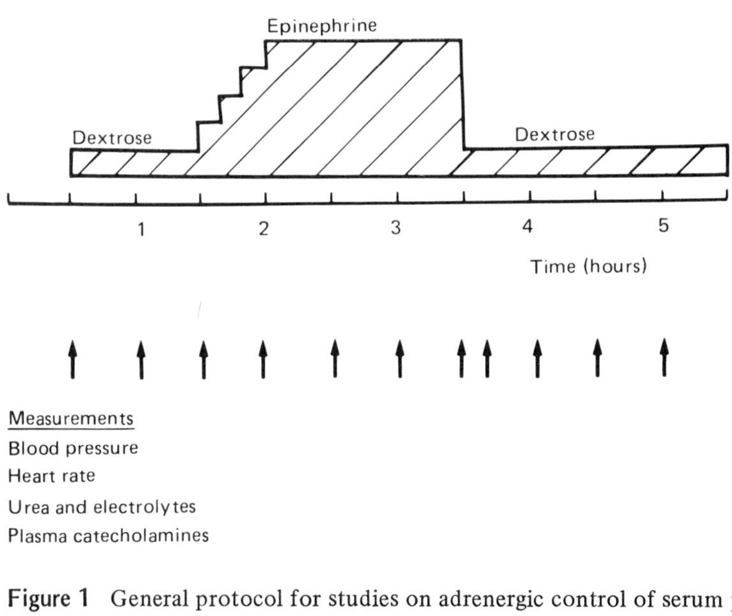

Figure 1 General protocol for studies on adrenergic control of serum potassium. Subjects were pretreated with placebo or active drug and received a series of stepwise intravenous infusions of epinephrine 0.01, 0.02, 0.04 μg/kg per min and, if tolerated, 0.06 μg/kg per min for 90 mins. Vehicle (5% dextrose) was infused at a similar rate before and after epinephrine infusion.

venously for a control period followed by an infusion for up to 90 mins with 0.06 μg/kg per min epinephrine. For safety reasons the epinephrine infusion is begun at a lower dosage (0.01 μg/kg per min) and increased in a stepwise manner to 0.02, 0.04, and 0.06 μg/kg per min at 10-min intervals. The higher dosage caused consistent but modest hemodynamic changes but no distress to the subjects (37). The electrocardiogram was continuously recorded from precordial leads and displayed on an oscilloscope. Blood pressure was recorded at intervals using a semiautomatic sphygmomanometer. Blood samples were collected from a cannula in the opposite arm from that into which epinephrine was being infused. After epinephrine infusion, during a recovery period of 2 hrs, 5% dextrose vehicle was infused once more. This protocol was followed in all our studies except the earlier one (38) in which, in addition to the 0.06 μg/kg per min dose of epinephrine, a lower dosage (0.01 μg/kg per min) was also given for 90 mins. In all the studies from our group reviewed here, the protocols were approved by the local ethics committee and followed a placebo-controlled random-order blind protocol so that neither subject, clinical observer, nor biochemical analyst were aware of whether placebo or drug pretreatment had been given. Plasma epinephrine and norepinephrine levels were measured by a sensitive radiometric assay (9). Infusions of epinephrine at a rate of 0.06 μg/kg per min increased plasma epinephrine levels 8-10-fold. Stable levels were achieved by at least 30 min after the infusion started and were maintained for the duration of the study. Levels fell to basal levels within minutes after the infusions were stopped. Concentrations achieved showed interindividual variation but were in the range of 2.5-4.5 nm. Epinephrine infusion increased systolic pressure by 10 mmHg, reduced diastolic pressure (14 mmHg), and this increased pulse pressure with little effect on mean arterial pressure (Figure 2). Heart rate increased by six to eight beats/min after administration of 0.06 μg/kg epinephrine. These modest hemodynamic effects were accompanied by a marked fall in serum potassium. Potassium levels fell rapidly within 15-20 min of infusion, reached a nadir which was maintained for the duration of the infusion, and recovered to baseline levels over 40-60 min after the infusion had been stopped (Figure 3). Hypokalemia was associated with electrocardiographic changes including prolongation of the QT interval and the rate-corrected QT (QT_c), reduced T wave amplitude, and, in some subjects, the appearance of U waves (37).

In a series of experiments we have established that hypokalemia after epinephrine infusion is mediated by beta-, not alpha-adrenoceptor mechanisms and that the beta receptor is probably $beta_2$ in type. Beta blockers with different selectivity and specificity were examined. Timolol, a nonselective ($beta_1$ + $beta_2$) antagonist was compared with atenolol, which is $beta_1$-selective (38), and with labetalol, which is a nonselective beta blocker that also blocks $alpha_1$ receptors (36). A new compound under development (ICI 11855) which is relatively $beta_2$-selective, was found in our own studies and by others to prevent the fall in potassium levels (4).

In brief, the hemodynamic effects were as would be predicted from results of animal and previous clinical studies (Figures 4 and 5A). Nonselective and $beta_2$-selective blockers caused "epinephrine reversal" with a rise in diastolic pressure and bradycardia. The former was a result of unopposed peripheral alpha-receptor activation and the latter was baroreflex-mediated. These interpretations are supported by the absence of diastolic pressure rise and bradycardia after the cardioselective $beta_1$ blocker atenolol and after labetalol which has alpha-receptor-blocking properties. Serum potassium changes are shown in Figure 5B. These changes make it likely that $beta_2$ receptors are predominant in mediating hypokalemia.

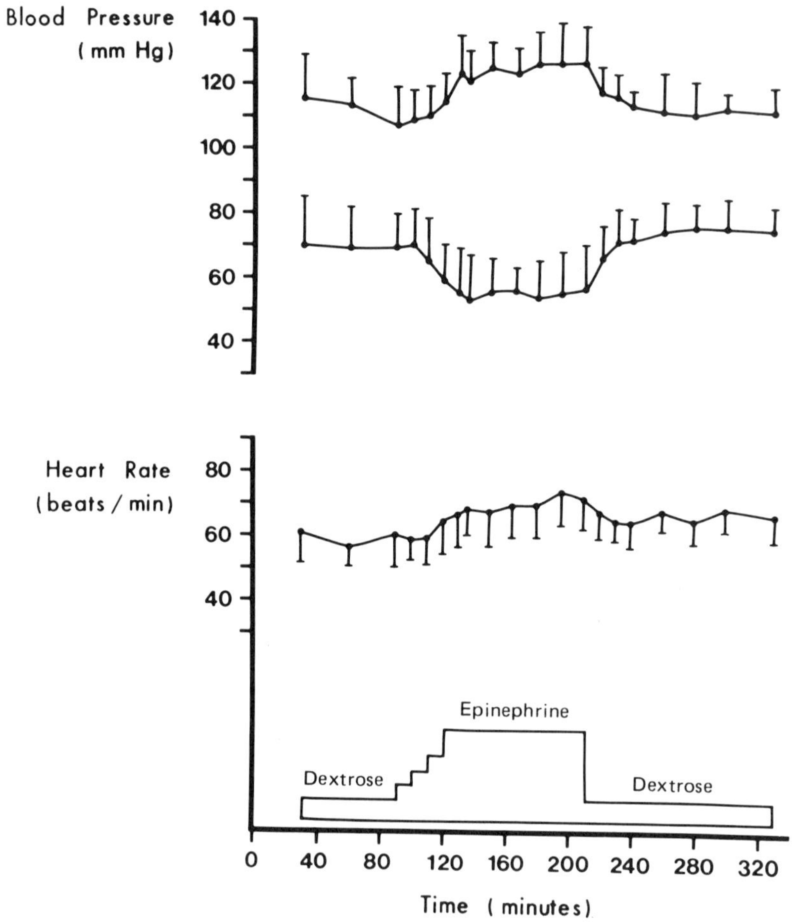

Figure 2 Blood pressure and heart rate (mean ± S.D.) in six normotensive subjects during intravenous administration of epinephrine 0.06 μg/kg per min.

In these studies there was no increase in urinary excretion of potassium to account for the fall in serum levels. In fact, urinary potassium fell (37). There was no increase in serum insulin levels concomitant with epinephrine infusion (37). In addition, pretreatment with nifedipine, the slow calcium channel blocker, did not modify the hemodynamic or hypokalemic effect of epinephrine, making it unlikely that receptor-operated calcium channels were involved (33).

Other groups have confirmed these observations using the same or other beta blockers and a range of beta receptor agonists (4,44). From our results and these studies it is likely that epinephrine-induced $beta_2$-receptor-mediated hypokalemia is a result of redistribution of potassium from extracellular to intracellular sites. It is encouraging that in the reports of Brown et al. (4) and Vincent et al. (44) the magnitude and duration of change in serum potassium after intravenous infusion of epinephrine and other $beta_2$ agonists were very similar to our observations. This unanimity unfortunately does not extend to the reports of effects of beta-agonist infusion on plasma norepinephrine levels. Vincent et al. have consistently observed increases in plasma norepinephrine during isoprenaline and

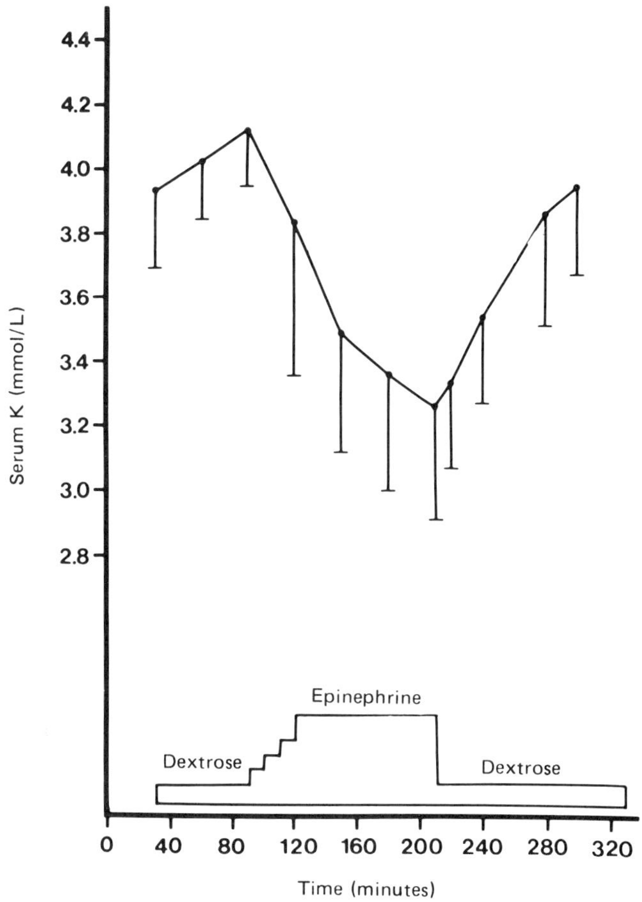

Figure 3 Serum potassium (mean ± S.D.) in six normotensive subjects before, during, and after intravenous administration of epinephrine 0.06 μg/kg per min.

salbutamol infusion and interpreted these changes as resulting from activation of facilitatory presynaptic beta receptors on sympathetic terminals (44). Brown and colleagues, who have also used isoprenaline by infusion, have not noted changes in plasma norepinephrine (4). In all our studies with epinephrine as the infused agonist we have been unable to confirm that plasma norepinephrine levels are significantly changed. The explanation for these discrepancies is not clear. They may partly reflect the dosages and receptor specificity of the agonists used, but different analytical techniques may also contribute.

Clausen and colleagues have characterized in rat soleus muscle a membrane-bound sodium potassium ATPase which appears to be linked to an adrenoceptor of the $beta_2$ type (6,7). Careful pharmacological studies have confirmed that this system transports potassium into cells and sodium out (7). It has been proposed that an abnormality of this mechanism is responsible for familial intermittent hyperkalemic paralysis (45). Patients with this condition show a marked improvement in muscle power accompanied by a fall in serum potassium when treated with $beta_2$ agonists. The $beta_2$ receptor linked to

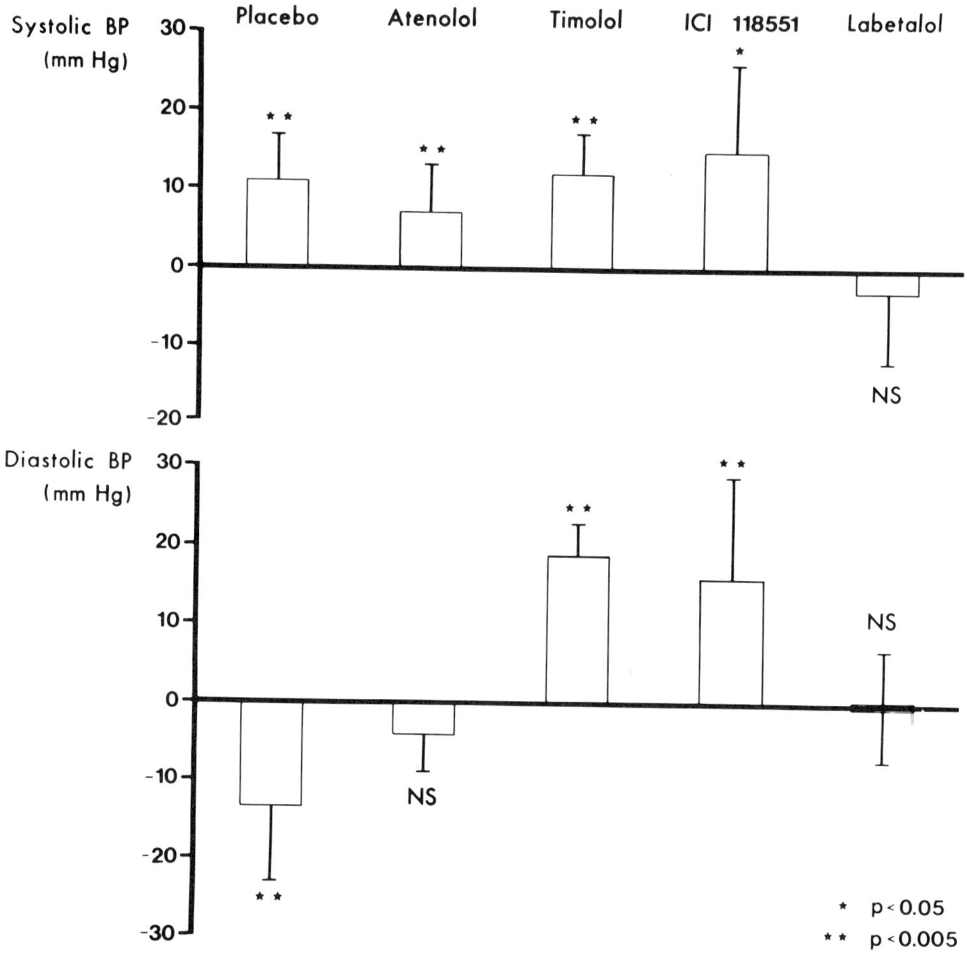

Figure 4 Systolic and diastolic blood pressure. Change (mean ± S.D.) in the last 30 min of a 90-min intravenous infusion of epinephrine 0.06 μg/kg per min. Adrenoceptor antagonists were given for a 5-day pretreatment period, except for ICI 118551 which was given as a single dose. See References 36 and 38 for details.

sodium potassium ATPase (Figure 6) may be an important mechanism of restoring intracellular ion concentration during heavy dynamic exercise. Stress-related increases in circulatory epinephrine without muscle contraction may lead to systemic hypokalemia. This pattern could underlie the hypokalemia of acute illness and acute myocardial infarction, both of which are indisputably stressful experiences that do not usually involve physical activity. It is further likely that blockade of this beta receptor during exercise is the mechanism of hyperkalemia of exercise (40) especially in patients taking beta blockers (23) and is a possible factor in the fatigue experienced by these patients. It is still not clear whether the beta receptor/sodium ATPase complex is only found in skeletal muscle or whether it is also active in vascular smooth muscle and cardiac muscle. The electrocardiographic (ECG) abnormalities we have observed during epinephrine infusion and

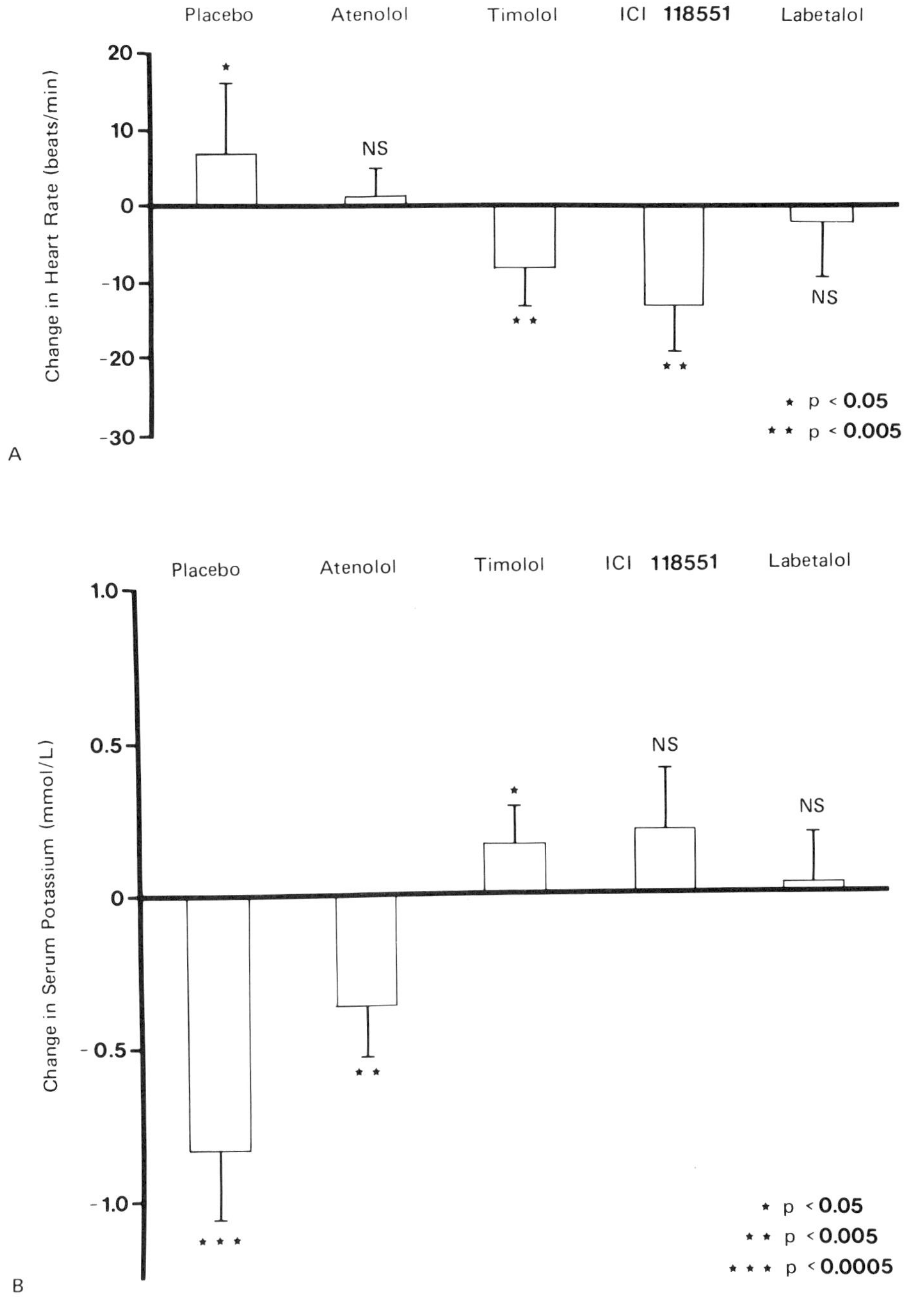

Figure 5 (A) Heart rate changes (mean ± S.D.). (B) Serum potassium changes (mean ± S.D.) in the last 30 min of a 90-min intravenous infusion of epinephrine 0.06 μg/kg per min. Adrenoceptor antagonists were given as described in Figure 4. See References 36 and 38 for details.

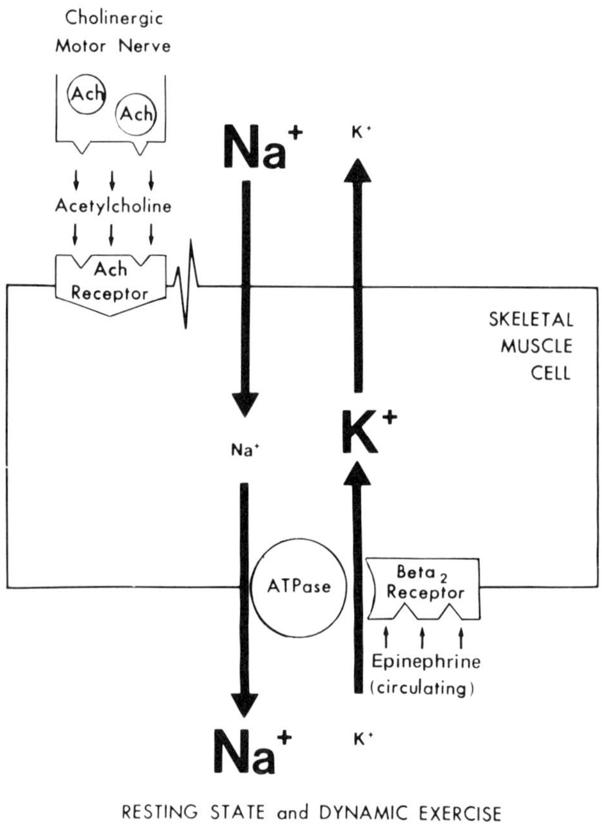

Figure 6 Schematic diagram of sodium potassium ATPase linked to a beta$_2$ adrenoceptor on the cell membrane of skeletal muscle. The pump restores intracellular potassium after depolarization and muscle contraction. Circulating epinephrine is not proposed to be the endogenous ligand for this receptor.

results from studies in animal hearts in vitro (5), suggest that there are important differences between cardiac muscle and other tissues. These remain to be further characterized and elucidated. There is thus good evidence that increases in circulating epinephrine within the pathophysiological range can cause rapid and reversible falls in serum potassium levels. Hypokalemia is a consequence of transport of potassium into cells. Skeletal muscle, both because of its specific beta$_2$ receptor mechanism and its considerable mass compared to total body mass, is the main site of potassium sequestration. Are the levels of circulating epinephrine in acute myocardial infarction high enough to cause hypokalemia by this mechanism?

PLASMA CATECHOLAMINES IN ACUTE MYOCARDIAL INFARCTION

Many published reports strongly suggest that sympathetic activity is increased after myocardial infarction (2,21,27,41,43). In uncomplicated infarcts without cardiogenic shock,

Table 1 Plasma Catecholamines in Acute Myocardial Infarction (Mean ± S.E.; ng/ml)

	n	Norepinephrine	Epinephrine
Uncomplicated acute myocardial infarction[a]	14	1.36±0.23	1.09±0.61
Myocardial infarction and cardiogenic shock[b]	12	2.94±0.32	1.13±0.19
Other acute medical illnesses[b]	10	0.46±0.06	0.58±0.09
"Normal" range	–	0.23–0.72	0.02–0.26

[a]Unpublished data, Reid et al. (1984).
[b]Data from Ref. 2.

sympathetic activity returns to normal over 3-5 days while in complicated cases, sympathetic activity remains high until death or recovery (2,21). Although the increase in sympathetic activity appears to involve increased sympathoneural tone, the marked increases in plasma epinephrine reported confirm that sympathoadrenal activity is also enhanced (Table 1). It is not clear how much the increase in sympathetic activity is a nonspecific response to stress (a very severe and life-threatening stress) and how much can be attributed to local release of norepinephrine from ischemic myocardium or by specific reflexes activated by myocardial ischemia or infarction. Previous studies have assumed that local cardiac release plays a prominent role. However, more recent insights into the relative contributions of various organs to plasma norepinephrine make it unlikely that the heart itself is the major source of increased plasma norepinephrine (15). Kinetic studies on organ and regional release and uptake of norepinephrine in humans, indicate that the heart may contribute less than 5% of the norepinephrine in plasma. The total contribution of heart, kidneys, and splanchnic bed is probably less than 25% (15). Thus, in those patients with uncomplicated infarcts, even when not in cardiac failure, a generalized increase in sympathetic nervous tone, and especially in adrenomedullary catecholamine release, occurs.

There is a wide interindividual range of changes in levels of both catecholamines in acute infarction (2,21). There are also difficulties in establishing an appropriate normal range or control group for comparison. Plasma catecholamines are a sensitive indicator of psychosocial stress (10). Rested, trained, normal subjects have lower levels of plasma norepinephrine than similarly rested hospital outpatients regardless of diagnosis (20). Admission to hospital with a suspected acute infarct is a stressful event to most people even if an infarct is subsequently excluded. Perhaps the most appropriate controls are patients admitted to hospital with other acute illnesses if a specific effect of cardiac infarction on sympathetic tone is to be explored. Plasma catecholamines in acutely ill patients are above the range observed in normal healthy resting subjects (Table 1) (21).

We have recently confirmed that in many patients plasma catecholamine levels are above resting normal levels on admission to a coronary care unit within 4-6 hr of symptoms of an acute infarct or suspected infarct. In patients without evidence of cardiac failure, epinephrine was elevated more prominently than norepinephrine. As observed by others in these patients, epinephrine usually fell to the normal range within a few days, although there was a wide range of responses.

In a prospective study which is part of a containing investigation into changes in catecholamines, potassium, and cardiac rhythm in acute myocardial infarction, we have studied 18 patients. All had characteristic clinical histories of acute myocardial infarction between 1 and 4 hr before admission. In all but three patients both measurements of serum enzymes and serial ECGs confirmed acute infarction. There was an inverse relationship between plasma epinephrine and serum potassium but no relation between plasma norepinephrine and the potassium levels. Higher epinephrine levels occurred in those patients with the lower serum potassium levels. There was a significant inverse relationship between the logarithm of epinephrine level and serum potassium ($r = -0.5207; p < 0.05$). The overall relationship was not altered if three patients with neither enzymatic nor ECG confirmation of recent acute infarction were excluded. There was no obvious relation between site of infarct or magnitude of enzyme rise and potassium or epinephrine levels. In most of these patients we do not have information on changes in potassium at present, since these subjects are currently taking part in a double-blind placebo-controlled study of the effects of intravenous beta blockade. These preliminary results, however, demonstrate a strong association between increases in plasma epinephrine and lower serum potassium levels. They are consistent with the hypothesis that increased sympathoadrenal activity could be an important cause of the transient hypokalemia of acute myocardial infarction.

CLINICAL RELEVANCE OF EPINEPHRINE-INDUCED HYPOKALEMIA

Retrospective analysis of coronary care unit experience indicates that hypokalemia is associated with an increased frequency of serious ventricular arrhythmias and a higher hospital mortality rate (11,13,30,39). If the beta receptor mechanisms described are a factor in causing hypokalemia and thus increasing the likelihood of arrhythmias and death, this would provide a further mechanism by which beta-adrenoceptor antagonists may reduce early and late mortality in acute myocardial infarction (17,29,31,47). There could be potential advantages for drugs such as propranolol (29) and timolol (31) which have both $beta_1$- and $beta_2$-blocking properties. Such advantages have not yet been established in clinical practice. However, $beta_1$ selectivity is relative. Even so-called cardioselective beta blockers do influence $beta_2$ receptors at the higher dosages used in practice, and there must be some doubt as to whether hypokalemia is entirely $beta_2$-mediated (38). In addition, the hemodynamic effects of $beta_2$ blockade may be undesirable in some patients with acute infarcts. The metabolic and hemodynamic profile of labetalol at least in experimental studies in normal subjects looks promising (36).

There are several other conditions in which epinephrine may cause hypokalemia, including the stress of acute illness (25), resuscitation, and open heart surgery (32). Beta blockers may have a role in reversing severe hypokalemia in these conditions.

We may speculate that epinephrine induced hypokalemia as a result of intermittent psychosocial stresses causes changes in serum potassium levels in everyday life. These changes in patients with underlying cardiac disease could precipitate or aggravate arrhythmias and may be a factor in sudden death in middle-aged and older persons.

We have found that thiazide diuretic treatment at relatively low dosages for 1 week in normal subjects causes a modest fall in serum potassium (35). Infusion of epinephrine 0.06 μg/kg per min, however, lowers serum potassium to below 3.0 mmol/L.

There is currently concern that drug regimens for hypertension which are based on thiazide diuretics have not been successful in reducing morbidity and mortality from coronary artery disease (28). Thiazide diuretic therapy has been associated with the finding of increased ventricular extrasystoles in several studies (18,26). However, a close relation between extrasystoles and serum potassium levels was not observed (26). This may implicate other factors, including serum magnesium. Alternatively, the rapid changes in potassium during and after increases in plasma epinephrine could result in blood samples taken at rest not reflecting the serum potassium during the ECG monitoring period when arrhythmias occurred. Further controlled studies are necessary to establish the mechanisms by which diuretics influence cardiac rhythm and their relevance to long-term morbidity. It is important to determine whether therapeutic maneuvers such as reduction of diuretic dosage, oral potassium supplementation, or potassium-sparing diuretics can help to avoid these problems. Coadministration of beta blockers with thiazides may be an alternative means of preventing epinephrine-induced changes in potassium.

Finally, $beta_2$-receptor-mediated hypokalemia may be a factor in sudden death in patients with asthma and chronic respiratory disease. The epidemic of asthma deaths in the 1960s was attributed to many factors including excessive use of beta-agonist aerosol inhalers (19). Hypokalemia was reported after high-dosage beta-agonist use in respiratory disease (22) and obstetrics (24). In New Zealand a further epidemic of asthma death has been reported following the widespread use of beta agonists, combined with a methylxanthine (16). We have observed that pretreatment with theophylline in healthy subjects increases the chronotropic effect of epinephrine 0.06 μg/kg per min infusion and also increased the magnitude of the fall in serum potassium occurring after epinephrine (46). Methylxanthines have several properties, including phosphodiesterase inhibitory activity, which could further potentiate the effects of epinephrine at beta adrenoceptors.

CONCLUSIONS

Epinephrine, a circulating hormone in plasma, has direct inotropic and chronotropic effects on the heart. It also acts on a $beta_2$ receptor on skeletal muscle to activate a membrane-bound sodium potassium ATPase which increases sodium efflux and potassium influx. The net result is systemic hypokalemia which is apparent during stress when physical activity is restricted. During the early stages of acute myocardial infarction, plasma catecholamines, particularly plasma epinephrine, are elevated associated with a reduction in serum potassium and increased ventricular fibrillation and higher mortality. Epinephrine or beta-agonist-induced hypokalemia may be a further mechanism contributing to cardiac arrhythmias in patients with acute myocardial infarction and severe asthma.

ACKNOWLEDGMENTS

The author thanks Dr. J.C. Rodger, Monklands Hospital, who stimulated the interest of our group in this area and also contributed data on some of the patients included. The studies described in this paper were conducted in association with Drs. Kenneth Whyte and Allan Struthers. The technical assistance of James McCulloch and Robert Whitesmith is gratefully acknowledged, as is the help of the staff of the Clinical Pharmacology Research Unit and the Coronary Care Unit at Stobhill Hospital. Mrs. M. Wood kindly typed the manuscript.

REFERENCES

1. Anonymous: Editorial: Adrenaline and potassium: everything in flux. *Lancet* 2: 1401–1403, 1983.
2. Benedict, C. R., and Grahame Smith, D. G.: Plasma adrenaline concentrations and dopamine beta hydroxylase activity in myocardial infarction with and without cardiogenic shock. *Br. Heart J.* 42:214–220, 1979.
3. Bia, M. J., and de Fronzo, R. A.: Extrarenal potassium homeostasis. *Am. J. Physiol.* 198:1066–1070, 1981.
4. Brown, M. J., Brown, D. C., and Murphy, M. B.: Hypokalemia from beta$_2$ receptor stimulation by circulating epinephrine. *N. Engl. J. Med.* 309:1414–1419, 1983.
5. Buckler, K. J., Bhattacharya, S. S., and Flear, C. T. G.: Actions of catecholamines and beta blockers on Na pump activity in heart and skeletal muscle. *Clin. Sci.* 63:38, 1982.
6. Clausen, T.: Adrenergic control of Na^+-K^+ homeostasis. *Acta Med. Scand.* Suppl. 672:111–115, 1983.
7. Clausen, T., and Flatman, J. A.: Beta$_2$ adrenoceptors mediate the stimulating effect of adrenaline on active electrogenic Na^+/K^+ transport in rat soleus muscle. *Br. J. Pharmacol.* 68:749–755, 1980.
8. Cryer, P. E.: Physiology and pathophysiology of the human sympathoadrenal neuroendocrine system. *N. Engl. J. Med.* 303:436–444, 1980.
9. da Prada, M., and Zurcher, G.: Simultaneous radioenzymatic determination of plasma and tissue adrenaline, noradrenaline and dopamine within the femtomole range. *Life Sci.* 19:1151–1174, 1975.
10. Dimsdale, J. E., and Moss, J.: Short term catecholamine response to psychological stress. *Psychosom. Med.* 42:493–497, 1980.
11. Donnelly, T., Gray, H., Simpson, E., and Rodger, J. C.: Serum potassium and acute myocardial infarction. *Scott. Med. J.* 25:176, 1980.
12. D'Silva, J. H.: Action of adrenaline on the perfused liver. *J. Physiol.* 87:181–188, 1936.
13. Dyckner, T., Helmers, C., Lundman, T., and Wester, P. O.: Initial serum potassium level in relation to early complications and prognosis in patients with acute myocardial infarction. *Acta Med. Scand.* 197:207–210, 1975.
14. Epstein, F. H., and Rosa, R. M.: Adrenergic control of serum potassium. *N. Engl. J. Med.* 309:1450–1451, 1983.
15. Esler, M., Jenning, G., Blomberg, P., Korner, P., and Leonard, P.: Measurement of total and organ specific noradrenaline release in humans (abstract). 5th Catecholamine Symposium, Goteborg, 1983.
16. Grant, I. W. B.: Asthma in New Zealand. *Br. Med. J.* 286, 374–377, 1983.
17. Hjalmarson, A., Elmfeldt, D., Herlitz, J., Holmberg, S., Malek, I., Wyberg, G., Ryden, L., Swedberg, K. J., Wedel, H., Wilhelmsen, L., and Wilhelmsson, C.: Effect on mortality of metoprolol in acute myocardial infarction. *Lancet* 2:823–827, 1981.
18. Hollifield, J. W., and Slaton, P. E.: Cardiac arrhythmias associated with diuretic induced hypokalaemia and hypomagnesaemia. In *Arrhythmias and Myocardial Infarction: The Role of Potassium. R. Soc. Med. Int. Congress Sympos. Series* 44:17–24, 1981.
19. Inman, W. M., and Adelstein, A. M.: Rise and fall of asthma mortality in England and Wales in relation to use of pressurised aerosols. *Lancet* 2:279–285, 1969.
20. Jones, D. H., Hamilton, C. A., and Reid, J. L.: Choice of control groups in the appraisal of sympathetic activity in essential hypertension. *Clin. Sci.* 57:339–344, 1979.
21. Karlsberg, R. P., Cryer, P. E., and Roberts, S.: Serial plasma catecholamine response

early in the course of acute myocardial infarction: relationship to infarct extent and mortality. *Am. Heart J.* 102:14–19, 1981.

22. Leitch, A. G., Clancy, L. J., Costello, J. R., and Flenley, D. C.: Effect of intravenous infusion of salbutamol on ventilatory response to carbon dioxide and hypoxia and on heart rate and plasma potassium in normal man. *Br. Med. J.* 1:365–367, 1976.
23. Lim, M., Lintan, R. A. F., Wolff, C. B., and Band, D. M.: Propranolol, exercise and arterial plasma potassium. *Lancet* 2:591, 1981.
24. Maravec, M. A., and Hurlbert, B. J.: Hypokalaemia associated with terbutaline administration in obstetrical patients. *Anesth. Analg.* 59:917–920, 1980.
25. Morgan, D. B., and Young, R. M.: Acute transient hypokalemia; new interpretation of a common event. *Lancet* 2:751–752, 1982.
26. M.R.C. Working Party on Mild to Moderate Hypertension: Ventricular extrasystoles during thiazide treatment: substudy of M.R.C. mild hypertension trial. *Br. Med. J.* 287:1249–1253, 1983.
27. Mueller, H. S., and Ayres, S. M.: Propranolol decreases sympathetic nervous activity reflected by plasma catecholamines during evolution of myocardial infarction in man. *J. Clin. Invest.* 65:338–346, 1980.
28. Multiple Risk Factor Intervention Trial: Risk factor changes and mortality results. *JAMA* 248:1465–1477, 1982.
29. National Heart Lung and Blood Institute Co-operative Trial: The beta blocker heart attack trial. *JAMA* 246:2073–2074, 1981.
30. Nordrehaug, J. E., and van der Lippe, G.: Hypokalemia and ventricular fibrillation in acute myocardial infarction. *Br. Heart J.* 50:525–529, 1983.
31. Norwegian Multicenter Study Groups: Timolol induced reduction in mortality and reinfarction in patients surviving acute myocardial infarction. *N. Engl. J. Med.* 304: 801–807, 1981.
32. Petch, M. C., McKay, R., and Bethune, D. W.: The effect of $beta_2$ adrenergic blockade on serum potassium and glucose levels during open heart surgery. *Eur. Heart J.* 2:123–126, 1981.
33. Struthers, A. D., and Reid, J. L.: Nifedipine does not influence adrenaline induced hypokalaemia in man. *Br. J. Clin. Pharmacol.* 16:342–343, 1983.
34. Struthers, A. D., and Reid, J. L.: The role of adrenal medullary catecholamines in potassium homeostasis. *Clin. Sci.* 66:377–382, 1984.
35. Struthers, A. D., Whitesmith, R., and Reid, J. L.: Prior thiazide diuretic treatment increases adrenaline induced hypokalaemia. *Lancet* 1:1358–1360, 1983.
36. Struthers, A. D., Whitesmith, R., and Reid, J. L.: Metabolic and haemodynamic effects of increased circulating adrenaline in man. Effect of labetalol on alpha and beta blocker. *Br. Heart J.* 50:277–281, 1983.
37. Struthers, A. D., Reid, J. L., Whitesmith, R., and Rodger, J. C.: Effect of intravenous adrenaline on electrocardiogram, blood pressure and serum potassium. *Br. Heart J.* 49:90–93, 1983.
38. Struthers, A. D., Reid, J. L., Whitesmith, R., and Rodger, J. C.: The effects of cardioselective and non selective beta adrenoceptor blockade or haemodynamic and hypokalaemic response to intravenous adrenaline in man. *Clin. Sci.* 65:143–147, 1983.
39. Soloman, R., and Cole, A.: Arrhythmias and myocardial infarction: role of potassium. *R. Soc. Med. Int. Congress Sympos. Series* 44:47–55, 1980.
40. Van Beaumont, W., Strand, J. C., Petroforky, J. S., Hipskind, S. G., and Greenleaf, J. E.: Changes in total plasma content of electrolytes and proteins with normal exercise. *J. Appl. Physiol.* 34:102–106, 1973.
41. Vetter, N. J., Strange, R. C., Adams, W., and Oliver, M. F.: Initial metabolic and hormonal response to acute myocardial infarction. *Lancet* 1:284–289, 1974.

42. Vick, R. L., Todd, E. P., and Luedke, D. W.: Epinephrine induced hypokalaemia: relation to liver and skeletal muscle. *J. Pharmacol. Exp. Ther.* 181:139–146, 1972.
43. Videback, J., Christensen, N. J., and Sterndorff, H.: Serial determination of plasma catecholamine in myocardial infarction. *Circulation* 46:846–855, 1972.
44. Vincent, H. H., Boomsma, F., Marrin t'Veld, A. J., Derkx, F. H. M., Wenting, G. J., and Schalekamp, M. A. D. H.: Effect of selective and non selective beta agonists on plasma potassium and norepinephrine. *J. Cardiovasc. Pharmacol.* 6:107–114, 1984.
45. Wang, P., and Clausen, T.: Treatment of attacks in hyperkalemia familial periodic paralysis by inhalation of salbutamol. *Lancet* 1:221, 1976.
46. Whyte, K., Addis, G. J., Whitesmith, R., and Reid, J. L.: Methylxanthines and adrenaline induced hypokalaemia–possible contribution to tachyarrhythmias in asthmatic patients. *Clin. Sci.* 66:57, 1984.
47. Yusuf, S., Ramsdale, D., Peto, R., Furse, L., Bennett, D., Bray, C., and Sleight, P.: Early intravenous atenolol treatment in suspected acute myocardial infarction. *Lancet* 2:273–276, 1980.

HYPOKALEMIA AND CARDIAC ARRHYTHMIAS DURING DIURETIC TREATMENT

16

Determinants of the Kaliuretic Action of Diuretic Drugs

GILBERT H. MUDGE
Dartmouth Medical School, Hanover, New Hampshire

Most diuretic drugs are used to increase the renal excretion of water, sodium, chloride, and sometimes bicarbonate. They have a variable tendency to increase the excretion of potassium. Since this may lead to hypokalemia this tendency is commonly considered an undesirable side effect. A subgroup of drugs, the aldosterone antagonists and the potassium-sparing diuretics (triamterene, amiloride), have a relatively minor effect on sodium, chloride, and water excretion, but they significantly reduce potassium loss.

With the chronic administration of diuretics, mild to moderate hypokalemia is a common clinical problem. In many instances early in treatment a slightly negative potassium balance occurs which fails to progress further (44). In studies conducted over a number of weeks the potassium deficit varies from zero to about 200 mEq (16). When diuretics are administered for as long as 2 years, total body potassium levels may be within normal limits (32). While these slight deficits are the common pattern, there is a small subgroup of patients in whom diuretics acutely produce severe hypokalemia associated with marked hyponatremia and, we have learned from somewhat indirect evidence, significant potassium depletion (1,21). Thorough studies are not available and the mechanisms are not understood. In addition, when diuretics are administered chronically in excessively high dosages a significant degree of potassium depletion may occur (33). Balance studies are rarely performed in clinical practice and the possibility of a rare instance of significant potassium depletion should be kept in mind. The degree of hypokalemia itself is an unreliable index of depletion (64). The tacit assumption that hypokalemia simply results from the urinary loss of potassium may also warrant reconsideration. Most common diuretics often produce metabolic alkalosis. If this is treated with ammonium chloride the diuretic-induced hypokalemia may be corrected without any change in external potassium balance (64).

This chapter will consider the factors involved in drug-induced kaliuresis; the drugs that conserve potassium will not be reviewed systematically.

RENAL TUBULAR TRANSPORT OF POTASSIUM

Potassium is not bound to plasma protein and hence is freely filterable at the glomerulus. Potassium excretion into the voided urine is the arithmetic sum of tubular transport in opposite directions: reabsorption and secretion. These terms refer to the direction of transport into or out of the tubular fluid without reference to mechanism. Although some organic compounds undergo bidirectional transport, among strong electrolytes the potassium ion is unique in exhibiting this property. Depending on the experimental condition, the amount of potassium excreted can range from about 2 to 200% of the amount filtered. Hence transport in either direction can involve large quantities of the ion. When the bidirectional nature of potassium transport was first being studied with the clearance technique, Gilman (11,45) suggested that the filtered potassium is completely reabsorbed proximally, that secretion occurs in the distal segment, and that this latter process is under homeostatic control. This hypothesis was consistent with the then available clearance studies but was by no means proven by them. Since that time many elegant micropuncture experiments have been carried out and in general have confirmed Gilman's speculation. However, not surprisingly, recent work has revealed a far more complicated mechanism than originally envisaged.

SEGMENTAL LOCALIZATION

On the basis of morphological and functional criteria, an increasing number of segments of the tubule have been identified. Figure 1 shows the major segments involved in potassium transport but does not include some of the minor subdivisions for which transport has not been characterized. For many tubular functions the nephron population may be classified into superficial cortical and deep juxtamedullary nephrons. In the case of potassium this separation is based primarily on technical rather than physiological considerations since the values shown in Figure 1 represent sites that are accessible to micropuncture. It is not known whether there are substantial functional differences. (For reviews, see References 11, 26-28, 58, 67, 68.)

As shown in Figure 1, filtered potassium is mainly reabsorbed in the proximal convoluted tubule (PCT), a process which probably continues into the pars recta (PR). In the descending limb of Henle's loop (DLH) potassium is secreted into the tubular fluid so that at the hairpin turn of the loop of Henle (L of H) net secretion is discernible during states of high potassium intake. In the descending limb, less secretion probably occurs with potassium deprivation. From the loop of Henle back to the cortex, potassium is again reabsorbed so that at the first accessible part of the early distal tubule (EDT) an amount equivalent to only about 10% of the filtered load remains within the tubular fluid. Undoubtedly large amounts of potassium are reabsorbed in the thick ascending limb (TAL) but the exact quantities are not known since neither TAL nor DLH is accessible for sampling. It has been proposed that potassium is recycled through the loop of Henle (2). This involves reabsorption from the medullary collecting duct (MCD) into the interstitium, secretion into DLH, and then reabsorption in TAL. With acute potassium loading, the potassium secreted into the loop may not be completely reabsorbed and may therefore contribute to final urinary excretion (63).

Nomenclature for the distal tubule has not been consistent but has gradually evolved as new cell types have been identified on the basis of studies of cytology and function. The early distal tubule (EDT) is convoluted and the cells are morphologically similar to

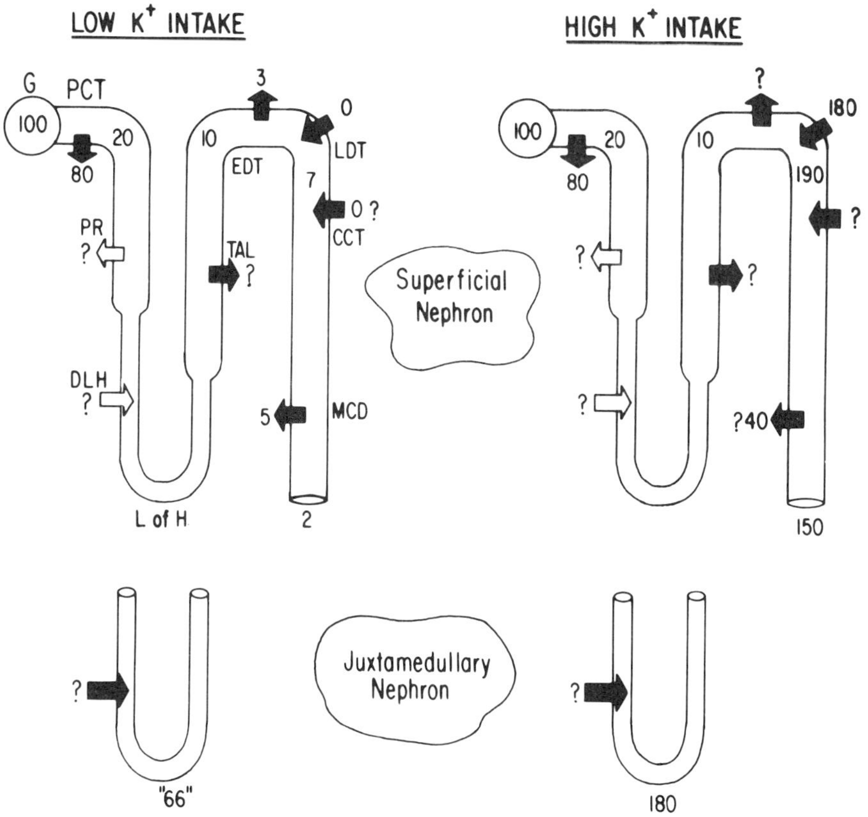

Figure 1 Schematic summary of segmental localization of transport in the nephron. All numerical values represent percentage of amount of potassium filtered. Values indicate either the amount within the tubular fluid or the amount transported at the adjacent arrows. Solid arrows indicate well-documented mechanisms; open arrows represent postulated mechanisms which have not been examined directly. Question marks indicate uncertainty as to quantity. Value of "66" at L of H was obtained with high water intake (2) but probably is in the right direction for low potassium intake. G, glomerulus; PCT, proximal convoluted tubule; PR, pars recta; DLH, descending limb of Henle; L of H, loop of Henle; TAL, thick ascending limb; EDT, early distal tubule; LDT, late distal tubule; CCT, cortical collecting tubule; MCD, medullary collecting duct. For discussion see text. (Modified from Ref. 58.)

those in TAL. During low intake the EDT reabsorbs small amounts of potassium; whether reabsorption persists during potassium loading is not known. The next segments down the tubule are the connecting tubule and the initial collecting tubule. In some studies these are considered together as the late distal tubule (LDT). However, the characteristics of the initial collecting tubule are similar to those of the cortical collecting tubule (CCT) for potassium secretion. The LDT is accessible to direct micropuncture in vivo. The CCT can not be punctured in vivo but must be studied as an isolated segment under in vitro conditions. Because of these differences in experimental techniques, under many circumstances it is not possible to differentiate the separate contributions of these two segments. For this reason the quantitative degree of secretion for CCT is indicated by a question mark in

Figure 1. Secretion is maximal with a high potassium intake and minimal with a low intake. Tubular secretion therefore plays an obvious role in regulating potassium balance.

According to some studies, potassium is either secreted or reabsorbed in the initial collecting tubule. The apparent coexistence of reabsorption and secretion in the same portion of the nephron has recently been resolved. Recent studies have revealed two different cell types which occur throughout the initial collecting tubule, the cortical collecting duct (CCT), and perhaps also in the medullary collecting duct (MCD). So-called *principal* cells are associated with secretion, *intercalated* cells with reabsorption (26,58). Beyond the cortical collecting tubule small amounts of potassium are usually reabsorbed, but secretion may at times occur, especially with maximal stimuli for kaliuresis (4,28,56).

In summary the major sites involving the transport of significant amounts of potassium are (for reabsorption) proximal tubule, thick ascending limb, early distal tubule, and medullary collecting duct and (for secretion) descending limb of Henle, late distal tubule, and cortical collecting tubule. Except for the proximal tubule, the magnitude of transport at each site is heavily influenced by potassium intake as well as a number of other factors which will be discussed below.

CELLULAR MECHANISMS OF POTASSIUM TRANSPORT

Figure 2 summarizes the major mechanisms of potassium reabsorption and secretion by the kidney. There are two general types of transport. *Active transport* occurs against an electrochemical gradient, is directly linked to cellular metabolism, and involves chemical mechanisms intimately associated with cell membranes (solid arrows, Figure 2). *Passive transport* occurs down an electrochemical gradient (dashed arrows, Figure 2). There are several types of passive transport: simple diffusion, mediated diffusion, and others. The present discussion is limited to differentiating active from passive transport as far as the site of diuretic action is concerned. The most important electrophysiological feature that directly influences passive transport is the potential difference. The electrophysiological mechanisms that generate these potential differences are beyond the scope of this review. Diuretic drugs affect active transport directly and passive transport secondarily. This may involve either both primary and secondary actions on the same tubular cell or a primary drug action on one cell type upstream with a secondary effect on other more downstream cells. The latter is mediated by changes in the volume or composition of the tubular fluid.

In the following text the numbered mechanisms refer to Figure 2. An active pump is located at the basolateral (i.e., peritubular) membrane of all segments of the nephron shown in Figure 2. In this respect the cells of the kidney are similar to those of many other organs. The active extrusion of sodium is linked to the inward uptake of potassium. The degree of linkage between these two cations and the activity of the pump itself vary from one cell type to another and for a given cell are subject to a number of physiological stimuli. The activity of this pump tends to keep the intracellular concentration of sodium low and that of potassium high. The pump is characterized by Na-K ATPase activity and an energy source depends on ATP generated elsewhere within the cell. This mechanism of potassium transport is identified as PCT: 4, TAL: 8, LDT: 12, LDT: 15, and CCT: 18 in Figure 2. These are considered to be qualitatively similar.

The passive transport of potassium from one compartment to another depends on two major factors: the electrochemical gradient between compartments and the permeability characteristics of the intervening membrane. In turn, the gradient between adjacent compartments is determined by two components: the concentrations of potassium and the

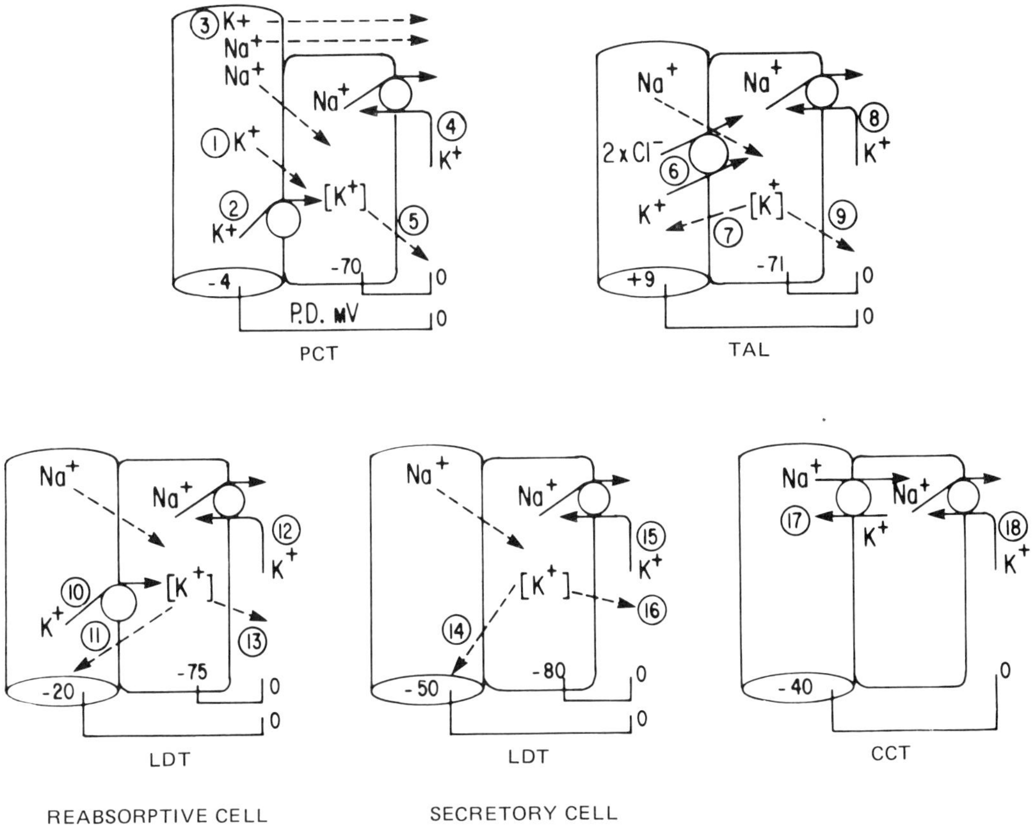

Figure 2 Schematic summary of cellular mechanisms of potassium transport for different segments of the nephron. Solid arrows indicate active transport, dashed arrows indicate passive. For clarity, most diagrams do not include hydrogen ions or anions. Potential differences are approximate averages. Abbreviations for tubule segments same as in Figure 1. See text for discussion of the numerically identified mechanisms.

potential difference. In Figure 2, the electrochemical gradients can be inferred from the direction of the dashed arrows. Consider, for example, the secretory cell of the late distal tubule (LDT). The high intracellular concentration of potassium tends to move potassium passively into both the lumen (LDT: 14) and the peritubular fluid (LDT: 16). However, the two surfaces of the cell are asymmetrical with respect to potential difference. The egress of the positively charged potassium cation tends to be counteracted by the intracellular negativity, but the magnitude of this potential is less across the luminal than across the basolateral membrane, and as a result potassium tends to move preferentially from cell to lumen (LDT: 14). The magnitude and direction of the electrochemical gradients vary from one segment to another. It should be reemphasized that probably all segments of the nephron have both active and passive mechanisms for potassium transport. By convention, the characterization of reabsorption or secretion as either active or passive refers to transport between tubular fluid and the cell. In all cell types at the basolateral membrane, transport between the cell and the peritubular fluid is active in one direction and passive in the other (Figure 2).

In the proximal tubule there are three mechanisms of potassium reabsorption. During the process of the isosmotic reabsorption of sodium and water, a significant amount of potassium undergoes passive reabsorption. This involves transcellular (PCT: 1) as well as paracellular (PCT: 3) transport. The latter occurs principally in the more distal portion of this segment (28). In addition, when proximal flow is increased by acetazolamide administration or osmotic diuresis the tubular fluid concentration of potassium decreases sufficiently to reveal an active component of potassium reabsorption (PCT: 2) (3,52).

In the thick ascending limb there is an unusual reabsorptive mechanism at the luminal membrane (TAL: 6) involving the cotransport of sodium, potassium, and chloride. This is sensitive to the high-ceiling, or loop, diuretics. This is driven by the basolateral extrusion of sodium (TAL: 8). In view of the recycling of potassium through the loop of Henle, large amounts of potassium almost certainly undergo net reabsorption by this mechanism. In addition, the cotransport mechanism involves the reabsorption of sodium and potassium in equivalent amounts. Since it is probable that the tubular fluid entering the TAL contains far higher concentrations of sodium than potassium, cotransport of these two cations in the reabsorptive direction (TAL: 6) would require the recycling of potassium from cell to tubular fluid (TAL: 7). Such a mechanism is supported by electrophysiological data (30). Because of the inaccessibility of the TAL, the exact amounts of potassium reabsorbed by this segment cannot be measured directly by micropuncture.

The early distal tubule only reabsorbs potassium. The mechanism is similar to that in the late distal tubule (LDT: 10), where potassium is either reabsorbed (LDT: 10) or secreted (LDT: 14) depending on the cell type. In this instance secretion is passive.

Farther on, in the cortical collecting tubule, active potassium secretion (CCT: 17) is linked to sodium reabsorption by a pump localized to the luminal membrane (29,53). This segment is sensitive to the action of cardiac glycosides, amiloride, and aldosterone, but insensitive to furosemide and thiazides. As indicated below, potassium secretion in the late distal tubule is dependent on the rate of tubular flow. In the cortical collecting duct, secretion is independent of flow rate (22).

Bidirectional transport across the same membrane of a given cell poses conceptual as well as semantic problems. In many instances transport in one direction may represent merely a backleak, having little net effect on the greater degree of transport in the opposite direction. As an example, consider the passive secretion at LDT: 11 which is overwhelmed by active reabsorption at LDT: 10. In other instances, within a given segment, bidirectional transport may be based on differences in cell type, for example, LDT-reabsorptive and LDT-secretory cells. A third possibility involves the coexistence of opposing mechanisms in the same cell in which an appropriate stimulus, such as a high potassium intake, inhibits transport in one direction thus unveiling net transport in the opposite. This has been proposed for the thick ascending limb (TAL: 6 and 9 vs. TAL: 8 and 7) (49). Such adaptations may involve the formation of new membrane elements which have a specific role in potassium transport (55,58).

FACTORS INFLUENCING POTASSIUM TRANSPORT IN THE DISTAL NEPHRON

The principal factors that modulate potassium transport are potassium intake (which, in turn, determines the levels of plasma and intracellular potassium), rate of fluid flow in the tubular lumen, sodium concentration of the tubular fluid, mineralocorticoid activity, pH, the excretion of unreabsorbable anions, and the level of antidiuretic hormone. Each of these factors has been well studied, many are interrelated, and all play a role in potassium homeostasis.

A high dietary intake of potassium, either acute or chronic, is a powerful stimulus for potassium excretion. Ingested or infused potassium raises the plasma level to a slight degree but the ion is principally distributed into intracellular fluid. Based on the finding of early clearances (5,47), it was postulated that tubular secretion was responsive to intracellular levels. This has been documented by direct measurements of intracellular concentrations or, more correctly, intracellular potassium activity (28).

Renal adaptation to high potassium intake is associated with a marked increase in Na-K ATPase activity (55) especially in the cortical and medullary collecting tubules (58). This tends to increase the intracellular pool of potassium by stimulating LDT: 15 or CCT: 18. The transepithelial difference may also increase, the lumen becoming more negative. These two factors in combination increase the electrochemical gradient from cell to lumen and enhance potassium secretion by LDT: 14. At the same time active secretion by the luminal membrane of the cortical collecting duct is also increased (CCT: 17). Diminished reabsorption of potassium in response to potassium loads has been described for the thick ascending limb of Henle (49,63); the extent to which this increases delivery of potassium to the distal segment is uncertain. Although high dietary potassium levels stimulate aldosterone production, this hormone is not directly involved in the adaptation response. In experiments in which all other factors known to affect potassium excretion were kept constant, the plasma potassium was elevated by stepwise increases in potassium intake. Below the normal level of plasma potassium this had little effect on potassium excretion, but above the normal plasma level slight changes had a powerful effect on excretion (69). This involves secretion by LDT: 14 (60). Presumably this is mediated by an expansion of the intracellular pool of the distal segments by the basolateral transport mechanism previously described.

In general, a reduction in potassium intake has an effect on excretion opposite to a high intake (41). With moderate potassium depletion, as little as 2% of the filtered load is excreted and all evidence for distal secretion vanishes.

The flow of tubular fluid in the distal nephron may be increased by saline loads or by diuretics which inhibit electrolytes and fluid reabsorption upstream. If other factors remain constant, the potassium concentration within the distal tubular fluid tends to remain unchanged and therefore total excretion becomes proportional to the rate of flow. In other words, tubular excretion by LDT: 14 is flow-dependent. This is an important mechanism underlying the kaliuresis induced by diuretics (17). Under the same conditions the distal secretion of potassium is also influenced by the concentration of sodium in the tubular fluid (39). Extremely low levels of sodium may completely inhibit potassium secretion. With normal or elevated concentrations of sodium, the distal reabsorption of sodium influences potassium secretion by two mechanisms. In reference to LDT: 14, increased sodium reabsorption contributes to the negativity of the lumen and increases the electrochemical gradient for potassium. This enhances passive secretion. In reference to CCT: 17, the reabsorption of sodium is linked to the active secretion of potassium at the luminal membrane. Potassium secretion at this site is inhibited by low concentrations of sodium (29).

Aldosterone acts on the distal area of the nephron to increase potassium secretion and sodium reabsorption. The cellular mechanisms are complex. In the late distal tubule the permeability characteristics of both the luminal and basolateral membranes may be altered to facilitate potassium secretion (26). In the cortical collecting tubule mineralocorticoids greatly increase the transepithelial potential difference (50). This stimulates those either luminal or basolateral pumps in which sodium reabsorption is linked to potassium secretion, CCT: 17 and CCT: 18. Aldosterone also stimulates Na-K ATPase activity, but in the absence of potassium loading the role of this mechanism for potassium homeostasis is uncertain (55).

Studies on aldosterone provide an interesting example of the manner in which multiple factors may interact to influence a given mechanism, in this instance the late distal tubule secretory cell. With the use of free-flow micropuncture methods, aldosterone reduces the flow of tubular fluid and appears to have only a negligible effect on potassium secretion. However when the same segment is perfused at a constant rate, aldosterone markedly stimulates potassium secretion by a direct tubular action. The overall effect of aldosterone is therefore the sum of the opposing effects of reduced tubular flow and direct tubular stimulation (23). This poses obvious difficulties in extrapolating from the experimental to clinical situation. Depending on a variety of factors, one might or might not expect a given level of aldosterone to influence potassium excretion.

Acid-base balance has a profound effect on potassium excretion. This is often complicated by changes in external fluid balance and by readjustments in segmental flow within the nephron. These may influence potassium transport independently of acid-base status. However, under controlled conditions, an increase in the peritubular pH (systemic metabolic alkalosis) stimulates the basolateral uptake of potassium and its secretion by acting on LDT: 15 (59). Systemic metabolic acidosis has the opposite effect. However not all segments of the nephron respond in the same manner. In the cortical collecting tubule, potassium secretion is responsive to the pH of the tubular fluid (8) while in the superficial late distal tubule it is responsive to the peritubular pH (59).

When one is considering clinical situations, metabolic alkalosis associated with fluid loss should be differentiated from alkalosis induced by the administration of alkalinizing fluids. In the former, aldosterone production may be stimulated by volume contraction; in the latter it may be inhibited by expanded volume and hypokalemia. As an example, consider patients who receive massive loads of isotonic sodium bicarbonate by duodenal tube for the treatment of ulcer disease (54). Despite significant systemic alkalosis there is only a slight potassium loss on the first day; thereafter renal excretion equals intake. This pattern reflects reduced aldosterone production. As far as potassium metabolism is concerned, it is proper to differentiate between two types of metabolic alkalosis; one occurring with volume expansion and the other with volume contraction.

Unreabsorbable anions must be excreted with an electrical equivalence of cations of which potassium is an important component. Such unreabsorbable anions increase the rate of urine flow and greatly increase potassium excretion (27). This probably involves decreased reabsorption in the proximal (PCT: 1, PCT: 2) as well as increased secretion in the late distal (LDT: 14) tubule. Unreabsorbable anions are also accompanied by sodium, and its concentration in the distal tubular fluid may facilitate potassium secretion. In addition, the distal transepithelial potential difference is increased by unreabsorbable anions (27). Since unreabsorbable anions are sometimes prescribed for therapeutic purposes (e.g., para-aminosalicylic acid and carbenicillin), the phenomenon has practical importance.

Although the kidney plays a major role in regulating potassium homeostasis, extrarenal nonsecretory organs have an important function in regulating the redistribution of potassium between the extracellular and intracellular compartments. A number of hormones are involved. These include sympathomimetic compounds. It has recently been shown that epinephrine and other $beta_1$ agonists inhibit potassium secretion by the renal tubule while $beta_1$ antagonists stimulate it (35). The renal mechanisms as well as their quantitative significance await further study.

The antidiuretic hormone of the posterior pituitary gland has recently been directly implicated in the renal regulation of potassium excretion. It has long been recognized that water diuresis is associated with a much lower potassium clearance rate than is seen with diuresis due to other causes (47). The antidiuretic hormone directly stimulates potassium secretion both in the late distal tubule and beyond (22). From a number of possible explanations, the most likely appears to be an increase in potassium permeability of the luminal membrane involved in passive secretion (LDT: 14).

EFFECT OF DIURETIC DRUGS ON POTASSIUM TRANSPORT IN THE KIDNEY

Diuretics may either increase or decrease the rate of potassium excretion in the voided urine by either inhibiting or stimulating either secretion or reabsorption or by combinations of these actions in different segments.

The following summary is based on reasonably firm evidence but in a number of instances the cellular mechanism is incompletely documented. For example, because of the bidirectional nature of potassium transport, complete documentation of drug effect would require measurement of net change and unidirectional fluxes in both directions. Data of this type are rarely available. In one instance in which radioactive potassium was used as a tracer, an increase in net secretion of potassium by the late distal tubule and cortical collecting duct was accompanied by a decrease in the unidirectional reabsorptive flux as well as an increase in the unidirectional secretory flux (25).

Osmotic Diuretics

Osmotic diuretics increase potassium excretion by decreasing reabsorption across the proximal tubule (PCT: 1) and probably also at the paracellular pathway (PCT: 3) (28,52). In addition, secretion of potassium is enhanced along the flow-dependent distal mechanism, LDT: 14 (39). Moderate dosages of mannitol also increase potassium secretion by the medullary collecting duct (56).

Mercurial Diuretics

These increase potassium excretion under normal circumstances but when excretion is initially high, as with potassium loading, excretion is then decreased (45). Increased excretion probably results from inhibition of reabsorption in the thick ascending limb (TAL: 6), which is the same site at which mercurials exert their major diuretic action on the reabsorption of sodium, chloride, and water (20). Mercurials inhibit potassium secretion when it is stimulated by high potassium intake (45), thiazides (31,51), or carbonic anhydrase inhibitors (6). In each of these situations, prior to the administration of the mercurial, potassium secretion is increased in the late distal tubule. Therefore mercurials inhibit transport at LDT: 15. Whether they also inhibit secretion in the cortical collecting duct is not known. It is of interest that the effect of mercurials on sodium reabsorption is additive to that of either acetazolamide or chlorothiazide, but at the same time the secretion of potassium stimulated by these drugs is sharply reduced (51).

Inhibitors of Carbonic Anhydrase

These are strongly kaliuretic (6). In the proximal convoluted tubule these drugs block sodium and water reabsorption and the sodium and potassium ions become dissociated as far as their relative concentrations in the tubular fluid are concerned. However, there is no net kaliuretic effect in this segment (3). These drugs also block sodium and water reabsorption in the distal tubule and in the more downstream collecting ducts (56). Thus, conditions are appropriate for passive potassium secretion (LDT: 14). However, probably the major effect of carbonic anhydrase inhibition is to increase potassium uptake at the basolateral membrane and thereby to increase the size of the intracellular pool. This leads to increased secretion of potassium (42). It is believed that the drugs initially inhibit carbonic anhydrase, that inhibition of this enzyme leads to local acid-base imbalance, and that this in turn increases cellular uptake of potassium and enhances potassium secretion (26). It is also possible that carbonic anhydrase inhibitors block coupled potassium reabsorption in the thick ascending limb (TAL: 6) but data for the mammalian tubule are incomplete. Potassium secretion is also increased in the medullary collecting duct (56).

Benzothiazides

The benzothiazides (or thiazides) regularly increase potassium excretion but their action within the nephron has been studied less well than that of other diuretics. There is no convincing evidence for an action on proximal reabsorption except for compounds that also have carbonic anhydrase inhibitory activity. Some studies show moderate inhibition of sodium and potassium reabsorption in the loop of Henle (i.e., prior to the earliest distal site) while other studies do not (15,66). Stop-flow analysis shows that the thiazides increase potassium secretion in the distal tubule (38). Some of their effect here may involve carbonic anhydrase inhibition. Isotope and micropuncture studies show that the secreted potassium is derived from the intracellular pool (24). This implicates actual secretion and not just decreased reabsorption as the underlying mechanism.

High-Ceiling Diuretics

The high-ceiling, or loop, diuretics increase potassium excretion. Furosemide has been studied the most widely but other compounds appear to have a similar action. Except with exceptionally high dosages, electrolyte transport in the proximal tubule remains unaffected. Inhibition of the reabsorption of sodium, chloride, and water in the thick ascending limb is principally responsible for the diuresis (TAL: 6). However, the mechanisms of kaliuresis are more complicated. By increasing the amount of fluid and sodium delivered to the late distal tubule, furosemide clearly increases the passive secretion of potassium at LDT: 14 (17). However, at the same time there is an increase in the delivery of potassium to this segment in amounts sufficient to account for about half of the potassium finally excreted. This probably is derived from inhibition of the furosemide-sensitive potassium reabsorption in the thick ascending limb (TAL: 6) (49). In the isolated perfused kidney furosemide stimulates potassium secretion (9), and may also inhibit reabsorption (65). It is of interest that in segments of isolated amphibian tubules, which are considered to be analogous to the mammalian thick ascending limb, furosemide converts net potassium reabsorption to net secretion (49). In the medullary collecting duct a slight increase in potassium secretion is induced by furosemide while at the same time sodium reabsorption in this segment is completely blocked (56).

Cardiac Glycosides

The cardiac glycosides act upon the kidney in high concentrations but, because of their toxicity, are not used for this purpose clinically. However, they have played an important role in the experimental analysis of renal function. Similarly to the mercurials they can either increase or decrease potassium excretion, depending on control conditions. Their dominant biochemical action is the inhibition of Na-K ATPase, the membrane-associated enzyme involved in active transport across the basolateral membrane. Under normal conditions or with slight potassium depletion the glycosides increase potassium excretion and at least three separate mechanisms may be involved. First, in species sensitive to the proximal action of these agents, the glycoside-induced diuresis increases the delivery of fluid and sodium to the late distal tubule. This enhances passive potassium secretion, LDT: 14 (13,62). Secondly, these drugs directly inhibit potassium reabsorption in amphibian nephrons in segments considered to be analogous to the mammalian thick ascending limb (28). And third, even in the absence of any action prior to the distal segment, the glycosides can increase potassium excretion in the potassium-depleted animal by inhibition of active distal reabsorption, LDT: 10 (17). When potassium excretion is initially increased by potassium loading or by furosemide, the glycosides then decrease potassium secretion (9,55,62). This has been interpreted as inhibition of either the basolateral pump (LDT: 15) or the luminal pump (CCT: 17), both of which drive potassium from the peritubular fluid to the lumen.

Potassium-Sparing Diuretics

Of the potassium-sparing diuretics, amiloride has been the most widely studied. Drugs of this class decrease the urinary excretion of potassium by reducing tubular secretion in the late distal and cortical collecting tubule. This is accomplished by inhibition of sodium reabsorption which in turn reduces the electronegativity of the tubular fluid and the electrochemical gradient for the passive secretion of potassium (LDT: 14) (17).

Diuretics in Combination

Combinations of diuretics are often unpredictable in terms of their effect on sodium, chloride, and water excretion. The same applies to potassium excretion though few systematic studies are available. One combination, however, warrants mention since severe potassium depletion may result. This involves carbonic anhydrase inhibitors, benzothiazides, and high-ceiling diuretics administered together with drugs that have mineralocorticoid activity (40). The available data are limited to case reports but the probable mechanisms may be surmised from the previous discussion.

FACTORS INFLUENCING DIURETIC ACTION

A number of factors influence the magnitude of diuretic-induced kaliuresis. Illustrative examples will be presented without attempting an inclusive review. The nature of the observations and their timing can affect the results and their eventual interpretation. For example, with the administration of intravenous furosemide and by the collection of urine samples at short intervals in the dog, the potassium/inulin ratio can rise from a control of 0.2 to over 2.0 at 5 min (46). When averaged over 1 hr the ratio is 0.9 and, when extended to 5 hr, it is about 0.5 despite persistence of drug action measured by other criteria.

Although aldosterone enhances potassium secretion in controlled experiments, it is difficult to evaluate its clinical contribution to kaliuresis quantitatively. When diuresis is produced in humans with the use of high-ceiling diuretics, the K/Na concentration ratio in the voided urine is directly proportional to the rate of aldosterone excretion on the control day (14,19). But since the degree of diuresis itself is often unpredictable, particularly in ill patients, there is no necessary relationship between aldosterone and kaliuresis when the latter is considered in absolute terms, that is, the amount of potassium excreted per unit time.

The relationship of aldosterone to diuretic-induced kaliuresis is further complicated by the changes in aldosterone production induced by the diuretic itself. Furosemide in the rat produces a 25-fold rise in the serum concentration of aldosterone within 30 min. This rise is completely blocked by indomethacin and is mediated through prostaglandins and renin (57). It is not possible to say whether such early changes in aldosterone have any effect on diuretic-induced kaliuresis. With repeated daily doses of hydroflumethiazide, the peak renal clearance of potassium is observed on about day 4 and is correlated with an increase in plasma aldosterone (12).

It should be emphasized that the interrelationship between modest changes in aldosterone production and the degree of kaliuresis induced by diuretic drugs has not been well established. This is not surprising in light of the observation that aldosterone can both decrease the rate of flow and directly stimulate the mechanism of potassium secretion in the late distal nephron. These actions have opposite effects on net secretion. In limited observations the combined effect of aldosterone and superimposed diuretics appears to be potentiation rather than simple addition (18), but detailed dosage-response curves are not available.

There are several examples in experimental animals in which the state of potassium balance directly influences diuretic action. Severe potassium depletion with extracellular alkalosis decreases the diuretic activity of acetazolamide but enhances that of mercurials. In both instances it has been proposed that the effect is related to intracellular acidosis within the cells of the nephron (43,48). In the dog the diuretic activity of cardiac glycosides is enhanced by prior potassium depletion and diminished by potassium loading (13). It has been postulated that this involves an interaction between potassium and the glycosides at the level of membrane-bound Na-K ATPase. An unusual effect of potassium loading has been described in the Amphiuma nephron for the transport mechanism involving sodium, potassium, and chloride (TAL: 6). With a normal potassium intake, potassium is reabsorbed at this site, but this is blocked by furosemide to such an extent that transport is converted to secretion. On the other hand, with potassium loading, potassium is secreted and furosemide no longer has any effect (49).

The above observations were made with rather extreme potassium loads. However, smaller changes in potassium intake may also influence diuretic efficacy. Modest loads of sodium chloride or potassium chloride decrease the electrolyte loss provoked by chronic administration of furosemide. In addition furosemide-induced kaliuresis is increased by a low chloride–normal sodium diet but decreased by a normal chloride–low sodium diet (34). The explanation for these findings is not clear but since sodium, potassium, and chloride are all involved it would be logical to consider the tubular site at which all three of these ions are cotransported (TAL: 6).

Water balance may also influence diuretic-induced kaliuresis. As described above, the antidiuretic hormone directly stimulates distal potassium secretion. During water diuresis, for example, during the physiological absence of antidiuretic hormone, furosemide is less kaliuretic than under control conditions. This occurs without any change in sodium excretion or aldosterone production (37).

RELATION OF DRUG DISPOSITION TO KALIURESIS

Pharmacokinetic studies should provide important information on the relationship of drug disposition to drug action, particularly to kaliuresis. However such studies are extremely limited in number. In micropuncture work and in many experiments on intact animals it is common practice to administer the diuretic in a dosage of known efficacy which in many situations is supramaximal. Relatively few dosage-response curves have been established.

The thiazides are secreted in the proximal tubule by the probenecid-sensitive organic anion transport system. Based on previous studies with mercurials, it was anticipated that probenecid would inhibit the tubular secretion of chlorothiazide and reduce its diuretic efficacy. However, in stop-flow experiments drug excretion was decreased, unexpectedly without impairment of diuresis (38). This effect can now be attributed to the use of supramaximal dosages of thiazide since it has subsequently been shown that diuresis can be blocked when smaller dosages of thiazide are employed (7). This also provides support for the concept that the thiazides act from the luminal border of the nephron. In another study hydroflumethiazide was administered in a constant single daily dose to healthy subjects for 1 week and urine was collected at three times each day (12). There was a positive correlation between the rate of thiazide excretion and the rate of sodium excretion (and its clearance). However, the slope of the regression line was considerably less steep on day 7 than day 1, indicating reduced diuretic efficacy. The rate of potassium excretion also correlated with that of thiazide excretion, but the potassium clearance diverged because of changes in plasma concentrations. The findings show a complex relationship between drug excretion, kaliuresis, natriuresis, and aldosterone levels (see above). The relationship of drug excretion to kaliuresis is not the same as for natriuresis.

With furosemide, the relationship of plasma concentration to urinary excretion is normally quite constant. Urinary excretion is inhibited by probenecid. This provides a means of dissociating plasma furosemide concentration from its rate of excretion. It can then be shown that furosemide-induced natriuresis depends on the amount of drug in the tubular fluid rather than the plasma concentration (10). No comparable data are available for kaliuresis. However, with oral administration, the 6-hr dosage-response curves for natriuresis are steeper than for kaliuresis (61). Presumably there would be the same response patterns if sodium and potassium excretion rates were related to rate of drug excretion rather than to drug dosage.

CONCLUSION

One might ask several questions to summarize these findings. First, why is it that diuretics (notably the thiazides and high-ceiling drugs) produce an initial kaliuresis which soon becomes self-limiting, so that significant potassium depletion rarely develops with chronic administration? What is the relationship of hypokalemia to potassium depletion, that is, negative potassium balance? And, as a therapeutic oddity, why is it that potassium supplements are recommended only when renal function is normal, that is, when the supplements can be excreted? And, as a second general question, to what extent in quantitative terms do the different renal mechanisms of potassium transport explain the phenomena that are observed clinically?

It is not surprising that it is difficult to extrapolate from laboratory experiments to the clinical situation. A number of factors are involved: the difference between acute and chronic observations, species differences, the problem of nephron heterogeneity, and others. Multiple factors influence distal secretion and at times may act in opposite directions. For example, acidosis inhibits secretion but the increased tubular flow which accompanies acidosis enhances it; aldosterone has a direct tubular action to increase secretion but it decreases flow rate which inhibits it; and antidiuretic hormone also directly increases tubular secretion but at the same time may decrease flow rate.

It is axiomatic that the effect of a drug is a function of its concentration. For drug-induced kaliuresis, relevant data are almost nonexistent. It is an understandable goal to employ a dosage of drug that will produce a clear and measurable end point. In clinical practice it is easy to know the dosage of drug as administered, but its concentration in the tubular fluid or urine remains, for the most part, unmeasured. The problem is complicated. The drugs studied act by virtue of their concentration within the tubular fluid. These drugs have a relatively high renal clearance as a result of which their concentration within the tubular fluid must rise progressively from glomerulus to papilla. And further, their concentrations within the tubular fluid may be secondarily modified by the drug-induced diuresis itself.

Why do the diuretic drugs produce an apparently self-limited kaliuresis? The question appears not to be answered by any of the factors known to modulate diuretic-induced kaliuresis in acute experiments. By way of speculation, three possibilities come to mind. First, since potassium secretion is driven in part by the intracellular concentration of potassium, is it possible that with a mildly negative balance for the total body a critical degree of intracellular depletion might develop in specific cells of the tubule which have a unique role in regulating potassium excretion? Despite obvious technical difficulties this might be subjected to experimental testing. Second, even when given on a daily basis, most diuretics do not exert a continuous action. Is it possible that in the intervals of nondiuresis potassium may be excessively conserved? In other words, apparent diminution of kaliuresis might represent the algebraic sum of essentially unaltered kaliuresis combined with periods of excessive potassium conservation. This is well documented with the mercuials administered on alternate days and one study has described a similar phenomenon for furosemide (36). Urine collections at less than the time-honored 24 hr might be helpful. And as a third possibility, nephrologists might well consider certain developments in neuropharmacology, namely the well-documented fact that chronic drug administration can change both the number and characteristics of drug receptors. Does this also apply to diuretics? There are no data. A simple approach might be to use some selected micropuncture procedures in animals that had been pretreated with diuretics for long periods of time. Would this significantly change the nature of transport within different segments of the nephron?

ACKNOWLEDGMENTS

I am indebted to Dr. I.M. Weiner for his critical review of the manuscript and to G. Giebisch and L. Stoner for making unpublished data available to me.

REFERENCES

1. Ashraf, N., Locksley, R., and Arieff, A. I.: Thiazide-induced hyponatremia associated with death or neurologic damage in outpatients. *Am. J. Med.* 70:1163–1168, 1981.

2. Battilana, C. A., Dobyan, D. C., Lacy, F. B., Bhattacharya, J., Johnson, P. A., and Jamison, R. L.: Effect of chronic potassium loading on potassium secretion by the pars recta or descending limb of the juxtamedullary nephron in the rat. *J. Clin. Invest.* 62:1093–1103, 1978.
3. Beck, L. H., Senesky, D., and Goldberg, M.: Sodium-independent active potassium reabsorption in proximal tubule of the dog. *J. Clin. Invest.* 52:2641–2645, 1973.
4. Bengele, H. H., McNamara, E. R., and Alexander, E. A.: Potassium secretion along the inner medullary collecting duct. *Am. J. Physiol.* 236:F278–F282, 1979.
5. Berliner, R. W., Kennedy, T. J. Jr., and Hilton, J. G.: Renal mechanisms for excretion of potassium. *Am. J. Physiol.* 162:348–367, 1950.
6. Berliner, R. W., Kennedy, T. J. Jr., and Orloff, J.: Relationship between acidification of the urine and potassium metabolism: effect of carbonic anlydrase inhibition on potassium excretion. *Am. J. Med.* 11:274–282, 1951.
7. Beyer, K. H., and Baer, J. E.: Physiological basis for the action of newer diuretic agents. *Pharmacol. Rev.* 13:517–562, 1961.
8. Boudry, J. F., Stoner, L. C., and Burg, M. B.: Effect of acid lumen pH on potassium transport in renal cortical collecting tubules. *Am. J. Physiol.* 230:239–244, 1976.
9. Bowman, R. H., Dolgin, J., and Coulson, R.: Interaction between ouabain and furosemide on Na and K excretion in perfused rat kidney. *Am. J. Physiol.* 224: 1200–1205, 1973.
10. Brater, D. C.: Pharmacodynamic considerations in the use of diuretics. *Annu. Rev. Pharmacol. Toxicol.* 23:45–62, 1983.
11. Brenner, B. M., and Berliner, R. W.: The transport of potassium. In *Handbook of Physiology Section 8, Renal Physiology,* edited by Orloff, J., and Berliner, R. W., Washington, American Physiological Society, 1973, pp. 497–519.
12. Brørs, O., Jacobsen, S., Foss, O. P., and Aakvaag, A.: Effect of repeated doses of hydroflumethiazide on renal excretion of electrolytes and uric acid in healthy subjects. *Acta Pharmacol. Toxicol.* 48:145–150, 1981.
13. Cade, J. R., Shalhoub, R. J., Canessa-Fischer, M., and Pitts, R. F. Effect of strophanthidin on the renal tubules of dogs. *Am. J. Physiol.* 200:373–379, 1961.
14. Cannon, P. J., Heinemann, H. O., Stason, W. B., and Laragh, J. H.: Ethacrynic acid. Effectiveness and mode of diuretic action in man. *Circulation* 31:5–18, 1965.
15. Costanza, L. S., and Windhager, E. E.: Calcium and sodium transport by the distal convoluted tubule of the rat. *Am. J. Physiol.* 235:F492–F506, 1978.
16. Davidson, C., Burkinshaw, L., McLachlan, M. S. F., and Morgan, D. B.: Effect of long-term diuretic treatment on body-potassium in heart disease. *Lancet* 2:1044–1047, 1976.
17. Duarte, C. G., Chomety, F., and Giebisch, G.: Effect of amiloride, ouabain, and furosemide on distal tubular function in the rat. *Am. J. Physiol.* 221:632–639, 1971.
18. Edmonds, C. J., and Wilson, G. M.: The action of hydroflumethiazide in relation to adrenal steroids and potassium loss. *Lancet* 1:505–509, 1960.
19. Espiner, E. A., Tucci, J. R., Jagger, P. I., Pauk, G. L., and Lauler, D. P.: The effect of acute diuretic-induced extracellular volume depletion on aldosterone secretion in normal man. *Clin. Sci.* 33:125–134, 1967.
20. Evanson, R. L., Lockhart, E. A., and Dirks, J. H.: Effect of mercurial diuretics on tubular sodium and potassium transport in the dog. *Am. J. Physiol.* 222:282–289, 1972.
21. Fichman, M. P., Vorherr, H., Kleeman, C. R., and Telfer, N.: Diuretic-induced hyponatremia. *Ann. Intern. Med.* 75:853–863, 1971.
22. Field, M. J., Stanton, B. A., and Giebisch, G. H.: Influence of ADH on renal potassium handling: a micropuncture and microperfusion study. *Kidney Int.* 25:502–511, 1984.

23. Field, M. J., Stanton, B. A., and Giebisch, G. H.: Differential acute effects of aldosterone, dexamethazone, and hyperkalemia on distal tubular potassium secretion in the rat kidney. *J. Clin. Invest.* 74:1792–1802, 1984.
24. Foulkes, E. C.: On the mechanism of chlorothiazide-induced kaliuresis in the rabbit. *J. Pharmacol. Exp. Ther.* 150:406–413, 1965.
25. Fowler, N., Giebisch, G., and Whittenbury, G.: Distal tubular tracer injection study of renal tubular potassium transport. *Am. J. Physiol.* 229:1227–1233, 1975.
26. Giebisch, G.: Effects of diuretics on renal transport of potassium. In *Methods in Pharmacology*, edited by Martinez-Maldonaldo, M., New York, Plenum, 1976, p. 121–164.
27. Giebisch, G., Klose, R. M., and Malnic, G.: Renal tubular potassium transport. *Bull. Swiss Acad. Med. Sci.* 23:287–312, 1967.
28. Giebisch, G., Malnic, G., and Berliner, R. W.: Renal transport and control of potassium excretion. In *The Kidney,* edited by Brenner, B. M., and Rector, F. C. Jr., Philadelphia, W. B. Saunders, 1981, pp. 408–439.
29. Grantham, J. J., Burg, M. B., and Orloff, J.: The nature of transtubular Na and K transport in isolated rabbit collecting tubules. *J. Clin. Invest.* 49:1815–1826, 1970.
30. Greger, R., and Schlatter, E.: Properties of the lumen membrane of the cortical thick ascending limb of Henle's loop of rabbit kidney. *Pflügers Arch.* 396:315–324, 1983.
31. Heinemann, H. O., Demartini, F. E., and Laragh, J. H.: The effect of chlorothiazide on renal excretion of electrolytes and free water. *Am. J. Med.* 26:853–861, 1959.
32. Hesp, R., Wilkinson, P. R.: Potassium supplementation of thiazide therapy. *Lancet* 2:1144, 1976.
33. Hollifield, J. W., and Slaton, P. E.: Cardiac arrhythmias associated with diuretic induced hypokalaemia and hypomagnesaemia. *R. Soc. Med. Int. Congress Sympos. Series* 44:17–24, 1981.
34. Kahn, T., Kaufman, A. M., and Mac-Moune, F. L.: Response to repeated frusemide administration on low chloride and low sodium intake in the rat. *Clin. Sci.* 64:565–572, 1983.
35. Katz, L. D., Jones, W., and DeFronzo, R.: Beta blockade and K secretion in the isolated perfused rat kidney. *Kidney Int.* 23:258, 1983.
36. Kelly, R., Wilcos, C. S., Mitch, W. E., Souney, P., Meyer, T., Skorecki, K., and Rayment, C.: Effects of increased urine flow and aldosterone on K balance during furosemide administration to man. *Kidney Int.* 23:128, 1983.
37. Kelly, R. A., Wilcox, C. S., Souney, P., and Mitch, W. E.: Effects of aldosterone and ADH on potassium excretion with furosemide. *Kidney Int.* 25:169, 1984.
38. Kessler, R. H., Hierholzer, K., Gurd, R. S., and Pitts, R. F.: Localization of action of chlorothiazide in the nephron of the dog. *Am. J. Physiol.* 196:1346–1351, 1959.
39. Khuri, R. N., Wiederholt, M., Strieder, N., and Giebisch, G.: Effects of flow rate and potassium intake on distal tubular potassium transfer. *Am. J. Physiol.* 228:1249–1261, 1975.
40. Knochel, J. P.: Rhabdomyolysis and effects of potassium deficiency on muscle structure and function. *Cardiovasc. Med.* 3:247–261, 1978.
41. Koch, A. R., Brazeau, P., and Gilman, A.: Role of renal tubular secretion in potassium homeostasis. *Am. J. Physiol.* 186:350–356, 1956.
42. Malnic, G., Klose, R. M., and Giebisch, G.: Micropuncture study of renal potassium excretion in the rat. *Am. J. Physiol.* 206:674–686, 1964.
43. Maren, T. H., Sorsdahl, O. A., and Dickhaus, A. J.: Renal action of acetazolamide in extracellular alkalosis of K+ deficiency. *Am. J. Physiol.* 200:170–174, 1961.
44. Maronde, R. F., Milgrom, M., and Dickey, J. M.: Potassium loss with thiazide therapy. *Am. Heart J.* 78:16–21, 1969.

45. Mudge, G. H., Ames, A., Foulks, J., and Gilman, A.: Effects of drugs on renal secretion of potassium in the dog. *Am. J. Physiol.* 161:151–158, 1950.
46. Mudge, G. H., Cooke, W. J., and Berndt, W. O.: Electrolyte excretion and free-water production during onset of acute diuresis. *Am. J. Physiol.* 228:1304–1312, 1975.
47. Mudge, G. H., Foulks, J., and Gilman, A.: Renal secretion of potassium in the dog during cellular dehydration. *Am. J. Physiol.* 161:159–166, 1950.
48. Mudge, G. H. and Hardin, B.: Response to mercurial diuretics during alkalosis: A comparison of acute metabolic and chronic hypokalemic alkalosis in the dog. *J. Clin. Invest.* 35:155–163, 1956.
49. Oberleithner, H., Giebisch, G., Lang, F., and Wang, W.: Cellular mechanisms of the furosemide sensitive transport system in the kidney. *Klin. Wochenschr.* 60:1173–1179, 1982.
50. O'Neil, R. G., and Helman, S. I.: Transport characteristics of renal collecting tubules: influences of DOCA and diet. *Am. J. Physiol.* 233:F544–F558, 1977.
51. Pitts, R. F., Kruck, F., Lozano, R., Taylor, D. W., Heidenreich, P. A., and Kessler, R. H.: Studies on the mechanism of diuretic action of chlorothiazide. *J. Pharmacol. Exp. Ther.* 123:89–97, 1958.
52. Rector, F. C. Jr., Bloomer, H. A., and Seldin, D. W.: Proximal tubular reabsorption of potassium during mannitol diuresis in rats. *J. Lab. Clin. Med.* 63:100–105, 1964.
53. Reineck, H. J., Osgood, R. W., and Stein, J. H.: Net potassium addition beyond the superficial distal tubule of the rat. *Am. J. Physiol.* 235:F104–F110, 1978.
54. Sanderson, P. H.: Renal response to massive alkali loading in the human subject. In *Ciba Foundation Symposium on the Kidney,* edited by Lewis, A. A. G., and Wolstenholme, G. E. W., Boston, Little, Brown, 1954, pp. 165–173.
55. Silva, P., Brown, R. S., and Epstein, F. H.: Adaptation to potassium. *Kidney Int.* 11:466–475, 1977.
56. Sonnenberg, H.: Effects of furosemide, acetazolamide, and mannitol on medullary collecting duct function in the rat. *Pflügers Arch.* 373:113–123, 1978.
57. Spät, A., Tarján, É., and Tóth, G.: Hyperaldosteronism in the sodium-depleted rat: Mode of aldosterone-stimulating action of frusemide. *J. Endocrinol.* 82:7–15, 1979.
58. Stanton, B. A., and Giebisch, G. H.: Regulation of potassium homeostasis. In *Functional Regulation at the Cellular and Molecular Levels,* edited by Corradino, R. A., New York, Elsevier North Holland, 1982, pp. 259–283.
59. Stanton, B. A., and Giebisch, G.: Effects of pH on potassium transport by renal distal tubule. *Am. J. Physiol.* 242:F544–F551, 1982.
60. Stanton, B. A. and Giebisch, G.: Potassium transport by the renal distal tubule: Effects of potassium loading. *Am. J. Physiol.* 243:F487–F493, 1982.
61. Stason, W. B., Cannon, P. J., Heinemann, H. O., and Laragh, J. H.: Furosemide. A clinical evaluation of its diuretic action. *Circulation* 34:910–920, 1966.
62. Strieder, N., Khuri, R., Wiederholt, M., and Giebisch, G.: Studies on the renal action of ouabain in the rat: effects in the non-diuretic state. *Pflügers Arch.* 349:91–107, 1974.
63. Sufit, C. R., and Jamison, R. L.: Effect of K replenishment on Na, Cl, and K reabsorption by Henle's loop. *Kidney Int.* 23:268, 1983.
64. Talso, P. J., and Carballo, A. J.: Effects of benzothidiazines on serum and total body electrolytes. *Ann. N.Y. Acad. Sci.* 88:822–840, 1960.
65. Tannen, R. L., and Gerrits, L.: Response of the renal K+ conserving mechanism to kaliuretic stimuli: evidence for a direct kaliuretic effect of furosemide. *Kidney Int.* 25:318, 1984.
66. Velazquez, H., and Wright, F. S.: Sodium, chloride, and potassium transport by the distal nephron: effect of bumetanide and chlorothiazide. *Kidney Int.* 25:319, 1984.
67. Wright, F. S.: Sites and mechanisms of potassium transport along the renal tubule. *Kidney Int.* 11:415–432, 1977.

68. Wright, F. S., and Giebisch, G.: Renal potassium transport: Contributions of individual nephron segments and populations. *Am. J. Physiol.* 235:F515–F527, 1978.
69. Young, D. B.: Relationship between plasma potassium concentration and renal potassium excretion. *Am. J. Physiol.* 242:F599–F603, 1982.

17

The Incidence of Hypokalemia and Hyperkalemia Associated with Diuretic Use

ANDREW WHELTON and ALAN J. S. WATSON
The Johns Hopkins University School of Medicine and The Johns Hopkins Hospital, Baltimore, Maryland

The adage that "common things occur commonly" is apt when applied to the incidence of diuretic-related disorders in potassium metabolism. Since the clinical introduction of the thiazide group of diuretics, the Literature has been replete with reports defining the incidence of hypokalemia in various subgroups of patients treated with these compounds. Shortly thereafter, as the potassium-sparing diuretics became popular, multiple reports of hyperkalemia associated with their use began to appear in the Literature. Between 1967 and the beginning of 1984 a total of 341 publications have appeared specifically related to the issue of diuretic-induced hyperkalemia and hypokalemia. This chapter represents a distillate of the latter publications together with a report of a diuretic trial at our institution.

Before we review specific quantitative data which define the prevalence or incidence of diuretic-related potassium disorders, some general observations are warranted. Several simple clinical events (Table 1) may significantly modulate the incidence of diuretic-induced hypo- or hyperkalemia. Hence, in any survey or study providing quantitative data pertinent to these electrolyte abnormalities, the modulating factors listed in Table 1 need to be taken into account. For example, in response to the apparently simple question "What is the incidence of hypokalemia when using a diuretic"? it is scientifically possible to respond with numbers that vary from a low of less than 2% associated with the use of low-dosage loop diuretics to a value of 100% associated with the use of high-dosage chlorthalidone. Therefore, there is something for everyone; any author can cite an incidence figure of hypokalemia that will fit with the concept he or she wishes to develop. In sorting out these issues, it would clearly be advantageous if an international clearing house could provide accurate information characterizing the incidence of hypo- and hyperkalemia secondary to diuretic use in the framework of the modifying features listed in Table 1. No such comprehensive service organization exists and it is unlikely to be developed in the foreseeable future.

Table 1 Clinical Factors that Modify the Incidence of Diuretic-Induced Hypokalemia

Definition: typically a serum level of 3.5 mEq/L or less
Initial potassium value and subsequent fall in serum concentration
Patient population and complications of underlying disease (i.e., CHF patients have a higher initial serum K^+ value than hypertensive or cirrhotic individuals)
Level of activity of the renin–angiotensin–aldosterone system
Presence and quantity of edema fluid that can be mobilized
Specific category of diuretic selected
Duration of diuretic therapy
Level of coexisting renal function

SPONTANEOUS REPORTING OF ADVERSE DRUG REACTIONS

In the United States all physicians and pharmaceutical manufacturers are required by federal regulation to report serious adverse drug reactions. The responsibility for collecting these "spontaneous" reports lies within the jurisdiction of the Federal Food and Drug Administration (FDA). Such data are then made available for appropriate dissemination within the medical community. Through the kind auspices of Dr. Jack Khalsa of the FDA it has been possible to retrieve and quantify all reports of diuretic-induced potassium disorders as reported from 1968 through May, 1984. In that 16-year period a total of 688 instances of diuretic-associated disorders of serum potassium concentration were reported from various sources. Of this total, 594 were hypokalemic events and 94 hyperkalemic in nature; 18 different diuretics or diuretic combinations were involved in these electrolyte abnormalities. The incidence of hypokalemia and hyperkalemia for any one diuretic was related entirely to the reporting source and did not reflect the incidence as seen in controlled prospective or retrospective clinical trials. Of particular interest was the finding that reports of the incidence of hypokalemia and hyperkalemia associated with the use of the potassium-sparing diuretics spironolactone or triamterene were almost identical. For example, in the case of triamterene and spironolactone there were 15 and 7 instances of hypokalemia and 14 and 5 incidences of hyperkalemia, respectively. Clinical details regarding the settings in which these divergent responses in potassium metabolism occurred were not available and the true reliability of these diuretic-induced side effects cannot therefore be assessed. Perhaps the most important inference that can be derived from this 16-year FDA experience report is that there is gross underreporting of diuretic-related potassium disorders.

Characteristically, when side effects of drugs are well known and are clearly defined in the drug packaging insert, although the toxic drug reactions may be severe and life-threatening, they are in general not reported to the FDA. It is also somewhat surprising to find that physicians are responsible for initiating less than 10% of all adverse drug reports filed with the FDA. It is apparent that we cannot rely upon any single national or international data source for the definition of the incidence of diuretic-induced potassium abnormalities. Hence, a detailed analysis of literature reports of individual trials and patient surveys will be necessary to provide scientific answers.

DIURETIC USE PATTERNS AND 10-YEAR TRENDS IN THE UNITED STATES

In 1984 approximately 100 million prescriptions for diuretic compounds were written by physicians (68). This indicates the enormous importance of diuretics in the overall dispensing trends of physicians. Approximately 75% of the time, physicians prescribe diuretics as part of the management of hypertension. It is therefore fascinating to recognize that only in the minority of instances are diuretics used for the mobilization of excess sodium and water.

A sizable number of diuretic compounds, many patented and many available in generic format, are readily available for prescription purposes. For example in the 1984 edition of the *Physician's Desk Reference*, 58 diuretics and diuretic combinations are listed together with 31 forms of potassium replacement therapy.

In view of the number of diuretics that have been available during the past several years and the extensive investigative efforts that have been reported defining electrolyte abnormalities associated with individual diuretics or diuretic classes, it is of interest to evaluate the impact of this information upon physician-prescribing trends during the 1970s and early 1980s. In most instances, prescriptions were written for patented rather than generic compounds. Table 2 lists the major diuretic compounds prescribed from 1973 throughout 1981. Numerous other compounds were also prescribed but the net amount for these miscellaneous diuretics did not influence prescribing trends and was not sufficient to warrant inclusion in these tables. Table 2 shows the use trends for thiazides and related compounds, for loop diuretics, and for combined potassium-losing and potassium-sparing formulations.

These national prescription audit data indicate that throughout the 1970s and into the 1980s there has been an increasing trend to prescribing generic hydrochlorothiazide, proprietary chlorthalidone, loop diuretics, and a marked interest in the use of combined potassium-losing and potassium-sparing compounds. On the other hand, there has been a reduction in the use of proprietary forms of chlorothiazide and ethacrynic acid.

GENERAL REPORTS AND CLINICAL RISK FACTORS

Definition of Hypokalemia

Because of the abundance of literature reports on diuretic-induced hypokalemia, for virtually all compounds there is an enormous spread of the numerical incidence of hypokalemia. Nonetheless, a solid pattern of hypokalemic events, for various diuretic compounds, and the high-risk clinical settings in which these side effects are likely to become manifest can be derived from the general literature reports. Special data sources such as the Boston Collaborative Study Group merit separate review and will be analyzed below.

Most authors define hypokalemia as a serum potassium level equal to or less than 3.5 mEq/L. This will be accepted as the definition of hypokalemia for this chapter. Table 3 summarizes select literature reports on the incidence of hypokalemia during the use of several different diuretics and during different dosing regimens for a number of these compounds.

The pattern that emerges from Table 3 and from the literature is that the highest incidence of diuretic associated hypokalemia is related to the use of thiazides and related

Table 2 National (USA) Prescription Audit for Diuretics: 10-Year Trend Number of Prescriptions in Thousands

Drug	1973	1974	1975	1976	1977	1978	1979	1980	1981
Thiazide-type									
Diuril	8768	8600	8071	7369	6316	5382	4470	3855	3461
Hydrodiuril	12681	13176	13720	14766	13953	12953	12938	11741	11113
Esidrix	3306	3362	3456	3618	3591	3303	2995	2837	2532
Hydrochlorothiazide	501	784	1159	1824	2764	4248	6296	6649	12547
Hygroton	5542	5438	6273	6765	7357	7442	8321	8518	8809
Zaroxolyn		131	392	809	1029	1208	1624	1753	1964
Loop Agents									
Lasix	16348	16249	18189	19616	19275	19310	20095	21675	23214
Edecrin	401	427	282	255	221	153	145	141	175
Potassium-sparing									
Aldactone	1903	1929	1979	2176	2021	2035	2078	2156	2114
Aldactazide	5656	5672	6593	6248	6194	5779	5400	5399	5394
Dyazide	8254	9500	10559	13340	16314	17740	19704	22657	26486

Source: Data copyright of National Drug and Therapeutic Index, Ambler, Pennsylvania, provided by R. Hampton.
Diuril, chlorothiazide; Hydrodiuril, hydrochlorothiazide; Esidrix, hydrochlorothiazide; Hygroton, chlorthalidone; Zaroxolyn, metolazone; Lasix, furosemide; Edecrin, ethacrynic acid; Aldactone, spironolactone; Aldactazide, spironolactone with hydrochlorothiazide; Dyazide, triamterene with hydrochlorothiazide.

Table 3 Hypokalemia and Diuretic Use: Differential Incidences in Various Reported Series ($K^+ < 3.5$ mEq/L)

Drug or category	Number of patients	% Incidence	References
Thiazide	16	62.5	86
Thiazide	16	25.0	7
Thiazide	50	6.0	54
Thiazide	53	10.0	3
Chlorthalidone	10	90.0	47
Chlorthalidone	16	25.0	25
Chlorthalidone	20	85.0	101
Furosemide	59	14.0	7
Furosemide	347	1.7 (40 mg)	57
Furosemide	160	6.3 (40–80mg)	57
Furosemide	78	6.4 (80+mg)	57
Furosemide	172	38.9	67
Furosemide	12	33.0	30
Bumetanide	742	14.7	104

compounds (1,3–49,51–91,94–104). For all of the potassium-losing diuretics the incidence of hypokalemia is dosage-related. The most kaliuretic member of the thiazide group is chlorthalidone. For typical clinical practice, including a cross-section of patients with hypertension and congestive heart failure treated for at least a month, one can develop a reasonable "projected range" for the incidence of hypokalemia. For chlorothiazide and hydrochlorothiazide the expected incidence is typically 5–30%; for chlorthalidone 50–100%, and for loop diuretics 5–15%. The clinical and pharmacological considerations that may be of importance in elucidating the mechanisms of action for these differences in incidence of hypokalemia are reviewed in Chapter 16 by Dr. Mudge.

It would appear that the most important issues promoting the high incidence of this problem associated with the thiazides, in particular chlorthalidone, are their predominant distal tubular site of action and their duration of effective action. Table 4 summarizes the onset of action of the major diuretic groups and the duration of their activity. Since thiazides and related compounds have a distal tubular site of action in their inhibition of the reabsorption of sodium chloride, this promotes distal tubular delivery of excess sodium to the aldosterone-mediated sodium-potassium exchange sites, in this segment of the tubule. This results in excess urinary potassium elimination in any circumstances in which there is a physiological or pathophysiological stimulus to activity of the renin-angiotensin-aldosterone axis. Clearly, with the long-acting potassium-losing diuretics, such as chlorthalidone, the delivery of excess amounts of sodium to the distal sodium-potassium exchange sites over an extended time promotes excessive urinary potassium losses and the often-observed high incidence of chlorthalidone-associated hypokalemia.

Enhanced Development of Hypokalemia During Mobilization of Edema Fluid

It is frequently observed that the development of hypokalemia associated with the use of any of the potassium-losing diuretics is greater in patients who are treated for the mobilization of edema fluid than those who are treated for hypertension alone. The explanation

Table 4 Comparative Action of Diuretics (in hours)

Drug	Hours		
	Onset	Peak	Duration
Acetazolamide	1–2	2–4	8–12
Hydrochlorothiazide	1–2	4–6	6–18
Chlorthalidone	2–3	4–24	48–72
Bumetanide	0.3–1	1–2	4–6
Furosemide	0.5–1	1–2	4–8
Amiloride	2–4	6–10	12–24
Triamterene	2–4	4–6	8–12
Spironolactone	8–24	24–48	48–72

for this clinical finding is related to the fact that the patient with edema states, such as congestive heart failure, the nephrotic syndrome or cirrhosis and ascites, has heightened activity of the renin-angiotensin-aldosterone systems. The latter system is activated as a result of decreased renal perfusion secondary to either decreased cardiac output or decreased intravascular oncotic pressure with resultant volume contraction and reduced renal blood flow. As the patient's edema fluid, typically containing isotonic concentrations of sodium, is mobilized by diuretics, massive delivery of sodium to the distal sodium-potassium exchange sites, which are then under a significant aldosterone stimulus to sodium retention and potassium loss, results in excessive urinary potassium elimination and resultant hypokalemia. By contrast, in the diuretic management of hypertensive patients, little change is induced therapeutically in their extracellular volume status. The quantitative delivery of sodium to their distal tubular sodium-potassium exchange site is substantially less than that in significant mobilization of edema.

HYPOKALEMIC ALKALOSIS AND TOTAL BODY EXCHANGEABLE POTASSIUM DURING DIURETIC THERAPY

Pathogenetic Sequences and Therapeutic Implications

The mechanism by which hypokalemic hypochloremic alkalosis develops secondary to the use of thiazide or loop diuretics is shown in Figure 1. The schema is somewhat simplified but emphasizes the fact that the saluretic diuretic effect of thiazide or loop diuretics promotes an equimolar loss of sodium and chloride. These losses come from an extracellular pool wherein the total amounts of sodium and chloride are not equal. The figure represents a simple but extreme clinical sample of the circumstances in which a 50-kg person with an extracellular fluid volume of 10 L was subjected to an isotonic sodium chloride diuresis of 2 L with associated enhanced distal tubular sodium-potassium exchange. As a result of the diuresis this patient's extracellular pool of sodium and chloride decreased by 280 mEq respectively. This was also accompanied by a small reduction in the patient's total body potassium secondary to enhanced distal tubular sodium-potassium exchange. Since the patient acutely lost 2 L of "isotonic" urine derived from the extracellular volume, the new extracellular fluid concentrations of sodium and chloride, derived by dividing the total extracellular sodium and chloride values by the reduced volume of 8 L, would be 140 mEq/L and 78 mEq/L respectively. In this patient, no bicarbonate losses

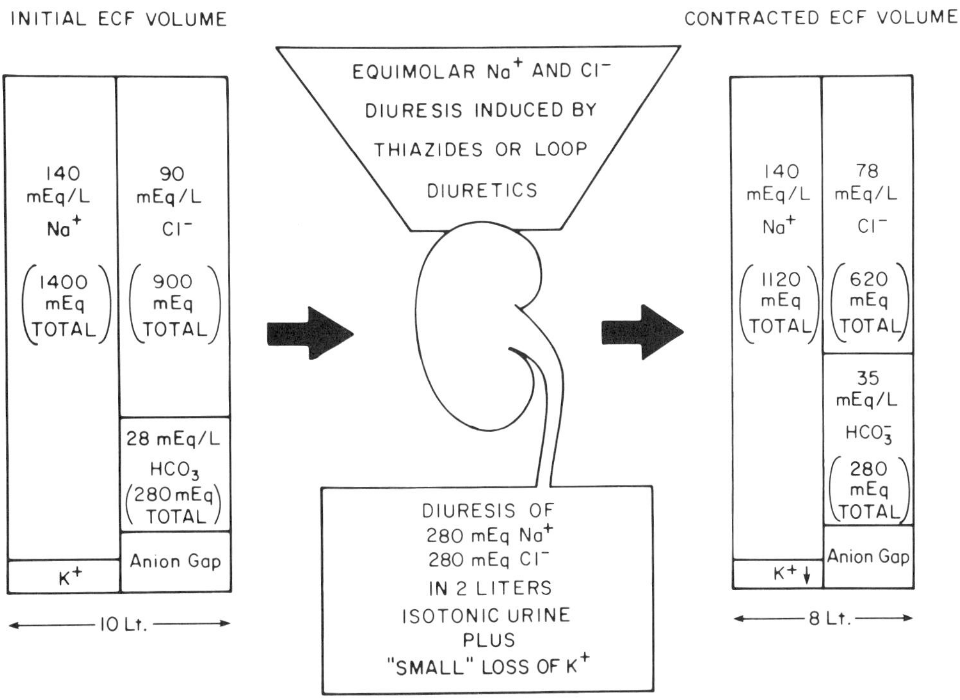

Figure 1 Conceptual schema for the development of hypokalemic, hypochloremic alkalosis secondary to the use of thiazide or loop diuretics.

occurred and the serum bicarbonate level therefore became elevated to 35 mEq/L. This hypochloremic alkalosis now induces some important intracellular and extracellular potassium exchange processes. The alkalosis stimulates a movement of hydrogen ion out of cells and an inward exchange of potassium thereby accentuating and maintaining the extracellular hypokalemic state. Without chloride replacement the alkalosis is perpetuated, with consequent maintenance of extracellular hypokalemia. Hence, in the replacement therapy of diuretic-induced hypokalemic alkalosis one must replace not only potassium but also chloride to ensure full replacement of the intracellular and extracellular potassium deficit. Chloride replacement leads to correction of the alkalosis. If one attempts to replace potassium as its alkaline salt form (for example, potassium gluconate, bicarbonate or acetate), in a patient with hypokalemic alkalosis it is possible to increase the extracellular levels of potassium but at the expense of accentuating the extracellular alkalosis. Clearly, diuretic-induced hypokalemia should therefore be treated with replacement potassium chloride.

The form in which this replacement should be administered (i.e., liquid potassium chloride, wax-matrix-imbedded potassium chloride, or microencapsulated potassium chloride is reviewed in Chapter 35). All of these modalities are satisfactory; the time-release forms of potassium replacement lead to a slower and more prolonged delivery of potassium into the extracellular fluid than is noted following the administration of liquid potassium chloride. Characteristically, the latter replacement therapy produces a more prompt increase in serum potassium levels, secondary stimulation of aldosterone production, and a more prompt urinary appearance of the administered potassium. If the patient undergoing potassium replacement therapy continues to have significant activity of the renin–angiotensin–aldosterone system, most of the administered potassium will promptly be excreted. In these circumstances the systemic potassium deficit is best treated by carefully monitoring concurrent administration of potassium and a potassium-sparing diuretic such as amiloride, spironolactone, or triamterene.

Long-Term Prevention of Diuretic-Associated Hypokalemia

The long-term prevention of diuretic-associated hypokalemia may be accomplished either by concurrent potassium chloride therapy or by the use of combined potassium-losing and potassium-sparing diuretics. This is one of the areas in clinical medicine in which it is logical to combine drugs in one formulation. The combination of a thiazide diuretic with amiloride, spironolactone, or triamterene is useful, popular, and clinically sound. Amiloride and triamterene will exert an effect on distal sodium–potassium exchange during or in the absence of aldosterone stimulation of the nephron whereas spironolactone will act specifically to inhibit aldosterone-mediated distal tubular sodium–potassium exchange. In patients with persistent hypokalemia, often those with a chronic stimulus to activity of their renin–angiotensin–aldosterone axis, the addition of potassium chloride alone to their management regimen will not satisfactorily prevent long-term hypokalemia. From the practical point of view these patients are best managed by administration of a potassium-sparing diuretic with potassium chloride and discontinuation of the potassium supplement once the total body deficit of potassium has been corrected. A small number of such patients may require long-term use of both potassium supplements and a potassium-sparing diuretic. The controversy associated with the routine use of potassium replacement therapy during diuretic use is reviewed by Dr. Harrington in Chapter 38.

Total Body Potassium Deficits Induced by Diuretics

Based on a knowledge of the mechanisms by which hypokalemia evolves in association with hypochloremic alkalosis, we can more logically assess the data defining the magnitude of total body potassium deficits induced by diuretics. Throughout the 1950s and 1960s it was repetitively reported that patients with heart failure who were treated with diuretics had 20–30% less exchangeable body potassium than comparable healthy persons (7,63). In 1976 Davidson and colleagues reported markedly divergent findings (7). They studied the effects of diuretic use on the total body potassium balance of patients with heart failure. In their investigations, potassium balance was measured by monitoring a naturally occurring isotope using a whole body counter. In 151 patients, 83 of whom were taking diuretics and potassium supplements, they found that the deficit in total body potassium was only 3–5% (100–150 mEq/L) in the diuretic group. Of their 13 patients with hypokalemia the potassium deficit was no greater than in the persons with normal serum potassium levels. These investigators found no relationship between the dosage of potassium supplement and either the plasma potassium or the total body potassium level. They concluded that potassium depletion is not a major problem in patients with heart failure treated with diuretics. Subsequently, Morgan and co-workers carefully reassessed the extant literature on diuretic-induced potassium depletion in heart failure and in a meticulous and thoughtful analysis noted that the widely accepted notion of a 20–30% body deficit of potassium in such a clinical setting could be explained, at least in part, by a failure to match patients in terms of age; the remaining differences could be explained by muscle wasting (63). A prevailing hypochloremic alkalosis, induced by thiazides or loop diuretics, would itself maintain an extracellular hypokalemic state by moving potassium into cells in an outward exchange for hydrogen ions, thereby sustaining low serum potassium levels but not necessarily a significant cellular depletion of potassium.

Most recent studies confirm that a significant diuretic-induced total body deficit of potassium is uncommon in patients with hypertension or heart failure (11,45,52,92).

SPECIFIC REPORTS DEFINING DIURETIC-ASSOCIATED HYPOKALEMIA AND HYPERKALEMIA

Hypokalemia

Four special reports defining diuretic induced hypokalemia merit separate commentary. In 1982 Lawson and associates reported, on behalf of the Boston Collaborative Drug Surveillance Program, their experience with drug-attributed alterations in potassium handling in congestive cardiac failure in some 25,000 monitored patients (52). Seventeen university teaching hospitals in seven countries provided the data for analysis. A total of 3,879 of the evaluated patients received diuretics for the treatment of their heart failure. Table 5 summarizes the study results. Hypokalemia was defined as a serum potassium level below 3.5 mEq/L and hyperkalemia if it was greater than 6.0 mEq/L. One hundred and seventy-five patients developed hypokalemia (4.5% of those treated with diuretics) and 144 developed hyperkalemia (3.7%). Seventeen patients had both hypokalemia and hyperkalemia during their hospitalization. Hypokalemia was more common in women, was unrelated to blood urea concentration on admission and was twice as common among recipients of potassium-losing diuretics who did not take potassium supplements than among those who received potassium-retaining diuretics. In direct contrast, the data indicated that hyperkalemia was strongly related to blood urea concentrations on admission and that it was also related to inhospital diuretic therapy, being three times as frequent among recipients of aldosterone antagonists than among those receiving potassium-losing diuretics without additional supplementation. Life-threatening hypokalemia and hyperkalemia were rare in this group of patients with heart failure and occurred with approxi-

Table 5 Hypokalemia/Hyperkalemia and Diuretic Use: Special Reports[a]

Hypokalemia
175 Developed hypokalemia (4.5%) 98 women/77 men
K^+-retaining: 28/862 (3.3%)
K^+-losing + KCL 69/1699 (4.1%)
K^+-losing alone 78/1318 (5.9%)
Solid dose relationship
Life-threatening in 5, death in 1, and arrhythmias in 2
Hyperkalemia
144 Developed hyperkalemia (3.7%) 81 men/63 women
Solid relationship to type of diuretic, KCL supplementation, and initial renal function
Life-threatening in 8

[a]17 Hospitals worldwide provided 25,000+ patients for review, of whom 3,879 received diuretics for CHF

Source: Ref. 52.

mately equal frequencies: 2: 1,000 patients treated. Lawson and colleagues also separately reported on the incidence of profound hypokalemia (<2.0 mEq/L) as seen at the Royal Infirmary in Glasgow, Scotland (51). In a 3-year period (1973-1975) 73 such patients were encountered. The authors noted that when compared with hospitalized subjects used as controls, these hypokalemic patients experienced a greater mortality, were substantially more likely to be female but were not more likely to have cardiovascular disease. In fact, use of the diuretic appeared to precipitate profound hypokalemia only infrequently, and when it did the clinical situation was extremely complex. More than 10% of the patients with hypokalemia had acute myeloid leukemia, an incidence 22 times greater than that expected.

Licht and colleagues have recently reported their experience with diuretic-induced hypokalemia in some 5,000 patients (55). Table 6 summarizes the prevalence of a serum potassium of less than 3.5 mEq/L in their clinic. Their data indicate that during the thiazide treatment of hypertension the addition of a potassium-sparing diuretic was more effective in reducing hypokalemia than simply adding a potassium supplement.

A thoughtful and painstaking analysis of publications on hypokalemia was reported in 1980 by Morgan and Davidson (64). Table 7 provides a synopsis of some of the important findings of their review. These authors concluded from their extensive analysis of publications that the average fall in serum potassium is less after the usual doses of loop diuretics than after the usual doses of thiazides and is little influenced by the dosage or duration of treatment. The fall with a given drug is the same in patients with heart failure and in those with hypertension, but the initial serum potassium concentration is higher in heart failure so that the final value is lower in hypertension. In standard dosages, potassium supplements were noted to be less effective than potassium-retaining diuretics in correcting hypokalemia. In a follow-up to this report, Hamdy and colleagues (30) reemphasized the importance of hypokalemia in the elderly since 37.4% of the latter population are receiving regular diuretic therapy. These investigators pointed out that apart from the well-known manifestations of hypokalemia in the elderly this electrolyte abnormality may also present in a nonspecific manner with lethargy, apathy, and easy fatigability. Although the latter manifestations may not be "harmful," the quality of life of older patients may be improved by preventing hypokalemia from developing in the first place.

Hyperkalemia

In singling out the most important studies pertinent to diuretic-related hyperkalemia, one must inescapably include an analysis of patients receiving potassium chloride in addition

Table 6 Hypokalemia and Diuretic Use: Special Reports

Prevalence of serum K^+ less than 3.5 mEq/L	%	N
Hydrochlorothiazide 50 mg/day	11.0	500
Hydrochlorothiazide 50 mg/day + KCL	11.6	328
Chlorthalidone 25 mg/day	8.1	37
Hydrochlorothiazide 50 mg + triamterene 100 mg/day	5.3	357
Hydrochlorothiazide 25 mg/day	2.2	183
Furosemide 40 mg/day	3.5	284

Source: Ref. 55.

Table 7 Hypokalemia and Diuretic Use: Special Reports

	Weeks				
	1	2	4	8	16
Mean fall in serum K^+ (mEq/L)	0.7	0.65	0.56	0.69	0.56
# Patients (# of studies)	52 (5)	96 (7)	136 (7)	255 (10)	141 (6)

Relationship to drug category

	Hydrochlorothiazide	Chlorthalidone	Furosemide
Mean fall in serum K^+ (mEq/L)	0.62±0.04	0.67±0.04	0.3±0.05

Effect of treatment on serum K^+ (mEq/L)

	K^+ Suppl	Amiloride	Triamterene	Spironolactone
Mean before	3.61	3.68	3.28	3.42
Mean rise	0.32	0.39	0.46	0.65
Mean dosage	36 mmol	15 mg	150 mg	75 mg

Fall in serum K^+ in congestive heart failure and hypertension similar but initial serum K^+ higher in congestive heart failure.

Source: Ref. 64.

to diuretics. A landmark report was made by Lawson on behalf of the Boston Collaborative Drug Surveillance Program in 1974 (50). In this report of adverse reactions to potassium chloride (Table 8) as monitored in 4,921 patients, 2,263 (46%) concurrently received diuretics. A total of 128 patients (2.6% of potassium recipients) received potassium-sparing diuretics (spironolactone or triamterene), 1,674 (34% received potassium-losing diuretics (thiazides, mercurials, and loop diuretics), and 461 patients (9.4%) received both potassium-sparing and potassium-losing diuretics together. The frequency of reported hyperkalemia in these three groups was 4.7%, 5.3%, and 7.4%. In this series of case analyses hyperkalemia was noted to be more frequent in elderly patients, in those with preexisting renal disease, in those who received potassium both orally and parenterally, and in those who died during the monitored admission. In addition, hyperkalemia was reported significantly more often in patients who received potassium chloride at the same time they were receiving diuretics.

It obviously bears repeating here that the potassium-sparing diuretics amiloride, spironolactone, and triamterene may all lead to life-threatening and or fatal hyperkalemia if they are not monitored carefully in high-risk patients who lack adequate renal function for any of several reasons.

Daily Cost Considerations

By comparison with many other drug categories that require a prescription prior to dispensing, diuretics are quite inexpensive. Table 9 lists the 1985 retail cost to patients of several popular diuretics or combination diuretic products, based on a cross-section of

Table 8 Hyperkalemia and Diuretic Use: Special Reports

16,048 Patients monitored and 4,921 (31%) received potassium chloride
Major clinical indication for potassium therapy was for *prophylaxis* against electrolyte depletion (87%); the remainder was for *therapy* of electrolyte depletion
Use pattern varied from 17 to 53% between hospitals (all medical services)
Of the 4,921 potassium recipients 2,263 received diuretics (K^+ given I.V. 1/3 of the time)

Type	#	Hyperkalemia (%)
K-depleting	1674	5.3
K-sparing	128	4.7
Both	461	7.4

In the 179 patients with hyperkalemia
Prior serum K^+ = 3.9 ± 0.1 mEq/L
Mean peak serum K^+ = 6.0 ± 0.1 mEq/L
in 7.3% (13 pts) $K^+ > 7.5$ mEq/L
Hyperkalemia was the major cause of fatal and life-threatening adverse effects: 6/7 deaths and 20/21 near fatalities
In the diuretic group *without* K^+ supplements 4.9% developed hypokalemia without apparent major consequence

Source: Ref. 50.

Table 9 Range of Cost of Various Diuretics[a]

	Dosage	$ Per 100	Number of tablets daily	$ Per day
Thiazide type				
Hydrochlorothiazide	50mg	2.47– 3.90	1	0.03
Hydrodiuril (hydrochlorothiazide)	50mg	8.65–14.00	1	0.11
Chlorthalidone	50mg	9.25– 9.95	1	0.10
Hygroton (chlorthalidone)	50mg	20.05–23.10	1	0.23
Zaroxolyn (metolazone)	5mg	17.75–22.80	1	0.20
Loop Agents				
Furosemide	40mg	9.05–10.25	1	0.10
Lasix (furosemide)	40mg	11.45–16.75	1	0.14
Bumex (bumetanide)	1mg	17.15–19.25	1	0.18
Potassium-sparing				
Midamor (amiloride)	5mg	20.25–25.90	1	0.23
Spironolactone	25mg	9.59–15.95	4	0.51
Aldactone (spironolactone)	25mg	23.00–28.60	4	1.03
Dyrenium (triamterene)	50mg	16.70–19.40	1	0.18
Combined agents				
Aldactazide (25mg spironolactone + 25mg hydrochlorothiazide)		22.00–33.25	1	0.28
Dyazide (50mg triamterene + 25mg hydrochlorothiazide)		17.29–25.40	1	0.21
Maxide (75mg triamterene + 50mg hydrochlorothiazide)		22.25–29.75	1	0.26
Moduretic (5mg amiloride + 50mg hydrochlorothiazide)		24.75–35.30	1	0.30

[a]Cost at retail pharmacies in Baltimore, Maryland, 1985.

pharmacies in the greater Baltimore area. Clearly, costs will differ in various regions of the United States and worldwide. Nonetheless, in all locations, the daily costs tend to be low. However, the global overview indicates that, although daily costs are low, so many patients tend to be on these drugs on a long-term basis that the 1985 national costs in the United States approach three-quarters of a billion dollars.

The major public health issues concerning the dietary intake of potassium, its relationship to the prevalence of hypertension, and the cost to the average individual if he or she needs to increase the intake of potassium-containing foods is reviewed in several other chapters in this text. The projected costs for this form of dietary manipulation of potassium intake is in the range of \$2-5 per day. In the subpopulation for whom it appears desirable to increase their total body potassium as a means of reducing the prevalence of hypertension, the cost data presented in Table 9 indicate that it is substantially less expensive to influence the quantity of body potassium by the administration of a potassium-sparing diuretic, than by dietary manipulation.

GENERAL CONCLUSIONS AND DEFINITIONS OF THE HIGH-RISK PATIENT

Diuretics are used extremely commonly: 100 million prescriptions are written for these compounds annually in the United States. They are an indispensable group of drugs for the management of both fluid and electrolyte overload and hypertension. Up to 11% of patients admitted to medical services can be expected to be on diuretics; this overall figure increases to approximately 35% in the elderly. Hypokalemia is variable in prevalence but in typical clinical practice one can expect an incidence of 5-30% in patients receiving potassium-losing diuretics. Thiazides, particularly chlorthalidone, are the most kaliuretic diuretics. The reduction in serum potassium consequent to diuretic therapy usually does not reflect a major intracellular deficit of potassium. This deficit is typically not more than 100-200 mEq/L of potassium.

During the thiazide management of hypertension, reduction of blood pressure tends to have a flat dosage-response curve whereas the induction of hypokalemia is enhanced as the dosage of the drug is increased. The reduction in serum potassium, if it occurs, will usually be seen in the first several days of therapy and does not progress over the long term. Patients with heightened activity of their renin-angiotensin-aldosterone axis and those who mobilize massive amounts of edema fluid tend to develop an obvious state of hypokalemia secondary to diuretic therapy. The elderly are also at high risk for the development of diuretic-induced hypokalemia and as a result of hypokalemia may be particularly at risk for the development of previously unidentified abnormalities in systemic glucose metabolism (2,29,103). In any person prone to hypokalemia, concurrent digitalis therapy needs to be monitored with extreme care. The issues of cardiac arrhythmia induced as a primary or secondary result of hypokalemia are fully reviewed in Chapter 14. There is an increasing awareness of the magnitude of extracellular hypokalemia that may be induced by circulating catecholamines in clinical settings with a stimulus to sympathoadrenergic activity (93). In such patients prior thiazide treatment importantly augments epinephrine-induced hypokalemia.

Hypokalemia induced by diuretics can be readily treated by potassium chloride administration, preferably with the concurrent use of a potassium sparing diuretic. However, it is perhaps wiser to consider the prevention of diuretic-induced hypokalemia by the use of potassium chloride supplements or, preferably, the use of combined formulations of potassium-losing and potassium-sparing diuretics. The latter combinations are scientifically sound, reliable, and appear to be better-tolerated and more effective than potassium supplements alone in the prevention of diuretic-associated hypokalemia. The clinical controversy concerning the routine use of potassium supplements is reviewed in detail elsewhere.

Hyperkalemic complications are seen in about 4% of patients receiving diuretics and typically are related to concurrent administration of potassium chloride. A reasonable clinical awareness of this complication should enable the clinician to avoid it completely.

ACKNOWLEDGMENTS

Supported in part by U.S.P.H.S. grants RR35 and RR722 for work performed in the General Clinical Research Centers of The Johns Hopkins University School of Medicine and The Johns Hopkins Hospital.

REFERENCES

1. Alberti, K. G. M. M., and Hockaday, T. D. R.: Thiazides and hypokalemia in diabetic ketoacidosis. *Postgrad. Med. J.* 49:29–31, 1973.
2. Amery, A., Berthaux, P., Bulpitt, C., Deruyterre, M., deSchafpdryver, A., Dollery, C., Fegard, R., Forette, F., Hellemans, J., Lund-Johansen, P., Mutsers, A. and Tuomilehto, J.: Glucose intolerance during diuretic therapy: Results of a trial by the European Working Party on Hypertension in the Elderly. *Lancet* 1:681–683, 1978.
3. Berglund, G., and Andersson, O.: Beta-blockers or diuretics in hypertension? A six year follow-up of blood pressure and metabolic side effects. *Lancet* 1:744–747, 1981.
4. Carney, S., Gillies, A. I., and Morgan, T.: Optimal dose of a thiazide diuretic. *Med. J. Aust.* 2:692–693, 1976.
5. Caruso, F. S., Szabadi, R. R., and Vukovich, R. A.: Pharmacokinetics and clinical pharmacology of indapamide. *Am. Heart J.* 106:212–220, 1983.
6. Cooper, I.: Potassium supplementation during diuretic therapy. *Curr. Ther. Res.* 17:555-563, 1975.
7. Davidson, C., McLachlan, M. S. F., Burkinshaw, L. and Morgan, D. B.: Effect of long term diuretic treatment on body-potassium in heart disease. *Lancet* 2:1044–1047, 1976.
8. Demanet, J. C.: Diuretics and hypokalemia: Aldosterone antagonists or potassium supplementation. *Acta. Clin. Belg.* 29:176–178, 1974.
9. Duke, M.: Thiazide-induced hypokalemia: Association with acute myocardial infarction and ventricular fibrillation. *JAMA* 239:43–45, 1978.
10. Dyckner, T., Helmers, C., and Wester, P. O.: Initial serum potassium level, early arrhythmias and previous diuretic therapy in acute myocardial infarction. *Int. J. Cardiol.* 2:147–148, 1982.
11. Editorial: Potassium in heart failure. *Br. Med. J.* 1:469–470, 1977.
12. Editorial: Diuretics in the elderly. *Br. Med. J.* 1:1092–1093, 1978.
13. Editorial: Slow-K, quick quick, slow. *Lancet* 2:1123–1124, 1974.
14. Editorial: Severe hypokalemia. *Lancet* 1:517–521, 1980.
15. Evans, E. R.: Potassium deficiency during treatment with Brinaldix K. *Br. Med. J.* 2:350, 1973.
16. Fichman, M. P., Vorherr, H., Kleeman, C. R., and Telfer, N.: Diuretic-induced hyponatremia. *Ann. Intern. Med.* 75:853-863, 1971.
17. Finnerty, F. A. Jr.: Diuretics as initial treatment for essential hypertension. *Br. J. Clin. Pharmacol.* 7 (suppl. 2):1858–1878, 1979.

18. Fischer, R. G.: Managing diuretic-induced hypokalemia in ambulatory hypertensive patients. *J. Fam. Pract.* 14:1029–1036, 1982.
19. Flamenbaum, W., and Friedman, R.: Pharmacology, therapeutic efficacy and adverse effects of bumetanide, a new "loop" diuretic. *Pharmacotherapy* 2:213–222, 1982.
20. Frolich, E. D.: Use and abuse of diuretics. *Am. Heart J.* 89:1–3, 1975.
21. Frolich, E. D., Mantell, G., Nancarrow, J. F., Stodden, C., and Walker, J. F.: Multiclinic comparison of amiloride, hydrochlorothiazide, and hydrochlorothiazide plus amiloride in essential hypertension. *Arch. Intern. Med.* 141:482–486, 1981.
22. Fujiwara, Y., Kikkawa, R., Nakata, K., Kitamura, E., Takama, T., and Shigeta, Y.: Hypokalemia and sodium retention in patients with diabetes and chronic hepatitis receiving insulin and glycyrrhizin. *Endocrinol. Jpn.* 20:243–249, 1983.
23. George, C. F., Breckenridge, A. M., and Dollery, C. T.: Comparison of the potassium-retaining effects of amiloride and spironolactone in hypertensive patients with thiazide-induced hypokalemia. *Lancet* 2:1288–1290, 1973.
24. Gifford, R. W. Jr.: A guide to the practical use of diuretics. *JAMA* 235:1890–1893, 1976.
25. Gray, J. M. B., Lawson, D. H., Boddy, K., and East, W.: Total body potassium in patients receiving chlorthalidone and metoprolol for hypertension. *Scott. Med. J.* 28:172–175, 1983.
26. Gray, M. J.: Use and abuse of thiazides in pregnancy. *Clin. Obstet. Gynecol.* 11: 568–578, 1968.
27. Greveson, G. C., and Lye, M.: Long-term thiazide diuretics. *Lancet* 1:941–942, 1981.
28. Griffing, G. T., Sindler, B. H., Aurecchia, S. A., and Melby, J. C.: Reversal of diuretic-induced secondary hyperaldosteronism and hypokalemia by enalapril (MK-421): A new Angiotensin-converting enzyme inhibitor. *Metabolism* 32:711–716, 1983.
29. Grunfeld, C., and Chappell, D. A.: Hypokalemia and diabetes mellitus. *Am. J. Med.* 75:553–554, 1983.
30. Hamdy, R. C., Tovey, J., and Perera, N.: Hypokalemia and diuretics. *Br. Med. J.* 280:1187, 1980.
31. Harrington, J. T., Isner, J. M., and Kassirer, J. P.: Our national obsession with potassium. *Am. J. Med.* 73:155–159, 1982.
32. Heffernan, A. G. A., Counihan, T. B., and Byrne, M.: Long-term studies with the new potassium-sparing diuretic, amiloride ("MK-870"). *Ir. J. Med. Sci.* 2:3–16, 1969.
33. Hettiarachchi, J. and Ramsay, L. E.: Diuretic-induced hypokalemia and the electrocardiogram (proceedings). *Br. J. Clin. Pharmacol.* 9:110P–111P, 1979.
34. Hollifield, J. W., and Slaton, P. E.: Thiazide diuretics, hypokalemia and cardiac arrhythmias. *Acta Med. Scand.* 647 (suppl 1):67–73, 1981.
35. Hulter, H. N., Licht, J. H., Glynn, R. D., and Sebastian, A.: Pathophysiology of chronic renal tubular acidosis induced by administration of amiloride. *J. Lab. Clin. Med.* 95:637–653, 1980.
36. Hume, L., and Forfar, J. C.: Hypertension and overdose of antihypertensive agents. *Lancet* 2:1182, 1977.
37. Imbs, J.-L., and Schwartz, J.: A propos d'hypokalimies survenues sous indapamide. *Nouv. Presse. Med.* 7:2477, 1978.
38. Jachuk, S. J.: Trial of mefruside. *Br. Med. J.* 2:590, 1972.
39. Jackson, P. R., Ramsay, L. E., and Wakefield, V.: Relative potency of spironolactone, triamterene and potassium chloride in thiazide-induced hypokalemia. *Br. J. Clin. Pharmacol.* 14:257–263, 1982.
40. Jelliffe, R. W., Hill, D., Tatter, D., and Lewis, E.: Death from weight control pills. *JAMA* 208:1843–1847, 1969.
41. Jensen, O. B., Mosdal, C., and Reske-Nielsen, E.: Hypokalemic myopathy during treatment with diuretics. *Acta Neurol. Scand.* 55:465–482, 1977.

42. Kassirer, J. P., and Harrington, J. T.: Diuretics and potassium metabolism: A reassessment of the need, effectiveness and safety of potassium therapy. *Kidney Int.* 11: 505–515, 1977.
43. Kleinfeld, M., and Rozanski, J. J.: Self-induced hypokalemia. *NY State J. Med.* 75:2229–2231, 1975.
44. Kohvakka, A., Eisaio, A., and Manninen, V.: Maintenance of potassium balance during diuretic therapy. *Acta Med. Scand.* 205:319–324, 1979.
45. Krakauer, R.: Potassium in heart failure. *Br. J. Med.* 1:1032–1033, 1977.
46. Kunau, R. T., and Stein, J. H.: Disorders of hypo- and hyperkalemia. *Clin. Nephrol.* 7:173–190, 1977.
47. Landmann-Suter, R., and Struyvenberg, A.: Initial potassium loss and hypokalemia during chlorthalidone administration in patients with essential hypertension: The influence of dietary sodium restriction. *Eur. J. Clin. Invest.* 8:155–164, 1978.
48. Laragh, J. H.: Amiloride, a potassium-conserving agent new to the U.S.A.: Mechanisms and clinical relevance. *Curr. Ther. Res.* 32:173–188, 1982.
49. Lawson, A. A. H.: Potassium replacement: When is it necessary? *Drugs* 21:354–361, 1981.
50. Lawson, D. H.: Adverse reactions to potassium chloride. *Q. J. Med. New Series* 43: 433–440, 1974.
51. Lawson, D. H., Henry, D. A., Lowe, J. M., Gray, J. M. B., and Morgan, H. G.: Severe hypokalemia in hospitalized patients. *Arch. Intern. Med.* 139:978–980, 1979.
52. Lawson, D. H., O'Connor, P. C., and Jick, H.: Drug attributed alterations in potassium handling in congestive cardiac failure. *Eur. J. Clin. Pharmacol.* 23:21–25, 1982.
53. Leiter, L.: Combinations of diuretics in the treatment of edema. *Am. Heart J.* 80: 422–426, 1970.
54. Lemieux, G., Beauchemin, M., Vinay, P., and Gougoux, A.: Hypokalemia during the treatment of arterial hypertension with diuretics. *Can. Med. Assoc. J.* 122:905–907, 1980.
55. Licht, J. H., Haley, R. J., Pugh, B., and Lewis, S. B.: Diuretic regimens in essential hypertension: A comparison of hypokalemic effects, B.P. control and cost. *Arch. Intern. Med.* 143:1694–1699, 1983.
56. Loewy, E. H.: Hypokalemia and arrhythmias in myocardial infarction. *JAMA* 239: 2113, 1978.
57. Lowe, J., Gray, J., Henry, D. A., and Lawson, D. H.: Adverse reactions to frusemide in hospital inpatients. *Br. Med. J.* 2:360–362, 1979.
58. MacLean, D., and Tudhope, G. R.: Modern diuretic treatment. *Br. Med. J.* 286: 1419–1422, 1983.
59. Manley, K. A.: Monitoring plasma potassium in patients on diuretics. *Lancet* 1:880, 1980.
60. McInnes, G. T., Shelton, J. R., Perkins, R. M., Harrison, I. R., and Clarke, J. M.: Use of a bioassay in healthy men to evaluate diuretic-spironolactone combinations. *Br. J. Clin. Pharmacol.* 15:564–566, 1983.
61. McKibbin, J. K., Pocock, W. A., Barlow, J. B., Millar, R. N. S., and Obel, W. P.: Sotalol, hypokalemia, syncope, and torsade de pointes. *Br. Heart J.* 51:157–162, 1984.
62. Merimee, T. J.: Potassium supplementation: Comparative studies in nonedematous and edematous patients. *J. Fla. Med. Assoc.* 68:37–39, 1981.
63. Morgan, D. B., Burkinshaw, L., and Davidson, C.: Potassium depletion in heart failure and its relation to long-term treatment with diuretics: A review of the literature. *Postgrad. Med. J.* 54:72–79, 1978.
64. Morgan, D. B., and Davidson, C.: Hypokalemia and diuretics: an analysis of publications. *Br. Med. J.* 2:905–908, 1980.
65. Morgan, T. O.: Potassium replacement: Supplements or potassium-sparing diuretics? *Drugs* 18:218–225, 1979.

66. Morgan, T., and Myers, J.: Potassium maintenance: Potassium supplements or potassium sparing agents. *Acta Med. Scand.* 647 (suppl):117–123, 1981.
67. Naranjo, C. A., Pontigo, E., Valdenegro, C., Gonzalez, G., Ruiz, I., and Busto, U.: Furosemide-induced adverse reactions in cirrhosis of the liver. *Clin. Pharmacol. Ther.* 25:154–160, 1979.
68. National Disease and Therapeutic Index: Ambler, Pennsylvania, 1984.
69. Nawar, T.: Hyperkalemia and overdose of antihypertensive agents. *Lancet* 1:717, 1978.
70. Nilsson, G.: Symptomatic diabetes mellitus cured by potassium and withdrawal of polythiazide in a hypokalemic hypertensive woman. *Acta Med. Scand.* 208:129–131, 1980.
71. Parker, M. S., Oster, J. R., Perez, O., and Taylor, A. L.: Chronic hypokalemia and alkalosis. *Arch. Intern. Med.* 140:1336–1378, 1980.
72. Pasquel, R., Tribble, P. W., and Simon, A.: Hypotensive effects of xipamide in essential hypertension. Crossover comparison with hydrochlorothiazide. *J. Clin. Pharmacol.* 21:316–322, 1981.
73. Penhall, R. K., and Frewin, D. B.: Plasma potassium levels in hypertensive patients receiving fixed-combinations diuretic therapy. *Med. J. Aust.* 1:376–378, 1980.
74. Perez-Stable, E., and Caralis, P. V.: Thiazide-induced disturbances in carbohydrate, lipid and potassium metabolism. *Am. Heart J.* 106:245–257, 1983.
75. Perez-Stable, E., and Materson, B.: Diuretic drug therapy of edema. *Med. Clin. North Am.* 55:359–372, 1971.
76. Poole-Wilson, P. A.: Hypokalemia induced by thiazide diuretics in the treatment of hypertension: A cause for concern, not nihilism. *Postgrad. Med. J.* 59 (suppl 3):137–139, 1983.
77. Rado, J. P., Marosi, J., Szende, L., and Tako, J.: Hyperkalemic changes during spironolactone therapy for cirrhosis and ascites, with special reference to hyperkalemic intermittent paralysis. *J. Am. Geriatr. Soc.* 16:874–886, 1968.
78. Ram, C. V. S., Holland, O. B., and Kaplan, N. M.: Attenuation of diuretic-induced hypokalemia by amiloride, a potassium-sparing agent. *J. Clin. Pharmacol.* 21:484–487, 1981.
79. Ramsay, L. E., Boyle, P., and Ramsay, M. H.: Factors influencing serum potassium in treated hypertension. *Q. J. Med.* 46:401–410, 1977.
80. Ramsay, L. E., and Hettiarachchi, J.: Spironolactone in thiazide-induced hypokalemia: Variable response between patients. *Br. J. Clin. Pharmacol.* 11:153–158, 1981.
81. Ramsay, L. E., Hettiarachchi, J., Fraser, R., and Morton, J. J.: Amiloride, spironolactone and potassium chloride in thiazide treated hypertensive patients. *Clin. Pharmacol. Ther.* 27:533–543, 1980.
82. Rodat, O., and Hamelin, J.-P.: Hypokalemie à 0.9 mEq au cours d'un traitement par l'indapamide. *Nouv. Presse. Med.* 7:3054, 1978.
83. Rodman, J. S., and Reidenberg, M. M.: Symptomatic hypokalemia resulting from surreptitious diuretic ingestion. *JAMA* 246:1687–1689, 1981.
84. Salonen, J. T., and Ylitalo, P.: Antihypertensive, saluretic and hypokalemic effects of cyclothiazide in comparison with hydrochlorothiazide with amiloride supplement. *Eur. J. Clin. Pharmacol.* 22:495–499, 1982.
85. Schifrin, B. S., Spellacy, W. N., and Little, W. A.: Maternal death associated with excessive ingestion of a chlorothiazide diuretic. *Obstet. Gynecol.* 34:215–220, 1969.
86. Shah, B. R., Shah, N. V., Sanghavi, N. G., Shah, C. P., Acharya, P. T., and Shukla, D. N.: Initial hypokalemia and hypokalemic effect of diuretic therapy in nutritional edema. *J. Indian Med. Assoc.* 54:144–150, 1970.
87. Sherlock, S., Walker, J. G., Senewiratne, B., and Scott, A.: The complications of diuretic therapy in patients with cirrhosis. *Ann. NY Acad. Sci.* 139:497–505, 1966.

88. Sopko, J. A., and Freeman, R. M.: Salt substitutes as a source of potassium. *JAMA* 238:608–610, 1977.
89. Steen, B.: Hypokalemia—clinical spectrum and etiology. *Acta Med. Scand.* 647 (suppl):61–66, 1981.
90. Steiness, E.: Diuretics, digitalis and arrhythmias. *Acta Med. Scand.* 647 (suppl): 75–78, 1981.
91. Steiness, E., and Olesen, K. H.: Cardiac arrhythmias induced by hypokalemia and potassium loss during maintenance digoxin therapy. *Br. Heart J.* 38:167–172, 1976.
92. Sterns, R. H., Cox, M., Feig, P. U., and Singer, I.: Internal potassium balance and the control of the plasma potassium concentration. *Medicine* 60:339–354, 1981.
93. Struthers, A. D., Whitesmith, R., and Reid, J. L.: Prior thiazide diuretic treatment increases adrenaline-induced hypokalemia. *Lancet* 1:1358–1360, 1983.
94. Sullivan, R. C., Freemon, F. R., and Caranasos, G. J.: Complications from diuretic therapy with ethacrynic acid and furosemide. *South. Med. J.* 64:869–872, 1971.
95. Sumiye, L., Vivian, A. S., Frisof, K. B., and Podany, E. C.: Potassium loss associated with hydrochlorothiazide versus chlorthalidone. *Clin. Ther.* 4:308–320, 1981.
96. Sweet, C. S., and Gaul, S. L.: Attenuation of hydrochlorothiazide-induced hypokalemia in dogs by a beta-adrenergic blocking drug, timolol. *Eur. J. Pharmacol.* 32:370–374, 1975.
97. Taylor, R. T., and Peaston, M. J. T.: Potassium deficiency during treatment with Brinaldix K. *Br. Med. J.* 2:48, 1973.
98. Vassallo, C. L., Gee, J. B. L., Raskin, P., and Robin, E. D.: The failure of organic potassium salts to repair diuretic-induced hypokalemia and alkalosis in chronic hypercapnia. *Am. Rev. Respir. Dis.* 97:804–809, 1968.
99. Viherkoski, M., Huikko, M., and Vajoranta, K.: The effect of amiloride/hydrochlorothiazide combination vs. furosemide plus potassium supplementation in the treatment of edema of cardiac origin. *Ann. Clin. Res.* 13:11–15, 1981.
100. Vincent, H. H., Boomsma, F., Man in't Veld, A. J., Derkx, F. H. M., Wenting, G. J., and Schalenkamp, M. A. D. H.: Effects of selective and nonselective beta-agonists on plasma potassium and norepinephrine. *J. Cardiovasc. Pharmacol.* 6: 107–114, 1984.
101. Whelton, A., Barnes, R. S., Stout, R. L., and Spilman, P. S.: A double-blind trial of chlorthalidone versus chlorthalidone and triamterene in renal edema. *J. Clin. Pharmacol.* (in press), 1985.
102. Whiting, G. F. M., McLaran, C. J., and Bochner, F.: Severe hyperkalemia with moduretic. *Med. J. Aust.* 1:409, 1979.
103. Yu, M. C.: Hypokalemic and hypoglycemia effects of ritodrine. *Am. J. Obstet. Gynecol.* 147:731–732, 1983.
104. Zempol, P. A.: Controlled, randomized studies of bumetanide (Bumex) in the treatment of edema secondary to cardiac, hepatic or renal disease. Data on file Roche Laboratories, Division of Hoffmann-LaRoche Inc., Nutley, New Jersey, 1984.

18

Diuretic-Induced Ventricular Arrhythmias

O. BRYAN HOLLAND
University of Texas Medical Branch at Galveston, Galveston, Texas

Until the last few years, the hazard of diuretic-induced ventricular arrhythmias in patients not receiving digitalis and in patients without overt cardiac disease was thought to be minimal. However, this previous opinion was based more on clinical impression than on careful studies. There have now been several clinical studies utilizing accurate techniques such as 24-hr ambulatory electrocardiographic (ECG) monitoring and ECG monitoring during exercise testing to evaluate the incidence of ventricular arrhythmias during diuretic therapy. These studies have included both hypokalemic and normokalemic patients treated with diuretics, and they have provided good evidence that diuretic-induced hypokalemia is associated with a significant incidence of ventricular arrhythmias, even in patients without overt cardiac disease.

STUDIES DEMONSTRATING AN ASSOCIATION OF DIURETIC THERAPY WITH VENTRICULAR ARRHYTHMIAS

Both 24-hr ambulatory ECG monitoring and exercise testing were utilized in one study (5) involving patients with mild to moderate uncomplicated essential hypertension and a history of diuretic-induced hypokalemia. These patients were taken off previous antihypertensive medications and given supplemental potassium chloride for 2-3 weeks during an initial 4-week placebo phase. Near the end of the placebo phase, baseline 24-hour ambulatory ECG monitoring was done to document that less than six unifocal ventricular premature beats (VPBs) per hour and no other types of ventricular ectopic activity (VEA) were present. In addition, an exercise test was done to evaluate the patient for occult coronary artery disease. Those patients who qualified for the study were then treated with hydrochlorothiazide (HCTZ, 100 mg/day) for 4 weeks to induce hypokalemia. At the end of this time, the ambulatory ECG monitoring, plasma potassium determination, and exercise testing were repeated. Seven of 21 HCTZ-treated patients showed an increase in the number of unifocal VPBs to greater than 30/hr or developed complex VEA (ventricular tachycardia, ventricular couplets, multifocal ventricular beats). These complex arrhythmias, which have been more clearly associated with sudden death, were seen in four of the seven patients. At the end of the HCTZ treatment phase, only two of these seven patients had ventricular arrhythmias provoked by exercise testing, demonstrating a greater sensitivity of ambulatory ECG monitoring in identifying ventricular arrhythmias. Those patients who showed VEA were then potassium-repleted with spironolactone, and the effect of potassium repletion was assessed by periodic additional 24-hr ambulatory ECG monitoring. Spironolactone therapy significantly reduced VEA in all patients. However, one patient had persistent unifocal VPBs after potassium repletion varying from 31 to 220 unifocal VPSs/hr during four ambulatory ECG monitorings done during 13 weeks. Even the addition of propranolol for an additional 6 weeks did not cause the ambulatory ECG monitoring to return to the normal baseline pattern. It thus appeared that this patient had undergone some kind of cardiac change as a result of HCTZ-induced hypokalemia that led to permanent ventricular irritability in spite of potassium repletion. This change might have been explained by focal cardiac lesions which have been observed with potassium depletion (4,9,11).

In this study, patients who were likely to develop VEA could not be identified by the usual clinical criteria. They did not complain spontaneously of symptoms compatible with VEA, though two patients who were told of their monitoring results noted that they had experienced occasional palpitations. Patients with and without VEA were essentially the same average age and had the same severity of HCTZ-induced hypokalemia, and they were not more likely to have left ventricular hypertrophy. Thus, usual clinical criteria would not have identified these patients with VEA. The suggestion has been made (3) that spontaneous variation in the ambulatory ECG monitoring might explain the study results, since more than one ambulatory ECG measurement was not made in the baseline phase to document the baseline pattern in greater detail. However, if this were true, the marked reduction in VEA during the phase of potassium repletion with spironolactone would not have been expected.

To allow evaluation of the problem of spontaneous variation, ambulatory ECG monitoring results were compared in those patients with diuretic-induced VEA (excluding the one patient just discussed with permanent change in the monitoring pattern after hypokalemia) during the time when the patients were hypokalemic and when they were normokalemic throughtout the entire study. Unifocal VPBs occurred with an average frequency of 14.7 beats/hr per 24-hr ECG monitoring while the patients were hypokalemic compared with an average of 0.5 unifocal VPBs/hr per 24-hr ECG monitoring while they were normokalemic. Furthermore, complex VEA was noted in only 1 hr of 19 ambulatory ECG monitorings done while the patients were normokalemic, but it was seen in 29 hr of 12 ambulatory ECG monitorings done while patients were hypokalemic. Both of the differences were statistically significant, and they indicated that the study results did not appear to be explained by spontaneous variation. Thus, diuretic-induced hypokalemia was associated with VEA, even in patients without apparent underlying cardiac disease.

Subsequently, we initiated another study to evaluate the genesis of diuretic-induced VEA. Two 24-hr ambulatory ECG monitorings as well as an exercise test were done in the baseline phase of this study. Patients were classified into one group treated with HCTZ (100 mg/day) and into another treated with a combination of HCTZ with amiloride to attempt to maintain normokalemia during diuretic therapy. As with our previous study, we noted more VEA in patients allowed to become hypokalemic with HCTZ treatment alone than in patients simultaneously treated with amiloride. Though hypomagnesemia has been noted with long-term diuretic treatment, we did not observe it with the shorter

4 weeks of HCTZ therapy. Unfortunately, one patient died suddenly 2 days before ambulatory ECG monitoring scheduled 2 weeks after initiation of HCTZ treatment. Autopsy did not reveal myocardial infarction, pulmonary emboli, cerebrovascular lesions, or other causes for the sudden death. Thus, even though this patient was not being monitored at the time of death, circumstantial evidence is highly suggestive of an arrhythmic death. When patients with VEA were switched from HCTZ to amiloride to provide potassium repletion, the frequency of VEA decreased. Interestingly, however, a small amount of VEA was noted in patients treated with HCTZ-amiloride to maintain normokalemia. This suggests that factors other than potassium depletion may also lead to VEA with diuretic therapy, unless potassium depletion is not being reflected by plasma potassium measurements. An alternative suggestion is that the VEA observed reflects a small amount of spontaneous variation in the ambulatory ECG monitoring pattern.

Hollifield and Slaton (6) have used exercise testing to document an increase in VEA during diuretic therapy. These studies are discussed in Chapter 19 in this book. Caralis et al. (2) withdrew previous antihypertensive therapy from a group of 16 patients during a baseline phase, and ambulatory ECG monitoring was performed before and after chlorthalidone treatment (100 mg/day) for 4-6 weeks to induce hypokalemia. Potassium chloride was then added to assess its influence upon VEA. A subgroup of these patients developed VEA when given chlorthalidone treatment, and it decreased in frequency with KCL supplementation. Patients with VEA were more likely to be older and to have ECG abnormalities, cardiomegaly on chest x-ray, or other subtle evidence of organic heart disease. Thus, this study provides additional documentation that ventricular arrhythmias may occur with diuretic therapy in patients without congestive heart failure or symptomatic cardiac disease.

In Chapter 20, Whelton discusses diuretic-induced ventricular arrhythmias in a study performed by the Medical Research Council Working Party on Mild to Moderate Hypertension (7). These investigators noted an increased incidence of ventricular arrhythmias in diuretic-treated patients. However, they concluded that diuretic-induced hypokalemia served as a marker for patients who would develop ventricular arrhythmias, but it did not satisfactorily explain the genesis of the arrhythmias. Nevertheless, several factors limit the ability to evaluate the role of hypokalemia in the genesis of these ventricular arrhythmias. First, this study was not confined to patients with a history of diuretic-induced hypokalemia, so the number of patients who might have developed ventricular arrhythmias secondary to potassium depletion was limited. A subgroup of 16 patients had satisfactory ambulatory ECG monitoring results before and after short-term diuretic therapy. However, the average serum potassium level at the end of diuretic therapy in this subgroup of patients only fell to 3.6 mEq/L, and the number of patients who became hypokalemic (K^+ less than 3.5 mEq/L) was not stated, though this was probably only about five to seven patients. Since other studies (5) have reported the occurrence of VEA in only about one-third of patients with hypokalemia (less than 3.5 mEq/L), the number of cases with hypokalemia studied would appear to have been inadequate for satisfactory statistical evaluation. In fact, the observation that these patients did not develop ventricular arrhythmias at a time when most of the patients remained normokalemic provides evidence against a major nonspecific effect of diuretic therapy in the genesis of ventricular arrhythmias.

A separate part of this MRC study involved a long-term study of 155 patients who had completed 3-50 months of placebo or diuretic therapy (average, 2 years). There was no correlation of the serum potassium values and the number of VPBs, though a significant increase in VPBs was noted in the diuretic-treated group. When all diuretic-treated patients in the study were evaluated, there was a significant correlation between the serum potassium concentration and the number of VPBs, and a subgroup of 16 patients with definite hypokalemia had a much greater incidence of multifocal VPBs and ventricular couplets compared with unselected placebo and diuretic-treated patients. A subgroup of eight of these hypokalemic patients were treated with supplemental KCL to raise their serum K^+ from 2.8 to 3.5 mEq/L. However, these patients were not withdrawn from previous diuretic therapy for baseline ambulatory ECG monitoring to make sure that they did not have VEA unrelated to diuretic therapy. In this group, three of four patients with greater than 10 VPBs/100,000 beats had a decrease in the number of VPBs with K^+ supplementation, but there was no correlation between changes in VPBs and changes in serum K^+ values. The investigators thus concluded that long-term diuretic therapy was associated with an increased incidence of VEA, but that potassium depletion could not satisfactorily explain the genesis of these arrhythmias. However, since serum K^+ levels were measured at random times during the day, some excess variation would be expected from variations in time of blood sampling in relation to eating and to administration of supplemental KCL. This factor, together with the small number (4) of patients with VEA treated with KCL and the lack of knowledge about VEA unrelated to diuretic therapy, seriously limits the ability to perform meaningful statistical evaluation of the effects of KCL supplementation. Thus, the power to evaluate the role which potassium depletion played in the genesis of ventricular arrhythmias in this study is limited.

STUDIES THAT HAVE NOT NOTED AN ASSOCIATION OF DIURETIC THERAPY WITH VENTRICULAR ARRHYTHMIAS

Though the four studies reviewed here have noted an increase in ventricular arrhythmias with diuretic therapy, other investigators have not been able to confirm this finding. Papademetriou et al. (8) evaluated 16 diuretic-treated patients with ambulatory ECG monitoring while they were hypokalemic and after potassium repletion with supplemental KCL or with triamterene. They noted no beneficial therapeutic effect of potassium repletion on observed ventricular arrhythmias. However, ambulatory ECG monitoring was not done while the patients were off diuretic therapy to determine if the patients had ventricular arrhythmias not attributable to diuretic therapy. In addition, other antihypertensive medications were being taken by 9 of these 16 patients, which may have influenced the study results.

These investigators have performed another study which is presented in Chapter 21. In this study they performed ambulatory ECG monitoring during an initial placebo phase before the initiation of diuretic therapy. Again, they did not note an increase in the number of ventricular arrhythmias during diuretic therapy. The reason for these different results is not evident. Perhaps the results may be explained by the fact that this study did not exclude patients with significant numbers of ventricular arrhythmias during the initial placebo phase. Calvert et al. (1) have reported that the reproducibility of ambulatory ECG monitoring is about 80% in patients with less than 30 unifocal VPBs/hr, whereas it decreases to only about 40% when more ventricular arrhythmias, including ventricular tachycardia, are present. Therefore, studies that include patients with significant numbers of ventricular arrhythmias while the patients are not taking diuretics may have a lesser ability to demonstrate ventricular arrhythmias attributable to diuretic therapy due to problems with spontaneous variation in ambulatory ECG monitoring. Thus, the majority of studies indicate that diuretic-induced hypokalemia may cause ventricular arrhythmias.

OTHER EVIDENCE SUGGESTING ADVERSE CARDIAC EFFECTS OF CHRONIC HYPOKALEMIA

In addition to the studies that have documented the occurrence of ventricular arrhythmias with diuretic therapy, other studies indicate that patients with mild diuretic-induced hypokalemia may become significantly more hypokalemic if they sustain a stressful event such as an acute myocardial infarction (10). This enhanced hypokalemia appears to result from epinephrine-mediated B_2 receptor stimulation. The fact that stress-induced epinephrine release may magnify considerably the severity of hypokalemia and thus the likelihood of fatal ventricular fibrillation may explain the failure to find a simple relationship between the severity of diuretic-induced hypokalemia and sudden death in the MRFIT study. This phenomenon may also be important in the association of an enhanced rate of malignant ventricular arrhythmias in hypokalemic patients undergoing a myocardial infarction. These studies are discussed in Chapters 12-15. In addition to the induction of ventricular arrhythmias, diuretic-induced potassium depletion may lead to adverse cardiovascular effects by interfering with glucose homeostasis (4). Even mild potassium depletion may have a prominent role in the diabetogenic effect of diuretics. This diabetogenic effect may lead to an enhanced rate of atherosclerosis.

IMPLICATIONS FOR THERAPY

Evidence is therefore good that diuretic therapy may lead to ventricular arrhythmias, even in patients without apparent underlying cardiac disease. Though potassium depletion appears to be important in the genesis of these ventricular arrhythmias, other factors may contribute. Other significant cardiovascular complications may be associated with chronic diuretic-induced potassium depletion. Since individual patient susceptibility to arrhythmias cannot be predicted using the usual clinical criteria, normokalemia should be maintained during chronic diuretic therapy.

ACKNOWLEDGMENTS

The assistance of Rebecca Hicks in the preparation of the manuscript is appreciated.

REFERENCES

1. Calvert, A., Lown, B., and Gorlin, R.: Ventricular premature beats and anatomically defined coronary heart disease. *Am. J. Cardiol.* 39:627–633, 1977.
2. Caralis, P. V., Materson, B. J., and Perez-Stable, E.: Potassium and diuretic-induced ventricular arrhythmias in ambulatory hypertensive patients. *Miner. Electrolyte Metab.* 10:148–154, 1984.
3. Harrington, J. T., Isner, J. M., and Kassirer, J. P.: Our national obsession with potassium. *Am. J. Med.* 73:155–159, 1982.
4. Holland, O. B.: Mild hypokalemia in non-edematous, non-digitalized patients. The case for routinely normalizing serum potassium. In *Controversies in Nephrology and Hypertension,* edited by Narins, R. G., New York, Churchill Livingstone, 1984.
5. Holland, O. B., Nixon, J. V., and Kuhnert, L.: Diuretic-induced ventricular ectopic activity. *Am. J. Med.* 70:762–768, 1981.

6. Hollifield, J. W., and Slaton, P. E.: Thiazide diuretics, hypokalemia and cardiac arrhythmias. *Acta Med. Scand.* Suppl. 647:67–73, 1981.
7. Medical Research Council Working Party on Mild to Moderate Hypertension: Ventricular extrasystoles during thiazide treatment: substudy of MRC mild hypertension trial. *Br. Med. J.* 287:1249–1253, 1983.
8. Papademetriou, V., Fletcher, R., Khatri, I. M., and Freis, E. D.: Diuretic-induced hypokalemia in uncomplicated systemic hypertension: effect of plasma potassium correction on cardiac arrhythmias. *Am. J. Cardiol.* 52:1017–1022, 1983.
9. Perkins, J. G., Petersen, A. B., and Riley, J. A.: Renal and cardiac lesions in potassium deficiency due to chronic diarrhea. *Am. J. Med.* 8:115–123, 1950.
10. Struthers, A. D., Whitesmith, R., and Reid, J. L.: Prior thiazide diuretic treatment increases adrenaline-induced hypokalemia. *Lancet* 1:1358–1361, 1983.
11. Welt, L. G., Hollander, W., Jr., and Blythe, W. B.: The consequences of potassium depletion. *J. Chron. Dis.* 11:213–254, 1960.

19

Potassium and Magnesium Abnormalities: Diuretics and Arrhythmias in Hypertension

JOHN W. HOLLIFIELD
Hypertension Center of Nashville, Nashville, Tennessee

Thiazide diuretics are widely used in antihypertensive therapy, both as initial monotherapy in some hypertensive patients and as a complement to other antihypertensive agents in combination therapy in others (4,11). They are so widely used because they are safe, effective, and well tolerated. Nonetheless, long-term thiazide diuretic therapy, particularly at higher dosages is associated with a number of undesirable metabolic side effects (3,6). One of these, hypokalemia (6), may be associated with cardiac arrhythmias, weakness, fatigue, and muscle cramps. Whether hypokalemia poses a real threat to health or is merely an inconsequential biochemical abnormality (3) is the subject of controversy.

In addition to hypokalemia, thiazides also cause hypomagnesemia, which complicates the relationship between the potassium ion and cardiac arrhythmias (2,5,7). Moreover, recent studies have shown that thiazide-induced hypokalemia and hypomagnesemia are associated with exercise-induced ventricular arrhythmia (5). Treatment of thiazide-treated patients with the combination of magnesium and potassium was more effective than either agent alone in reducing the incidence of ventricular ectopy induced by thiazides (7).

In our studies, outpatients aged 35-57 years were evaluated to exclude secondary forms of hypertension (5,7). Serum potassium and magnesium levels were measured by standard laboratory techniques (5) and blood pressure was measured weekly with a mercury manometer according to a previously published protocol (12).

COMPARATIVE STUDIES OF THIAZIDE DIURETICS

Study 1

Hydrochlorothiazide 50 mg a day was initially administered in two divided doses (25 mg twice daily). The dosage was increased at 4-week intervals to 100 mg (50 mg twice daily), 150 mg (75 mg twice daily), and 200 mg (100 mg twice daily) until either diastolic blood pressure levels were reduced to 90 mmHg or less or a dosage of 200 mg a day hydrochlorothiazide was reached. At this point hydrochlorothiazide was continued for an additional 24 weeks at the maximum dosage used during the dosage escalation phase of the

Table 1 Effects of Hydrochlorothiazide on Blood Pressure and Serum Potassium and Magnesium

	Hydrochlorothiazide (mg)	Percentage mean arterial pressure change	Potassium (mEq/L)	Magnesium mEq/L)
Short-term effects	0	–	4.5±0.2	2.10±0.2
	50	40±3.1	4.2±0.3	2.06±0.1
	100	51±10.4	4.0±0.3	1.99±0.1
	150	59±11.4	3.7±0.2	1.97±0.1
	200	70±12.8	3.5±0.3	1.92±0.2
Long-term effects	0	–	4.5±0.2	2.10±0.2
	50	38±5.0	3.92±0.3	1.87±0.2
	100	47±8.9	3.38±0.2	1.72±0.15
	150	55±10.1	2.91±0.2	1.61±0.2
	200	59±13.2	2.44±0.3	1.56±0.1

experiment. Electrolytes, urea, creatine, and magnesium levels were measured at the conclusion of each 4-week interval during dosage escalation and during the 24-week long-term maintenance therapy.

Table 1 shows the effect of hydrochlorothiazide therapy on blood pressure and serum cation levels during study 1. In general, the greater the dosage of thiazide, the greater the fall in serum potassium and magnesium levels. Potassium and magnesium did not show as impressive changes during the dosage ranging portion of the protocol as at the end of the long-term continuous dosing portion of the protocol (Table 1). In addition, patients whose blood pressure levels normalize with lower dosages of hydrochlorothiazide exhibit smaller decreases in potassium and magnesium levels during hydrochlorothiazide therapy. Those who require higher dosages exhibit greater decreases in serum potassium and magnesium.

Study 2

Thirty-eight patients aged 40–55 years (different from those in the first study) were selected from the same outpatient population. All patients had normal or borderline results on resting electrocardiograms (none exhibited more than one paroxysmal ventricular contraction/min during rhythm monitoring) and cardiac physical examinations. None exhibited ischemic changes during exercise tolerance testing. Nonetheless, all patients in this study were selected because they had previous evidence of marked hypokalemia during thiazide treatment (potassium 3.0 mEq/L or less) or had complained of palpitations, cardiac awareness, or arrhythmia. All patients underwent exercise testing with electrocardiographic monitoring. Paroxysmal ventricular contractions were counted during 5 min of standing rest before exercising on the treadmill. Dynamic exercise was conducted on a treadmill at 1.7 miles/hr, 10% grade (Bruce stage 1). Premature ventricular contractions were counted from 6 to 10 min into the exercise protocol. The frequency of premature ventricular contractions at rest (control periods) was compared with the frequency during exercise. All patients were studied twice: once before hydrochlorothiazide therapy and again during hydrochlorothiazide administration. Hydrochlorothiazide, 50 mg a day, reduced blood pressure to normal in 17 patients who subsequently underwent exercise

Table 2 Effect of Exercise on Occurrence of Premature Ventricular Contractions (PVCs) During Long-Term Treatment with Thiazides

	Pretreatment		Hydrochlorothiazide treatment	
	Heart rate (bpm)	PVCs (bpm)	Heart rate (bpm)	PVCs (bpm)
Rest	68±3	0.6±0.08	79±4	1.4±0.1
Static exercise	90±3	0.6±0.06	114±5	3.6±0.7
Dynamic exercise	156±12	0.8±0.15	166±10	5.7±0.8

studies. All other patients were studied during the administration of hydrochlorothiazide, 100 mg a day. Serum for potassium determination was collected without a tourniquet at sitting rest immediately prior to exercise studies both before and during hydrochlorothiazide therapy.

Table 2 shows the effect of exercise and hydrochlorothiazide on the occurrence of paroxysmal ventricular contractions in 38 patients. Exercise itself did not increase paroxysmal ventricular contractions in the absence of hydrochlorothiazide treatment. During hydrochlorothiazide therapy, however, the frequency of exercise-induced paroxysmal ventricular contractions increased from 1.4 to 5.7 beats/min. During dynamic exercise, multifocal paroxysmal ventricular contractions occurred in 4 of 38 patients, and short salvos of ventricular tachycardia (three- to seven-beat runs) were noted in one patient. There was a significant correlation between the fall in serum potassium levels (ΔK^+) during hydrochlorothiazide therapy and the occurrence of paroxysmal ventricular con-

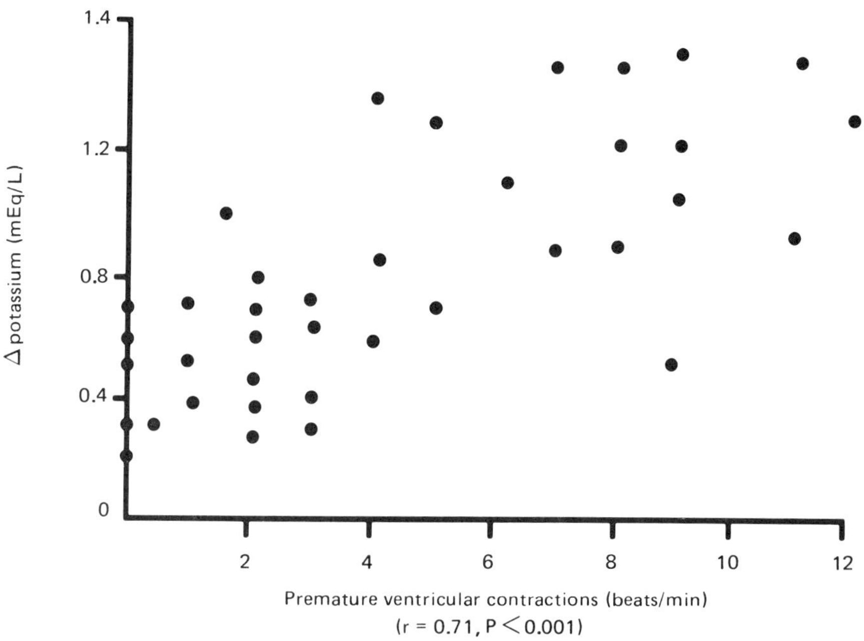

Figure 1 Correlations between change in serum potassium and frequency of premature ventricular contractions in 38 patients with mild-to-moderate hypertension.

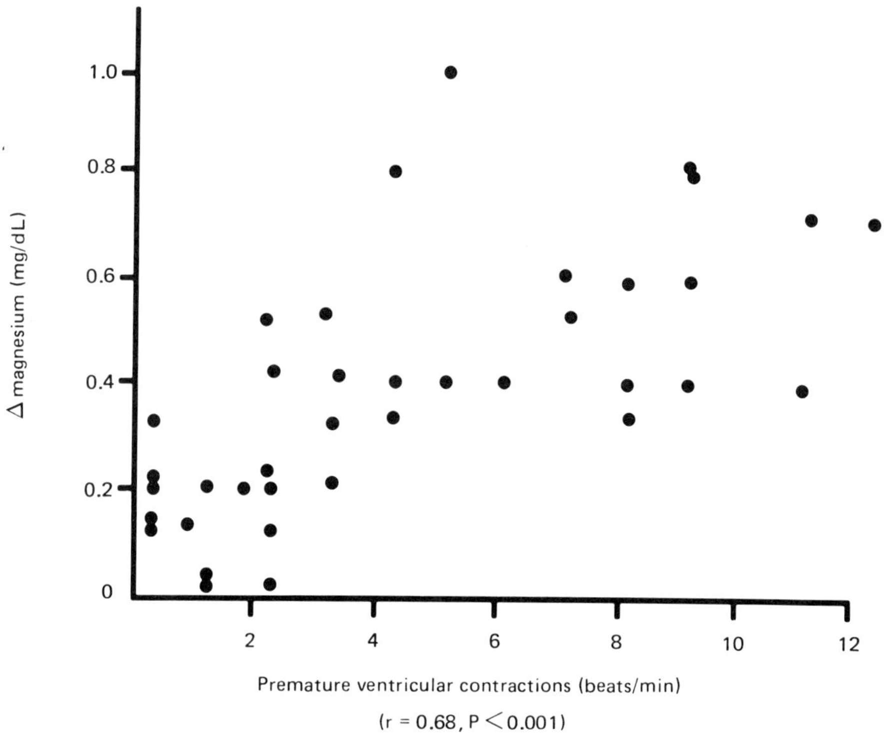

Figure 2 The significant decrease in serum magnesium during thiazide therapy correlated with the occurrence of premature ventricular contractions.

tractions (r=0.71; p>0.001) (Figure 1). Decreases in serum magnesium levels also occurred during thiazide therapy and correlated with the occurrence of paroxysmal ventricular contractions and were significant (r=0.68; p<0.001) (Figure 2). Serum potassium level before exercise correlated with the frequency of paroxysmal ventricular contractions to a lesser degree of significance (r=0.54; p<0.02).

Table 3 Effects of Potassium and Magnesium with Hydrochlorothiazide Therapy

Therapy	Dosage	Number of patients	Potassium (mEq/L)	PVCs (bpm)
Hydrochlorothiazide	100 mg	21	-1.1	+4.3
Hydrochlorothiazide and potassium chloride	100 mg/60 mEq	11	-0.8	+2.7
Hydrochlorothiazide and magnesium oxide	100 mg/20 mEq	6	-1.0	+3.5
Hydrochlorothiazide, potassium chloride, and magnesium oxide	100 mg/60 mEq/20 mEq	7	-0.3	+0.7

Study 3

Potassium chloride, magnesium oxide, or both were administered to a group of patients who had received hydrochlorothiazide 100 mg a day for 6 weeks and who developed hypokalemia, hypomagnesemia, and ventricular ectopy during exercise on the treadmill.

Table 3 shows the results of the addition of 60 mEq/day potassium chloride (20% solution) to hydrochlorothiazide therapy. After 6 weeks of therapy with supplemental potassium, a 0.3 mEq/L increase in the serum level was noted. Similarly, little change was seen when 20 mEq/day of magnesium oxide was added to the hydrochlorothiazide therapy. However, the combination of potassium chloride and magnesium oxide significantly altered the hypokalemia, hypomagnesemia, and ventricular arrhythmia.

COMMENTS

Hypertension affects more than 50 million adults in the United States today. The initial treatment commonly recommended for patients with mild to moderate hypertension (diastolic blood pressure 90–119 mmHg) is a thiazide diuretic (11). However, one of the major side effects of thiazide therapy is hypokalemia (6). The Veterans Administration Cooperative Study showed that serum potassium levels between 2.5 and 3.4 mEq/L were sustained over a 2-year period in 23% of patients who were given thiazide diuretic alone or in combination with reserpine and hydralazine (12). Some investigators speculate that this hypokalemia is of little consequence to health. On the other hand, sinus arrythimia, first- or second-degree atrioventricular block, atrial flutter, paroxysmal atrial tachycardia with block, atrioventricular dissociation, and atrial fibrillation have all been observed in patients with hypokalemia alone (14). Brater and Morelli (1) reported a high frequency of arrhythmias in patients with therapeutic digitalis levels, normokalemia, and diuretic-induced alkalosis.

The Veterans Administration Cooperative Study of Mild Hypertension (diastolic blood pressure, 90–114 mmHg) observed that the major cause of death in a group of patients treated with thiazide diuretics was sudden cardiac death (13). In fact, four of eight deaths observed in this study were sudden, an occurrence associated most often with ventricular fibrillation and usually not associated with coronary occlusion. In the multicenter Veterans Administration Cooperative Study of the effect of antihypertensive therapy on stroke recurrence, there were eight unexplained, sudden deaths in the drug-treated group, compared with only four in the placebo-treated group (8). In addition, the effects of antihypertensive therapy on morbidity and mortality in patients with mild hypertension (diastolic blood pressure less than 105 mmHg) are of great interest. Mean serum potassium levels in the treatment group that received a combination of reserpine and chlorthalidone fell by 0.8 mEq/L to a mean of 3.5 mEq/L. In a substantial number of the patients, serum potassium levels were less than 3.5 mEq/L. Many arrhythmias, including frequent supraventricular ectopic beats per minute, bundle branch block, and atrioventricular conduction abnormalities, were observed in the drug-treated group. In contrast, the placebo-treated group had only one incident of an atrioventricular conduction abnormality. Overall, there was a higher incidence of sudden cardiac death in the drug-treated group compared with no sudden deaths in the placebo-treated group. However, this difference is not significant because of the small number of sudden deaths.

The Multiple Risk Factor Intervention Trial study (10) included a group of mildly hypertensive patients with cardiac abnormalities who were treated with regimens that included large dosages of thiazide diuretics. These patients experienced an increased occurrence of sudden cardiac death when compared with patients who were treated less intensively.

On the other hand, Lown et al. (9) showed that in 24% of patients with sudden cardiac death, frank hypokalemia was associated with thiazide diuretic therapy for hypertension. Thus, although there is insignificant evidence from any single study to make a definite conclusion, the data suggest that sudden cardiac death is a major cause of death in hypertensive patients treated with thiazide diuretics; and that when the prominence of sudden cardiac death in the thiazide-treated group is viewed in light of the known effects of potassium deficiency on cardiac rhythm, we must at least question whether the treatment may be contributing to the sudden cardiac death.

Little has been written about the effects of thiazide diuretics on cations other than potassium, although Dyckner and Wester (2) have documented changes in both serum and muscle magnesium during treatment with hydrochlorothiazide and a relationship to ventricular arrhythmias. Our studies were carried out to evaluate the effects of hydrochlorothiazide on serum potassium and magnesium in relation to its ability to lower blood pressure. Hydrochlorothiazide causes a decrease in blood pressure and results in a decrease in the serum potassium and magnesium levels.

Although use of hydrochlorothiazide does produce hypokalemia and hypomagnesemia, this clearly does not answer the question: Do hypokalemia and hypomagnesemia predispose certain persons to malignant arrhythmias? In study 2 we attempted to answer this by studying the effects of exercise on cardiac rhythm in thiazide-treated patients. These studies were performed during treatment with ordinary dosages of hydrochlorothiazide (50 mg/day in 17 patients and 100 mg/day in 21 patients) that produced a modest degree of potassium and magnesium depletion. Nonetheless, an increased frequency of paroxysmal ventricular contractions developed during dynamic exercise compared with the pretreatment studies. The fact that the frequency of these extra systolic beats correlates well with the decrease observed in serum potassium and magnesium from pretreatment and preexercise values suggests a relationship that should be explored further.

Study 3 demonstrated that treatment of the hypokalemic, hypomagnesemic, hypertensive patient with exercise-induced ventricular ectopy can be affected by the combined administration of potassium chloride and magnesium oxide, but not by either of these agents singly. Unfortunately, these agents are unpalatable and cumbersome to take. The use of other agents, such as potassium-sparing diuretics (which also spare magnesium), beta blockers, and angiotension-converting enzyme inhibitors may prove more useful than combinations of minerals in the management of patients who require potassium/magnesium supplementation during thiazide therapy.

Our data demonstrated that thiazides do result in hypokalemia and hypomagnesemia and that thiazide therapy results in ventricular ectopy. There is an inverse correlation between the occurrence of paroxysmal ventricular beats and the level of serum potassium and magnesium, and correction of this arrhythmia requires a combination of both cations. But which thiazide-treated patients require careful attention to their potassium and magnesium level? Certainly, those in whom larger amounts of thiazides are required to achieve successful blood pressure control are prime candidates since there appears to be a dosage-dependent relationship between thiazide diuretics and hypokalemia. Those patients who are taking digitalis, who have ischemic heart disease or left ventricular enlargement, or perhaps even those who show asymptomatic abnormalities on their electrocardiogram should be strongly considered for therapy that prevents (as well as treats) hypokalemia and hypomagnesemia. Finally, while our data show a relationship between thiazide therapy and ventricular ectopy, neither our data nor any other single study clearly demonstrates that the hypertensive patient is predisposed to malignant ventricular arrhythmia and instantaneous death. This hypothesis, while certainly likely, remains to be proven.

SUMMARY

Thiazide diuretics are generally considered to be the cornerstone of antihypertensive therapy and are suggested as the initial step in treatment of uncomplicated essential hypertension. Nonetheless, there are many metabolic consequences of long-term thiazide therapy. Among these, hypokalemia is well known, but the effect of thiazide on serum magnesium is less well known. Thirty-eight patients (22 with low renin, 16 with normal renin levels) with mild to moderate diastolic hypertension were treated with hydrochlorothiazide administered twice a day. The initial daily dosage was 50 mg; this was increased at 4-week intervals to 100 mg, 150 mg, and 200 mg. The increasing dosage schedule was terminated when either blood pressure was normalization or the 200-mg dosage level was reached. Patients were maintained on that maximum dosage of hydrochlorothiazide they received during the dosage escalation phase of the study and continued receiving this dosage for 24 continuous weeks of diuretic monotherapy. The serum potassium level during the control period was 4.5±0.2 mmol/L. During dosage escalation and long-term maintenance therapy, the serum potassium and magnesium levels fell in a stepwise, dosage-dependent fashion. In another study, the effects of hydrochlorothiazide therapy (50 or 100 mg daily) on the occurrence of premature ventricular contractions were observed during both rest and dynamic exercise. During rest, 0.6±0.08 paroxysmal ventricular contractions/min (mean ± SEM) were observed, and during dynamic exercise the rate was 0.8±0.15 paroxysmal ventricular contractions/min. During hydrochlorothiazide therapy (50 or 100 mg per day) paroxysmal ventricular contractions per minute were 1.4 and 5.7, respectively. The occurrence of paroxysmal ventricular contractions correlated significantly with the decrease observed in serum potassium ($r=0.71$, $p<0.001$) and in serum magnesium ($r=0.68$, $p<0.001$). Thiazide therapy appears to cause both potassium and magnesium depletion, and decreases in both correlate well with the appearance of the ventricular ectopic depolarizations.

REFERENCES

1. Brater, D. C., and Morelli, M. N.: Digitalis-induced arrhythmias associated with normokalemia, potassium depletion and alkalosis. *Clin. Res.* 24:253A, 1976.
2. Dyckner, T., and Wester, P. O.: Diuretic treatment and magnesium losses in electrolytes and cardiac arrhythmias. *R. Soc. Med. Int. Sympos. Series*, 145–152, 1981.
3. Harrington, J. T., Isner, J. M., and Kassiener, J. B.: Our national obsession with potassium. *Am. J. Med.* 73:155–159, 1982.
4. Hollifield, J. W., and Slaton, P. E.: A demographic approach to initiating antihypertensive therapy. In *Management Strategies in Hypertensive Therapies*, edited by Weber, M., New York, 1980, pp. 51–57.
5. Hollifield, J. W., and Slaton, P. E.: Thiazide diuretics, hypokalemia and cardiac arrhythmia. *Acta Med. Scand.* 647 (suppl):67–73, 1980.
6. Hollifield, J. W., Slaton, P. E. Jr., and Liddle, G. W.: Some biochemical consequences of diuretic therapy of low renin essential hypertension. Proceedings of the Third Symposium of Hypertension by UCLA, at Boca Raton, 1975. In *Systemic Effects of Antihypertensive Agents,* edited by Sambhi, M. P., New York, Stratton Intercontinental Medical Books, 1976, pp. 131–149.

7. Hollifield, J. W., Slaton, P. E. Jr., and Moore, L. C.: Thiazide diuretics, hypokalemia, and cardiac arrhythmias. In *Electrolytes and the Heart*, edited by Wester, P. O., New York, Transmedica, 1983, pp. 111–119.
8. Hypertension Stroke Cooperative Study Group: Effect of antihypertensive treatment on stroke resurrence. *JAMA* 229:409–418, 1974.
9. Lown, B., et al.: Monitoring for serious arrhythmias and high risk of sudden death. *Circulation* 51, 52 (suppl 3):189–198, 1975.
10. Multiple Risk Factor Intervention Trial Research Group: Multiple risk factor intervention trial: Risk factor changes and mortality results. *JAMA* 248:1465–1477, 1982.
11. U. S. Department of Health, Education and Welfare: Blood pressure of adults as by race and area, U.S. 1960–1962. National Health Survey, National Health Survey, National Center Center of Health Statistics Series 2 (5), 1964.
12. VA Cooperative Study: Effects of treatment on morbidity in hypertension. *JAMA* 202:1028–1034, 1967.
13. VA Cooperative Study: Effects of treatment on morbidity in hypertension. *JAMA* 213:1143–1150, 1970.
14. VA Cooperative Study: Effects of treatment on morbidity in hypertension. *Circulation* 45:991–1004, 1972.

20

Thiazide-Associated Cardiac Arrhythmias: Experience in the General Population

PAUL K. WHELTON
The Johns Hopkins University School of Hygiene and Public Health, The Johns Hopkins University School of Medicine, and The Johns Hopkins Hospital, Baltimore, Maryland

Treatment of high blood pressure is usually a lifelong process. Antihypertensive drug therapy has progressively been advocated for persons with less severe forms of hypertension and thus slighter increases in risk. For this reason, a desire to recognize and prevent adverse effects during therapy is now more appropriate than ever. Indeed, side effects that may not have seemed important when only those with moderate or severe hypertension were being treated are worthy of serious consideration in the present setting where the majority of those being treated in most Western countries have mild hypertension.

Thiazide diuretics are among the most frequently prescribed drugs in clinical practice. Their introduction in the mid-1950s revolutionized the treatment of common disorders such as hypertension and congestive heart failure. A recent survey of physician opinion within the state of Maryland suggests that many U.S. physicians continue to consider thiazides as the drugs of choice during treatment of essential hypertension (1). In this survey 90% of a representative sample of physicians in general/family, internal medicine, and specialty (cardiology, nephrology, and endocrinology) practice recommended thiazides for first-step therapy of essential hypertension. Based on the well-proven effectiveness, favorable hemodynamic profile, and low cost of thiazides this favorable response among practitioners is not surprising.

Despite the undoubted beneficial attributes of thiazides a variety of complications can occur during administration of these agents. Such untoward effects include thiazide-induced symptomatic, biochemical, and electrocardiographic alterations. This chapter will briefly review the potential for symptomatic and biochemical changes during thiazide treatment. Information on the relationship between thiazide administration and cardiac arrhythmias will be reviewed in more detail.

SYMPTOMATIC AND BIOCHEMICAL EFFECTS OF THIAZIDE THERAPY

The largest body of information on symptomatic complaints and reasons for discontinuation of thiazides comes from the Medical Research Council trial of treatment in patients with mild to moderate hypertension (9). Principal reaons for withdrawal from randomized therapy encountered during 23,582 patient years of treatment in men and women are outlined in Table 1. As can be seen, withdrawal from thiazide therapy was almost twice as common in men as in women. Most of this difference was accounted for by the increased frequency of impotence, gout, impaired glucose tolerance, and lethargy in men. The impressive incidence of sexual dysfunction noted during thiazide therapy in men was surprising. However, questionnaire results also documented an increased frequency of impotence in men following 12 weeks and 2 years of diuretic treatment and a similar experience had previously been noted during a smaller Veterans Administration-National Heart, Lung, and Blood Institute study (10). It should be stressed that the overall rate of withdrawal from thiazide treatment in men and women (58.7 and 28.3 per 1,000 patient years, respectively) was low. The corresponding rates per 1,000 patient years encountered during active treatment with propranolol was 44.6 and 63.9 for men and women, respectively.

In addition to the symptomatic effects outlined above a variety of diuretic-induced laboratory abnormalities have been reported. Biochemical changes include hypokalemia, hyperglycemia, hyperuricemia, hypomagnesemia, hypertriglycemidemia, and hypercholesterolemia. The reported prevalence of these abnormalities has varied dramatically depending on (a) the criteria used for case-definition; (b) the type, duration, and dosage of diuretic treatment; (c) the composition of the group being studied; (d) the techniques used for specimen collection and analysis; and (e) whether prevalence is being measured

Table 1 Principal Reasons for Withdrawal From Randomized Therapy During 23,582 Patient Years of Follow-Up in the Medical Research Council Trial of Treatment in Mild to Moderate Hypertension (Expressed as Rates per 1,000 Patient Years of Follow-Up)[a]

	Thiazide		Propranolol		Placebo	
	Men	Women	Men	Women	Men	Women
Years of Follow-up	2,452	2,827	2,738	2,667	6,776	6,122
Reason for withdrawal						
Impotence	19.6	–	5.5	–	0.9	–
Gout	12.2	1.1	2.6	0	1.0	0
Impaired glucose tolerance	9.4	6.0	3.7	1.1	2.5	0.8
Lethargy	6.9	2.1	10.2	15.0	0.3	0.3
Constipation	1.6	2.1	0.4	0	0	0
Dyspnea	0	0	8.0	6.4	0.1	0.3
Raynaud's phenomenon	0	0.3	5.5	5.6	0.1	0
Skin disorder	0.4	0.3	2.2	1.9	0.1	0
Nausea, dizziness, or headache	8.6	16.3	6.6	13.9	1.2	2.1
Total	58.7	28.3	44.6	43.9	6.3	3.8

[a]Thiazides were administered in a fixed dosage as bendrofluazide 5 mg twice daily and propranolol in a variable dosage up to 320 mg per day.
Source: Adapted from Ref. 2.

at one point (point prevalence) or over a period in time (period prevalence). Despite the difficulties in determining exact prevalences, it is clear that diuretic-induced biochemical changes such as hypokalemia and lipid/lipoprotein abnormalities are common problems in clinical practice (16). In addition, mild biochemical abnormalities, however defined, are always far more common than more severe alterations.

ELECTROCARDIOGRAPHIC CHANGES IN HOSPITAL-BASED STUDIES

ST-T wave depression, T wave inversion, and prominent U waves are well-known findings on the resting electrocardiograms of thiazide recipients who develop hypokalemia (2,3,11). Likewise, it has long been known that cardiac arrhythmias may develop in those whose hypokalemia is severe or occurs in the setting of concurrent digitalis administration (11-13). With the advent of more sensitive methods, such as exercise and ambulatory monitoring of the electrocardiogram, it has become possible to study the relationship between thiazide administration and cardiac arrhythmias more carefully. Holland et al. and Hollifield et al. were the first investigators to utilize these techniques in a study setting (4,5). Both groups reported that ventricular ectopy during thiazide therapy was considerably more common than previously recognized. The experience of these two investigators is discussed in more detail in Chapters 18 and 19. Although both provided substantial evidence in favor of a close association between thiazide administration and cardiac arrhythmias, some investigators, including Papademetriou and Freis (whose experience is detailed in Chapter 21) have failed to identify the association.

CARDIAC ARRHYTHMIAS DURING THIAZIDE TREATMENT IN A COMMUNITY-BASED STUDY

The previously mentioned studies detailing the relationship between thiazide administration and cardiac arrhythmias have provided valuable information which greatly increased our fund of knowledge. However, each of these reports was based on results obtained from relatively small and selected hospital-based patient samples. In addition, none provided comparative information from a concurrent placebo control group. The framework of the Medical Research Council (MRC) trial of treatment in mild to moderate hypertension provided an excellent and unusual opportunity to study a relatively large and more representative sample of patients with essential hypertension being treated in general practice. Moreover, since the trial participants were being randomly assigned to placebo or active treatment, one could, with considerable confidence, identify associations between active therapy and an outcome variable such as ventricular ectopy.

During the 9 months between November, 1980, and July, 1981, 324 subjects enrolled in the MRC trial participated in a substudy of ambulatory electrocardiographic patterns during thiazide and placebo treatment. Of these, 110 trial participants were studied before and approximately 10 weeks after random assignment to placebo or to potassium-chloride-supplemented or unsupplemented thiazide therapy. A second group of 194 participants were studied approximately 2 years after random assignment to placebo (n=99) or unsupplemented thiazide (n=95) treatment. The remaining 20 patients were a selected group of hypokalemic (serum potassium $\leqslant$ 2.7 mEq/L) participants who had been treated with unsupplemented thiazide for an average of almost 4 years. Ambulatory monitoring of the electrocardiogram (ECG) was performed with a small, easily portable, frequency-modulated recorder (Medilog II, Oxford Instruments). Both direct visual and semiautomatic (performed by Hertford Medical Ltd. using Reynold's Medical Pathfinder System) forms of analysis were used to interpret the ambulatory ECG records (8). Detailed results of both forms of analysis have previously been published (14,15).

Results Following Short-Term Treatment

Short-term (approximately 10 weeks) thiazide treatment was associated with an overall reduction in serum potassium and increase in serum urate levels. As indicated in Table 2, the average reduction in serum potassium was less for those receiving potassium chloride supplementation (0.3 mEq/L) than for persons not receiving supplements (0.6 mEq/L). Although the number of paired observations available for analysis was small (n=16), the frequency of ventricular ectopic beats appeared to be unaffected by short-term treatment with unsupplemented thiazide. However, there was a statistically significant ($p<0.05$) reduction in ventricular ectopy following potassium-supplemented thiazide therapy. Indeed, the posttreatment rate of ventricular ectopy was reduced in each of the nine potassium-supplemented participants with ventricular ectopic beats before treatment.

Results During Chronic Treatment

The 194 unselected trial participants studied during chronic therapy had been on a stable regimen of either placebo or unsupplemented bendrofluazide given in a dosage of 5 mg twice daily. As expected, the thiazide takers had a significantly lower level of serum potassium ($p<0.001$) and higher level of serum urate ($p<0.001$) than those observed in the placebo group. Of greater importance, there were impressive differences in the rate of ventricular ectopy in each group. With either form of ECG interpretation, ventricular ectopic beats were significantly more common during thiazide treatment. For instance, 34% of the thiazide group as opposed to only 21% of their placebo counterparts had 100 or more ventricular ectopic beats per 100,000 beats during semiautomatic analysis of the ECG (Table 3). In addition, the thiazide group had a significantly ($p<0.006$) higher overall prevalence (38% vs. 14%) of special forms of ventricular ectopy such as multifocal beats, R on T beats, bigeminy, and couplets during the direct visual interpretation (Table 4).

All of the patients selected for study on the basis of previously recognized hypokalemia had been treated with bendrofluazide (5 mg twice daily) for a minimum of 2 years (mean ± SEM = 45 ± 5 months). As expected, each member of the group was hypokalemic (serum potassium ≤3.6 mEq/L) at the time of the electrocardiographic substudy and the average serum potassium level for the group was 2.7 mEq/L. In keeping with the previously mentioned findings in the unselected bendrofluazide takers, there was a high prevalence of ventricular ectopy in the hypokalemic group (Table 5). For instance, on semiautomated analysis 44% had more than 100 ventricular ectopic beats per 100,000 beats and on direct visual analysis 45% had one or more of the previously mentioned special forms of ventricular ectopy.

Sixteen of the hypokalemic patients were restudied after a 5-week interval. Between the first and second studies each continued receiving bendrofluazide 5 mg twice daily but 8 of the 16 were randomly assigned to receive supplemental oral potassium in a dosage of 48 mEq/day. By the time of the second study the supplemented group had increased their serum potassium (mean ± SEM) by 0.7 ± 0.1 mEq/L but in this small study there was little evidence of a decrease in the rate of ventricular ectopic beats in the supplemented group.

Table 2 Serum Potassium, Serum Urate, and Ambulatory Electrocardiographic Results in 73 Medical Research Council Trial Participants With Technically Satisfactory Studies Before and Approximately 10 Weeks After Treatment With Placebo, Thiazide, or a Thiazide–Potassium Chloride Combination[a]

	Placebo group		Unsupplemented thiazide group		Potassium-supplemented thiazide group	
	Before	After	Before	After	Before	After
No. of participants	38	38	16	16	19	19
Serum potassium (SD), mEq/L	4.1 (0.3)	4.0 (0.3)	4.2 (0.4)	3.6 (0.3)	4.2 (0.6)	3.9 (0.5)
Serum urate (SD), mg/dl	6.1 (1.2)	6.0 (1.1)	6.0 (1.0)	7.2 (1.4)	6.1 (1.1)	6.9 (1.5)
% with ventricular ectopic beats/100,000 beats						
<10	63	71	69	63	53	74
10–99	21	18	13	19	16	21
100–999	13	8	13	13	21	5
⩾1000	3	3	6	6	10	0

[a]Participants in the thiazide groups received 5 or 10 mg bendrofluazide with or without 16.8 or 33.6 mEq potassium chloride per day.

Source: Adapted from Ref. 14.

Table 3 Semiautomatic Analysis of 24-hr Ambulatory Electrocardiographic Monitoring in 155 MRC Trial Participants with Technically Satisfactory Studies During Chronic Placebo and Thiazide Treatment[a]

	Placebo group	Thiazide group
No. of participants	81	74
Serum potassium (SD), mEq/L	4.1 (0.3)	3.6 (0.4)
Serum urate (SD), mg/dl	5.5 (1.1)	7.0 (1.5)
% with ventricular ectopic beats/100,000 beats		
<10	58	39
10–99	21	27
100–999	15	19
⩾1000	6	15

[a]Participants in the thiazide group were treated with unsupplemented bendrofluazide in a dosage of 5 mg twice daily.

Source: Adapted from Ref. 14.

Table 4 Direct Visual Interpretation of a Standard Daytime (5 p.m. to 6 p.m.) and Nighttime (5 a.m. to 6 a.m.) Hour of Ambulatory Electrocardiographic Monitoring in 164 Trial Participants Studied During Chronic Placebo and Thiazide Treatment

	Placebo group		Thiazide group	
No. of participants	82		82	
Months in trial (SD)	24 (9.0)		24 (9.0)	
Serum potassium (SD), mEq/L	4.1 (0.4)		3.6 (0.5)	
Serum urate (SD), mg/dl	5.4 (1.2)		7.1 (1.9)	
	Day	Night	Day	Night
% with daytime (D) or nighttime (N) ventricular ectopic beats				
0–4	80	90	68	77
5–9	4	2	10	8
⩾10	16	7	22	15
	Day or night		Day or night	
% with special forms of ventricular ectopy				
Multifocal beats	10		17	
R on T beats	1		9	
Bigeminy	1		7	
Couplets	2		5	

Source: Adapted from Ref. 15.

Table 5 Electrocardiographic Findings in Hypokalemic Patients Studied During Chronic Thiazide Treatment

Semiautomated 24-hr analysis (n=16)		Direct visual 1-hr analysis (n=17)				
Ventricular ectopic beats per 100,000 beats	% of group	Ventricular ectopic beats per hr	% of group: Day	% of group: Night	Special forms of ventricular ectopy	% of group: Day or night
<10	43	0–4	55	80	Multifocal	35
10–99	13	5–9	5	5	R on T	10
100–999	25	$\geqslant 10$	40	15	Bigeminy	5
$\geqslant 1000$	19				Couplets	15

Source: Adapted from Refs. 14, 15.

Relationships Between Ventricular Ectopy and Other Study Variables

No significant ($p<0.05$) relationships were noted between the frequency of ventricular ectopic beats and other study variables during subgroup analysis. Examination of pooled data identified several statistically significant associations. The relationship between serum potassium and ventricular ectopy was highly significant ($p=0.003$ for the semi-automatic analysis). However, on the basis of the results from either form of ECG analysis, less than 4% of the variance in ventricular ectopy could be accounted for by differences in the value of serum potassium. During multivariate analysis the partial correlation coefficients between ventricular ectopy and serum potassium (−0.158) and serum urate (0.154) were quite similar.

IMPORTANCE OF HYPOKALEMIA IN THIAZIDE-INDUCED CARDIAC ARRHYTHMIAS

Although a considerable body of evidence supports the proposal that cardiac arrhythmias occasionally occur as a result of thiazide treatment, the role of hypokalemia in this relationship is less well defined. Ventricular ectopy is a recognized complication of severe hypokalemia. Indeed, "torsade de pointe" is a form of ventricular tachycardia classically seen in patients with severe hypokalemia and hypomagnesemia (7). However, severe hypokalemia is the exception rather than the rule during diuretic administration. Hypokalemia, even when mild, is a well-known precipitant of cardiac arrhythmias in patients who are also receiving digitalis therapy (12,13). However, concurrent digitalis therapy is also the exception rather than the rule during diuretic treatment.

Holland et al. reported an impressive relationship between the presence of hypokalemia and thiazide-associated cardiac arrhythmias. However, the group of patients studied had been chosen on the basis of previously recognized hypokalemia and so the likelihood of identifying an association between a diuretic-induced outcome variable such as cardiac arrhythmias and hypokalemia was increased. Hollifield et al. reported a strong relationship between diuretic-related cardiac arrhythmias and hypokalemia as well as hypomagnesemia. Both groups reported an impressive reduction in the frequency of diuretic-associated ventricular ectopy following short-term administration of potassium-sparing agents.

In contrast with the previously mentioned findings, the relationship between diuretic-induced cardiac arrhythmias and hypokalemia was less impressive in the MRC substudy. No associations between ventricular ectopy and the absolute value of, or changes in, serum potassium were noted in any of the subgroups studied. Examination of pooled data revealed a highly significant association between absolute values in serum potassium and the rate of ventricular ectopy, but differences in the level of serum potassium accounted for little of the variance in cardiac arrhythmia frequency. The rate of ventricular ectopy appeared to be diminished by potassium supplementation during short-term treatment but no such effect was noted during therapy of the chronically hypokalemic subjects. The power to recognize a beneficial effect of potassium supplementation in the hypokalemic participants was limited since the number of subjects available for study was small. It must also be stated that the impressive degree of day-to-day variability known to exist for measurements of both serum potassium and cardiac arrhythmias tends to ensure that any true biological association between diuretic-induced hypokalemia and ventricular ectopy will be underestimated. Last, but not least, it must be recognized that the changes that occur in potassium metabolism during diuretic administration are complex. Thus, alterations in intraskeletal muscle and, to an even greater extent intracardiac muscle, potassium content are not clearly related to changes in serum potassium levels. In addition, the ability of potassium to enter cells is influenced by a variety of factors including some, such as the level of magnesium, acid-base balance, and adrenergic activity, which are affected by diuretic administration as well.

THERAPEUTIC IMPLICATIONS

The belief that diuretic-induced ventricular ectopy may occasionally take the form of ventricular tachycardia, ventricular fibrillation, and sudden death is controversial and commentary on the subject is often emotionally charged. Any such discussion must be deliberated in a context in which the overwhelming body of epidemiological and clinical trial experience suggests an overall benefit for antihypertensive treatment with thiazide diuretics. Likewise it must be recognized that the evidence linking diuretic administration to sudden death is circumstantial and inconclusive. Despite the indecisive nature of the evidence, the available data are substantial enough to warrant some caution on the part of the therapist (17), especially when caring for older men, patients with known electrocardiographic abnormalities, and those who are being treated concurrently with digitalis.

Diuretics should be administered at the lowest dosage necessary to achieve the desired reduction in blood pressure (6). In addition, simple recommendations such as a reduction in dietary salt and saturated fat intake may help to reduce the likelihood of diuretic-induced hypokalemia and hypercholesterolemia. As discussed in Chapters 34 and 35, diuretic-induced hypokalemia can also be treated or prevented by concurrent administration of potassium supplements or potassium-sparing agents. The latter appear to spare magnesium as well as potassium (see Chapter 2) and are the agents most frequently reported to decrease the prevalence of diuretic-associated ventricular ectopic beats. Concurrent therapy with antihypertensive agents which interfere with the renin-angiotensin system or the andrenergic beta 2 receptor-mediated capability to shift potassium intracellularly provides an alternative to potassium sparing which may be appropriate in selected instances. For instance, nonselective beta blockers such as propranolol have been reported to increase serum potassium levels by 0.2-0.5 mEq/L. Converting enzyme inhibitors such as captopril are even more potent potassium sparing agents. Last, but not least, monotherapy with nondiuretic agents should be considered. None of the nondiuretic approaches represents a panacea as each is known to be a potential cause of undesirable symptoms and/or laboratory abnormalities. Moreover, none has been evaluated as carefully as diuretics for the possibility of side effects.

SUMMARY

Little doubt exists as to the overall benefit of antihypertensive treatment with thiazide diuretics. However, a number of symptomatic, biochemical, and electrocardiographic alterations can occur during thiazide administration. Hypokalemic changes on the resting electrocardiogram such as an increased rate of ventricular ectopic beats during concurrent digitalis administration and the occurrence of ST-T wave depression, T wave inversion, and prominent U waves are well-known findings. Recent studies employing exercise and ambulatory monitoring of the electrocardiogram have suggested that diuretic-induced ventricular ectopy may be far more common than was previously recognized. Findings in the ambulatory electrocardiographic monitoring substudy of the MRC trial suggest that diuretic-induced ventricular ectopy is relatively common even in "low-risk" patients with essential hypertension being treated in the general community. The mechanism by which thiazide diuretics induce ventricular ectopy is less certain and may be complex. However, it seems likely that hypokalemia plays a role. For this and other reasons, therapists should take precautions to prevent or, if necessary, treat hypokalemia during the administration of thiazide diuretics. This is especially true in subgroups of the population who are at greatest risk for the arrhythmiagenic complications of thiazide diuretics.

ACKNOWLEDGMENTS

Supported in part by grants from the Outpatient Department Clinical Research Center (RR00722) and the Milbank Memorial Fund. Computing performed on The Johns Hopkins Clinical Research Center CLINFO computer system.

REFERENCES

1. Cloher, T. P., and Whelton, P. K.: Physician approach to the recognition and initial management of hypertension: Results of a statewide survey of Maryland physicians. *Arch. Intern. Med.* (in press).
2. Davidson, S., and Surawicz, B.: Ectopic beats and atrioventricular conduction disturbances in patients with hypopotassemia. *Arch. Intern. Med.* 120:280–285, 1967.
3. Fisch, C., Knoebel, S. B., Feigenbaum, H., and Greenspan, K.: Potassium and the monophasic action potential, electrocardiogram, conduction and arrhythmias. *Prog. Cardiovasc. Dis.* 8:387–418, 1966.
4. Holland, O. B., Nixon, J. V., and Kuhnert, L.: Diuretic-induced ventricular ectopic activity. *Am. J. Med.* 70:762–768, 1981.
5. Hollifield, J. W., and Slaton, P. E.: Thiazide diuretics, hypokalemia and cardiac arrhythmias. *Acta Med. Scand. (Suppl)* 647:67–73, 1981.
6. Joint National Committee on Detection, Evaluation, and Treatment of High Blood Pressure: The 1984 Report of The Joint National Committee on Detection, Evaluation, and Treatment of High Blood Pressure. *Arch. Intern. Med.* 144:1045–1057, 1984.
7. Kellman, K., and Singh, B. N.: Serum electrolytes and the heart. In *Clinical Disorders of Fluid and Electrolyte Metabolism* (3rd ed.), edited by Maxwell, M. H., and Kleeman, C. R., New York, McGraw-Hill, 1980, pp. 145–180.
8. McLeod, A., Kitson, D., McComish, M., and Jewitt, D.: Role of ambulatory electrocardiographic monitoring: Accuracy of quantitative analysis system. *Br. Heart J.* 39:347, 1977.
9. Medical Research Council Working Party on Mild to Moderate Hypertension: Adverse reactions to bendrofluazide and propranolol for the treatment of mild hypertension. *Lancet* 2:539–543, 1981.
10. Perry, H. M., Goldman, A. I., Lavin, M. A., Schnaper, H. W., Fitz, A. E., Frohlich, E. D., Steele, B., and Richman, H. G.: Evaluation of drug treatment in mild hypertension: VA-NHLBI Feasibility Trial. *Ann. NY Acad. Sci.* 304:267–292, 1978.
11. Surawicz, B., Braun, H. A., Crum, W. B., Kemp, R. L., Wagner, S., and Bellet, S.: Quantitative analysis of the electrocardiographic pattern of hypopotassemia. *Circulation* 16:750–763, 1957.
12. Steiness, E., and Oleson, K. H.: Cardiac arrhythmias induced by hypokalemia and potassium loss during maintenance digoxin therapy. *Br. Heart J.* 38:167–172, 1976.

13. Steiness, E.: Diuretics, digitalis and arrhythmias. *Acta Med. Scan.* 647 (Suppl):75–78, 1981.
14. Whelton, P. K., Brennan, P. J., Greenberg, G., Miall, W. E., Raftery, E. B., and Subramanian, B., for The Medical Research Council Working Party on Mild to Moderate Hypertension: Ventricular extrasystoles during thiazide treatment: Sub-study of MRC mild hypertension trial. *Br. Med. J.* 287:1249–1253, 1983.
15. Whelton, P. K.: Diuretics and arrhythmias in the Medical Research Council Trial. *Drugs* 28(Suppl 1):54–65, 1984.
16. Whelton, P. K.: Thiazide induced hypokalemia—an epidemiologic prospective. In *Electrolytes and the Heart,* edited by Wester Per, O., New York, Transmedica, 1983, pp. 77–81.
17. Whelton, P. K.: Systemic hypertension, diuretic drugs, arrhythmias and death. *Am. J. Cardiol.* 55:221–222, 1985.

21

Diuretic-Induced Hypokalemia and Cardiac Arrhythmias: Effect of Potassium Repletion

VASILIOS PAPADEMETRIOU and EDWARD D. FREIS
Veterans Administration Medical Center and Georgetown University School of Medicine, Washington, D.C.

Diuretic compounds have been widely used in the management of systemic hypertension for more than 25 years. However, certain side effects of diuretics (mostly biochemical) have recently become subjects of concern. Although there is some concern about side effects such as hyperuricemia, hyperglycemia, or increase in cholesterol, hypokalemia concerns the practicing physician the most.

Fears that mild to moderate hypokalemia may impair renal function, decrease intestinal mobility, or, most importantly, aggravate cardiac arrhythmias, led to the widespread use of potassium salts or potassium-sparing diuretics. As will be shown, these concerns are not based on convincing evidence.

Despite the lack of evidence, however, that mild to moderate hypokalemia due to diuretic therapy is harmful to the patient with benign essential hypertension, hundreds of millions of dollars are spent annually for potassium supplements or potassium-sparing diuretics and thousands of patients have to cope daily with the inconveniences associated with the consumption of these compounds.

Several published studies indicated that routine administration of potassium supplements or potassium-sparing diuretics not only may be unnecessary (7,9,23,48) but also may even be dangerous (26). Lawson (26) found that among 4,900 hospitalized patients treated with diuretics and potassium supplements, 176 developed hyperkalemia which was fatal in 7 and life-threatening in 21 others. Harrington et al. (21) in a recent review of the literature, concluded that there is no convincing evidence that fatal arrhythmic activity results from thiazide-induced hypokalemia per se.

This chapter will discuss the following aspects of diuretic-induced hypokalemia in patients with essential hypertension: (a) potassium loss with thiazide diuretics, (b) cardiac arrhythmias in diuretic-induced hypokalemia, and (c) the effect of potassium supplements on cardiac arrhythmias.

POTASSIUM LOSSES WITH THIAZIDE DIURETICS

Hypokalemia, defined as plasma potassium concentration below 3.5 mEq/L, occurs in 20 to 40% of patients with systemic hypertension treated with diuretics (19,46). Although the degree of plasma potassium reduction depends on the dosage and the duration of action of the diuretic, severe hypokalemia with conventionally used diuretics is encountered only rarely (23,38).

Whether a decrease in plasma potassium reflects a significant change in total body potassium stores is questionable. Although Edmonds and Jasani (13) found a significant decrease in total body potassium with diuretic therapy most investigators found minimal or no change in total body potassium stores with long-term diuretic therapy (7,9,28,48). In addition, when potassium supplements were added to diuretic therapy, they failed to increase total body potassium stores (9,28).

While diuretic treatment results initially in an increased loss of potassium in the urine (18,33), the excess kaliuresis is transient and prolonged losses resulting in biologically significant potassium depletion do not occur with the use of thiazides alone. Although numerous studies examining the effects of diuretic therapy on plasma and total body potassium have been published, data from patients who develop overt hypokalemia on diuretics are scarce. Therefore, studies were conducted in our laboratory to assess potassium changes with diuretic therapy in 11 patients known to develop significant hypokalemia with the use of diuretics.

Diuretic therapy was discontinued for an adequate period of time to allow blood pressure and plasma potassium to return to pretreatment levels. Baseline data were then obtained, including plasma and 24-hr urinary electrolyte levels. Hydrochlorothiazide 50 mg twice daily was then begun and the patients were seen on days 1, 3, 7, 14, and 28 of diuretic therapy. Plasma and 24-hr urinary electrolyte levels were measured at each visit. The average (± SEM) baseline plasma potassium was 3.9 ± 0.1 mEq/L and 24-hr urinary potassium was 58 ± 7 mEq (Table 1). Following hydrochlorothiazide treatment, the plasma potassium decreased significantly within 24 hr. By day 3 the decrease from baseline was 1.0 mEq/L and stabilized thereafter. The 24-hr urinary excretion of potassium increased by an average of 26 mEq in the first 24 hr, 41 mEq by day 3, and returned to baseline by day 14. The estimated cumulative loss of potassium did not exceed 300 mEq. Since the total body potassium is approximately 4,000 mEq (1) this loss represents only 7% of the total body potassium, which is biologically insignificant. From these data and data from other studies it becomes apparent that in patients with thiazide-induced hypokalemia there is a relatively greater decrease in extracellular potassium than intracellular potassium.

An average decrease of 1 mEq/L in plasma potassium represents a reduction of 25% in extracellular potassium while an average loss of 300 mEq/L represents a decrease of only

Table 1 Mean (±SEM) Plasma and Urinary Potassium Changes with Hydrochlorothiazide

	Baseline	Changes from baseline				
		Day 1	Day 3	Day 7	Day 14	Day 28
PK (mEq/L)	3.9±0.1	-0.4±0.1[a]	-1.0±0.2[a]	-1.1±0.1[a]	-1.0±0.1[a]	-1.0±0.1[a]
UK (mEq/24hr)	58±7	26±8[a]	41±8[a]	27±14	5±5	6±8

PK, plasma potassium; UK, urinary potassium.
[a]$p < 0.01$.

7% of intracellular potassium. The unequal losses probably are the result of the following influences. First, the sodium potassium pump on the cell membrane that is responsible for the maintenance of much higher intracellular than extracellular potassium concentrations maintains control and prevents diffusion of potassium from the intracellular space despite the decrease in the extracellular concentration. Second, diuretics induce volume contraction and mild metabolic alkalosis that favor the shift of extracellular potassium intracellularly.

VENTRICULAR ARRHYTHMIAS IN DIURETIC-INDUCED HYPOKALEMIA

Following the introduction and wide use of diuretics in the late 1950s and early 1960s it was recognized that diuretic-related hypokalemia increased cardiac arrhythmias in patients taking digitalis. This association was later well documented (16,17,31) and is now widely accepted.

An association, however, between hypokalemia and cardiac arrhythmias in patients with hypertension uncomplicated by heart disease who are not receiving digitalis has not been documented. Although numerous studies have been published on the subject (2,6,8, 14,25,45,47) severe shortcomings in the design of most of them limit their value. Harrington and co-workers (21), in their review of the pertinent literature, pointed out explicitly the limitations of these studies. In brief, most studies failed to establish a firm relationship between the level of serum potassium and the observation of ventricular arrhythmias. In some studies (25,47) ventricular ectopy was only observed retrospectively on random electrocardiograms and was related to any potassium value obtained within 24 hr of the tracing. The study most often quoted as establishing an association between diuretic-induced hypokalemia and ventricular ectopic activity is that by Holland et al. (22). Although in some respects the design of this study was adequate, it also had serious limitations.

As previously indicated (40) the most important problems of this study are the following. All patients with any baseline arrhythmias were excluded from the study. Therefore, because of the wide spontaneous fluctuation in day-to-day arrhythmic activity a second ambulatory electrocardiographic (ECG) monitoring during hypokalemia was likely to show increased ectopy, simply on the basis of spontaneous variation. Of the 21 patients included in the study only the 7 who developed more than minimal ventricular ectopic activity during hypokalemia were remonitored after receiving spironolactone. Once again, the possibility of observing more ectopy after correcting hypokalemia, due to spontaneous variability (37,39), in the remaining 14 patients, could not be excluded. Finally, hydrochlorothiazide was either decreased in dosage or discontinued in the seven patients who received spironolactone for potassium repletion.

In our laboratory, therefore, further studies were conducted to determine the relationship between diuretic-induced hypokalemia and cardiac arrhythmias. Eighteen patients with systemic hypertension uncomplicated by heart or renal disease were included in the study. These patients were known to develop hypokalemia with diuretic therapy. Initially, all medications including the diuretic were discontinued for at least 3 weeks to allow blood pressure and plasma potassium to return to pretreatment levels. Forty-eight-hour ambulatory ECG monitoring was performed at baseline and after 4 weeks of treatment with hydrochlorothiazide (HCTZ) 100 mg daily. Plasma potassium was measured at the beginning and at the end of each 48-hr monitoring and the average of the two represented the plasma potassium at each phase.

Table 2 Findings in 18 Patients with Hypokalemia on Hydrochlorothiazide (HCTZ)

	Baseline	HCTZ	Change	P Value
PK (mEq/L)	4.03 ± 0.06[a]	3.06 ± 0.07	0.97	< 0.001
BW (kg)	92.9 ± 4.1	91.5 ± 4.1	1.4	< 0.01
PCVs (/hr)	6.9 ± 2.7	6.4 ± 4.0	–	NS
Couplets (total)	29	10	–	NS
VT (no. of episodes)	1 (4)[b]	0	–	NS
AV Grade/hr	0.78 ± 0.18	0.70 ± 0.18	–	NS

[a]Mean ± SEM
[b]Number of consecutive premature contractions.
PK, plasma potassium; BW body weight; PVC, premature ventricular contractions; VT, ventricular tachycardia.

As shown in Table 2, the baseline plasma potassium level was 4.03 mEq/dl and decreased to 3.07 with hydrochlorothiazide treatment ($p<0.001$). The average number of premature ventricular contractions was 6.9 ± 2.7/hr at baseline and 6.4 ± 4.0/hr (p=NS) following hydrochlorothiazide. The total number of couplets in all patients was 29 at baseline and 10 after hydrochlorothiazide. One four-beat run of ventricular tachycardia occurred at baseline but not after the diuretic. The average grade, which is an index of severity and frequency of ectopy (32,41) was also decreased from 0.78 ± 0.18/hr at baseline to 0.70 ± 0.18/hr after diuretic therapy. When patients' results were tabulated according to their highest grade of arrhythmias (32) nine patients had more than minimal (grade 2 or more; Table 3) ventricular ectopic activity at baseline, while only six patients had more than minimal ventricular ectopic activity following hydrochlorothiazide treatment (Table 3). The results indicate that in these patients even overt hypokalemia did not result in increased ventricular ectopic activity. In fact, there was a trend towards decreased ectopic activity following diuretic administration and hypokalemia although this activity did not reach the level of significance.

Similar results have been published by Lief and co-workers in an abstract (29). They performed 48-hr ambulatory ECG monitoring in 13 patients with uncomplicated hypertension before and after treatment with hydrochlorothiazide. Mean (±SEM) plasma potassium levels decreased from 4.0 ± 0.1 mEq/L to 3.0 ± 0.1 mEq/L, but no change in ventricular ectopic activity was noted between the two phases.

Although the results of the Medical Research Council's mild hypertension trial (35) will be discussed elsewhere, a brief comment is relevant here. In this trial the relationship between ventricular extrasystoles and thiazide treatment was studied in two groups of

Table 3 18 Patients with Hypokalemia Taking Hydrochlorothiazide: Highest Grade of Arrhythmias

	Arrhythmia grade					
	0 (No PVC)	1 (≤29/hr)	2 (≥30/hr)	3 (mult.)	4 (couplets)	5 (VT)
Baseline	4	5	2	5	1	1
HCTZ	2	10	0	2	4	0

PVC, premature ventricular contractions; mult, multifocal; VT, ventricular tachycardia.

patients, those assigned to the short-term study and those assigned to the long term study. In the short term study 110 patients were randomly assigned to one of three groups, to receive placebo, bendrofluazide, alone or bendrofluazide with potassium supplements. Twenty-four-hour ambulatory electrocardiographic monitoring was performed before treatment and 9–10 weeks later while the patients were still taking their assigned treatment. Although serum potassium level was decreased after thiazide therapy, no significant increase in the number of ventricular extrasystoles was noted.

The long-term study included patients who have been treated with either bendrofluazide or placebo for an average of 2 years. Twenty-four-hour ambulatory electrocardiographic monitoring was conducted in 74 patients receiving thiazide therapy and in 81 patients receiving placebo. Although counts of ventricular extrasystoles were significantly higher in the patients receiving thiazide treatment than in those receiving placebo, there was no correlation between the number of ventricular extrasystoles and serum potassium level in the treated group. However, there was a significant correlation with the serum uric acid concentration. Therefore, it appears justified to conclude that the results of our studies and data available in the literature do not disclose any evidence that diuretic-related hypokalemia causes cardiac arrhythmias.

EFFECTS OF POTASSIUM SUPPLEMENTS ON CARDIAC ARRHYTHMIAS

The potential association between diuretic-induced hypokalemia and cardiac arrhytymias was also studied using a different approach. Studies were conducted to assess the effects of potassium repletion on cardiac arrhythmias in diuretic treated hypokalemic patients. Holland and co-workers (22) performed 24-hr ambulatory ECG monitoring during hypokalemia induced by diuretics and following normalization of plasma potassium using spironolactone. They noted a significant decrease in ventricular ectopic activity following potassium repletion. However, as indicated above, the method of selecting subjects made the result of questionable significance. In the MRC trial (35) in the short-term group 19 patients were monitored prior to bendrofluazide therapy and after 9-10 weeks of treatment with bendrofluazide plus potassium supplements. A significant decrease in ventricular extrasystolic counts was noted during combined treatment with potassium supplements despite a concurrent decrease in the group's mean serum potassium level, from 4.2 to 3.9 mEq/L. Therefore, a correlation between the improvement and plasma potassium levels was not established.

Studies to assess the effectiveness of potassium replacement in controlling cardiac arrhythmias in diuretic-treated hypokalemic patients, were also conducted in our laboratory (40). Sixteen patients with essential hypertension uncomplicated by heart disease who were known to develop overt hypokalemia with diuretic therapy were studied. All patients required potassium supplements or a potassium-sparing diuretic to maintain near-normal serum potassium levels before the study. Potassium supplements or the potassium sparing diuretic were discontinued in all patients. Antihypertensive therapy, including a diuretic, was continued and patients were seen every 2 weeks until plasma potassium level was reduced to < 3.2 mEq/L. Once hypokalemia was confirmed, 24-hr ambulatory ECG monitoring was performed and the patients were given potassium supplements. Hypokalemia was corrected to < 3.5 mEq/L and at least 0.5 mEq/L higher than the unsupplemented value using potassium chloride, triamterene, or a combination of the two. Thereafter, 24-hr ambulatory ECG monitoring was repeated. The antihypertensive therapy

Table 4 Average Number of Hours Each Group of Arrhythmias Was Observed During 24-hr ECG Monitoring

VEA	Hypokalemic phase	K Repletion phase
O	17.31 ± 1.62	14.06 ± 2.05
Unifocal PVC 1-9/hr	3.75 ± 0.87	4.50 ± 1.33
Unifocal PVCs ⩾10/hr	0.13 ± 0.09	0.50 ± 0.33
Multifocal PVCs 1-9/hr	1.19 ± 0.44	1.75 ± 0.58
Multifocal PVCs ⩾10/hr	1.38 ± 1.13	2.00 ± 1.39
Couplets	0.25 ± 0.25	0.63 ± 0.24
VT	0	0

Values are mean ± SEM.
K, potassium; PVC, premature ventricular contractions; VEA, ventricular ectopic activity; VT, ventricular tachycardia.

remained unchanged throughout the study. Arrhythmias noted on the 24-hr ECG monitoring were classified in the following groupings: unifocal PVCs 1-9/hr, >10/hr, multifocal PVCs 1-9/hr, >10/hr, couplets or runs of ventricular tachycardia.

Following potassium repletion, ventricular ectopic activity improved in 5 patients and worsened in 10. No change was observed in one patient. Although not significant, there was a trend towards more complex arrhythmias after correction of hypokalemia (Table 4). Multifocal premature ventricular contractions or couplets were present in six patients during hypokalemia and in 10 patients following correction of hypokalemia

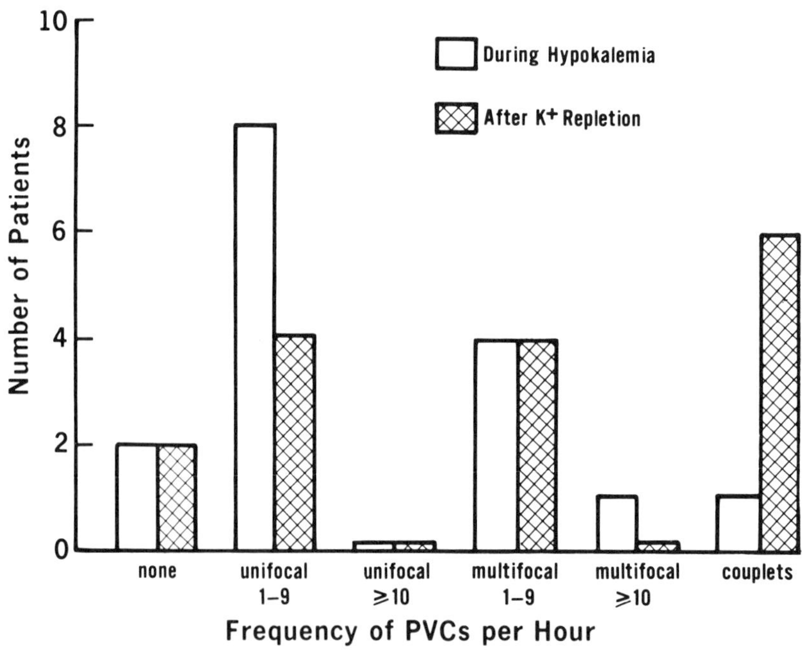

Figure 1 Distribution of patients according to the most severe or complex type of ventricular arrhythmia during hypokalemia and after plasma potassium (K) correction. Changes are not statistically significant. PVCs, premature ventricular contractions.

(Figure 1). It is clear from the results of this study that neither the frequency nor the complexity of ventricular arrhythmias decreased after correction of hypokalemia and that the most probable explanation for this observation was that there was no casual association between the observed arrhythmias and hypokalemia.

Ventricular arrhythmias occur in apparently normal individuals without cardiovascular disease. Brodsky (4) and co-workers found that one-half of 50 healthy medical students with normal findings on electrocardiograms exhibited premature ventricular contractions on ambulatory electrocardiographic monitoring. One medical student even had couplets and another had a brief episode of ventricular tachycardia. Clarke et al. (5) found ventricular ectopy on 63 of 86 normal subjects. Thirteen subjects had multiform premature ventricular contractions, three had bigeminy, two had R on T phenomenon, and two eshibited episodes of ventricular tachycardia.

Dyckner and Wester (10–12) reported that correction of hypokalemia did not result in an improvement in either the frequency or the type of ventricular arrhythmias. These authors implicated magnesium depletion for the lack of response. In our studies, however, plasma magnesium levels were within the normal range both before and after correction of hypokalemia. Other investigators (15) believe that magnesium depletion can only induce arrhythmias at concentrations that are unphysiological and even incompatible with life.

ELECTROPHYSIOLOGICAL CONSIDERATIONS

Although a great deal has been published about the association of hypokalemia and cardiac arrhythmias, no satisfactory physiological explanation has been proposed. It has simply been assumed that a decrease in serum potassium levels would cause electrical instability and induction of cardiac arrhythmias. However, our present knowledge of electrophysiological mechansisms indicates that less rather than more electrical instability would result from diuretic-induced hypokalemia. The role of potassium concentration on myocardial arrhythmogenicity is probably best defined by its effect on resting membrane potential (RMP).

The Goldman equation defines the dependence of RMP on intracellular and extracellular ion concentrations (20). Although other ions such as calcium, sodium, or magnesium are playing a role, under clinical conditions the RMP is primarily determined by the concentration gradient for potassium across the cell membrane (1). The equation therefore can be validly simplified as follows:

$$\text{RMP} = -65.5 \log \frac{\text{intracellular potassium}}{\text{extracellular potassium}}$$

From this equation it becomes clear that relatively greater decrease in intracellular potassium compared to extracellular potassium will result in a less negative RMP, with a consequent increase in automaticity. This effect on the RMP also results in a decreased rate of rise and diminished amplitude of the action potential with consequent slowing of conduction throughout the heart. The latter effect may result in partial blocks and promote reentrant circuits. The opposite is true with relatively greater decrease in extracellular than intracellular potassium concentrations. The RMP will become more negative, automaticity will diminish, and reentrant arrhythmias should be less likely to appear.

The impression that hypokalemia per se is arrhythmogenic was originally derived from observations made in hypokalemic patients taking digitalis. The electrophysiological

Table 5 Changes in Total Body (TBK) and Plasma Potassium Level (PK) with Diuretics: Summary of Literature

	TBK	PK
Baseline	4,000 mEq	4.0 mEq/L
Change with diuretics	200–300 mEq	0.6–1.0 mEq/L
Percentage change	5–7.5	15–25

Source: Data from Refs. 7, 23, 28, 48.

mechanisms involved, however, are quite different. Digoxin is known to exert its activity by blocking the sodium-potassium "pump" on the cell membrane which is responsible for the maintenance of high intracellular potassium concentrations. Inhibition of the "pump" results in decreased intracellular potassium and increased intracellular sodium levels. Conversely, there is a slight increase in extracellular potassium and slight decrease in extracellular sodium (27,30,34). The RMP becomes less negative, resulting in a decreased rise and diminished amplitude of the action potential with resulting slowing of atrioventricular and intraventricular conduction. These changes are reflected on the electrocardiogram as an increase in the P-R interval, a decrease in the frequency of conduction through the A-V node, and widening of the QRS complex (3). The same ionic changes also result in an increased automaticity of Purkinje's fibers (24,27,34).

Hypokalemia affects digitalis kinetics by at least two mechanisms. Low-serum potassium results in increased binding of digitalis to the myocardial tissue (36,42) and decreased secretion of digitalis in the urine (43,44). The resulting increased myocardial/serum ratio of digitalis may account for the increased arrhythmias observed in hypokalemic patients treated with the drug.

Contrary to the changes associated with digitalis therapy, diuretic-induced hypokalemia is not associated with overt intracellular potassium depletion. With few exceptions, many studies have shown that there is only minimal change in total body potassium even in the presence of significant decrease in extracellular potassium associated with diuretic therapy (7,23,28,48). Even patients with overt diuretic-induced hypokalemia have a greater relative decrease in extracellular than intracellular concentrations of potassium. The available data from the literature (7,23,28,48) in this regard are summarized in Table 5. An average decrease in extracellular potassium of 15-25% is associated in most studies with only 5-7% decrease in intracellular potassium. Therefore the change in the ratio will result in a more negative RMP which, as indicated above, should decrease the arrhythmogenicity of the myocardial cells.

CONCLUSION

Considering both the evidence from the literature and our own data with regard to diuretic-induced hypokalemia in patients with uncomplicated hypertension we conclude that (a) diuretic therapy results in a relatively greater decrease in extracellular than in intracellular potassium and this change will result in a more negative resting membrane potential; (b) even overt diuretic-induced hypokalemia is not associated with increased ventricular arrhythmias; (c) correction of diuretic-related hypokalemia does not result in improvement of cardiac arrhythmias; and (d) complex arrhythmias, including breif episodes of ventricular tachycardia, may occur in otherwise asymptomatic hypertensive patients but are unrelated to diuretic therapy.

These findings indicate that in nondigitalized patients with uncomplicated hypertension, diuretic-induced hypokalemia is a benign process that does not require treatment.

REFERENCES

1. Anderson, K. E.: The heart cell: electrophysiological aspects. *Acta Med. Scand.* 647:7–13, 1981.
2. Bellet, S., Nadler, C. S., Gazes, P. C., and Lanning, M.: The effect of vomiting due to intestinal obstruction on the serum potassium. *Gastroenterology* 12:49, 1949.
3. Brater, D. C., and Morelli, H. F.: Systemic alkalosis and digitalis related arrhythmias. *Acta Med. Scand.* 647:79, 1981.
4. Brodsky, M., Wu, D., Denes, P., Kanakis, C., and Rosen, K.: Arrhythmias documented by 24-hour continuous electrocardiographic monitoring in 50 male medical students without apparent heart disease. *Am. J. Cardiol.* 39:390–395, 1977.
5. Clarke, J. M., Hamer, J., Shelton, J. R., Taylor, S., and Venning, G. R.: The rhythm of normal human heart. *Lancet* 2:508–512, 1976.
6. Curry, P., Stubbs, W., Fitchett, D., and Krikler, D.: Ventricular arrhythmias and hypokalemia. *Lancet* 2:231, 1976.
7. Dargie, H. F., Bobby, K., Kennedy, A. C., King, P. C., Read, P. R., and Ward, D. M.: Total body potassium in long-term frusemide therapy: is potassium supplement necessary? *Br. Med. J.* 2:316, 1974.
8. Davidson, S., and Surawicz, B.: Ectopic beats and atrioventricular conduction disturbances in patients with hypopotassemia. *Arch. Intern. Med.* 120:280, 1967.
9. Down, P. F., Polak, A., Rao, R., and Mead, J. A.: Fate of potassium supplements in six outpatients receiving long-term diuretics for oedematous disease. *Lancet* 2:721, 1972.
10. Dyckner, T., and Wester, P. O.: Ventricular extrasystoles and intracellular electrolytes in hypokalemic patients before and after correction of the hypokalemia. *Acta Med. Scand.* 204:357–359, 1973.
11. Dyckner, T., and Wester, P. O.: Intracellular potassium after magnesium infusion. *Br. Med. J.* 1:822–823, 1978.
12. Dyckner, T., and Wester, P. O.: Ventricular extrasystoles and intracellular electrolytes before and after potassium and magnesium infusion in patients on diuretic treatment. *Am. Heart J.* 97:12–18, 1979.
13. Edmonds, C. J., and Jasani, B.: Total body potassium in hypertensive patients during prolonged diuretic therapy. *Lancet* 2:8, 1972.
14. Eliel, L. P., Pearson, O. H., and Rawson, R. W.: Postoperative potassium deficit and metabolic alkalosis. *N. Engl. J. Med.* 243:478, 1950.
15. Fisch, C.: Relation of electrolyte disturbances to cardiac arrhythmias. *Circulation* 47:408–419, 1973.
16. Fisch, C., Greenspan, K., Knoebel, S. B., and Feigenbaum, H.: Effect of digitalis on conduction of the heart. *Prog. Cardiovasc. Dis.* 6:343, 1964.
17. Fisch, C., and Surawicz, B.: *Digitalis*. New York, Grune & Stratton, 1969.
18. Freis, E. D., Wanko, A., Wilson, I. M., and Parrish, A. E.: Chlorothiazide in hypertensive and normotensive patients. *Ann. N.Y. Acad. Sci.* 71:450, 1958.
19. Gifford, R. W., Masttox, V. R., Orvis, A. L., Sones, D. A., and Rosevaer, J. W.: Effects of thiazide diuretics on plasma volume, body electrolytes and excretion of aldosterone in hypertension. *Circulation* 24:1197, 1961.
20. Goldman, D. E.: Potential impedance and rectification in membranes. *J. Gen. Physiol.* 27:37, 1943.
21. Harrington, J. T., Isner, J. M., and Kassirer, J. P.: Our national obsession with potassium. *Am. J. Med.* 73:155, 1982.

22. Holland, O. B., Nixon, J. V., and Kuhnert, L.: Diuretic-induced ventricular ectopic activity. *Am. J. Med.* 70:762, 1981.
23. Kassirer, J. P., and Harrington, J. T.: Diuretics and potassium metabolism: a reassessment of the need, effectiveness and safety of potassium therapy. *Kidney Int.* 11: 505, 1977.
24. Koerpel, B. J., and Davis, L. D.: Effects of lidocaine, propranolol and sotalol on ouabain-induced changes in transmembrane potentil on canine Purkinje fibers. *Circ. Res.* 30:681, 1972.
25. Kunin, A. S., Surawicz, B., and Sims, E. A. H.: Decrease in serum potassium concentrations and appearance of cardiac arrhythmias during infusion of potassium with glucose in potassium-depleted patients. *N. Engl. J. Med.* 266:228, 1962.
26. Lawson, D. H.: Adverse reaction to potassium chloride. *Q. J. Med.* 43(171):433–440, 1974.
27. Lee, K. S., and Klaus, W.: The subcellular basis for the mechanism of inotropic action of cardiac glycosides. *Pharmacol. Rev.* 23:193, 1971.
28. Leemhuis, M. P., Van Damme, K. H., and Struyrenberg, A.: Effects of chlorthalidone on serum and total body potassium in hypertensive patients. *Acta Med. Scand.* 200:37, 1976.
29. Lief, P. D., Belizou, I., Matos, J., and Bank, N.: Diuretic-induced hypokalemia does not cause ventricular ectopy in uncomplicated essential hypertension. American Society of Nephrology, 16th Annual Meeting, 1983.
30. Lown, B., Black, H., and Moore, F. D.: Digitalis, electrolytes and the surgical patient. *Am. J. Cardiol.* 6:309, 1960.
31. Lown, B., and Levine, H. D.: *Atrial Arrhythmias, Digitalis and Potassium.* New York, Lansberger, 1958.
32. Lown, B., and Wolf, M. A.: Approaches to sudden death from coronary heart disease. *Circulation* 44:30, 1971.
33. Maronde, R. F., Milgrom, M., and Dickey, J. M.: Potassium loss with thiazide therapy. *Am. Heart J.* 78:16, 1969.
34. Mason, D. T., Zelis, R., Lee, G. et al.: Current concepts and treatment of digitalis toxicity. *Am. J. Cardiol.* 27:546, 1971.
35. Medical Research Council Working Party On Mild To Moderate Hypertension: Ventricular extrasystoles during thiazide treatment: substudy of MRC Mild Hypertension Trial. *Br. Med. J.* 287:1249, 1983.
36. Meldgaard, L., Steiness, E., and Waldorff, S.: Dependence on extracellular potassium and calcium concentration. *Br. J. Pharmacol.* 73:341–345, 1981.
37. Michelson, E. L., and Morganroth, J.: Spontaneous variability of complex ventricular arrhythmias detected by long-term electrocardiographic recording. *Circulation* 61:690–695, 1980.
38. Morgan, D. B., and Davidson, C.: Hypokalemia and diuretics: an analysis of publications. *Br. Med. J.* 1:905, 1980.
39. Morganroth, J., Michelson, E. L., Horowitz, L. N., Josephson, M. E., Pearlman, A. S., and Dunkman, W. B.: Limitations of routine long-term electrocardiographic monitoring to assess ventricular ectopic frequency. *Circulation* 58:408–414, 1978.
40. Papademetriou, V., Fletcher, R., Khatri, I. M., and Freis, E. D.: Diuretic-induced hypokalemia in uncomplicated hypertension: effect of plasma potassium correction on cardiac arrhythmias. *Am. J. Cardiol.* 52:1017–1022, 1983.
41. Singh, S. N., DiBianco, R., Davidov, M. E., Gottdiener, J. S., Johnson, W. L., Laddu, A. R., and Fletcher, R. D.: Comparison of acebutolol and propranolol for treatment of chronic ventricular arrhythmia: a placebo-controlled, double-blind, randomized crossover study. *Circulation* 65(7):1356, 1982.
42. Steiness, E.: Digoxin toxicity compared with myocardial digoxin and potassium concentration. *Br. J. Pharmacol.* 63:233–237, 1978.

43. Steiness, E.: Suppression of renal excretion of digoxin in hypokalemic patients. *Clin Pharmacol. Ther.* 23:511–514, 1978.
44. Steiness, E.: Diuretics, digitalis and arrhythmias. *Acta Med. Scand.* 647:75, 1981.
45. Tamura, K., Tamura, T., Yoshida, S., Inui, M., and Fukuhara, N.: Transient recurrent ventricular fibrillation due to hypopotassemia with special note on the U wave. *Jpn. Heart J.* 6:652, 1967.
46. Veterans Administration Cooperative Study Group on Antihypertensive Agents: Effects of treatment on morbidity in hypertension; influence of age, diastolic pressure and prior cardiovascular disease; further analysis of side effects. *Circulation* 45: 991, 1972.
47. Weaver, W. F., and Burchell, H. B.: Serum potassium and the electrocardiogram in hypokalemia. *Circulation* 21:505, 1960.
48. Wilkinson, P. R., Hesp, R., Issler, H., and Raftery, E. B.: Total body and serum potassium during prolonged thiazide therapy for essential hypertension. *Lancet* 1:759, 1975.

22

Diuretics, Serum Potassium, and Mortality in the Multiple-Risk Factor Intervention Trial

ROGER SHERWIN
University of Maryland School of Medicine, Baltimore, Maryland

PROTOCOL

Population

The Multiple Risk Factor Intervention Trial (MRFIT) was a randomized clinical trial of the preventibility of fatal first heart attacks by intervention on major risk factors in men with one or more such factors. The protocol has been described in detail previously (10). A total of 361,662 men aged 35-57 years attended the first screening visit conducted by 22 clinical centers throughout the United States. At this visit, blood pressure was measured, blood was drawn for the measurement of serum cholesterol, and a short questionnaire was used to explore smoking habits, and to elicit any history of treated diabetes or hospitalization for heart attacks, both of which were grounds for exclusion from the trial. An estimate of the future risk of coronary heart disease (CHD) was based on the levels of serum cholesterol, diastolic blood pressure (DBP), and amount of cigarettes smoked, using a multiple logistic function with coefficients derived from the Framingham experience (6). Of the 25,545 men from the upper end of the risk spectrum who attended the first screening and were invited to return, 22,080 (86.4%) attended a second screening examination which included a detailed medical history, physical examination, resting electrocardiogram (ECG), and measurement of blood electrolytes, lipids, and lipoproteins. Of the 6,289 (28.5%) men excluded at the second screening examination, about one-half had evidence of cardiovascular (primarily coronary) disease and only about one-quarter were unwilling to participate in the trial. Thus 15,791 apparently eligible men were invited to the third screening examination which included a baseline exercise ECG (not used for exclusion), a 24-hr dietary recall, formal consent to the trial, and randomization into study groups. Of the 14,111 attending the third screening examination, 12,866 gave written consent and were randomized. Therefore,

This chapter was prepared under the auspices of the Multiple Risk Factor Intervention Trial Research Group. See credit roster at end of chapter for membership of the group.

among the 25,545 eligible by risk factors, approximately 20% were ineligible by reason of existing disease and a further 30% either actively or passively declined to participate. These figures speak against any high level of motivational selection of the participants in the trial. The 12,866 men were randomized either to receive either special intervention (SI) or usual care (UC).

All men in the SI group were invited to attend, together with their spouses, a series of group meetings designed to facilitate the reduction of their risk factors. A moderate cholesterol-lowering diet was recommended to all participants regardless of the serum cholesterol level. Cigarette smokers were urged to quit smoking and offered a variety of techniques and modes of support to assist them. Men whose DBP remained ⩾ 90 mmHg on two consecutive visits after the second screening examination had antihypertensive medication prescribed (unless a trial of weight loss resulted in a reduction of DBP below 90 mmHg).

Men assigned to the UC group were referred to their usual source of medical care with full disclosure of their risk factors and the results of their screening examinations. No direct advice about changing their risk factors was given by MRFIT personnel, but UC men were encouraged to discuss these factors with their own physicians. They were invited to return once each year for a comprehensive examination, which included a resting ECG and measurement of their risk factors.

Hypertension

The protocol for the treatment of high blood pressure is outlined in Table 1. This protocol was adapted from that developed for the Hypertension Detection and Follow-Up Program (HDFP) which was initiated several years before MRFIT (4). There were only two potentially important differences between the HDFP and MRFIT protocols. Either hydrochlorothiazide or chlorthalidone could be used as a step 1 diuretic in MRFIT, at the discretion of the clinic physician, whereas chlorthalidone was the primary diuretic recommended in HDFP. Propranolol was also added as an alternative step 2 drug early in the course of MRFIT, whereas it was never adopted as a recommended drug in the HDFP protocol. The prescription of potassium chloride (10% liquid solution) was optional when serum potassium levels were 3.0-3.4 m Eq/L and mandatory at levels below 3.0 mEq/L. Goal blood pressure was established at 89 mmHg for those with DBP ⩾ 100 mmHg and 10 mmHg less than the DBP at the initiation of treatment for those with DBP 90-99 mmHg. Men who were already taking antihypertensive medication at entry to MRFIT and whose DBP was ⩾ 90 mmHg were assigned a goal of 80 mmHg. The protocol for the

Table 1 Summary of Special Intervention Protocol for the Drug Treatment of Hypertension in MRFIT

Step	Preferred drug(s)	Dosage (mg/day)	Other drugs	Dosage (mg/day)
1	Hydrochlorothiazide	50–100	Spironolactone	50–100
	Chlorthalidone	50–100	Triamterene	100–200
2	Reserpine	0.1–0.25	Methyldopa	500–2000
			Propranolol	140–320
3	Hydralazine	30–200	–	–
4	Guanethidine	10–200	–	–

management of hypertension and its implementation has been described in detail by Cohen et al. (1). Men in the SI group were asked to return at least three times each year for assessment of their risk factors and for further intervention on factors that persisted above goal levels; many of the men were actually seen more frequently.

In 1979, data suggesting an adverse response to hypertension intervention were noted. Because of these data and the recently reported positive results of the HDFP, which had used chlorthalidone as the primary diuretic drug (3), it was decided to designate chlorthalidone as the single diuretic to be used in MRFIT. At the same time a lower maximum dosage (50 mg) of chlorthalidone was advised. These changes in the protocol were implemented about 2 years before the end of the study.

RESULTS OF INTERVENTION

Changes in Risk Factors

The changes in risk factors that occurred in the SI and UC groups over the course of the trial are shown in Table 2. In the SI group, intervention goals were exceeded by a wide margin for smoking cessation and by a smaller margin for reduction in blood pressure, but reduction in serum cholesterol never reached the goal established from the results of the National Diet-Heart Study 10 years before (9). This was apparently attributable to changes in the American diet resulting in a doubling of the ratio of polyunsaturated to saturated fat over the previous decade, on the one hand, and the cholesterol-raising effect of the two diuretics used in MRFIT, on the other. Changes in all three risk factors of the UC group much exceeded expectation. The net calculated risk (based on the same logistic function that was used to assess eligibility) was about 22% lower in the SI group than in the UC group, rather than the 28% reduction predicted in the design.

Mortality

The mortality observed in the UC and SI groups by the end of the study, after an average participation of about 7 years, was reported in 1982 (7) and is shown in Table 3. The 7% lower incidence of death from CHD (the primary endpoint of the trial) in the SI group has a 90% confidence interval of −15%–+25% and falls, therefore, some way short of formal statistical significance. There was an excess of deaths from causes other than CHD in the SI group and similar numbers of deaths from all causes in the two groups. Perhaps the most striking result of all was the low mortality from CHD in both groups: in the UC group the rate was little more than half of that predicted from Framingham experience.

Table 4 shows mortality rates from CHD and all causes for SI and UC participants when they are classified according to both the blood pressure and the presence or absence of abnormalities on the resting ECG at baseline. Among those who had ECG abnormalities and who also met the MRFIT definition of baseline hypertension (average of second and third screen DBP $\geqslant$ 90 mmHg or use of antihypertensive medications), there was a substantial excess of deaths from all causes. Table 5 shows that most of the excess deaths from CHD occurred within 60 min of the onset of symptoms and that there was also an excess of deaths of unknown cause and chronology (which could have occurred within 60 min of the onset of symptoms) among these patients who were hypertensive and who also had abnormalities of the resting ECG at baseline. The prevalence of the various types of ECG abnormality is shown in Table 6; none of them appears to be specifically associated with sudden death.

Table 2 Average Risk Factor Levels in Special Intervention (SI) and Usual Care (UC) Groups

	Group	Screening S_1	Screening S_2/S_3	Years after Randomization 1	2	3	4	5	6
No. of participants attending	SI	6,428	6,428	6,112	5,995	5,883	5,791	5,682	5,754
visit	UC	6,438	6,438	6,080	5,919	5,793	5,711	5,615	5,639
Diastolic blood pressure	SI	99	91	85	83	82	82	81	81
(mm Hg)	UC	99	91	88	87	86	86	85	84
Reported cigarette smoking	SI	64	59	36	35	35	34	33	32
(%)	UC	64	59	56	52	51	48	47	46
Serum cholesterol (mg/dl)	SI	254	–	238	238	237	235	235	236
	UC	254	–	247	246	244	243	241	240
Plasma cholesterol (mg/dl)	SI	–	240	–	230	228	227	227	228
	UC	–	241	–	237	235	235	232	233

Table 3 Number of Deaths (and Mortality per 1,000 Men) from Several Causes in Special Intervention and Usual Care Groups of MRFIT

Cause of death	Special Intervention	Usual Care
Coronary heart disease	115 (17.9)	124 (19.3)
Cardiovascular disease	138 (21.5)	145 (22.5)
All causes	265 (41.2)	260 (40.4)

Role of Hypokalemia in Mortality Rate

Because thiazide and thiazide-derived diuretics are known to induce hypokalemia, and because of the known association of hypokalemia with cardiac dysrhythmia and sudden death, it is of interest to explore the possible role of hypokalemia in explaining the excess of sudden death among the MRFIT SI participants with abnormalities of the resting ECG at baseline. Table 7 shows that more SI than UC men were treated with diuretics and that, among those so treated, twice as many SI as UC men had serum potassium levels below 3.5 mEq/L. As a result, almost three times as many SI as UC men from the whole study sample had serum potassium levels below 3.5 mEq/L. Table 8 shows that for given doses of either chlorthalidone or hydrochlorothiazide, average serum potassium levels were approximately equal, but the more frequent use of either drug and the use of higher doses in the SI group resulted in an average serum potassium of 3.8 mEq/L in the SI group compared with an average level of 4.0 mEq/L in the UC group. However, Table 9 shows that levels of serum potassium below 3.5 mEq/L were in fact more frequently observed among survivors taking diuretics than among those who died of CHD.

DISCUSSION

While subgroup hypotheses relating to baseline blood pressure and to baseline ECG abnormalities had been separately stated before the data were analysed, no such hypothesis relating to their interaction had been formulated; nor was sudden death identified as a specific end point. It is therefore necessary to regard the apparent excess risk of sudden death among those with both baseline DBP $\geqslant 90$ mmHg and abnormalities of the resting ECG as a hypothesis suggested by the data, which should only be subjected to a formal statistical test on data that are independent of those from which the hypothesis was derived.

The data of two other completed randomized controlled trials of antihypertensive therapy have been reanalyzed to test this hypothesis. In the relatively small Oslo study of mild hypertension there was a moderate excess of events of CHD in the treated group among those without abnormalities in the resting ECG at baseline (4.4% vs. 3.6%) and a larger excess in those with ECG abnormalities (6.0% vs. 3.2%) but it was not statistically significant (2). Although there was an excess of sudden coronary deaths in the entire treated group compared with the entire control group (1.5% vs. 0.5%), the published reanalysis based on ECG abnormalities did not address sudden or CHD death per se. The Oslo study used 50 mg hydrochlorothiazide as the step 1 medication except in 11 men with elevated fasting blood glucose levels who received the step 2 drugs methyldopa or propranolol alone. Higher dosages of hydrochlorothiazide were not used and potassium supplements were used only "in a few patients." The much larger data set of the HDFP has also been reanalyzed (5) as an independent test of the hypothesis formulated from

Table 4 Number of Deaths (and Death Rates per 1,000 Men) from CHD and All Causes by Baseline Blood Pressure and Electrocardiographic (ECG) Among Special Intervention (SI) and Usual Care (UC) MRFIT Participants

Baseline blood pressure status	Baseline resting ECG	Number of participants		Cause of death: Coronary heart disease		Cause of death: All causes	
		SI	UC	SI	UC	SI	UC
Hypertensive	Positive	1,233	1,185	36 (29.2)	21 (17.7)	74 (60.0)	47 (39.7)
	Negative	2,785	2,808	44 (15.8)	58 (20.7)	100 (35.9)	122 (43.4)
Nonhypertensive	Positive	592	583	11 (18.6)	15 (25.7)	20 (33.8)	28 (48.0)
	Negative	1,817	1,862	24 (13.2)	30 (16.1)	71 (39.1)	63 (33.8)

Table 5 Number of Deaths (and Death Rates per 1,000 Men) Definitely or Possibly Occurring Within 60 min of the Onset of Symptoms Among Special Intervention (SI) and Usual Care (UC) MRFIT Participants

Baseline blood pressure status	Baseline resting ECG	Cause of death: Coronary heart disease < 60 min after symptoms, SI	Coronary heart disease < 60 min after symptoms, UC	Unknown, SI	Unknown, UC
Hypertensive	Positive	21 (17.0)	8 (6.8)	4 (3.2)	0 (0.0)
	Negative	19 (6.8)	23 (8.2)	2 (0.7)	3 (1.1)
Nonhypertensive	Positive	5 (8.4)	8 (13.7)	0 (0.0)	1 (1.7)
	Negative	9 (5.0)	17 (9.1)	5 (2.8)	2 (1.1)

Table 6 Frequency Distribution of Nonmutually Exclusive Abnormalities in the Baseline Resting Electrocardiograms Among MRFIT Participants

Type of abnormality	Minnesota code	Percentage of all participants
High R waves	3.1–3.3	11.0
IV conduction defects	7.1–7.8	6.8
Negative T waves	5.1–5.3	4.0
Arrhythmias	8.1–8.6	3.8
Left axis deviation $< -30^\circ$	–	3.0
ST elevation	9.2	1.9
ST depression	4.1–4.3	1.8
Q-QS waves	1.1–1.3	1.4
AV conduction defects	6.1–6.8	1.4
Right axis deviation $\geq 120^\circ$	–	0.1
Low QRS amptitude	9.1	0.1
Any abnormality		27.9

Table 7 Use of Diuretics,[a] and Prevalence of Low Serum Potassium at Fourth Annual Visit in Special Intervention and Usual Care MRFIT Participants

	Special Intervention	Usual Care
Percentage of men treated with diuretics	53	35
Percentage of those men treated with diuretics with serum potassium < 3.5 mEq/L	23	12
Number of men with serum potassium < 3.5 mEq/L	715	248

[a]Includes diuretics other than hydrochlorothiazide and chlorthalidone.

Table 8 Mean Levels of Serum Potassium in Special Intervention and Usual Care MRFIT Participants Who Were Being Treated With Diuretics at the Fourth Annual Visit

	Special Intervention	Usual Care
Chlorthalidone ⩽ 50 mg/day	3.7	3.8
Chlorthalidone > 50 mg/day	3.6	3.6
Hydrochlorothiazide ⩽ 50 mg/day	4.0	4.1
Hydrochlorothiazide > 50 mg/day	3.8	3.7
Mean serum potassium of all men treated with diuretics[a]	3.8	4.0

[a]Includes diuretics other than hydrochlorothiazide and chlorthalidone.

the MRFIT data. Among HDFP participants with baseline DBP of 90-104 mmHg, not on antihypertensive medication at entry, and free of major target organ damage, but with abnormalities of the resting ECG at baseline, there was an excess of deaths from CHD in the experimental (Stepped Care) group compared with the control (Referred Care) group. Despite this excess (which was not significant) there was an excess of deaths from all causes in the Referred Care group. Among a similar subgroup free of abnormalities of the resting ECG at baseline, there was an excess of deaths from CHD and from all causes in the Referred Care group (as there was in the complete Referred Care group). Unfortunately, the HDFP protocol did not call for classification of the chronology of death and it is not therefore possible to explore the extent to which the MRFIT findings are replicated in HDFP with respect to sudden death. It is also important to recognize that a smaller proportion of HDFP Stepped Care participants (24%) than SI men in MRFIT (36%) were receiving more than 50-mg doses of diuretic. However, none of the studies cited, including MRFIT, had sufficient power to detect subgroup effects with a reasonable degree of reliability. The question of possible adverse effects of certain antihypertensive medications in individuals with abnormalities of the resting ECG remains an open one. A more detailed presentation of the MRFIT data relating to these possible adverse effects has recently been published (8).

In summary it can be said that MRFIT raised the suspicion that hydrochlorothiazide and chlorthalidone may increase the risk of CHD death, especially sudden death, and that some further (but far from conclusive) support for this hypothesis was provided by reanalysis of the Oslo study and the HDFP. Although hypokalemia is theoretically attractive as a mechanism for this apparent increase in risk, the data do not support this explanation.

Table 9 Percentage Prevalence of Serum Potassium 3.5 mEq/L Among MRFIT Special Intervention Participants Who Were Being Treated with Diuretics and Who Either Died of CHD or Survived

Diuretic being taken at time of measurement	CHD deaths (last annual visit)	Survivors (fourth annual visit)
Hydrochlorothiazide	9	17
Chlorthalidone	23	36

CREDIT ROSTER

The principal investigators and senior staff of the clinical, coordinating, and support centers, the National Heart, Lung, and Blood Institute, and members of the MRFIT Policy Advisory Board and Mortality Review Committee are:

American Health Foundation, New York: Charles Arnold, M.D., M.P.H. (principal investigator), Rebecca Mandriota, M.S., M.Ed., Richard Ames, M.D., Joan Ruff Eisenbach, R.N.

Boston University, Boston: H. Emerson Thomas, Jr., M.D. (principal investigator), William Kannel, M.D. (co-principal investigator), L. Ken Smith, M.D., Charles Deckman.

Cox Heart Institute, Kettering, Ohio: Paul Kezdi, M.D. (principal investigator), Edwin Stanley, M.D. (co-principal investigator), Frederick Ernst, Ph.D., E. Jean Case, R.N., M.S.

Dade County Department of Public Health, Miami: George Christakis, M.D., M.P.H. (principal investigator), Janice Burr, M.D. (co-principal investigator), Terence Gerace, Ph.D. (co-principal investigator), Mary Ellen Wilcox, R.D., M.Ed.

Dalhousie University Halifax, Nova Scotia (MRFIT ECG Center), Pentti Rautaharju, M.D., Ph.D. (principal investigator), Hermann Wolf, Ph.D.

Harvard University, Boston: Robert Benfari, Ph.D. (principal investigator), Kevin McIntyre, M.D., J.D. (co-principal investigator), Oglesby Paul, M.D. (co-principal investigator; former chairperson, Steering Committee), Elinor Danielson, M.A., Judith Ockene, Ph.D.

Kaiser Foundation Research Institute, Portland, Oregon: John Wild, M.D. (principal investigator), M. R. Greenlick, Ph.D. (co-principal investigator), John Grover, M.D. (co-principal investigator), Sara Lamb, Jeffry Bailey, Judith Dyer, M.S.Hyg, R.D., Barbara Brokop, R.N., Victor Stevens, Ph.D., Geraldine Bailey, R.N.

Lankenau Hospital, Philadelphia: William Holmes, Ph.D. (principal investigator), J. Edward Pickering, M.D. (co-principal investigator), James Allaire, M.Ed., Diane Fellon, R.N., Barbara Feinstein, M.S.A., Diana Hutchins, M.D.

National Center for Disease Control, Atlanta: Gerald Cooper, Ph.D., M.D. (principal investigator).

New Jersey Medical School, Newark: Norman Lasser, M.D., Ph.D. (principal investigator), Norman Hymowitz, Ph.D. (co-principal investigator).

Northwestern University, Chicago: Jeremiah Stamler, M.D. (principal investigator), Dorothy Moss, M.S., R.D., Victoria Persky, M.D., Linda Van Horn, Ph.D., R.D., Kay Shannon, M.A., David Meyers, M.D.

University of Chicago, Chicago: Louis Cohen, M.D. (principal investigator), Juliet Morgan, Ph.D. (co-principal investigator), Gayle Grundmann, M.S., R.D., Thomas Vestal, P.A., Ben Huang.

St. Joseph's Hospital, Chicago: David Berkson, M.D., (principal investigator), Gary Lauger, M.S., Stevan Grujic, M.D., David Obradovic, M.D.

Institutes of Medical Sciences–University of California, San Francisco and Berkeley: James Billings, Ph.D., M.P.H. (principal investigator), Stephen Hulley, M.D., M.P.H. (co-principal investigator), W. McFate Smith, M.D., M.P.H. (co-principal investigator), Richard Cohen, M.S., Lisa Dzvonik, M.A., R.D., Leslie Ross, Mary Kahn, R.N.

Institutes of Medical Sciences–San Francisco Central Laboratory: Graham Widdowson, Ph.D. (co-principal investigator), George Williams, M.D. (co-principal investigator), Stephen Hulley, M.D., M.P.H. (co-principal investigator).

Rush-Presbyterian–St. Luke's Medical Center, Chicago: James Schoenberger, M.D. (principal investigator), Joseph Schoenenberger, Ph.D., Richard Shekelle, Ph.D., Gilberto Neri, M.D., Therese Dolecek, Ph.D., R.D.

Rutgers Medical School, Piscataway, New Jersey: Nicholas Wright, M.D., M.P.H. (principal investigator), Steven Kopel, Ph.D. (co-principal investigator), Kenneth Suckerman, Ph.D., Marilyn Schorin, M.P.H., R.D.

St. Louis Heart Association, St. Louis: Nathan Simon, M.D. (principal investigator), Jerome Cohen, M.D. (co-principal investigator), Elizabeth Bunkers, R.D.

University of Alabama in Birmingham: Harold Schnaper, M.D. (principal investigator), Glenn Hughes, Ph.D. (co-principal investigator), Ralph Allen, P.A., Phillip Johnson.

University of California, Davis: Nemat Borhani, M.D. (principal investigator), Carolyn Sugars, R.D., Karen Kirkpatrick, Marshall Lee, M.D., Frances LaBaw, R.N.

University of Maryland, Baltimore: Roger Sherwin, M.B., B.Chir. (principal investigator), Mary McDill Sexton, Ph.D., M.P.H. (co-principal investigator), Quely de Barros, M.S., Patricia Dischinger, Ph.D., Jutta Heiner, M.D., Mary Pilkington, R.N., M.S.N. Barbara Scanlon, M.A.

University of Minnesota, Minneapolis: Richard Grimm, Jr, M.D., M.P.H. (principal investigator), Henry Blackburn, M.D. (co-principal investigator), Richard Crow, M.D. (co-principal investigator), Maurice Mittelmark, Ph.D. (co-principal investigator), Mary McDonald, R.N., M.S.

University of Minnesota ECG Coding Center, Minneapolis: Ronald Prineas, M.B., Ph.D. (director), Richard Crow, M.D. (associate director).

University of Minnesota Nutrition Coding Center, Minneapolis: Ida Buzzard, Ph.D. (director), Joyce Wenz, M.S., R.D. (associate director).

University of Minnesota Coordinating Center, Minneapolis: Marcus Kjelsberg, Ph.D. (principal investigator), Glen Bartsch, Sc.D. (co-principal investigator), James Neaton, Ph.D. (co-principal investigator), Steven Broste, M.S., John Connett, Ph.D., Alain DuChene, Diane Gorder, M.S., Gregory Grandits, M.S., Kenneth Svendsen, M.S.

University of Pittsburgh, Pittsburgh: Lewis Kuller, M.D., D.P.H. (principal investigator), Robert McDonald, M.D. (co-principal investigator), Lorita Falvo-Gerard, M.N., M.P.H. (co-principal investigator), Arlene Caggiula, Ph.D., R.D. (co-principal investigator), Elizabeth Gahagan, R.N., Roberta Moyer, R.N., Mary Alman, R.N., Karen Southwick, A.S.C.P.

University of South Carolina, Columbia: Warren Giese, Ph.D. (principal investigator), J. Frank Martin, M.D. (co-principal investigator), James Keith, Ph.D. (co-principal investigator), Harriet Harrison, R.N.

University of South California, Los Angeles: Eugene Fishman, M.D. (principal investigator), Laurence Wampler, Ph.D., Gretchen Newmark, M.A., R.D., Shahida Siddiqui, M.D., Lauren Paquet, R.N.

Policy Advisory Board: William Insull, Jr., M.D. (chairperson), John Farquhar, M.D., C. David Jenkins, Ph.D., Elliot Rapaport, M.D., Donovan Thompson, Ph.D., Herman Tyroler, M.D., Park Willis III, M.D., William Friedewald, M.D. (ex officio), William Zukel, M.D. (ex officio).

Mortality Review Committee: Joseph Doyle, M.D. (chairman), Howard Burchell, M.D., Paul Yu, M.D., Park Willis III, M.D. (former member).

National Heart, Lung, and Blood Institute Staff, Bethesda, Maryland: William Friedewald, M.D. (program director), Curt Furberg, M.D. (project office director), Jeffrey Cutler, M.D. (scientific project officer), William Zukel, M.D. (former program director), Eugene Passamani, M.D. (former scientific project officer), Charles Kaelber, M.D. (former scientific project officer), Joel Verter, Ph.D., Margaret Wu, Ph.D.

REFERENCES

1. Cohen, J. D., Grimm, R. H., and Smith, W. M.: The Multiple Risk Factor Intervention Trial (MRFIT)–VI. Intervention on blood pressure. *Prev. Med.* 10:501–518, 1981.
2. Holme, I., Helgeland, A., Hjermann, I., Leren, P., and Lund-Larsen, P.G.: Treatment

of mild hypertension with diuretics. The importance of ECG abnormalities in the Oslo Study and in MRFIT. *JAMA* 251:1298–99, 1984.

3. Hypertension Detection and Follow-Up Program Cooperative Group: Five-year findings of the Hypertension Detection and Follow-up Program. I. Reduction in mortality of persons with high blood pressure, including mild hypertension. *JAMA* 242:2562–2571, 1979.
4. Hypertension Detection and Follow-up Program Cooperative Group: Therapeutic control of blood pressure in the Hypertension Detection and Follow-up Program. *Prev. Med.* 8:2–13, 1979.
5. The Hypertension Detection and Follow-up Program: The effect of antihypertensive drug treatment on mortality in the presence of resting ECG abnormalities at baseline: the HDFP experience. *Circulation* 70:996–1003, 1984.
6. Multiple Risk Factor Intervention Trial Research Group: Statistical design considerations in the NHLBI Multiple Risk Factor Intervention Trial (MRFIT). *J. Chron. Dis.* 30:261–275, 1977.
7. Multiple Risk Factor Intervention Trial Research Group: Multiple Risk Factor Intervention Trial: risk factor changes and mortality results. *JAMA* 248:1465–1477, 1982.
8. Multiple Risk Factor Intervention Trial Group: Baseline rest electrocardiographic abnormalities, antihypertensive treatment, and mortality in the Multiple Risk Factor Intervention Trial. *Am. J. Cardiol.* 55:1–15, 1985.
9. The National Diet-Heart Study Research Group: The National Diet Heart Study trial report. *Circulation* 37/38 (suppl. I):1–428, 1968.
10. Sherwin, R., Kaelber, C. T., Kezdi, P., Kjelsberg, M., and Thomas, H. E.: The Multiple Risk Factor Intervention Trial (MRFIT). II. The development of the protocol. *Prev. Med.* 10:402–424, 1981.

23

Risk Implications of Ventricular Premature Beats

SIMON W. RABKIN
University of British Columbia, Vancouver, British Columbia, Canada

Risk has a dictionary definition of the possibility or chance of loss, injury, disadvantage, or destruction and is usually coupled with a statement of the probability of such an event. In medicine, this means the chance or probability of death or of a major morbid event. The factor under consideration, ventricular premature beats (VPBs), may indicate or be responsible for the occurrence of the adverse outcome. An extension of the concept of risk is the determination of high- and low-risk groups based on the use of other clinical features, population factors, or characteristics of the variable under consideration. For VPBs, many other considerations enter into the equations assessing risk. Thus, this chapter will deal with the nature of VPBs, factors affecting their occurrence and recognition; possible models that relate VPBs to the serious outcome of death, and the risk implications of VPBs in the absence of heart disease and in the presence of different kinds of heart disease.

DEFINITION

Ventricular premature beats (VPBs) is the name most frequently used to refer to a ventricular depolarization beginning from a site in the ventricle. Although the term ventricular premature depolarization is more precise because the event is detected on the electrocardiogram (ECG) which records electrical and not mechanical events, nevertheless, tradition has preferred the word "beat" so it will be used herein. Tradition has also accepted the adjectives simple or complex to describe VPBs. There are no consistent criteria for the definition of these terms in the literature. Simple VPBs refers to VPBs of one form and which are infrequent. The exact definition of infrequent, however, is not consistent between studies. Complex VPBs refer to VPBs that are repetitive (two or more in a row), bigeminal or trigeminal, have different forms, are of high frequency, or occur in the T wave of the preceding complex. Again, consistency is not always apparent between studies. Furthermore, there is considerable controversy about whether these criteria truly identify major differences in VPB characteristics. For example, VPBs that occur long after the preceding T wave may represent a more serious and, therefore, more complex VPBs than those occurring on the T wave (20,54). Thus, when the term complex VPBs is used in a study described here, the definition will be provided.

CONSIDERATIONS

Understanding the risk implications of VPBs cannot be accomplished without considering a number of factors such as the nature of VPBs, the method used to detect them, the individual or population under study, the presence or absence of heart disease, the nature and severity of heart disease, and the underlying causative factor or factors (Table 1).

VPBs are more complex than the usual clinical variable used to determine risk. Blood pressure, for example, is a continuous variable. Despite the complexities of blood pressure regulation and the mechanisms responsible for hypertension, epidemiological evidence has consistently shown that the higher the blood pressure the greater the risk of cardiovascular morbidity and mortality. VPBs are not simply a continuous variable as the discussion in the "Definition" section indicates. VPBs can occur in one or more forms or be present alone or two in a row or three in a row, and so on. This has risk implications. The use of a quantitative or semiquantitative grading system to assess the "seriousness" of VPBs is an important approach but there is no general agreement on a classification system. The Lown grading system for VPBs is a hierarchical one: grade 0, no VPBs; grade 1, VPBs less than 30/hr; grade 2, VPBs 30 or more/hr; grade 3, multiform VPBs; grade 4A, two

Table 1 Factors to be Considered in Assessing the Risk Implications of Ventricular Premature Beats (VPBs)

Characteristics of ventricular premature beat
Frequency
Form
Number in a row
Prematurity
Method used to detect VPBs
Routine ECG
Continuous ambulatory ECG monitoring
Circumstances during which VPB detected: exercise, anxiety
Presence or absence of heart disease
Nature of heart disease
Ischemic
Cardiomyopathy
Mitral valve prolapse
Severity of heart disease
Precipitating (causative) factor(s)
Electrolyte imbalance
Blood gas imbalance
Infection
Autonomic nervous system effects
Central nervous system effects
Psychogenic effects
Coffee, tea, alcohol, cigarette smoking
Drugs

consecutive VPBs; grade 4B, three or more consecutive VPBs; and grade 5, R on T (41). Bigger and Weld (5) have found serious problems with this classification in predicting the risk of cardiac death in patients after myocardial infarction. It gives too much weight to R on T VPBs and too little to repetitive VPBs. Furthermore, there is a lack of homogeneity in the three highest Lown grades as exemplified by the identification of 16 subgroups in grade 5 with a mortality risk which varied from 0 to 75%. Clearly, improved quantification classification systems are necessary.

Another consideration is the method used to detect VPBs. The standard ECG may sample the individuals ECG for 30 sec or less. Continuous ECG monitoring usually records the ECG for 24 hr but can also monitor for 1 hr, or 48 hr, or longer. Continuous ambulatory monitoring is of great value in increasing the sensitivity of VPB detection. This is illustrated in a study of 101 patients with stable coronary heart disease (81). Ten hours of ambulatory ECG monitoring detected VPBs in 77 patients, of which 50% were considered serious and 9% had ventricular tachycardia. By comparison, 1,414 standard ECGs had been done on the same patients and VPBs were detected in only 49 patients of which 25% were considered serious and 1% had ventricular tachycardia. On the other hand, if ECG monitoring is prolonged long enough, VPBs could be detected in most individuals, which would thereby reduce the specificity of VPBs for risk assessment.

VPBs can also be detected during or immediately after exercise. Because of the neurohumeral and circulatory changes during exercise, the risk implications of exercise-induced VPBs will be discussed separately.

The individuals or populations under study are another important consideration in assessing the risk implications of VPBs. The prognosis of urban subjects with a high prevalence of hypertension and taking antihypertensive medications is undoubtedly quite different from that of a rural population in a less industrialized nation with a low prevalence of hypertension. The presence, nature, and severity of cardiac disease are both major determinants of prognosis and critical factors that influence the impact that VPBs have upon prognosis. Thus, the risk implications of VPBs must be discussed within the context of the presence or absence of heart disease as well as the nature and severity of the heart disease.

The cause or causes of VPBs are also important determinants of their risk implications. For example, emotional factors maybe responsible for VPBs. If the psychological stress is transient and does not recur then there may be little if any long-term adverse risk from those VPBs. The causes of VPBs are quite extensive and a detailed discussion is beyond the scope of this chapter, however, some must be mentioned. Electrolyte abnormalities, which are a focus of this book, as well as alterations in blood pH, alkalosis, and acidosis have been linked to the occurrence of VPB (17,36,73). VPBs can be induced by the autonomic nervous system with the afferent stimulus originating in the heart, vasculature, gastrointestinal tract, biliary tract, or genitourinary tract (3). The stimulus for sympathetic overactivity may also come from central nervous system disease (44), or be psychological in origin (45). Emotions, especially anxiety, are the most frequent emotional concomitants in patients whose VPBs were induced by emotional states (72). In some individuals, the interaction between a sensitive myocardium and powerful psychological stimuli can produce serious ventricular arrhythmias (42). VPBs can be precipitated by bradycardia from any cause, presumably due to inhomogenity of conduction at slow rates (28). The role of caffeine-containing beverages and cigarettes is not resolved although clearly some individuals are extremely sensitive to the effects of caffeine to induce VPBs. In population studies, some investigators have found a direct relationship between heavy coffee consumption (9 cups/day or more) and VPBs (53). Other investigators have not found a relationship between coffee and VPBs (39). The relationship between VPB and cigarettes is said to exist (19). Its importance has been considered too overrated (3) or nonexistent (11,39). A number of drugs have been linked to the occurrence of VPB. Of interest is the potential for antiarrhythmic drugs to precipitate the same condition they are used to cure (71). This brief overview of factors inducing VPBs should make the reader aware of the problems of sensitivity, specificity, or signal-to-noise ratio that may be present in many studies that simply relate VPB occurrence to the risk of morbidity and mortality from cardiovascular disease.

MODELS TO BE CONSIDERED

The mechanism(s) that links VPBs to a particular outcome is often not known. A number of different models or mechanisms may be operative and are crucially important for our understanding of the risk implications of VPBs. Figure 1 illustrates three examples of how VPBs may be related to sudden death. In one model (A), the cause of sudden death can also cause VPBs. A statistically significant association between VPBs and sudden death would be found but in the absence of a direct relationship between VPBs and sudden death. In another potential model (B), the cause or causes of VPBs are not linked to sudden death directly; rather there is a direct causal relationship between VPB and sudden death. In yet another model (C), the causes of sudden death also cause VPBs and VPBs themselves play a causative role in sudden death. In all models, the various causative factors may lead to VPBs when there is a low level or intensity of these factors present. With a greater severity of these factors, then more frequent and/or complex VPBs will be found. A further increase in severity of these factors leads to sudden death. These models have great importance both for establishing the scientific "truth" of the presence or absence of a causative relationship between VPB and sudden death and also for determining whether antiarrhythmics are of value. Let us assume that diuretics are a causative factor. If model A were operative then VPB occurrence with diuretics is of interest but there is no point using antiarrhythmic drugs because the cause of sudden death is the

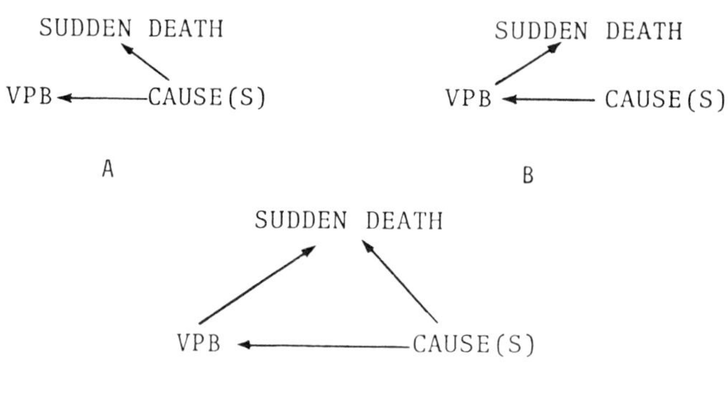

Figure 1 Three models (A, B, and C) that could govern the relationship between ventricular premature beats (VPBs), death, and the causative factor(s).

diuretic. If model B were operative then complete suppression of VPB with antiarrhythmic agents should prevent sudden death. If model C were operative then complete suppression of VPB would only partially prevent sudden death.

The next kind of model to be considered relates to the nature of the outcome. The various kinds of heart disease have to be considered. When myocardial infarction is the outcome, it is unlikely that VPBs cause the infarction. Thus, model A or C is more likely. VPBs in those models are indicators of the processes in the myocardium. When sudden death is the outcome under consideration, any of the three models is possible.

CAUSATIVE RELATIONSHIP BETWEEN VPB AND CARDIOVASCULAR DISEASE MORBIDITY AND MORTALITY?

A number of criteria should be met to provide sufficient evidence that a causal relationship exists between a factor and a disease (56). These include (a) experimentation: demonstration that exposure to the factor under experimental circumstances produces the outcome and the removal of the factor prevents the outcome; (b) strength of association: the relative risk of the disease occurrence in those with the factor as compared to those without it; (c) consistency: the repeated demonstration of the association using different approaches in different settings; (d) gradient of risk: the association of increasing risk of or severity of disease with increasing intensity or duration of exposure to the potential cause; (e) specificity: the limitation of the association to a specific type of exposure and to a specific disease entity. Some evidence supports each of these criteria in the VPBs and cardiovascular disease. I will briefly review some of the evidence and concepts as they relate to the first criteria. The others will be discussed below.

Experimental Evidence

The risk implication of VPBs that immediately comes to mind is sudden death. The two are linked because both VPBs and ventricular fibrillation, the major arrhythmia responsible for sudden death (67), are ventricular arrhythmias. The experimental evidence for a causal relationship between VPBs and sudden death is that premature ventricular depolarization delivered during electrophysiological studies in humans can induce ventricular tachycardia and fibrillation (35,79). This does not happen in all individuals, so other factors, such as a vulnerable myocardium, must also exist. This is in part similar to the situation in persons with VPBs: not all individuals with VPBs die suddenly; other factors must act in concert with VPBs. Thus, high-risk groups for sudden death must also have other abnormalities such as myocardial ischemia, ventricular hypertrophy, hypertension, or abnormalities of cardiac rate such as bradycardia or tachycardia, obesity, or be cigarette smokers. Similarly, there is no simple relationship between the production of cardiac electrical instability that produces sudden cardiac death and VPBs. Sudden death undoubtedly results from a complex interplay of cardiac factors and extracardiac factors. Cardiac factors include altered automaticity and/or conduction, areas of myocardial ischemia or infarction that, in turn, may be a function of coronary blood flow which is dependent on the degree of atherosclerosis, spasm, or platelet aggregation. Extracardiac factors to be considered include the role of the central nervous system, neuroreflex, hypoxia, acidosis, electrolyte disturbance, and catecholamines, to name a few.

Another element of the criteria of experimentation is to determine if there is a reduction in observed outcome (sudden death, for example), in individuals who have had VPBs reduced in frequency or eliminated; within the context of present approaches, this is usually pharmacological suppression of VPBs with antiarrhythmic drugs. A discussion of management of VPBs and its implications is beyond the scope of this chapter. However, it is appropriate for the reader to consider the questions that must be asked of such an intervention trial for VPBs. Is (are) the underlying mechanism(s) responsible for the VPBs in each case known and is the intervention appropriate? Could the adverse effects of the intervention (drug) be responsible for a failure of a trial to show a meaningful difference or is it evident that VPBs are not a causative factor? Is the intervention aimed at the underlying problem or the precipitating factor? What are the other effects of the drug and could they be responsible for the observation? The latter may be especially relevant for studies of antiarrhythmic drugs which themselves have the potential for serious adverse effects including induction of arrhythmias (71).

Coronary Heart Disease

Coronary atherosclerotic heart disease consists of a number of clinical entities such as myocardial infarction, angina pectoris, and coronary insufficiency that are further classified according to temporality of their occurrence, that is, recent or old myocardial infarction. Sudden cardiac death in the absence of other cardiac conditions is also considered to be a manifestation of coronary artery disease. Each of these clinical entities is important when we are considering risk implications of VPBs.

The frequency and severity of VPBs in patients with coronary artery disease are indicators of increased severity of disease. In acute myocardial infarction, the frequency and severity of VPBs are related to the extent of the infarction as assessed by enzyme release (59). Patients in the late hospital phase of acute myocardial infarction (10-24 days after onset of symptoms), with complex VPBs (multiform, coupled R on T, or ventricular tachycardia) on 24-hr ambulatory ECG recording have a greater number of proximally narrowed major coronary arteries, a lower ejection fraction, and a greater percentage of abnormal left ventricular segments compared to patients with unifocal or no VPBs (68). In a sample of patients undergoing coronary angiography, the majority of whom had old myocardial infarction, the prevalence and grade (Lown classification) of VPBs was greater in those with greater extent of coronary atherosclerosis, or elevated left ventricular end diastolic pressure, or ventricular asynergy (10,69). Thus, the risk implications of VPBs in patients with coronary artery disease are the presence of more severe coronary artery disease and left ventricular dysfunction.

These findings have important prognostic implications, because the severity of coronary disease and ventricular dysfunction are each significant determinants of prognosis. Assessment of the risk implications of VPBs, therefore, must take into account these two factors. To obtain such data, patients have had to have cardiac catheterization so that they represent those with angina pectoris or coronary insufficiency with or without previous myocardial infarction. Hammermeister et al. reported on the risk implications for 2,603 patients with VPBs on resting ECG, 733 of whom received medical treatment only and 1,870 of whom had coronary artery bypass surgery (27). For the medically treated patients, the presence of VPBs was associated with a threefold greater mortality than patients without ventricular arrhythmias. In a multivariate analysis that included 46 variables, VPBs, left ventricular ejection fraction, number of stenotic coronary arteries, and patients' age were the only significant predictors of survival. For the surgically treated patients, VPBs were the variable most predictive of survival in multivariate analysis, followed by ejection fraction, heart murmur, left main stenosis, and the use of diuretics (27). A preliminary communication on 611 medically treated patients suggested that VPBs classified by the Lown grading system are not an independent predictor of survival after one considers ejection fraction (9). Pending full publication of the report, this study has already been criticized for the probable bias or errors in arrhythmia detection, grading system, and the few number of deaths upon which conclusions were based (4).

RISK IMPLICATIONS IN SPECIFIC DISEASES

Survivors of Myocardial Infarction

The risk implications of VPBs in patients who have survived myocardial infarction are an increased probability for coronary mortality and especially sudden cardiac death in those with VPB compared to those without VPBs (40,49,58,62,80) (Table 2). Some of the studies on which this conclusion is based will be discussed in detail to indicate the factors considered to be independent of the relationship between VPB and sudden death. In the Coronary Drug Project, 235 of 2,035 male survivors of myocardial infarction had one or more VPBs on their resting baseline ECG (13). During a 3-year follow-up, deaths were about twice as frequent in those with any VPB compared to those with no VPBs. Excess long-term risk of death, including sudden death, was associated with the frequency of VPB and VPBs in pairs or runs. This excess risk of VPBs was independent of the risk associated with a variety of clinical and ECG factors such as age, body weight, cholesterol, triglycerides, blood pressure, cigarette smoking, blood glucose level, digitalis or diuretic use, cardiomegaly and previous myocardial infarction, heart failure, or angina pectoris. A subsample of this population underwent 12-hr ECG monitoring; sudden death occurred in 13.8% of those with complex VPBs (frequent multiform or repetative) but in only 3% of those with infrequent or no VPBs (40). The relationship between VPBs and sudden death was examined in 1,739 male survivors of myocardial infarction enrolled in the Health Insurance Plan of Greater New York who had 1 hr of ECG monitoring at a baseline examination (62,64). The presence of simple VPB was associated with a very slight increased mortality rate, while complex VPBs (interrupting the preceeding T wave, runs of two or more, multiform (two or more morphological types), and bigeminy were associated with a considerable increase in mortality. The relative risk for sudden death (3.5) was higher than for mortality from all causes (2.5) evident after adjustment was made for such factors as heart failure, diuretic or digitalis usage, blood pressure, heart rate, and other ECG variables (62). In a subsequent study that included data on repeated ECG monitoring at 6-month intervals for a maximum of four monitorings, patients with complex VPBs had three times the risk of mortality in the 3½ years after each monitoring (64). Moss et al. (49) found that VPBs on 6-hr ECG monitoring before hospital discharge from acute myocardial infarction were associated with an increased risk of cardiac, sudden, and nonsudden death. Complex VPBs (bigeminy, multiform, repetitive or R on T) were associated with a greater risk than simple VPBs, which resulted in a greater mortality than the absence of VPBs. This relationship was evident even after adjusting for such clinical variables as age, education, social class, cigarette smoking, New York Heart Association functional class, history of angina or previous myocardial infarction, or clinical evidence of left ventricular dysfunction.

The major criticism of these (early) studies was that the critical factor of left ventricular function was only assessed clinically, usually by the clinical evidence of heart failure.

Table 2 Data from Studies Indicating Risk of Ventricular Premature beats in Survivors of Myocardial Infarction

Author	Population	VPB Detection	Follow-up	Outcome
The Coronary Drug Project (13)	2,789 men	Routine	3 yrs	SD: 21.7% VPBs vs. 11.4% no VPBs
Kotler et al. (40)	160 men (sample CDP)	12-hr ECG	30–54 mos	SD: 13.8% VPBs vs. 3% no or infrequent VPBs
Vismara et al. (80)	64 men and women	10-hr ECG	25.8 mos	SD: 24.5% VPBs vs. 0% no VPBs
Moss et al. (49)	978 men and women	6-hr ECG	36 mos	Cardiac death rate: 23% complex VPB; 15% simple; 8% no VPBs
Health Insurance Plan New York (62)	1,739 men	1-hr ECG	24.4 mos	Mortality: 15.5% VPBs (complex) vs. 4.2% no or simple VPBs
Rehnquist et al. (58)	127 men, 33 women	6-hr ECG	1 yr	SD and reinfarction: 28.1% VPB vs. 14.8% no or infrequent VPBs

SD, sudden death.

Schulze et al. (68) using radionuclide determination of left ventricular ejection fraction, found that all 8 deaths in their 81 patients occurred in the group with high-grade VPBs on 24-hr ECG and with ejection fraction below 40%. Despite the inability to assess the independent contribution of these two factors, because all deaths were in one subset, this study raised the concern or possibility that the risk implications of VPBs were only due to severe left ventricular dysfunction. Recent studies have shown this is not the case. The multicenter postinfarction research group collected 452 variables on 766 patients who were under 70 years of age and had survived a recent myocardial infarction (51). Univariate analysis showed a progressive and significant increase in cardiac mortality when the number of VPBs exceeded one/hr during 24-hr ECG monitoring. Only four factors among eight prespecified variables were independent predictors of mortality: 10 VPBs or more/hr, ejection fraction below 0.40, advanced New York Heart Association functional class before infarction, and rales heard in the upper two-thirds of the lung fields during the patients stay in the coronary care unit. Various combinations of these four factors were able to identify subgroups with different risks of mortality from 3% (no factors) to 60% (all four factors) (51). Further study of the relationship between VPBs, left ventricular dysfunction, and mortality in this group showed that for all levels of reduction in ejection fraction, increasing numbers of VPBs per hour were associated with increasing mortality. In multivariate analysis, ejection fraction was a better predictor of early mortality (less than 6 months) and VPB a better predictor of late mortality (after 6 months). Thus, VPB and left ventricular dysfunction were considered independent predictors of risk of death after myocardial infarction. Preliminary results of the Multicentre Investigation of the Limitation of Infarct Size (MILIS) also suggest that the association of VPB and mortality after myocardial infarction is independent of left ventricular dysfunction (50).

Angina Pectoris

Ruberman et al. (63) reported the prognosis of VPBs occurring during 1 hr of ECG monitoring in 416 men with effort angina who had never had a myocardial infarction. The relative risk of death over a 5-year period was considerably greater in those with one or more VPBs compared to those without VPBs (Figure 2). There was little difference in survival between those with complex VPBs (runs of two or more, bigeminy, multiform, or R on T) and those with simple VPB. In multivariate analysis, after such factors as presence of heart failure, blood pressure elevation, diabetes, heart rate, diuretic and digitalis use, age, and presence of ST depression were considered, VPBs were seen to contribute significantly to predicting sudden cardiac death and mortality from all causes.

Cardiomyopathy

Cardiomyopathy refers to a group of diseases affecting only cardiac muscle. Idiopathic dilated cardiomyopathy is one of the most frequent kinds in the classification of cardiomyopathy. Many patients with this disease die suddenly. A high frequency and severity of ventricular arrhythmias have been identified in patients with this condition. In a prospective study of 74 patients with idiopathic dilated cardiomyopathy, 35% had frequent PVCs (>1,000/24 hr) and 87% had complex VPBs (Lown grade 3 and 4). Patients who died suddenly had significantly more VPBs and more ventricular pairs compared with survivors and those who died of heart failure (Figure 3). The arrhythmias were sig-

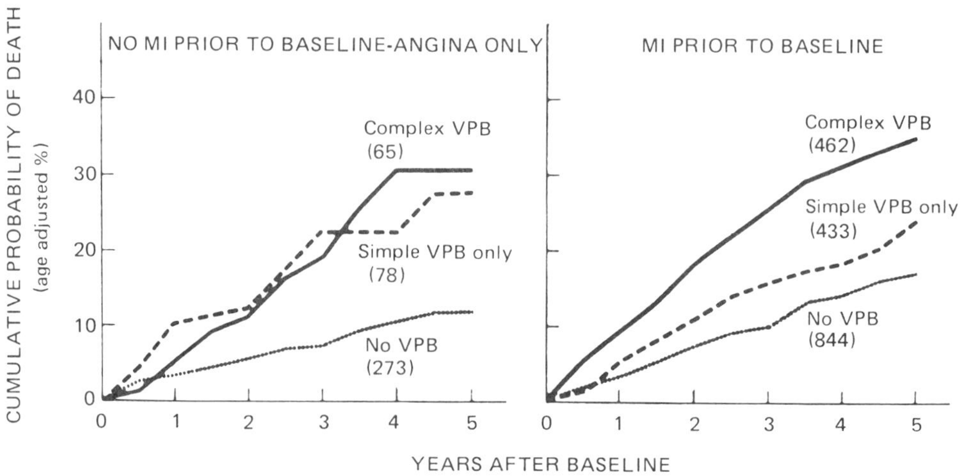

Figure 2 Mortality over 5 years after baseline monitoring in relation to VPB in the monitoring hour. Complex VPB are multiform, bigeminy, runs of two or more in a row, and R on T phenomenon. (From Ref. 63.)

nificantly related to sudden death even in multivariate analysis after taking into account the severity of hemodynamic dysfunction (48).

Hypertrophic cardiomyopathy is another form of cardiomyopathy in which the abnormality is myocardial hypertrophy in the absence of a definable cause such as hypertensive or valvular heart disease. Hypertrophic cardiomyopathy may result in obstruction to left ventricular outflow if there is focal or septal hypertrophy or may result in

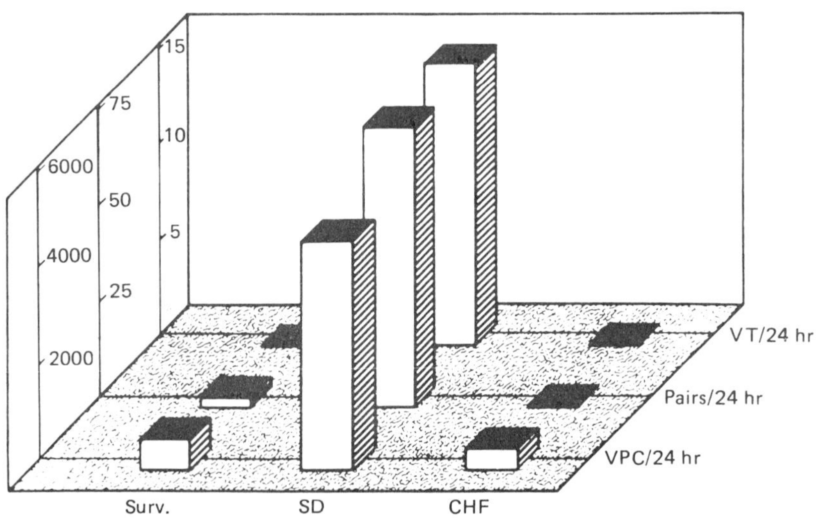

Figure 3 Frequency and complexity of VPBs in patients with idiopathic congestive cardiomyopathy. (From Ref. 48.)

generalized abnormalities of filling or contraction if the hypertrophy is generalized. VPBs have been detected on 24-hr ECG monitoring in 83% of patients with either obstructive or nonobstructive hypertrophic cardiomyopathy (66). There is a high frequency of complex VPBs (multiform, repetitive: two or more in a row) in this condition even in asymptomatic individuals. Sudden (unexpected) cardiac death occurs frequently (1,29). This has been attributed to arrhythmias, since death can occur in persons who have mild or no symptoms from outflow tract obstruction. In contrast to studies of myocardial infarction, there is no large-scale detailed prospective study on the relationship of VPBs and sudden death in patients with hypertrophic cardiomyopathy, probably because of the low prevalence of hypertrophic cardiomyopathy. Nevertheless, there is the strong clinical impression of a definite association between VPB occurrence and sudden cardiac death in patients with this condition (25).

Mitral Valve Prolapse

Mitral valve prolapse is a frequent condition, especially in women, where a prevalence may be as high as 17%. VPBs occur relatively frequently in persons with mitral valve prolapse (83). Despite the high prevalence of VPBs in individuals with mitral valve prolapse, sudden death is rare (33,34). The low frequency of sudden death has led Jeresaty (33,34) to conclude that it is not worth alarming patients with mitral valve prolapse about this possibility. While VPBs in mitral valve prolapse do not per se imply a high risk of sudden death, a subset at high risk of sudden death can be defined. It consists mainly of women with a mean age of 40 years with marked mitral valve prolapse on clinical, echocardiographic, or angiographic examination, ST segment and T wave changes on the ECG, and frequent VPBs. The female preponderance (75%) for sudden death occurrence may reflect the excessive proportion of women with mitral valve prolapse. Similarly, the age of patients at high risk may be an indicator of the prevalence of the syndrome because sudden cardiac death has been reported in patients 60 years of age and older with mitral valve prolapse with normal coronary arteries and ventricular arrhythmias (38). Thus, VPBs in the presence of severe mitral valve prolapse identify a group at high risk of sudden cardiac death.

Survivors of Cardiac Arrest

Although this is a small population of patients, it does have bearing on the question of the relationship of VPB to sudden death. Weaver et al. reported on 24-hr ambulatory ECG monitoring of 144 patients with coronary heart disease who had been previously resuscitated from out-of-hospital ventricular fibrillation (82). The recordings were made an average of 5 months after the cardiac arrest. Ninety percent of 129 patients had VPBs and in two-thirds these were complex VPBs (bigeminy, trigeminy, repetitive forms, or frequent multiforms). VPBs were significantly related to mortality over the next 2½ years. Complex VPBs were related to subsequent mortality after the presence of other clinical factors such as congestive heart failure was adjusted for.

No Clinically Apparent Heart Disease

VPBs often occur in apparently healthy individuals (8,31). The subject of risk implications of VPBs in the absence of clinically apparent heart disease has generated a great deal of controversy. This is in part due to the population under study, its sample size, and the nature of the outcome or end point examined. The occurrence of a cardiovascular disease event, especially the major outcome–sudden death–is much less common in persons without apparent heart disease than in those who have survived a recent myocardial infarction. Thus, a much larger sample of apparently healthy persons must be studied. Another issue is the population under study. For example, a clinical study could select a population with VPBs of long duration so that those with an adverse risk would have been already excluded (37). The choice of end points other than cardiovascular disease could obscure a possible relationship between VPBs and cardiovascular events. For example, data from some insurance companies or clinical studies data do not support an adverse prognosis for VPB based on all-cause mortality (16,60) although an excessive number of sudden cardiac deaths was observed (60).

VPBs occurring in apparently healthy men suggest an increased risk of cardiovascular disease (7,43,55,77) (Table 3). However, the age at occurrence of VPBs is an important prognostic factor. For men younger than 40 years, with VPBs, no excess coronary heart disease or sudden death risk is apparent. The increased risk is found for men 40 years of age and older (54). The kind of coronary heart disease is also an important factor. The risk is greatest for sudden death followed in order by myocardial infarction, coronary insufficiency. and angina pectoris (54).

A comparison of the risk implications of VPBs in apparently healthy individuals and those who have survived acute myocardial infarction is given in Figure 4. The occurrence of sudden death is much greater in persons after myocardial infarction as is the prevalence of simple and complex VPBs. Fewer individuals experience VPBs and sudden death (overlap) if they have no apparent heart disease than if they have had myocardial infarction. The large number of persons with VPBs who remain free of disease does not invalidate the group that does die suddenly. Rather it stresses the need to identify those at high risk

Table 3 Relationship Between Ventricular Premature Beats on Routine ECG in Apparently Healthy Men and Risk of Sudden Death, Coronary Heart Disease, Cardiovascular Disease and All-Cause Mortality

		Relative Risk or Mortality Ratio			
Study	Population	Sudden death	CHD death	CV death	All causes
Aetna Life Ins. Co. (7)	Insurance applicants				1.4
Prudential Life Assur. Co. (43)	11,000 employees				2.1
Equitable Life Assur. Co. (60)	712 insured men				1.0[a]
Seven-Country (6)	12,770 men in six European and one U.S. cohort		2.0[b]		
Canton All ages	1,224 men	1.3	0.9		
50–59 yrs. (22)	319 men	2.4[b]	1.8[b]		
U.K. Civil Servant (61)	18,403 men		2.0		
Manitoba (55)	3,983 men	3.1[b]			

[a]Those with elevated BP excluded; many experienced cardiac sudden death.
[b]Statistically significant.

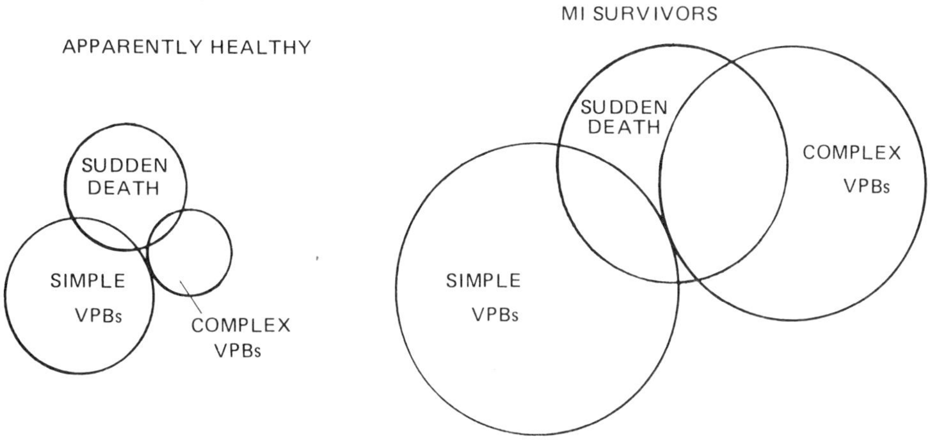

Figure 4 Possible relationship of simple and complex VPBs to occurrence of sudden death in persons without apparent heart disease (left) and survivors of myocardial infarction (right).

of disease. This can be done by considering other ECG factors. The association of VPBs and ST-segment and T-wave abnormalities identifies a group with almost three times the risk of either abnormality alone (Figure 5). The combination of ventricular extrasystoles and left ventricular hypertrophy increased the sudden death risk over four times that of either abnormality alone.

Pathophysiological mechanisms responsible for the predictive value of ST-segment and T-wave abnormalities for the occurrence of sudden death are unknown. There are a number of possibilities. These include the obvious one that these electrocardiographic findings indicate subclinical myocardial damage from coronary atherosclerosis that later becomes clinically manifested as sudden death. An intriguing possibility relates to the observation that the ST-T-wave form in the electrocardiogram can reflect inequalities in ventricular recovery and disparity in recovery of excitability in cardiac muscle, which reflect an increased vulnerability to arrhythmias (78). The pathophysiological mechanism(s) responsible for the predictive value of left ventricular hypertrophy with VPBs is also unknown. Possible explanations could be that the abnormal (thickened) myocardium is more vulnerable to ventricular fibrillation induced by an irritable myocardium as indicated by VPBs. Characteristics of the VPB do not clearly identify high-risk groups (54). QRS duration, conformation of the VPB, or its coupling interval do not identify those at increased risk. The occurrence of T wave changes in the beat following the VPBs is suggestive of a group at slightly higher risk. More complex assessment of VPBs may be developed which will improve risk assessment (57).

There is little multivariate data analysis to determine the independent contribution of VPBs. Blackburn et al. have suggested that the relationship between VPBs and coronary heart disease incidence may become weak when age, blood pressure, and coronary risk factors are accounted for. However, in the 16-year follow-up of an Australian cohort, VPBs on a routine electrocardiogram as part of a mass health examination were a significant predictor of coronary heart disease mortality in women and total cardiovascular but not coronary heart disease mortality in men; after multivariate analysis that included age, blood pressure, cigarette smoking, and levels of cholesterol and blood sugar (14).

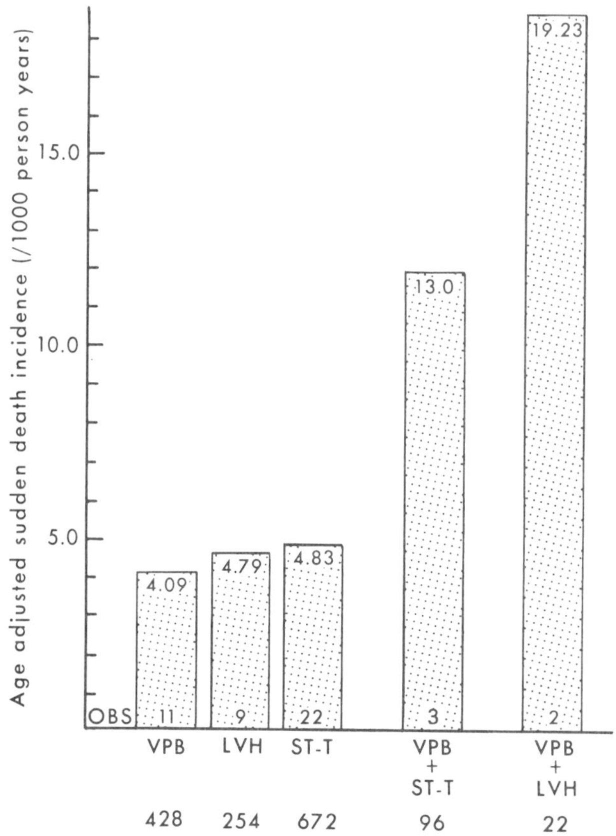

Figure 5 Age-adjusted incidence of sudden death in apparently healthy men with VPBs, left ventricular hypertrophy (LVH), and ST-T-wave changes alone or the combination of VPBs and LVH or ST-T changes. (From Ref.55.)

EXERCISE-RELATED VPBs

One of the problems with defining the risk implications of exercise VPBs is the problem of their reproducibility. The reproducibility of VPBs on exercise testing is about 50% with a range of about 20-75%. Reproducibility rates are higher with older age groups and patients with cardiovascular disease (2,32). In patients who have survived acute myocardial infarction, VPB reproducibility rates are better if the exercise tests are done closer together (65). However, even exercise tests done within 45 min in persons with previously identified VPBs can show considerable differences and a significant reduction in VPB frequency has been found by exercise stress testing during and after the second test (70). Although the reproducibility of VPBs on exercise testing is statistically significant, there is serious doubt that the reproducibility rate is high enough to permit it to be useful for assessing the risk of future cardiovascular disease.

In persons with no apparent heart disease exercise VPBs are not of value for predicting risk of coronary disease (Table 4). In patients referred for chest pain syndromes, some of whom have definite coronary artery disease, exercise VPBs indicate minimal or no increase in incidence of coronary disease. In patients who have survived a recent myocardial

Table 4 Studies Indicating Risk Ventricular Premature Beats in Exercise Testing

Author	Population	Follow-Up	Outcome
Froelicher et al. (23)	1,390 asymptomatic men (aircrew)	6.3 yr	Very low sensitivity of predictive value and risk ratio for development of coronary disease events
Udall and Ellestad (76)	6,500 patients: 80% men referred for chest pain (57%), history of MI (22%), hypertension (22%), or previous cardiac surgery (6%)	5 yr	Slight increased annual coronary disease occurrence in with VPBs vs. no VPBs in those with ST depression 11.4% vs. 9.5%) and without ST depression (6.4% vs. 1.7%)
Dagenais et al. (15)	202 men, 18 women, 5 yr ST segment depression on exercise; medical treatment only	5 yr	No significant difference between survivors and nonsurvirors for exercise VPBs
Nair et al. (52)	197 men, 83 women, normal resting ECG, no prior MI, referred for chest pain	4 yr	No significant difference in subsequent occurrence coronary events in those with (9%) or without VPBs (8%)

infarction, exercise VPBs indicate an increased risk of mortality, although the predictive value of other exercise factors such as ST changes is much better than VPBs (75). Another risk implication of VPBs on exercise testing is a greater probability of severe or moderately severe coronary artery stenosis in patients with known coronary artery disease (3,12,30). VPBs are not, however, indicative of clinically significant disease when persons with or without symptoms of coronary disease (7) are compared.

CONCLUSION

VPBs reflect a complex phenomenon or interplay of a considerable number of cardiac and extracardiac factors. An understanding of the risk implications of VPBs requires identification of the precipitating cause, presence of heart disease, nature and severity of the heart disease, and associated factors. The risk of an adverse prognosis is much greater in a person who has survived a myocardial infarction than one who has no apparent heart disease. In patients who have survived myocardial infarction, VPBs indicate a high risk of sudden death. In the same patient population, VPBs, with reduced ejection fraction, and heart failure, identify a group at higher risk. In apparently healthy men, the association of VPBs with ST-segment or T-wave changes or left ventricular hypertrophy identifies a high-risk group. Although much has been learned about the risk implications of VPBs, there remains much to be learned before we can precisely identify persons and conditions in which VPBs indicate a large or small risk of adverse prognosis. However, the presence of VPBs should prompt a search for their cause and presence of heart disease and other factors which together are of value to determine the risk implications of VPBs.

REFERENCES

1. Adelman, A. G., Wigle, E. D., Ranganathan, N., Webb, G. D., Kidel, B. S. L., Bigelow, W. G., and Silver, M. D.: The clinical course in muscular subaortic stenosis. A retrospective and prospective study of 60 hemodynamically proved cases. *Ann. Intern. Med.* 77:515–525, 1972.
2. Astrand, I.: Exercise electrocardiograms recorded twice with an 8 year interval in a group of 204 women and men 48–63 years old. *Acta Med. Scand.* 178:27–39, 1965.
3. Bellet, S.: *Clinical Disorders of the Heart Beat*, 3rd ed. Philadelphia, Lea and Febiger. 1971, pp. 251–309.
4. Bigger, J. T., Fleiss, Y., Fleiger, R., Miller, J. P., Rolnitsky, L. M., and the Multicentre Post-Infarction Research Group: The relationships among ventricular arrhythmias, left ventricular dysfunction and mortality in the 2 years after myocardial infarction. *Circulation* 60:250–258, 1984.
5. Bigger, J. T., and Weld, F. M.: Analysis of prognostic significance of ventricular arrhythmias after myocardial infarction. Shortcomings of 'Lown' grading system. *Br. Heart J.* 45:717–724, 1981.
6. Blackburn, H., Taylor, H. L., and Keys, A.: The electrocardiogram in prediction of five year coronary heart disease incidence among men aged forty through fifty-nine. *Circulation* 41 & 42 suppl 1:154–161, 1970.
7. Brandon, K. F., Neill, M. H., and Streeter, G. S.: The use of the electrocardiogram in twenty-five years of insurance selection. *Trans. Assoc. Life Insur. Med. Dir. Am.* 34: 143–156, 1950.
8. Brodsky, M., Wu, D., Denes, P., Konakis, C., and Rosen, K. M.: Arrhythmias documented by 24 hour continuous electrocardiographic monitoring in 50 male medical students without apparent heart disease. *Am. J. Cardiol.* 39:390–395, 1977.

9. Calif, R. M., Wagner, G. S., and Rosati, R. A.: Prognostic value of ventricular arrhythmias (abstract). *Am. J. Cardiol.* 47:397, 1981.
10. Calvert, A., Lown, B., and Gorlin, R.: Ventricular premature beats and anatomically defined coronary heart disease. *Am. J. Cardiol.* 39:627-634, 1977.
11. Cellina, G. O., Honour, A. J., and Littler, W. A.: Direct arterial pressure, heart rate and electrocardiogram during cigarette smoking in unrestricted patients. *Am. Heart J.* 89:18-25, 1975.
12. Cohn, K., Kanm, G., Feteih, N., Brand, R., and Goldschlager, N.: Use of treadmill score to quantify ischemic response and predict extent of coronary disease. *Circulation* 59:286-296, 1979.
13. Coronary Drug Project Research Group: Prognostic importance of premature beats following myocardial infarction. *JAMA* 223:1116-1154, 1973.
14. Cullen, R., Wearne, K. L., Stenhouse, N. S., and Cumpston, G. N.: Q-waves and ventricular extrasystoles in resting electrocardiogram: A 16 year follow up in Busselton Study. *Br. Heart J.* 50:465-468, 1983.
15. Dagenais, G. R., Rouleau, J. R., Christen, A., and Fabia, J.: Survival of patients with a strongly positive exercise electrocardiogram. *Circulation* 65:452-456, 1982.
16. Desai, D. C., Hershberg, P. I., and Alexander, S.: Clinical significance of ventricular premature beats in an outpatient population. *Chest* 64:564-569, 1973.
17. Davidson, S., and Surawicz, B.: Ectopic beats and atrioventricular conduction disturbance. *Arch. Intern. Med.* 120:280-285, 1967.
18. De Busk, R. F., Davidson, D. M., Houston, N., and Fitzgerald, J.: Serial ambulatory electrocardiography and treadmill exercise testing after uncomplicated myocardial infarction. *Am. J. Cardiol.* 45:547-554, 1980.
19. Dreifus, L. S., and Watanabe, Y.: Tension, drugs and premature systole. *Am. Heart J.* 70:291-294, 1965.
20. Engel, T. R., Meister, S. G., and Fronkle, W. S.: The "R-on' T" phenomenon; an updated and critical review. *Ann. Intern. Med.* 88:221-225, 1978.
21. Farrs, J. V., McHenry, P. L., Jordan, J. W., and Morris, S. N.: Prevalence and reproducibility of exercise induced ventricular arrhythmias during maximal exercise testing in normal men. *Am. J. Cardiol.* 37:617-622, 1976.
22. Fisher, F. D., and Tyroler, H. A.: Relationship between ventricular premature contractions on routine electrocardiography and subsequent sudden death from coronary heart disease. *Circulation* 47:712-719, 1973.
23. Froelicher, V. F., Thomas, M. M., Pilloue, C., and Lancaster, M. C.: Epidemiologic study of asymptomatic men screened by maximum treadmill testing for latent coronary artery disease. *Am. J. Cardiol.* 34:770-776, 1974.
24. Goldschlager, N., Cake, D., and Cohn, K.: Exercise-induced ventricular arrhythmias in patients with coronary artery disease. Their arrhythmias in patients with coronary artery disease. Their relation to angiographic findings. *Am. J. Cardiol.* 31:434-440, 1973.
25. Goodwin, J. F., and Krikler, D. N.: Arrhythmias as a cause of sudden death in hypertrophic cardiomyopathy. *Lancet* 2:937-940, 1973.
26. Grossman, M. A.: Cardiac arrhythmias in acute central nervous system disease. *Arch. Intern. Med.* 136:203-207, 1976.
27. Hammersmeister, K. E., De Rouen, T. A., and Doge, H. T.: Variables predictive of survival in patients with coronary disease. Selection by univariate and multivariate analyses from the clinical, electrocardiographic, exercise, arteriographic and quantitative angiographic evaluation. *Circulation* 59:421-429, 1979.
28. Han, J., De Traglia, J., and Moe, G. K.: Incidence of ectopic beats as a function of basic rate in the ventricle. *Am. Heart J.* 72:632-639, 1966.
29. Hardarson, T., de la Calzoda, C. S., Curiel, R., and Goodwin, J. F.: Prognosis and mortality of hypertrophic obstructive cardiomyopathy. *Lancet* 2:1462-1467, 1973.

30. Helfant, R. H., Pine, R., Kabde, V., and Banka, V. S.: Exercise related ventricular premature complexes in coronary heart disease: correlations with ischemic and angiographic severity. *Ann. Intern. Med.* 80:589-592, 1974.
31. Hiss, R. G., and Lamb, L. E.: Electrocardiographic findings in 122,043 individuals. *Circulation* 45:947-958, 1962.
32. Jelenek, M. U., and Lown, B. Exercise stress testing for exposure of cardiac arrhythmias. *Prog. Cardiovasc. Dis.* 13:497-522, 1974.
33. Jeresaty, R. M.: Sudden death in the mitral valve prolapse-click syndrome. *Am. J. Cardiol.* 37:317-318, 1976.
34. Jeresaty, R. M. *Mitral Valve Prolapse.* New York, Raven Press, 1979.
35. Josephson, M. E., Spielman, S. R., Greenspan, A. M., and Horowitz, L. N.: Mechanism of ventricular fibrillation in man. Observations based on electrode catheter recordings. *Am. J. Cardiol.* 44:623-631, 1979.
36. Karis, J. H., Harmel, M. H., and Hoffman, B. F.: Effects of pH and pCO2 on the sensitivity of Purkinje fibers to digitalis. *Circulation* 22:770-779, 1960.
37. Kennedy, H. D., and Underhill, S. J.: Frequent or complex ventricular ectopy in apparently healthy subjects. A clinical study of 25 cases. *Am. J. Cardiol.* 38:141-148, 1976.
38. Kolibash, A. J., Bush, C. A., Fontana, M. B., Ryan, J. M., Kilman, J., and Wooley, C. F.: Mitral valve prolapse syndrome analysis of 62 patients aged 60 years and older. *Am. J. Cardiol.* 52:534-539, 1983.
39. Kostis, J. B., McCrone, K., Moreyra, A. E., Gotzoyannis, S., Aglitz, N. M., Natarajan, N., and Kuo, P. T.: Premature ventricular complexes in the absence of identifiable heart disease. *Circulation* 63:1351-1356, 1981.
40. Kotler, M. N., Tabatznik, B., Mower, M. M., and Tominaga, S.: Prognostic significance of ventricular ectopic beats with respect to sudden death in the postinfarction period. *Circulation* 47:959-966, 1973.
41. Lown, B., Calvert, A. F., Armington, R., and Ryan, M.: Monitoring for serious arrhythmias and high risk of sudden death. *Circulation* 51 & 52 Suppl 3:189-198, 1975.
42. Lown, B., Temte, J. V., Reich, P. et al. Basis for recurring ventricular fibrillation in absence of coronary heart disease and its management. *N. Engl. J. Med.* 294:263-267, 1976.
43. Lyle, A. M.: A study of premature beats be electrocardiogram. *Trans. Soc. Actuar.* 14:493-508, 1950.
44. Lynch, J. J., Paskewitz, D. A., Gimbel, K. S., and Thomas, S. A.: Psychological aspects of cardiac arrhythmias. *Am. Heart J.* 93:645-657, 1977.
45. Malliani, A., Schwartz, P. J., and Zanchetti, A.: Neural mechanisms in life threatening arrhythmias. *Am. Heart J.* 100:705-715, 1980.
46. Maron, B. J., Savage, D. D., Wolfson, J. K., and Epstein, S. E.: Prognostic significance of 24 hour ambulatory electrocardiographic monitoring in patients with hypertrophic cardiomyopathy: a prospective study. *Am. J. Cardiol.* 48:252-257, 1981.
47. McHenry, P. L., Fisch, C., Jordan, J. W., and Corya, B. R.: Cardiac arrhythmias observed during maximal treadmill exercise testing in clinically normal men. *Am. J. Cardiol.* 29:331-336, 1972.
48. Meinertz, T., Hofmann, T., Kasper, W., Treese, N., Bechtold, H., Stienen, U., Pays, T., Leitner, E. R. V., Andresen, D., and Meyer, J.: Significance of ventricular arrhythmias in idiopathic dilated cardiomyopathy. *Am. J. Cardiol.* 53:902-907, 1984.
49. Moss, A. J., Davis, H. T., De Camila, J., and Bayer, L. W.: Ventricular ectopic beats and their relation to sudden and non-sudden death after myocardial infarction. *Circulation* 60:998-1003, 1979.

50. Mukharji, J., Rude, R. E., Poole, K., Croft, C., Thomas, L. J., Strauss, H. W., Roberts, R., Roobe, D. S., Braunwald, E., Willerson, J. T., and cooperating investigators: Multicenter investigation of the limitation of infarct size (MILIS). Late sudden death following acute myocardial infarction: importance of combined presence of repetitive ventricular ectopy and left ventricular dysfunction (abstract). *Clin. Res.* 30:108A, 1982.
51. Multicenter Postinfarction Research Group: Risk stratification and survival after myocardial infarction. *N. Engl. J. Med.* 309:331–336, 1983.
52. Nair, C. K., Aronoue, W. S., Sketch, M. H., Pagans, T., Lynch, J. D., Moss, A. N., Esterbrooks, D., Runco, V., and Ryschan, K.: Diagnostic and prognostic significance of exercise-induced premature ventricular complexes in men and women: a four year follow up. *J. Am. Coll. Cardiol.* 5:1201–1206, 1983.
53. Prineas, R. J., Jacobs, D. R., Crow, R. S., and Blackburn, H.: Coffee, tea and VPB. *J. Chron. Dis.* 33:67–72, 1980.
54. Rabkin, S. W., Mathewson, F. A. L., and Tate, R. B.: Relationship of ventricular ectopy in men without apparent heart disease to occurrence of ischemic heart disease and sudden death. *Am. Heart J.* 101:135–142, 1981.
55. Rabkin, S. W., Mathewson, F. A. L., and Tate, R. B.: The electrocardiogram in apparently healthy men and the risk of sudden death. *Br. Heart J.* 47:546–552, 1982.
56. Rabkin, S. W., and Sackett, D. S.: Epidemiology of arterial thrombo-embolism. In *Textbook of Hemostasis,* edited by Colman, R. W., Hirsh, J., Marder, V. J., and Salzman, E. W., Philadelphia, J. B. Lippincott, 1982, pp. 873–888.
57. Rabkin, S. W., and Ohmae, M.: A classification of ventricular ectopic beats. *J. Electrocardiol.* 15:55–60, 1982.
58. Rehnquist, N., Lundman, T., and Sjogren, A.: Prognostic implications of ventricular arrhythmias registered before discharge and one year after acute myocardial infarction. *Acta Med. Scand.* 204:203–209, 1978.
59. Roberts, R., and Sobel, B.: Relationship between infarct size and ventricular arrhythmias. *Br. Heart J.* 37:1169–1175, 1975.
60. Rodstein, M., Wolloch, L., and Gubner, R. S.: Mortality study of the significance of extrasystoles in an insured population. *Circulation* 44:617–625, 1971.
61. Rose, G., Baxter, P. J., Reid, D. D., and McCartney, P.: Prevalence and prognosis of electrocardiographic findings in middle-aged men. *Br. Heart J.* 40:636–643, 1978.
62. Ruberman, W., Weinblatt, E., Goldberg, J. P., Frank, C. W., and Shapiro, S.: Ventricular premature beats and mortality after myocardial infarction. *N. Engl. J. Med.* 279:750, 1970.
63. Ruberman, W., Weinblatt, E., Goldberg, J. D., Frank, C. W., Shapiro, S., and Chaudhary, B. S.: Ventricular premature complexes in prognosis of angina. *Circulation* 61:1172–1178, 1980.
64. Ruberman, W., Weinblatt, E., Frank, C. W., Goldberg, J. D., and Shapiro, S.: Repeated 1 hour electrocardiographic monitoring of survivors of myocardial infarction at 6 month intervals: arrhythmia detection and relation to prognosis. *Am. J. Cardiol.* 47:1197–1204, 1981.
65. Sami, M., Kraemer, H., and De Busk, R. F.: Reproducibility of exercise-induced ventricular arrhythmia after myocardial infarction. *Am. J. Cardiol.* 43:724–730, 1979.
66. Savage, D. D., Seides, S. F., Maron, B. J., Myers, D. J., and Epstein, S. E.: Prevalence of arrhythmias during 24 hour electrocardiographic monitoring and exercise testing in patients with obstructive and non-obstructive hypertrophic cardiomyopathy. *Circulation* 59:866–875, 1979.
67. Schaffer, W. A., and Cobb, L. A.: Recurrent ventricular fibrillation and modes of death in survivors of out of hospital ventricular fibrillation. *N. Engl. J. Med.* 293: 260–262, 1975.

68. Schutze, R. A., Humphries, J. O'N., Griffith, L. S. C., Ducci, H., Achuff, S., Baird, M. G., Mellits, E. D., and Pitt, B.: Left ventricular and coronary angiographic anatomy. Relationship to ventricular irritability in the late hospital phase of acute myocardial infarction. *Circulation* 55:839-843, 1977.
69. Sharma, S. D., Ballantyne, F., and Goldstein, S.: The relationship of ventricular asynergy in coronary artery disease to ventricular premature beats. *Chest* 66:358-362, 1974.
70. Sheps, D. S., Ernst, J. C., Briese, F. R., Lopez, L. V., Conde, C. A., Castellanos, A., and Myerbury, R. J.: Decreased frequency of exercise-induced ventricular ectopic activity in the second of two consecutive treadmill tests. *Circulation* 55:892–895, 1977.
71. Singh, B. N.: Side effects of antiarrhythmic drugs. *Pharmacol. Ther.* 2:151–166, 1977.
72. Stevenson, I. P., Duncan, C. H., Wolf, S., Ripley, H. S., and Wolff, H. G.: Life situations, emotions and extrasystoles. *Psychosom. Med.* 11:257–272, 1949.
73. Surawicz, B.: Role of electrolytes and management of cardiac arrhythmias. *Prog. Cardiovasc. Dis.* 8:364–380, 1966.
74. Swartz, M. H., Teichholz, L. E., and Donoso, E.: Mitral valve prolapse: a review of associated arrhythmias. *Am. J. Med.* 62:377-389, 1977.
75. Theroux, P., Waters, D. D., Halphen, C., Debaisieux, J. C., and Mizgalla, H. F.: Prognostic value of exercise testing soon after myocardial infarction. *N. Engl. J. Med.* 301:341–345, 1979.
76. Udall, J. A., and Ellestad, M. H.: Predictive implications of ventricular premature contractions associated with treadmill stress testing. *Circulation* 56:985-989, 1977.
77. Ungerleider, H. E.: The prognostic implications of the electrocardiogram. *Am. J. Cardiol.* 2:35–44, 1960.
78. Urie, P. M., Burgess, M. J., Lux, R. L., Wyatt, R. F., and Abildskore, J. A.: The electrocardiographic recognition of cardiac states at high risk of ventricular arrhythmias. An experimental study in dogs. *Circ. Res.* 42:350–358, 1978.
79. Vandepol, C. J., Farshidi, A., Spielman, S. R., Greenspan, A. M., Horowitz, L. N., and Josephson, M. E.: Incidence and clinical significance of induced ventricular tachycardia. *Am. J. Cardiol.* 45:725–731, 1980.
80. Vismara, L. A., Amsterdam, E. A., and Mason, D. T.: Relation of ventricular arrhythmias in the late hospital phase of acute myocardial infarction to sudden death after hospital discharge. *Am. J. Med.* 59:6–10, 1975.
81. Vismara, L. A., Pratt, C., Price, J. E., et al.: Correlation of the standard electrocardiogram and continuous ambulatory monitoring in the detection of ventricular arrhythmias in coronary patients. *J. Electrocardiol.* 10:299-304, 1977.
82. Weaver, W. D., Cobb, L. A., and Hallstrom, A. P.: Ambulatory arrhythmias in resuscitated victims of cardiac arrest. *Circulation* 66:212–218, 1982.
83. Winkle, R. A., Lopes, M. C., Fitzgerald, J. W., et al.: Arrhythmias in patients with mitral valve prolapse. *Circulation* 52:73–81, 1975.

24

Ventricular Ectopic Beats: Are They Important?

PAUL K. WHELTON
The Johns Hopkins University School of Hygiene and Public Health, The Johns Hopkins University School of Medicine, and The Johns Hopkins Hospital, Baltimore, Maryland

The "intermittent pulse" has been a recognized physical finding since the second century B.C. Observers such as Galan (132-201 A.D.) identified an intermittent pulse as an ominous prognostic indicator long before it was known that extrasystoles accounted for most such cases (15). Following the introduction of string galvanometry by Einthoven in 1906, it became practical to classify cardiac rhythm disturbances into those that are supraventricular in origin and those that result from ventricular irritability. The latter disturbance was identified as being primarily due to the occurrence of ventricular ectopic beats (VEBs) and these were electrocardiographically characterized by the presence of (a) a premature, bizarre QRST complex with a widened QRS, and a T wave which points in the opposite direction; (b) no associated preceding P wave; and (c) a compensatory pause until the emergence of the next normal sinus beat. With the advent and widespread utilization of resting and, more recently, exercise and ambulatory electrocardiography there has been an explosion in the number of publications related to ventricular ectopy. The following chapter reviews some of the most important studies and an attempt will be made to summarize opinion about the risk implications of VEBs in different clinical settings.

PREVALENCE

Ventricular ectopy is a common rhythm disturbance, present in 1-15% of resting 12-lead electrocardiograms performed in apparently healthy subjects (2,6,26,34,36,41) and approximately 80% of myocardial infarction survivors monitored in the cardiac care unit (23). In addition to the duration and circumstances of electrocardiographic monitoring, a variety of factors influence the prevalence of VEBs. The most important of these are age, sex, the presence or absence of coronary heart disease, medication use, and certain environmental exposures such as cigarette smoking, caffeine consumption, and alcohol intake (2,4,6,10,38,41,51). Age is a dominant variable which results in an exponential rate of rise in VEB prevalence after the fourth to fifth decade. Sex has an important but somewhat less dominant effect which becomes most apparent in middle-aged and elderly subjects. A two- to fourfold increase in the prevalence of VEBs has been reported in subjects with overt coronary heart disease. Medication may either increase or decrease the prevalence of VEBs depending on which drug is being administered. Some environmental exposures such as cigarette smoking, coffee drinking, and alcohol intake are positively related to VEB prevalence but these effects are usually only recognized in large studies.

RISK IMPLICATIONS

The prognosis of VEBs occurring during resting or ambulatory electrocardiography is an important and controversial issue. The previously mentioned factors which influence VEB prevalence must be taken into account during any interpretation of risk. This is particularly the case for dominant variables since a VEB risk association could easily be confounded by the effects of age, sex, or the presence of coronary heart disease. In this instance VEBs might be a useful marker of risk but make no independent contribution to the risk. In the following sections the overall and independent risk contributions of VEBs in varying clinical circumstances will be reviewed.

Myocardial Infarction Survivors

Much of the early interest in VEB-related risk evolved from experience in coronary care units. Continuous monitoring of hospitalized acute myocardial infarction survivors facilitated the detection of electrocardiographic changes prior to subsequent morbidity or mortality. Experience in this setting identified ventricular ectopic beats as a precursor of more serious cardiac arrhythmias and sudden death (24). Likewise, suppression of ventricular ectopic beats in such patients was reported to prevent a subsequent progression to ventricular tachycardia, ventricular fibrillation, and sudden death. Since many subjects who died soon after an acute myocardial infarction were noted to have a paucity of pathological changes, it was suggested that ventricular ectopy might be a forerunner of sudden death in a large number of patients with acute myocardial infarction. This view was supported by information gathered during the early days of electrocardiographic monitoring in ambulatory and coronary care unit settings (8).

Following these initial inpatient studies, interest shifted to the larger group of ambulatory subjects with known coronary heart disease. This issue was addressed in considerable detail by the Coronary Drug Project Research Group (4). They reported on the relationship between VEBs recorded on a resting 12-lead electrocardiogram and subsequent mortality in ambulatory acute myocardial infarction survivors. Slightly more than 2,000 placebo-treated men aged 30–65 years were studied after a minimum postinfarction survival period of 3 months. Each participant had New York Heart Association functional class 1 or 2 heart disease and was free of recent worsening of symptoms at the time of study. A baseline 12-lead electrocardiogram was recorded in the conventional manner at the first visit and participants were subsequently evaluated for 3-years. Two hundred and thirty-five (11.5%) of the 2,035 studied had one or more ventricular ectopic beats in their baseline electrocardiogram (Table 1). During the 3-year follow-up period the men with baseline ventricular ectopy had almost twice the death rate (21.7%) experienced by those with no apparent ventricular ectopic beats (11.4%). Likewise, as shown in Table 1, baseline ventricular ectopy was associated with close to a doubling in sudden death mortality (9.8% vs. 4.9%). The excess in mortality risk was apparent during each of the 3 years of

Table 1 Three-Year Mortality in 2,035 Placebo-Treated Myocardial Infarction Survivors

12-Lead ECG findings	% Prevalence (number of men)	% Total mortality	% Sudden death
No VPB	88.5 (1,800)	11.4	4.9
Any VPB	11.5 (235)	21.7[a]	9.8
⩾VPB/100 complexes	2.2 (45)	24.4[b]	15.6[a]
VPB pairs or runs	0.5 (10)	40.0	10.0
VPB T-R interval			
<0.20 sec	0.2 (51)	31.4	11.8
⩾0.20 sec	8.4 (171)	19.3	11.7

[a]<0.01
[b]<0.05
Source: Adapted from Ref. 4.

follow-up. Multivariate analyses with up to 31 other factors suggested an independent relationship between ventricular ectopy and subsequent mortality risk. Certain characteristics, including the frequency of VEBs, the presence of VEB pairs or runs, and possibly the presence of early cycle VEBs appeared to be useful in the identification of infarct survivors with the greatest risk of subsequent mortality. In keeping with results of most other studies, supraventricular ectopic beats did not appear to be associated with any increase in overall or cause-specific mortality.

In a substudy of 160 coronary drug project patients, Kotler et al. performed Holter monitoring on four to five occasions at one center (21). Eighty percent of the patients had ventricular ectopic beats on at least one tape recording. In keeping with the previously described results, these authors reported an impressive relationship between VEBs and sudden death especially in the presence of ventricular ectopy that was frequent, multifocal, or accompanied by runs of ventricular tachycardia. Thus 12 of 87 patients (13.8%) with frequent (⩾ 10 VEBs/hr) or complex ventricular ectopy as compared to only 2 of 66 patients (3%) with absent or infrequent VEBs were sudden death victims ($p<0.03$). The risk of ventricular ectopy appeared to be independent of other known cardiovascular risk predictors.

In a more recent study of 1,739 male survivors of myocardial infarction, Rubermann et al. reported that ventricular ectopy recorded during 1 hr of electrocardiographic monitoring was associated with an increase in overall and sudden death mortality (38). As in the previously mentioned reports, ventricular ectopy was an independent contributor to the risk of overall or sudden death. However, in this study all of the risk appeared to result from an excess of deaths in patients with complex ventricular ectopy (runs, bigeminy, multifocal, or R-on-T beats). After 3 years of follow-up the cumulative all-causes and sudden death mortality was increased by 90% and 156%, respectively, in patients with frequent (⩾10/hr) and complex VEBs. Other studies that have employed longer periods of ambulatory monitoring in myocardial infarction survivors have almost uniformly identified VEBs as a useful risk predictor in the individual patient (40,44). Data on the implications of ventricular ectopy in patients with nonischemic disorders are limited but tend to suggest that VEBs are a risk predictor in subjects with cardiomyopathy and congestive heart failure (7,27,39).

Insured Persons

The prognosis of VEBs in less-selected samples than those described above is less clear. Some of the earliest relevant information comes from the insurance industry (25). In 1963 Lyle reported on a 27-year follow-up of 11,000 Prudential home-office employees (26). Premature beats (supraventricular and ventricular beats) were noted in approximately 10% of the employees. Of these, almost three-quarters had simple premature beats while the remainder had one or more variant characteristics (pairs, runs, bigeminy, multifocal beats, post-extrasystolic T-wave inversion, or abnormal conduction of supraventricular beats). During the follow-up period a total of 258 employees died. When compared to Prudential's standard insurance experience, those with premature beats were noted to have a slight but definite increase in mortality risk. The risk was higher in employees with variant beats and in persons with other cardiovascular risk factors. The risk of premature beats was apparent in female patients, albeit at a lower level than in male patients. A similar trend had previously been reported in somewhat smaller groups of insured persons by both Brandon et al. and Kirkland et al. (1,20).

In a subsequent study, Rodstein et al. examined the insurance experience of 712 persons with premature beats who were evaluated for an average of 18 years (37). These authors reported no appreciable increase in the observed/expected mortality ratio of the 604 persons who were considered to have a normal life expectancy except for the presence of extrasystoles. This overall finding was true both for those with ventricular as well as supraventricular arrhythmias and for those above and below the age of 40 years. However, the finding of ventricular ectopy in subjects with other abnormalities was associated with an increase in the observed/expected mortality ratio. For instance a mortality ratio of 223% was noted in the 42 subjects with VEBs in the setting of an insurance rating of high blood pressure or cardiac disease, whereas the corresponding ratio for those without the rating was 131% ($p<0.05$). The trend toward an increase in mortality ratio for subjects with other insurance abnormalities was more apparent in those with complex (pairs, bigeminy or trigeminy, multifocal beats, R-on-T beats, or postextrasystolic T-wave inversion) than simple VEBs. There were too few cases to allow the authors to determine with certainty which forms of complexity were most dangerous. The mortality ratio was also increased in those with frequent extrasystoles, particularly in subjects aged ≥45 years. Supraventricular beats appeared to play little if any role in the increased mortality of high-risk persons with premature beats. Thus 34 patients who died from acute myocardial infarction had a record of ventricular ectopic beats whereas supraventricular ectopics were only noted in 4. Likewise only 2 of 24 sudden death victims had antecedent supraventricular ectopic beats.

Selected and Unselected Community Samples

Additional information on the risks of VEBs has been generated in a variety of community settings. One of the earliest and best known community-based reports was published by Chiang et al. (2). Between 1959 and 1960 they obtained a resting 12-lead electrocardiogram on 85% of the residents of Tecumseh, Michigan. Morbidity and mortality of the 5,129 persons examined were carefully tracked over the next 4-6 years and the relationship of premature beats to such events was identified. At the initial examination coronary heart disease was found to be significantly more prevalent in subjects >30 years with ventricular ectopy than in their age-matched counterparts without VEBs ($p<0.05$). Likewise, the 6-year age-adjusted incidence of sudden death was significantly increased ($p<0.01$) in those with (61/1,000 persons) compared to those without (21/1,000 persons) VEBs. Multiple regression suggested that the presence of VEBs identified a sudden death risk in addition to and independent of that identified by more traditional cardiovascular risk factors. It must be stressed that more than three-quarters of the sudden deaths occurred in the larger group without VEBs on their baseline electrocardiogram. In addition, the risk of VEBs was most apparent in patients in the oldest age ranges studied. Six of the 10 sudden deaths in the group with antecedent VEBs occurred in subjects older than 70 years. It has also been suggested that only 1 of the 45 sudden death victims was in entirely normal health before death (15). Thus, while VEBs appeared to be an overall predictor of risk, this risk seemed to vary considerably depending on other covariables such as age, sex, and general health and VEBs per se may not have been important cardiovascular risk predictors (3). By implication, the risk experience encountered in Tecumseh may not be representative of that which might apply to subjects whose sole cardiovascular abnormality is the incidental finding of VEBs.

Hinkle et al. performed 6-hr ambulatory monitoring on an organizationally stratified sample of 301 actively employed men who were randomly selected from a 6-year age cohort born between 1902 and 1908 (11). When the men were initially examined in 1963–1964 their median age was 58 years. Sixty-two percent had one or more VEBs on their 6-hr recording and almost 9% had ⩾10 VEBs/1,000 complexes. There was a significant relationship ($p<0.01$) between the frequency of VEBs and the presence of coronary heart disease or risk of developing coronary heart disease. A similar trend was apparent for those with complex forms of VEBs (bigeminy, trigeminy, pairs, multifocal beats, and paroxysmal ventricular tachycardia). However, because of the small numbers involved, this latter trend was only significant for the presence of bigeminy. During a 6-year period of follow-up there were a total of 32 (11%) deaths of which 17 (6%) were due to coronary heart disease and 9 (3%) occurred suddenly. Coronary deaths were significantly more common ($p<0.01$) among the men with antecedent VEBs, especially for those with ⩾10 VEBs/1,000 beats. Complex forms of VEBs were also associated with an increase in risk, and in the case of ventricular bigeminy this was significant ($p<0.005$). It is not clear how much of the apparent increase in risk due to ventricular ectopy could be ascribed to the demonstrated increase in coronary heart disease prevalence in those with VEBs.

In a more recent publication, Rabkin et al. reported on the relationship between VEBs during routine electrocardiography and subsequent cardiovascular disease in a cohort of 3,983 male Canadian air pilots free of overt heart disease who were followed for 29 years (34). These investigators noted a relationship between ventricular ectopy and overall ischemic heart disease incidence, especially in subjects whose VEBs were noted in the fourth and fifth decades of life (Table 2). The relationship between ventricular ectopy and cardiovascular disease was strongest for sudden death where the age-adjusted relative risk for the entire cohort was 3.96 (33). VEB frequency and the configuration characteristics studied did not appear to influence the risk of ischemic heart disease or sudden death. However, the combination of VEBs with either ST-T wave abnormalities or left ventricular hypertrophy was associated with an impressive increase in relative risk (13.0 and 19.23, respectively), although the estimates were based on rather small numbers. Fifty (71%) of the seventy sudden death victims had antecedent abnormalities on one or more of their resting electrocardiograms. ST-T wave changes (71%), ventricular ectopy (23%), and left ventricular hypertrophy (19%) accounted for the vast majority of the anomalies noted. The study has been criticized because a 24-hr rather than a 1-hr interval was used to define sudden death, and because important covariables such as blood

Table 2 Relative Risk of Ischemic Heart Disease During 2526 Person-Years of Follow-Up After Detection of Ventricular Ectopy in Apparently Health Men

	Age (years)		
	40–49	50–59	60–69
Any ischemic heart disease[a]	1.65	1.80	0.87
Sudden death	1.05	4.20	3.28

[a]Includes myocardial infarction, suspected myocardial infarction, coronary insufficiency, angina pectoris, and sudden death.
Source: Adapted from Ref. 34.

pressure, blood lipid levels, cigarette smoking, physical activity, behavioral type, and certain electrocardiographic abnormalities were not included in multivariate analyses (15). Thus, the results obtained strongly support the concept that VEBs are important predictors of cardiovascular risk even in apparently healthy middle-aged men. However, the value of VEBs as independent risk predictors in otherwise healthy subjects remains controversial.

In contrast to the experience of Chiang, Hinkle, and Rabkin, several investigators have reported an inability to recognize ischemic heart disease or sudden death risk in otherwise healthy subjects with VEBs. For instance, Fisher and Tyroler could find no overall VEB risk association during an 11-year follow-up of 1,214 white factory employees aged 35-69 years (16). This was the case for sudden death victims, whether a 1- or 24-hr period was used for classification, and also for an analysis of all coronary heart disease deaths. Subgroup analysis did suggest that the mortality risk was increased for those with baseline VEBs and aged 50–59 years at the initial examination. This was especially the case for those with VEBs and other electrocardiographic changes. However, these subgroup analyses were based on small numbers. In keeping with the experience of Fisher and Tyroler, Rose et al. could find little evidence of a relationship between frequent premature beats (⩾10% of all beats; Minnesota Code 8_1) and coronary heart disease deaths in a group of 18,403 male civil servants aged 40-64 years at their initial exam (36). This was true for both symptomatic (N=49) and asymptomatic (N=200) subjects classified with an 8_1 code. In a further analysis these authors compared the prevalence of VEBs in a selected group of 165 civil servants who died from coronary heart disease and 165 age-matched survivors. The selection criteria excluded subjects with symptomatic coronary heart disease and those with Q/QS, ST, T, or left bundle branch block changes identified by use of the Minnesota code. Among these "low-risk" subjects there was no difference in the prevalence of VEBs in either group. As with other population-based investigations, this study indicated that the predictive value of an electrocardiographic change is usually highly dependent on the presence or absence of other indicators of coronary heart disease. Thus, one must be cautious about generalizing risk results obtained in free-living asymptomatic "normals" to the clinical care setting (where one is often treating subjects with a more abnormal cardiovascular system) or vice versa.

The importance of the clinical setting was also emphasized in a report by Tunstall-Pedoe (41). In this study a variety of baseline electrocardiographic findings were related to the rate of sudden death in three groups of subjects: (a) 311 myocardial infarction survivors; (b) a relatively unselected sample of 9,166 employed men, and (c) a subsample composed of the 8,228 employed men who were asymptomatic. There was, as expected, a strong tendency toward better prognosis in asymptomatic subjects. The primary electrocardiographic predictors of sudden death were those commonly accepted as indicators of ischemia such as Q, ST, and T wave changes. However, disturbances of rhythm and rate as well as ventricular conduction defects appeared to be important in the presence of established coronary heart disease.

Kannel et al. have recently reported on the epidemiological features of sudden death during a 26-year follow-up of 5,209 Framingham residents (18). No prior coronary heart disease was apparent in 50% of 147 male and 70% of 50 female sudden death victims. In persons of both sexes, the overall risk of sudden death was impressively influenced by traditional cardiovascular risk factors. In respect to electrocardiographic changes, VEBs appeared to be less important than other commonly associated findings such as left ventricular hypertrophy and intraventricular block. However, in the presence of overt coronary heart disease the risk of sudden death increased ninefold and arrhythmias, other electrocardiographic changes, and poor cardiac function became important risk predictors.

Frequent/Complex VEBs in Apparently Healthy Subjects

The previously cited insurance and community-based studies, as well as a considerable body of additional evidence, indicate that VEBs sometimes occur in apparently healthy young subjects and that the prognosis in this setting is quite different from that when the host is older and sicker (11,18,36,37,41). In an interesting study, Horan and Kennedy evaluated a group of 72 asymptomatic subjects with frequent (>100/hr) and complex (multifocal or repetitive) VEBs for up to 8 years (16). Despite the frequency and complexity of the ventricular ectopy observed, no deaths occurred during the follow-up period. The results of this study again indicate that ventricular ectopy, even if frequent and complex, is not necessarily associated with a dramatic increase in sudden death risk when it occurs in young and healthy persons.

VEBs DURING DIURETIC THERAPY

Several investigators have reported an increased frequency of ventricular ectopy during diuretic treatment of otherwise healthy patients with essential hypertension. The relationship has been reported during treatment of average patients in the community (47,50) as well as in more selected samples treated in hospital outpatient departments (12,13). Circumstantial evidence supporting the presence of a thiazide-related risk has also surfaced from two recently completed large clinical trials (14,30). Despite these reports, several investigators have failed to identify an increase in VEB frequency during diuretic therapy, and the proposed association remains controversial (9). Evidence for and against the association is presented in more detail in Chapters 18-22 and 38.

Although the public health implications of such an association are substantial, any adverse effects during chronic thiazide administration are probably subtle and can only be recognized in a large placebo-controlled trial. The overall and sudden death rate experience in the Medical Research Council Trial of treatment in mild to moderate hypertension may be helpful in defining such implications (28).

The possibility that VEBs may result from thiazide diuretic administration is an appropriate cause for concern but several points should be emphasized. First, diuretics have been the mainstay of drug therapy in each of the large trials of antihypertensive treatment performed to date (17,35,42,43). In every one of these trials active, mainly thiazide,

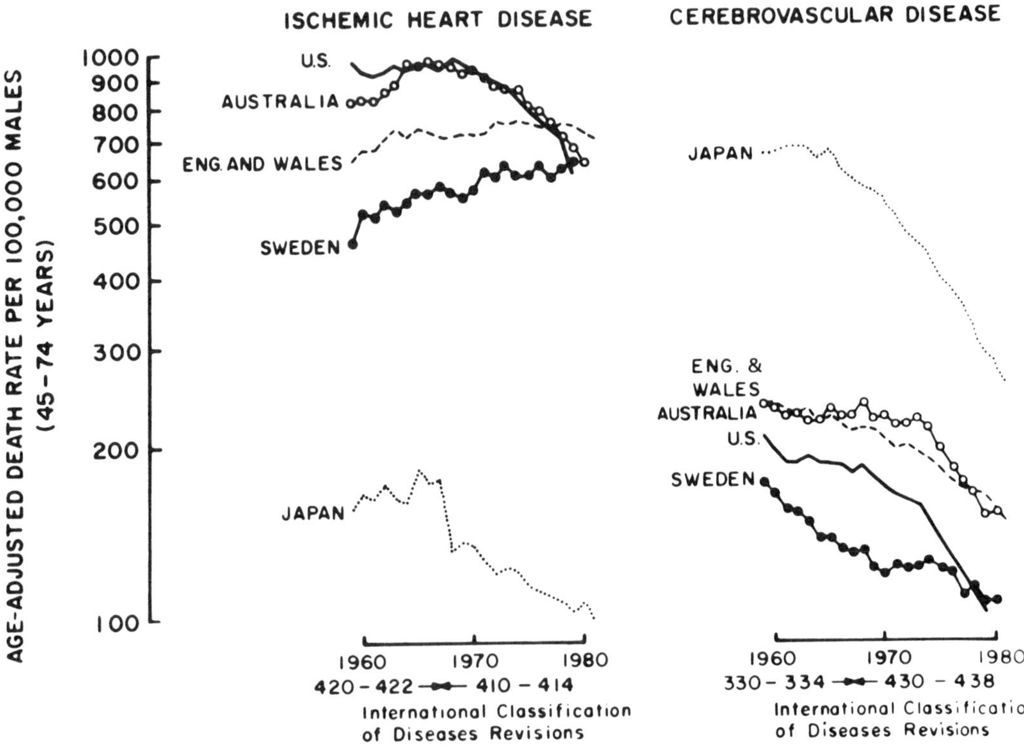

Figure 1 Secular trends in age-adjusted (45–74 years) mortality from coronary heart disease and stroke in men. Because of the well-known difficulties associated with interpretation of vital statistics (45), the trends presented can only serve as a rough approximation of the true changes in coronary heart and cerebrovascular disease mortality.

therapy has appeared to result in a substantial overall benefit. In a more general sense, the increasing use of antihypertensive therapy, primarily thiazide diuretics, probably accounts for an acceleration in the decline of stroke mortality in Western countries during the last two decades (45). Likewise, in some countries, including the United States and Japan, the death rate from coronary heart disease has decreased over the same time period, albeit to a lesser extent (48). The dramatic nature of the reduction in age-adjusted stroke and ischemic heart disease mortality in the United States is graphically outlined in Figure 1. Thus, while concern related to an arrhythmic potential of thiazides is appropriate, it must be viewed in a context where there is little doubt as to the overall benefit of antihypertensive therapy with thiazide diuretics (49).

SUMMARY

VEBs are a relatively common finding during routine electrocardiography especially in older men and those with underlying coronary heart disease. The risk implications of VEBs vary tremendously depending on the clinical setting in which they are recognized. Ventricular ectopy is an important predictor of overall cardiovascular and sudden death risk in subjects with established or presumed coronary heart disease. However, the risk of

VEBs in apparently healthy subjects is much more controversial and less important than other clinical findings or electrocardiographic indicators of myocardial ischemia and left ventricular hypertrophy. The existence and risk of diuretic-induced ventricular ectopy are also controversial. The risk, if any, is probably greatest for those with underlying coronary heart disease.

REFERENCES

1. Brandon, K. F., Neill, M. H., and Streeter, G. C.: The use of the electrocardiogram in twenty-five years of insurance selection. *Trans. Assoc. Life Insur. Med. Dir. Am.* 34:143–150, 1951.
2. Chiang, B. N., Perlman, L. V., Ostrander, L. D., Jr., and Epstein, F. H.: Relationship of premature systoles to coronary heart disease and sudden death in the Tecumseh epidemiologic study. *Ann. Intern. Med.* 70:1159–1166, 1969.
3. Chiang, B., Perlman, L., Fulton, M., Ostrander, L., and Epstein, F.: Predisposing factors in sudden cardiac death in Tecumseh, Michigan. *Circulation* 41:31–38, 1970.
4. Coronary Drug Project Research Group: Prognostic importance of premature beats following myocardial infarction: Experience in the Coronary Drug Project. *JAMA* 223:1116–1124, 1973.
5. Crow, R., Prineas, R., and Blackburn, H.: The prognostic significance of ventricular ectopic beats among the apparently healthy. *Am. Heart J.* 101:244–248, 1981.
6. Fisher, F. D., and Tyroler, H. A.: Relationship between ventricular premature contractions on routine electrocardiography and subsequent sudden death from coronary heart disease. *Circulation* 47:712–719, 1973.
7. Follansbee, W. P., Michaelson, E. L., and Morganroth, J.: Nonsustained ventricular tachycardia in ambulatory patients: Characteristics and association with sudden cardiac death. *Ann. Intern. Med.* 92:741–747, 1980.
8. Han, J.: Mechanisms of ventricular arrhythmias associated with myocardial infarction. *Am. J. Cardiol.* 24:800–813, 1969.
9. Harrington, J. T., Isner, J. M., and Kassirer, J. P.: Our national obsession with potassium. *Amer. J. Med.* 73:155–159, 1982.
10. Hennekens, C. H., Lown, B., Rosner, B., Grufferman, S., and Dalen, J.: Ventricular premature beats and coronary risk factors. *Am. J. Epidemiol.* 112:93–99, 1980.
11. Hinkle, L. E., Jr., Carver, S. T., and Stevens, M.: The frequency of asymptomatic disturbances of cardiac rhythm and conduction in middle-aged men. *Am. J. Cardiol.* 24:629–650, 1969.
12. Holland, O. B., Nixon, J. V., and Kuhnert, L.: Diuretic-induced ventricular ectopic activity. *Am. J. Med.* 70:762–768, 1981.
13. Hollifield, J. W., and Slaton, P. E.: Thiazide diuretics, hypokalemia and cardiac arrhythmias. *Acta Med. Scand.* (Suppl.) 647:67–73, 1981.
14. Holme, I., Helgeland, A., Hjermann, I., Leren, P., and Lund-Larsen, P. G.: Treatment of mild hypertension with diuretics. The importance of ECG abnormalities in the Oslo Study and in MRFIT. *JAMA* 251:1298–1299, 1984.
15. Horan, M. J., and Kennedy, H. L.: Ventricular ectopy. History, epidemiology, and clinical implications. *JAMA* 251:380–386, 1984.
16. Horan, M., Kennedy, H.: Characteristics and prognosis of apparently healthy patients with frequency and complex ventricular ectopy: Evidence for a relatively benign new syndrome with occult myocardial and/or coronary disease. *Am. Heart J.* 102:809–810, 1981.
17. Hypertension Detection and Follow-up Program: Five-year findings of the hypertension detection and follow-up program. *JAMA* 242:2562–2577, 1979.
18. Kannel, W. B., McGee, D. L., and Schatzkin, A.: An epidemiological perspective of

sudden death: 26-year follow-up in the Framingham Study. *Drugs* 28 (Suppl 1):1-16, 1984.

19. Kaplan, N. M.: Therapy of mild hypertension: An overview. *Am. J. Cardiol.* 53: 2A-8A, 1984.
20. Kirkland, H. B., Kiessling, C. E., and Lyle, A. M.: The evaluation of certain fundamental electrocardiographic patterns in the selection of insurance risks. *Trans. Am. Life Insur. Med. Dir. Am.* 35:86-134, 1951.
21. Kotler, M. N., Tabatznik, B., Mower, M. M., and Tominaga, S.: Prognostic significance of ventricular ectopic beats with respect to sudden death in the late post-infarction period. *Circulation* 47:959-966, 1973.
22. Lief, P. D., Belizon, I., Matos, J., and Bank, N.: Diuretic-induced hypokalemia does not cause ventricular ectopy in uncomplicated essential hypertension. *Kidney Int.* 25:203, 1984.
23. Lown, B., Vassaux, C., Hood, W. B. Jr., Fakhro, A. M., Kaplinsky, E., and Roberge, G.: Unresolved problems in coronary care. *Am. J. Cardiol.* 20:494-508, 1967.
24. Lown, B., and Wolf, M.: Approaches to sudden death from coronary heart disease. *Circulation* 44:130-142, 1971.
25. Lyle, A. M.: A study of premature beats by electrocardiogram. *Trans. Soc. Actuaries* 14:493-507, 1953.
26. Lyle, A. M.: Coronary disease as an underwriting problem. *Trans. Soc. Actuaries* 15:324-350, 1963.
27. Maron, B. J., Savage, D. D., Wolfson, J. K., and Epstein, S. E.: Prognostic significance of 24 hour ambulatory electrocardiographic monitoring in patients with hypertropic cardiomyopathy: A prospective study. *Am. J. Cardiol.* 48:252-257, 1981.
28. Medical Research Council Working Party on Mild to Moderate Hypertension: Randomized controlled trial of treatment for mild hypertension: Design and pilot trial. *Br. Med. J.* 1:1437-1440, 1977.
29. Morgan, T. O., Adam, W. R., Hodgson, M., and Gibberd, R. W.: Failure of therapy to improve prognosis in elderly males with hypertension. *Med. J. Aust.* 2:27-31, 1980.
30. Multiple Risk Factor Intervention Trial Research Group: Multiple Risk Factor Intervention Trial. Risk factor changes and mortality results. *JAMA* 248:1465-1477, 1982.
31. Papademetriou, V., Fletcher, R., Khatri, I. M., and Freis, E. D.: Diuretic-induced hypokalemia in uncomplicated systemic hypertension: Effect of plasma potassium correction on cardiac arrhythmias. *Am. J. Cardiol.* 52:1017-1022, 1983.
32. Poole-Wilson, P. A.: Potassium, diuretics and heart muscle. In *Electrolytes and the Heart,* edited by Wester Per, O., New York, Transmedica, 1983, pp. 57-62.
33. Rabkin, S. W., Mathewson, F. A. L., and Tate, R. B.: The electrocardiogram in apparently healthy men and the risk of sudden death. *Br. Heart J.* 47:546-552, 1982.
34. Rabkin, S. W., Mathewson, F. A. L., and Tate, R. B.: Relationship of ventricular ectopy in men without apparent heart disease to occurrence of ischemic heart disease and sudden death. *Am. Heart J.* 101:135-142, 1981.
35. Reader, R.: The Australian therapeutic trial in mild hypertension: Report by the management committee. *Lancet* 1:1261-1267, 1980.
36. Rose, G., Baxter, P. J., Reid, D. D., and McCartney, P.: Prevalence and prognosis of electrocardiographic findings in middle-aged men. *Br. Heart J.* 40:636-643, 1978.
37. Rodstein, M., Wolloch, L., and Gubner, R. S.: Mortality study of the significance of extrasystoles in an insured population. *Circulation* 44:617-625, 1971.
38. Ruberman, W., Weinblatt, E., Goldberg, J. D., Frand, C. W., and Shapiro, S.: Ventricular premature beats and mortality after myocardial infarction. *N. Engl. J. Med.* 297:750-757, 1977.

39. Stapleton, J. F., Segal, J. P., and Harvey, W. P.: The electrocardiogram of myocardipathy. *Prog. Cardiovasc. Dis.* 13:217–239, 1970.
40. Taylor, G. J., Humphries, J. O., Mellits, E. D., Pitt, B., Schulze, R. A., Griffith, L. S. C., and Achuff, S. C.: Predictors of clinical course, coronary anatomy and left ventricular function after recovery from acute myocardial infarction. *Circulation* 62:960–970, 1980.
41. Tunstall Pedoe, H. D.: Predictability of sudden death from resting electrocardiogram: Effect of previous manifestations of coronary heart disease. *Br. Heart J.* 40: 630–635, 1978.
42. Veterans Administration Cooperative Study Group on Antihypertensive Agents: Effects of treatment on morbidity in hypertension. I. Results in patients with diastolic blood pressures averaging 115 through 129 mmHg. *JAMA* 202:1028–1034, 1967.
43. Veterans Administration Cooperative Study Group on Antihypertensive Agents: Effects of treatment on morbidity in hypertension. II. Results in patient with diastolic blood pressure averaging 90 through 114 mmHg. *JAMA* 213:1143–1152, 1970.
44. Vismara, L. A., Amsterdam, E. A., and Mason, D. T.: Relation of ventricular arrhythmias in the late hospital phase of acute myocardial infarction to sudden death after hospital discharge. *Am. J. Med.* 59:6–12, 1975.
45. Whelton, P. K.: Declining mortality from hypertension and stroke. *South. Med. J.* 75:33–38, 1982.
46. Whelton, P. K.: Thiazide induced hypokalemia—an epidemiologic prospective. In *Electrolytes and the Heart,* edited by Wester Per, O., New York, Transmedica, 1983, pp. 77–81.
47. Whelton, P. K.: Diuretics and arrhythmias in the Medical Research Council Trial. *Drugs* 28 (Suppl 1):54–65, 1984.
48. Whelton, P. K.: Essential hypertension—therapeutic implications of epidemiologic risk estimation. *Hypertension* 2 (Suppl 2):3–8, 1984.
49. Whelton, P. K.: Systemic Hypertension, Diuretic Drugs, Arrhythmias and Death. *Am. J. Cardiol.* 55:221–222, 1985.
50. Whelton, P. K., Brennan, P. J., Greenberg, G., Miall, W. E., Raftery, E. B., and Subramanian, B., for Medical Research Council Working Party on Mild to Moderate Hypertension: Ventricular extrasystoles during thiazide treatment: Sub-study of MRC mild hypertension trial. *Br. Med. J.* 287:1249–1253, 1983.
51. Winkle, R. A.: Ambulatory electrocardiography and the diagnosis, evaluation, and treatment of chronic ventricular arrhythmias. *Prog. Cardiovasc. Dis.* 23:99–128, 1980.

POTASSIUM IN BLOOD PRESSURE HOMEOSTASIS

25

Hypokalemia in the Surgical and Anesthetized Patient

RICHARD J. SOLOMON
Brown University Program in Medicine, Roger Williams General Hospital, and Veterans Administration Medical Center, Providence, Rhode Island

The routine preoperative evaluation of patients scheduled for surgery includes an assessment of serum electrolytes. This practice is based on the generally accepted understanding that severe electrolyte abnormalities increase the risks associated with anesthesia and surgery and interfere with the postoperative recovery of patients. Despite the widespread acceptance of this position, there is relatively little literature on the relative risks of mild electrolyte disturbances. This review will focus on the importance of *hypokalemia* in the management of the surgical and anesthetized patient.

Hypokalemia represents a common occurrence in both medical and surgical patients. An incidence as high as 50% has been reported in some series of acutely ill patients (24). Such hypokalemia may occur as a result of chronic gastrointestinal losses or renal losses secondary to diuretic therapy. However, of equal clinical significance is the hypokalemia that results from shifts of potassium from the extracellular to the intracellular compartment, an effect mediated by catecholamines (3,28,38,41). This effect accounts for the observation that the hypokalemia, observed in many acutely ill patients at the time of admission, gradually returns to normal levels over the first few days of hospitalization even in the absence of potassium replacement (24). Catecholamines are released during all kinds of stress, including physical pain and trauma (36) and surgery (10). The shift of potassium to intracellular stores usually produces a fall of 0.5 mEq/L or less in the serum level of potassium. The reduction in serum potassium is maintained until the stress levels of catecholamines return to normal. However, in more stressful situations, such as myocardial infarction (15,27) or head trauma (6,26), the fall in serum potassium can be as great as 1.0 mEq/L.

These shifts result from specific stimulation of the β_2 adrenoceptors, predominately on skeletal muscle, and can be reproduced by the administration of exogenous β_2 agonists (28,41). For example, salbutamol and terbutaline, both of which are used to delay premature labor, have been associated with the development of significant hypokalemia (2,5,7,18,21,25,40,41). While the serum potassium usually returns to normal as the serum levels of β-agonist fall, hypokalemia persisted for up to 3 hr following termination of infusions of terbutaline (14). This effect on serum potassium may be clinically useful.

For example, salbutamol has been found to be effective in lowering the elevated serum potassium of dialysis patients. Following 0.5 mg of intravenous salbutamol, serum potassium levels fell from 5.5 to 4.4 mEq/L within 30 min, an effect similar to that obtained with insulin and glucose infusions (23).

The movement of potassium into the cell is opposed by α-adrenoceptor stimulation (44). The net effect on serum potassium in any given circumstance in which catecholamines are elevated will depend upon the relative stimulation of β and α adrenoreceptors (45). For example, in the presence of elevated circulating catecholamines, blockade of the β_2 adrenoceptor may actually lead to hyperkalemia (28).

Hypokalemia may be an important contributor to the development of arrhythmias in many patients. It is not within the scope of this paper to discuss the evidence for this. It should be appreciated, however, that not all patients are at equal risk. Patients with underlying ischemic heart disease, cardiomyopathies, and who use digitalis represent a group most at risk and therefore the group in which particular efforts should be made to correct the electrolyte disturbance prior to surgery (vide infra). Efforts to prevent further falls in serum potassium are thus important. Discontinuation of diuretics prior to surgery may be helpful. Hypokalemia can be exacerbated by mechanical ventilation. A 0.5-mEq/L fall in serum potassium for each 10-torr decrease in $PaCO_2$ is observed acutely (46). Serious cardiac arrhythmias have been described during prolonged mechanical ventilation (17). These arrhythmias can be particularly refractory to treatment (47). Arrhythmias are also more common during the postoperative period in the presence of hypokalemia, particularly when alkalosis is also present (34,37).

However, the potential hazard of an arrhythmia during anesthesia and surgery is but one of the consequences of hypokalemia. The postoperative course of patients may also be adversely affected even in the absence of arrhythmias. Severe hypokalemia ($K = <3.0$ mEq/L) may produce weakness of respiratory muscles, contributing to atelectasis and/or difficulties in weaning patients from ventilatory support (16). Even if clinically not debilitated, patients with hypokalemia are probably more sensitive to the paralyzing properties of the nondepolarizing muscle relaxants (11,43). This conclusion is drawn from animal studies that have shown a direct correlation between D-tubocurarine ED50 (43) or pencuronium ED90 (22) and the extracellular potassium concentration.

Smooth muscle function is likewise impaired. Decreases in gastrointestinal peristalsis may contribute to postsurgical ileus and prolong the need for parenteral nutritional support (16). Furthermore, gastric atony and dilation may predispose to pulmonary aspiration of gastric contents. Similar impairment in bladder smooth muscle may produce incontinence or urinary retention, which will complicate the postsurgical recovery of the patient (30). Severe and prolonged hypokalemia may interfere with the kidneys' ability to conserve water (31). The resultant polyuria will complicate fluid management in the critically ill patient. Glucose homeostasis is also adversely affected by hypokalemia (29). Insulin release is diminished in response to a glucose load, and the resulting hyperglycemia will contribute further to polyuria and fluid imbalance. Hypokalemia also impairs the pressor response to catecholamines and angiotensin, which will interfere with the postural maintenance of blood pressure (4). This may interfere with the patient's ability to ambulate in the postoperative period.

HYPOKALEMIA AND INTERACTION WITH ANESTHETIC AGENTS

As noted above, hypokalemia is associated with increased sensitivity to the paralyzing properties of muscle relaxants (43). Additionally, more anticholinesterase is necessary to satisfactorily reverse the nondepolarizing neuromuscular-blocking drugs (22). In the event that administration of epinephrine is necessary, the complex interactions with potassium should be recalled. Epinephrine not only reduces serum potassium further (28,41), but hypokalemia per se reduces the threshold for epinephrine-induced arrhythmias (1), particularly in the presence of digitalis (12). It should be remembered that succinylcholine produces a transient increase in serum potassium (9). This increase is enhanced and prolonged in the presence of nonselective β-blockade (20). Particular care must therefore be given to the administration of potassium-containing solutions when succinylcholine is to be used.

MANAGEMENT

It is important to stress that despite the evidence that hypokalemia is associated with an increased risk for the development of arrhythmias, there is little literature in the anesthetized-surgical patient to indicate the relative risks (42,48). For example, hypokalemia is a frequent occurrence during cardiopulmonary bypass and hemodilution, and electrocardiographic abnormalities as well as arrhythmias have been described (19,49). However, there is little evidence that hypokalemia occurring in this setting adversely affects the hospital course of such patients (49).

Nevertheless, a conservative approach, particularly in patients at risk for arrhythmias, is warranted. If administration of potassium salts is considered necessary, potassium chloride rather than any of the alkaline salts should be used. When potassium is administered as the alkaline salt, more potassium ions will move intracellularly then when potassium is given as the chloride salt. This difference is probably related to the fact that the cell membrane is not very permeable to chloride. The maximum recommended rate of replacement is 0.5-0.7 mEq/kg per hr given in a concentration of 80-120 mEq/L (39). The rate of infusion must be carefully monitored so as not to accidently flush a large amount of potassium into the patient with the consequence of sudden hyperkalemia. It should be remembered that there are only 63 mEq of potassium in the entire extracellular space. A sudden infusion of 63 mEq could quickly double the serum level of potassium. Because β agonists and insulin both play an important role in the movement of potassium into cells, deficiencies of either of these humoral systems will result in higher serum potassium levels for a given rate of potassium infusion (28). Thus, patients with insulin-dependent diabetes and those receiving nonselective β blockers are particularly susceptible to hyperkalemia during potassium infusions. Endogenous release of norepinephrine during surgery would also tend to antagonize the movement of potassium into cells through stimulation of α adrenoceptors (44). This might further increase the risks associated with the administration of potassium-containing solutions during surgery (35).

Once the serum potassium level exceeds 3.0 mEq/L and the electrocardiographic indexes have returned to normal, it is safe to proceed with general anesthesia. When potassium-containing solutions are to be continued during surgery, they should be given through a secondary intravenous line to avoid sudden bolus injections of potassium. Monitoring of the electrocardiogram and urine output are considered particularly important in this setting.

While there are no specifically indicated anesthetic techniques for dealing with the hypokalemic patient, it is best to avoid those techniques and drugs that are associated with a higher incidence of arrhythmias, e.g., halothane, exogenous catecholamines, atropine. The dose of muscle relaxant must be adjusted for the expectation of increased sensitivity (43). Excessive hyperventilation should be avoided to limit respiratory alkalosis and a possible exacerbation of the hypokalemia (46). Careful replacement of

Table 1 Electrolyte Concentration in Gastrointestinal Fluids

Gastrointestinal fluid	Sodium (mEq/L)	Potassium (mEq/L)
Gastric	20–80	10–15
Pancreatic	140	5
Biliary	148	5
Small bowel	80–110	5
Large bowel	120	25

fluid losses in the postoperative period and monitoring of the serum potassium levels will minimize the adverse effects of potassium disturbances on metabolic and smooth muscle function. Typical electrolyte contents of gastrointestinal fluids are noted in Table 1. The deficit of total body potassium in chronic hypokalemia is approximately 200 mEq for each 1 mEq/L decrease in the serum level (32). Potassium replacement should not exceed 150–200 mEq per day. In the patient with long-standing hypokalemia resulting from diuretic therapy or gastrointestinal losses, concomitant replacement therapy with magnesium may be necessary. Magnesium is a cofactor for the enzyme Na+K ATPase, which pumps potassium into the cell (33). Supplemental magnesium (20 mEq/d) is often necessary to replete intracellular stores of potassium (8) and to raise the serum level of potassium (13).

SUMMARY

Hypokalemia is a common finding in the acutely ill surgical patient. While the etiology of the hypokalemia may be multifactorial, the consequences are similar. An increased risk for arrhythmias both during and after surgery is noted, particularly in patients with concomitant alkalosis, digitalis usage, and ischemic heart disease. Postoperative recovery may be adversely affected by sustained hypokalemia because of impairment in smooth muscle function and metabolic homeostasis. Where feasible, hypokalemia should be corrected prior to surgery particularly in high-risk patients. A normal serum potassium level in the postoperative period should be maintained by careful attention to fluid replacement.

REFERENCES

1. Azar, I., Thiagarajah, S., and Lear, E.: The arrhythmogenic dose of epinephrine in chronic hypokalemic dogs. *Anesth. Analg.* 61:221, 1982.
2. Berend, N., and Marlin, G. E.: Characterization of beta-adrenoceptor subtype mediating the metabolic actions of salbutamol. *Br. J. Clin. Pharmacol.* 5:207–211, 1978.
3. Brown, M. J., Brown, D. C., and Murphy, M. B.: Hypokalemia from beta-receptor stimulation by circulating epinephrine. *N. Engl. J. Med.* 309:1414–1419, 1983.
4. Biglieri, E. G., and McIlroy, M. D.: Abnormalities of renal function and circulatory reflexes in primary aldosteronism. *Circulation* 303:78–86, 1966.
5. Chew, W. C., and Lew, L. C.: Ventricular ectopics after salbutamol infusion for preterm labour. *Lancet* 2:1383–1384, 1979.
6. Conci, F., Procaccio, F., and Boselli, L.: Hypokalemia from β_2-receptor stimulation by epinephrine. *N. Engl. J. Med.* 310:1329, 1984.

7. Corea, L., Bentivoglio, M., and Verdecchia, P.: Hypokalaemia due to salbutamol overdosage. *Br. Med. J.* 283:500, 1981.
8. Dyckner, T., and Wester, P. O.: Ventricular extrasystoles and intracellular electrolytes before and after potassium and magnesium infusions in patients on diuretic treatment. *Am. Heart J.* 97:12–18, 1979.
9. Gronert, G. A., and They, R. A.: Pathophysiology of hyperkalemia induced by succinylcholine. *Anesthesiology* 43:89–99, 1975.
10. Halter, J. B., Pflug, A. E., and Porte, D., Jr.: Mechanism of plasma catecholamine increases during surgical stress in man. *J. Clin. Endocrinol. Metab.* 45:936–944, 1977.
11. Hill, G. E., Wong, K. C., Shaw, C. L., and Blatnick, R. A.: Acute and chronic changes in intra- and extracellular potassium and responses to neuromuscular blocking agents. *Anesth. Analg.* 57:417–421, 1978.
12. Hoffman, S. A., Wallace, H. W., Baue, A. E., Blakemore, W. S., and Zinsser, H. F.: Postoperative ventricular arrhythmias caused by isoproterenol. Conversion with insulin. *J. Thoracic Cardiovasc. Surg.* 58:664–667, 1969.
13. Hollifield, J. W.: Potassium and magnesium abnormalities: diuretics and arrhythmias in hypertension. *Am. J. Med.* 77:28–32, 1984.
14. Hurlbert, B. J., Edelman, J. D., and David, K.: Serum potassium levels during and after terbutaline. *Anesth. Analg.* 60:723–725, 1981.
15. Karlsberg, R. P., Cryer, P. E., and Roberts, R.: Serial plasma catecholamine response early in the course of clinical acute myocardial infarction: relationship to infarct extent and mortality. *Am. Heart J.* 102:24–29, 1981.
16. Knochel, J. P.: Diuretic induced hypokalemia. *Am. J. Med.* 77:18–27, 1984.
17. Lawson, N. W., Butler, G. H., and Ray, C. T.: Alkalosis and cardiac arrhythmias. *Anesth. Analg.* 52:951–964, 1973.
18. Leitch, A. G., Clancy, L. J., Costello, J. F., and Flenley, D. C.: Effect of intravenous infusion of salbutamol on ventilatory response to carbon dioxide and hypoxia and on heart rate and plasma potassium in normal men. *Br. Med. J.* 1:356–357, 1976.
19. Marcial, M. B., Vendoya, R. C., Zerbini, E. J., Verginelli, G., Bittencourt, D., and doAmaral, R. G.: Potassium in cardiac surgery with extracorporeal perfusion. *Am. J. Cardiol.* 23:400–408, 1969.
20. McCammon, R. L., and Stoelting, R. K.: Exaggerated increase in serum potassium following succinylcholine in dogs with beta blockade. *Anesthesiology* 61:723–725, 1984.
21. McInnes, G. T., and Davies, D. L.: Hypokalaemia due to salbutamol overdosage. *Br. Med. J.* 283:500–501, 1981.
22. Miller, R. D., and Roderick, L. L.: Diuretic-induced hypokalemia, pancuronium neuromuscular blockade and its antagonism by neostigmine. *Br. J. Anaesth.* 50: 541–544, 1978.
23. Montoliu, J., Marinez-Vea, A., Lopez-Pedret, J., and Revert, L.: Hypokalemia from $beta_2$-receptor stimulation by epinephrine. *N. Engl. J. Med.* 310:1329–1330, 1984.
24. Morgan, D. B., and Young, R. M.: Acute transient hypokalaemia: new interpretation of a common event. *Lancet* 2:751–752, 1982.
25. O'Brien, I. A. D., Fitzgerald-Fraser, J., Lewin, I. G., and Corrall, R. J. M.: Hypokalemia due to salbutamol overdosage. *Br. Med. J.* 282:1515–1516, 1981.
26. Robertson, C. S., Clifton, G. L., Taylor, A. A., and Grossman, R. G.: Treatment of hypertension associated with head injury. *J. Neurosurg.* 59:455–460, 1983.
27. Rolton, H., Simpson, E., Connelly, T., and Rodger, J. C.: Plasma potassium in acute myocardial infarction. *Eur. Heart J.* 2(Suppl)A:21, 1981.

28. Rosa, R. M., Silva, P., Young, J. B., et al.: Adrenergic modulation of extrarenal potassium disposal. *N. Engl. J. Med.* 302:431–434, 1980.
29. Sagild, U., Andersen, V., and Andreasem, P. B.: Glucose tolerance and insulin responsiveness in experimental potassium depletion. *Acta Med. Scand.* 169:243–251, 1961.
30. Samellas, W., and LeVeen, H. H.: Effect of alterations in serum potassium on ureteral peristalsis. *JAMA* 188:76–78, 1964.
31. Schwartz, W. B., and Relman, A. S.: Effect of electrolyte disorders on renal structure and function. *N. Engl. J. Med.* 276:383–289, 1967.
32. Scribner, B. H., and Burnell, J. M.: Interpretation of the serum potassium concentration. *Metabolism* 5:468–479, 1956.
33. Skou, J. C.: The influence of some cations on the adenosine triphosphatase from peripheral nerve. *Biochim. Biophys. Acta* 23:394–401, 1957.
34. Sliwinski, M., Hoffman, M., Biederman, A., Wangin, H., and Holdrowicz, M.: Association between hypokaliaemic alkalosis and development of arrhythmia in early postoperative period. *Anaesth. Resus. Inten. Therap.* 2:193–204, 1974.
35. Smiler, B. G.: Hyperkalemia during anesthesia. *N. Engl. J. Med.* 311:1187, 1984.
36. Smith, J. S.: Hypokalemia in resuscitation from multiple trauma. *Surg. Gynecol. Obstet.* 147:18–20, 1978.
37. Streisand, R. L., Gourin, A., and Stuckey, J. H.: Respiratory and metabolic alkalosis and myocardial contractility. *J. Thor. Cardiovasc. Surg.* 62:431–435, 1971.
38. Struthers, A. D., Reid, J. L., McLean, K., and Rodger, J. C.: Adrenaline, hypokalaemia and cardiac arrhythmias: effects of beta adrenoceptor antagonists. *Clin. Sci.* 62:1P, 1982.
39. Surewicz, B.: Role of potassium in cardiovascular therapy. *Med. Clin. North Am.* 52:1103–1113, 1968.
40. Thomas, D. J., and Dove, A. F.: Metabolic effects of salbutamol infusion during premature labor. *Br. J. Obstet. Gynecol.* 84:494–499, 1977.
41. Vincent, H. H., Boomsma, F., Man in't Veld, A. J., et al.: Effects of selective and nonselective beta agonists on plasma potassium and norepinephrine. *J. Cardiovasc. Pharmacol.* 6:107–114, 1984.
42. Vitez, T. S., Soper, L. E., and Soper, P. G.: Chronic hypokalemia does not increase anesthetic dysrhythmias. *Anesth. Analgesia* 61:221, 1982.
43. Waud, B. E., Mookerjee, A., and Waud, D. R.: Chronic potassium depletion and sensitivity to tubocurarine. *Anesthesiology* 57:111–115, 1982.
44. Williams, M. E., Rosa, R. M., Silva, P. S., et al.: Impairment of extrarenal potassium disposition by alpha adrenergic stimulation. *N. Engl. J. Med.* 311:145–149, 1984.
45. Williams, M. E.: Hyperkalemia during anesthesia. *N. Engl. J. Med.* 311:1187, 1984.
46. Winnie, A. P., and Edwards, R.: Anesthesia, alkalosis, and arrhythmias. *Surg. Ann.* 9:75–82, 1977.
47. Wright, B. D., and DiGiovanni, A. J.: Respiratory alkalosis, hypokalemia, and repeated ventricular fibrillation associated with mechanical ventilation. *Anesth. Analg.* 48:467–473, 1969.
48. Wong, K. C., Tseng, C. K., Puerto, B. A., and Puerto, A. X.: Chronic hypokalemia on epinephrine-induced dysrhythmias during halothane, enflurane or methoxyflurane with N_2O anesthesia. *Anesthesiology* 51:S118, 1979.
49. Yokoyama, M., Fujikura, I., Yokoyama, K., and Sakakibara, S.: Transient hypopotassemia and ECG changes following hemodilution perfusion. *Arch. Surg.* 104: 640–643, 1972.

26

Relationship Between Potassium and Blood Pressure in Normotensive and Untreated Hypertensive Subjects

W. GORDON WALKER
The Johns Hopkins University School of Medicine and The Johns Hopkins Hospital, Baltimore, Maryland

We previously reported (23) that patients with high blood pressure (essential hypertension) excreted less potassium, and therefore had a diminished potassium intake. This report focused attention upon the possible role of potassium in the development and progression of essential hypertension. This was the first report calling attention to a relationship between potassium and high blood pressure in humans with untreated hypertension, but it followed upon extensive animal studies demonstrating the importance of potassium in modulating their response to a number of procedures designed to produce experimental hypertension. In particular, Meneely showed that potassium ingestion reduced the adverse effects of blood pressure elevation produced in rats by increased sodium intake (20). Dahl subsequently identified the relationship between the blood pressure response of his genetically developed salt-sensitive rats to sodium and the ratio of sodium to potassium in the diet the animals were fed (6). These experimental studies are all consistent in showing that increased potassium intake in animals reduces the adverse effects from sodium-induced hypertension and provide a strong case for the study of potassium metabolism in essential hypertension in humans. Langford et al. (16) reported a significantly higher urine Na/K ratio in hypertensive subjects. Addison had identified a therapeutic benefit attributable to potassium administration in severe hypertension more than 50 years earlier and he proposed that a potassium deficit may underlie the development of high blood pressure (2). McQuarrie subsequently reported that potassium administration ameliorated the hypertensive effects of acute administration of large quantities of sodium to three young diabetic patients (19).

Several investigators have recently published data that corroborate our initial report and further substantiate the existence of a relationship between potassium and high blood pressure (3,4,9,14). These include several reports demonstrating that potassium administration lowers blood pressure of patients with essential hypertension (12,15,18). A brief review of our more relevant findings and of further data dealing with this subject is presented here.

RELATION OF POTASSIUM EXCRETION TO BLOOD PRESSURE

Our report that urinary potassium excretion correlates negatively with blood pressure in "free-living" subjects was based upon data from studies done on 574 ambulatory subjects whose blood pressures ranged from a low of 94/55 mmHg to a high of 250/145 mmHg. This group of subjects included hypertensive patients who were recruited for the study from the emergency room of the Johns Hopkins Hospital by a screening procedure reported in detail elsewhere (22), plus a group of volunteers from a U.S. Air Force reserve unit who represented normotensive subjects from the same area. Untreated hypertensive patients were entered into the study after a total of six separate blood pressure measurements that demonstrated diastolic blood pressure exceeding 90 mmHg. Potential candidates were excluded if they were taking any type of medication, including oral contraceptives. Patients exhibiting evidence that the blood pressure elevation had been associated with any significant vascular damage such as renal impairment indicated by abnormal urinalyses or elevated blood urea nitrogen or creatinine levels, history of heart attack, stroke, or other evidence of vascular disease were also excluded. Three-hundred subjects were recruited in this manner and an additional 274 subjects were recruited from among the Air Force Reserve personnel. Although this was not a population-based sample, the two groups were remarkably similar with respect to age, sex, weight, and race.

All subjects at the time of study were ambulatory and were on their usual unrestricted diet. None had received previous dietary instruction of any type. Thus every effort was made to study them with as little change in their standard dietary pattern as possible. Studies were performed between 9 and 11 a.m., and urine specimens obtained between 9 and 10 a.m. Written consent was obtained following a detailed explanation of the nature and hazards of the study. Subjects were ambulatory for at least 2 hr before collection of venous blood for measurement of plasma renin activity, aldosterone, and angiotensin II. Urinary sodium, potassium, and creatinine were measured by techniques previously described.

Sodium and potassium excretion rates were assessed from the sodium/creatinine (Na/Cr) ratio and the potassium/creatinine (K/Cr) ratio measured on the urine collected between 9 and 10 a.m. Reliability of this index of sodium excretion was evaluated as previously described (23). In studies performed with three groups of individuals, the spot morning urine was compared with the 24-hr urine specimen and data analyzed from 18 normal subjects on an ad lib salt diet ($R=+0.62$; $p<0.025$); 37 patients were studied similarly while on varying salt intake ($r=+0.56$; $p<0.005$). Further validation was obtained by comparing spot urine collections obtained both at 6:30 a.m. and at 10:30 a.m. with 24-hr sodium/creatinine ratios. These yielded virtually identical correlations. In addition, the sodium/creatinine ratio was demonstrated to correlate with simultaneously measured plasma renin activity in 22 subjects studied on both a low- and high-salt diet ($r=-0.42$; $p<0.025$), further validating use of this index.

Blood pressure measurements were recorded by three different individuals, each of whom recorded a supine and standing blood pressure. Intraindividual blood pressure data, obtained by different observers, correlated closely ($r=+0.9$; $p<.0001$).

This discussion focuses upon the data on electrolyte excretion and the patterns of excretion in relation to blood pressure and related variables. Table 1 shows the mean values for the entire study group and also compares subsets of data representing individual subjects whose diastolic pressure exceeded 90 mmHg and those with a diastolic blood pressure

Table 1 Comparison of Urinary Electrolytes and Related Variables in Normotensive and Hypertensive Individuals

Variable	Total study population (n=574) mean+SD	Diastolic BP ⩽90 mmHg (n=277) mean+SEM	Diastolic BP >90 mmHg (n=297) mean+SEM
Age (yrs)	31.8±6.7	31±.4	32±.4
Weight (lbs)	175±33	173±1.6[a]	178±2.2
Systolic blood pressure	142±21	129±.8	154±1.1
Diastolic blood pressure	94±15	81±.5	105.8±.6
Urine K (mEq/L)	60±29	65.8±1.7[a]	54.7±1.8
Urine Na (mEq/L)	129±5.0	128±3	129±3
Urine Na/K	2.65±1.7	2.24±.07[a]	3.07±.13
Urine creatinine (mg/dl)	164±81	164±5.1	165±4.7
Plasma renin activity (mg/ml/hr)	0.296±.19	0.31±.01[b]	0.28±.01
Plasma aldosterone (mg/dl)	12.7±10	15.6±.7[a]	9.9±.5

[a]$p<0.0001$
[b]$p<0.05$

⩽90 mmHg. No significant difference was evident in the age of the two subsets grouped according to blood pressure. Individuals with the higher blood pressure were significantly heavier than individuals within the low blood pressure group but the mean difference of 2.25 kg was of questionable clinical significance. There was no difference in the urinary sodium concentration, creatinine concentration, or the sodium/creatinine ratio. In contrast, a highly significant difference was observed in urinary potassium with the rate of potassium excretion among the subjects with a higher blood pressure being 20% less than that exhibited by the normotensive population (<0.0001).

When these variables were examined for correlation with the recumbent diastolic blood pressures the data presented in Table 2 were obtained. The most remarkable

Table 2 Correlations Between Recumbent Diastolic Blood Pressure, Electrolyte Excretion, and Plasma Aldosterone

Variables	Bivariate correlation coefficient	p Value
Diast. BP vs. urine [Na]	0.000	>0.99
Diast. BP vs. urine Na/Cr	0.004	>0.92
Diast. BP vs. urine [K]	-0.24	<0.0001
Diast. BP vs. urine K/Cr	-0.12	<0.008
Diast. BP vs. urine Na/K	+0.26	<0.0001
Diast. BP vs. plasma aldosterone	-0.20	<0.001
Plasma aldosterone vs. urine [Na]	-0.09	=0.05
Plasma aldosterone vs. Ur Na/Cr	0.03	>0.5
Plasma aldosterone vs. urine [K]	+0.23	<0.0001
Plasma aldosterone vs. urine K/Cr	+0.25	<0.0001
Plasma aldosterone vs. Na/K	-0.20	<0.0001

findings were a highly significant negative correlation between the urinary potassium and blood pressure (particularly recumbent diastolic blood pressure), a similar negative correlation between plasma aldosterone and blood pressure, and a strong *positive* correlation between plasma aldosterone and urinary potassium. It was of equal interest that no correlation could be demonstrated between aldosterone and urinary sodium levels nor between urinary sodium levels and diastolic blood pressure.

The regression equations for these bivariate correlations that define the relationship of diastolic blood pressure as dependent variable for urinary potassium, the sodium/potassium ratio, and plasma aldosterone are displayed in Figure 1. Though the correlations can only be described as moderate, the relationships are highly significant ($p<0.001$). Urinary sodium as an independent variable was not included here because no significant correlation between sodium and blood pressure could be demonstrated. Hence the relationship shown for blood pressure and the urinary Na/K ratio is due to the correlation between

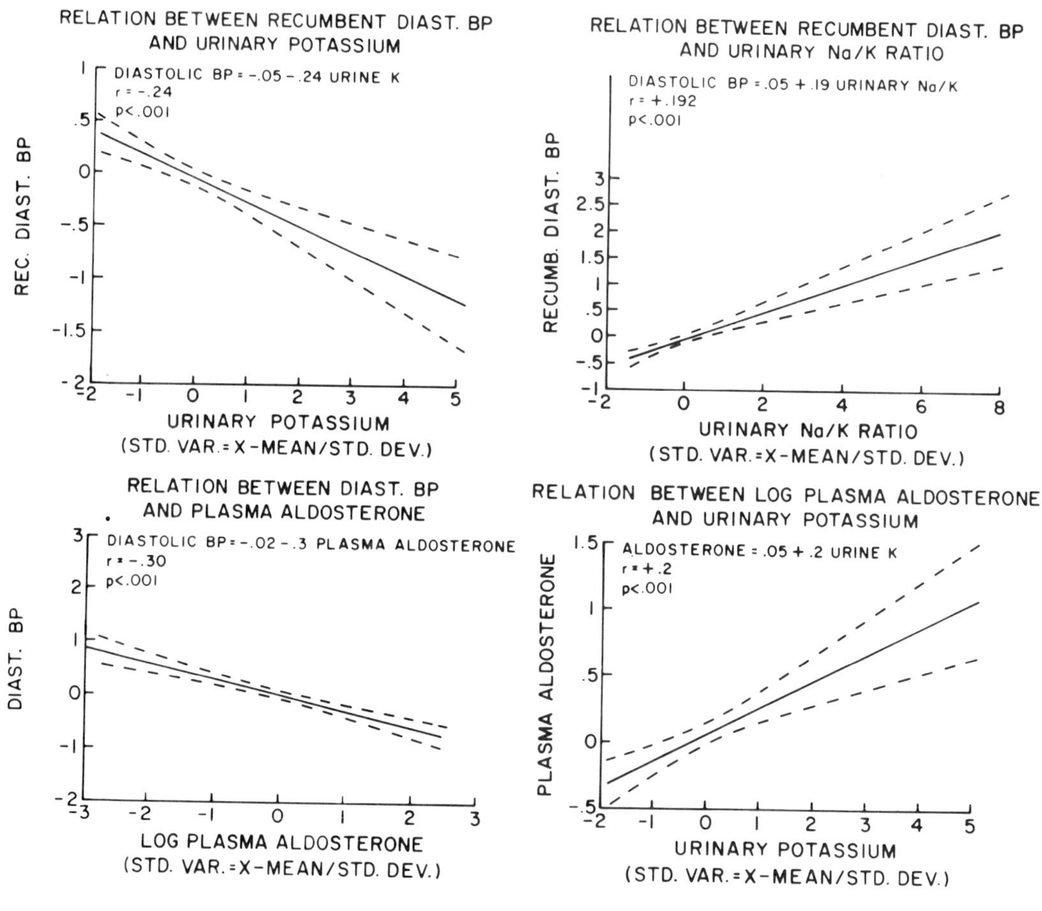

Figure 1 Interrelationship between recumbent diastolic blood pressure, urinary potassium, urinary Na/K ratio, and aldosterone. No significant correlation between Na and blood pressure could be demonstrated. Solid lines in each graph identify the regression equation, with dashed lines representing the 95% confidence limits of the regression equation. All coordinates are expressed in standard variable notation (mean=0; ±SD).

blood pressure and urinary potassium. Similar relationships were demonstrable when either systolic blood pressure or mean arterial pressure was substituted for diastolic pressure, but diastolic blood pressure tended to yield slightly higher values for the correlation coefficients.

The variables tested against blood pressure are themselves intercorrelated and this introduces a potential confounding influence that may yield spurious correlations. For this reason, it is more instructive to use multiple linear regression analysis to assess the relative influence of these variables upon the observed variance in blood pressure and to minimize the introduction of spurious correlations. When recumbent diastolic blood pressure is taken as the dependent variable and the influence of potassium excretion, sodium excretion, plasma aldosterone and age are evaluated the results are shown in Table 3. Equations 1 and 1a in Table 3 establish that the sodium/potassium ratio and aldosterone correlate significantly with diastolic blood pressure and that this correlation is influenced virtually not at all by age. The multiple correlation coefficient of 0.32 which is obtained for equation 1a is virtually identical to equation 1, indicating that omission of age as a variable does not alter this relationship. It is of interest that the standardized regression coefficients, which are identical to partial correlation coefficients, indicate that the influence of the level of plasma aldosterone on the blood pressure is at least as great as that exhibited by the sodium:potassium ratio. In similar fashion, equation 2 and 2a reveal that this correlation between sodium/potassium ratio and diastolic blood pressure can be attributed virtually completely to the influence of potassium, the relationship being relatively little altered by omission of the sodium data as illustrated by equation 2a. This relationship between blood pressure, urine sodium, urine potassium, and aldosterone is virtually identical whether K/Cr and Na/Cr are used as indices of the rate of electrolyte

Table 3 Standardized Multiple Linear Regression Equations

Dependent variable = Diastolic blood pressure
Independent variables = Urine Na, urine K, urine Na/K, urine Na/Cr, urine K/Cr, aldosterone, age

	Equation	Multiple correlation coefficient	p Value
1	Diast. BP=−0.05+0.12 age+0.22 Na/K−0.25 aldosterone	0.35	<0.0001
1a	Diast. BP=−0.05+0.14 Na/K−0.27 aldosterone	0.32	<0.0001
2	Diast. BP=−0.06+0.1 Na/Cr−0.22 K/Cr−0.26 aldosterone	0.34	<0.0001
2a	Diast. BP=−0.06−0.16 K/Cr−0.27 aldosterone	0.33	<0.0001
3	Diast. BP=−0.07+0.03 [Na]−0.21 [K]−0.26 aldosterone	0.35	<0.001
3a	Diast. BP=−0.07−0.20 [K]−0.27 aldosterone	0.35	<0.001

Dependent variable = Plasma aldosterone
Independent variables = Urine Na, urine K, urine Na/K, plasma renin activity, age

	Equation	Multiple correlation coefficient	p Value
4	Pl. aldosterone 0.06−0.02 age−0.18 Na/K+0.11 PRA	0.25	<0.0001
4a	Pl. aldosterone 0.06−0.18 Na/K+0.11 PRA	0.25	<0.0001
5	Pl. aldosterone = 0.07−0.110 Na+0.20 K+0.11 PRA	0.25	<0.0001
5a	Pl. aldosterone = 0.07−0.14 Na+0.22 K	0.22	<0.0001
5b	Pl. aldosterone = 0.07−0.01+0.17 PRA	0.17	<0.001

excretion obtained from the spot urines or whether urinary concentrations are used, as illustrated in equation 3 and 3a. In both groups the multiple correlation coefficients are indistinguishable, and in neither instance does sodium play a significant role in accounting for any of the observed variance in the diastolic blood pressure. Thus, fluctuations in diastolic blood pressure in the present study population can be much more readily associated with fluctuations in potassium excretion (and, by inference, intake) and plasma aldosterone than with sodium intake. Moreover when the data are controlled for age, these relationships persist essentially unchanged, indicating that age has not played a significant role in this observed association despite the well-recognized association between changes in the plasma renin-angiotensin-aldosterone system and age (10).

DISCUSSION

Because of the remarkably strong correlation between aldosterone and diastolic blood pressure, it was instructive to see what other variables correlated with plasma aldosterone and whether there was any evidence that sodium could be exerting an indirect effect on blood pressure through its control of plasma aldosterone. It is important to point out that the correlation between diastolic blood pressure and aldosterone was a negative one and hence it is not reasonable to suppose that aldosterone can be assigned a primary role in the pathogenesis of hypertension analogously to that seen with experimentally induced steroid hypertension as in the DOC rat model (5). Nevertheless the plasma aldosterone could be inappropriately high for a given level of sodium intake. Since no significant correlation could be demonstrated between sodium and the blood pressure, we undertook to examine the influence of urinary sodium, urinary potassium, and plasma renin activity on the observed values of plasma aldosterone. These data are also included in Table 3 where equation 4 and 4a identify the relationship between aldosterone as a dependent variable and age, sodium and potassium ratio in the urine, and plasma renin activity as independent variables. Age plays virtually no role since the correlation coefficient is unchanged when age is omitted (equation 4a). It is interesting, and unexpected, that plasma aldosterone exhibited a stronger correlation with potassium than with either sodium or plasma renin activity (equation 5). Equation 5a, b and c establish that variations in potassium correlate more closely with plasma aldosterone than do either sodium or plasma renin activity.

These findings indicate that blood pressure can be correlated much more closely with potassium intake and excretion than with corresponding data for sodium. It must be stressed that it is not possible to explain the differences in urinary potassium by supposing that they arise solely from differences in K transport at the cellular level in hypertensive subjects. Even though such differences have been demonstrated to exist (8), the reduction in urinary potassium can only be explained by a reduction in potassium intake. If the difference was attributable to some altered physiological transport of the potassium within the individual, lowered excretion must nevertheless reflect decreased intake, since otherwise a normal excretion rate with a lowered component of the body's changeable potassium would be expected. It seems unlikely that this could represent decreased gastrointestinal absorption of K with increased fecal losses since the only circumstances in which such a difference has been documented has been in the presence of severe aldosterone excess and renal failure (11) or chronic diarrhea.

This relationship between blood pressure and potassium intake or excretion has been confirmed by a number of subsequent investigators who have repeated the studies on a population-based sample (4,7,9,13,14). For the most part they have all shown that the primary alteration among hypertensive subjects is a reduction in potassium intake and or excretion. In at least one instance however the study suggests that the same relationship can be identified in circumstances where the sodium/potassium ratio is altered by fluctuations in sodium intake. The study of Ueshima and associates (21) is of particular interest since these workers showed a remarkably strong correlation between the prevalence of high blood pressure and the level of serum potassium based upon data from six separate population samples from various regions in Japan where sodium intake varied greatly. When the prevalence of hypertension in each of these population samples is compared with the corresponding mean plasma potassium value, a correlation coefficient of 0.99 is obtained with a p value of <0.001 even though the data set has only 5 degrees of freedom. Moreover their data on sodium and potassium intake based upon recall of food ingested in the preceding 24 hr suggested that this fluctuation in plasma potassium was accounted for by variations in sodium intake, and they postulated that the hypokalemia was related to the kaliuretic properties of a high-sodium diet. Most importantly, the observed prevalence of hypertension could be demonstrated to correlate as closely with the level of plasma potassium as with the sodium/potassium ratio in the diet. Thus both lowered potassium and decreased aldosterone levels are encountered in patients with essential hypertension, and the magnitude of the increase in blood pressure can be related quantitatively to the magnitude of decrease in both plasma and urinary potassium as well as the decrease in plasma aldosterone.

The suggestion has been made repeatedly that altered potassium balance in hypertension can be explained adequately as the result of sodium induced kaliuresis, but this is inadequate to explain the reported urinary findings. Even if increased sodium intake produced a sustained kaliuresis that significantly reduced body potassium, the resulting daily urinary loss of potassium would reflect this continuing loss of body K in addition to excretion of the usual daily intake. The result would be a daily urinary potassium output among hypertensives that exceeded values observed in normal subjects; reported data are exactly the opposite of this and cannot be explained without a decreased dietary potassium intake being posited.

The mechanism whereby decreased potassium intake predisposes a subject to or aggravates a tendency for the blood pressure to rise is unclear. The possibility that this could be merely a secondary phenomenon or an alteration associated with hypertension, but unrelated pathogenetically, must be considered. The impressive experimental data associating decreased potassium intake with aggravation of high blood pressure and the easily demonstrable therapeutic benefit of K administration to hypertensive rats (including the remarkable effects in stroke-prone rats as presented by Tobian in Chapter 29) together represent compelling evidence for a role of decreased potassium intake in the development of hypertension (6,20, and Chapter 29).

It is perhaps relevant that Abbrecht and others have demonstrated that moderate potassium depletion in the dog and in the rat results in a significant elevation in systemic vascular resistance (1,17). This elevated resistance tends to increase progressively, at least in the dog, over a period of weeks as the potassium deficit increases. Though these animals did not show an increase in blood pressure, and indeed the cardiac output decreased when examined in this circumstance, the progressive elevation in systemic vascular resistance was the most impressive finding. Potassium repletion lowered the systemic vascular resistance in extrarenal vascular beds in these animals before reduction of renal vascular resistance was demonstrable. Given such an apparent differential influence upon vascular resistance within the kidney, it is possible that such an alteration could result in impairment of the ability of the kidney to excrete a sodium load and may in fact initiate progressive blood pressure elevation as a mechanism for facilitating the excretion of sodium. While this possibility has not been examined carefully it may prove an important avenue for further investigation.

Finally, the consistency with which various investigators have succeeded in establishing an association between elevated blood pressure and reduced potassium intake, taken together with the several reports of a beneficial effect of potassium administration in mild hypertension, merit careful consideration in relation to treatment of hypertension. At the very least, it prompts one to question whether dietary modification designed to increase potassium intake and reduce sodium intake may not be more important in reducing the prevalence and severity of high blood pressure than present efforts to provide drug treatment for all subjects with recognizable hypertension.

ACKNOWLEDGMENTS

This work supported in part by NIH grants HL03303, RR00035, RR00722, AM07145, The Irving Blum Fund, and The Jane Hilder Harris Foundation.

REFERENCES

1. Abbrecht, P. H.: Cardiovascular effects of chronic potassium deficiency in the dog. *Am. J. Physiol.* 223:555, 1972.
2. Addison, W. L. T.: The use of sodium chloride, potassium chloride, sodium bromide and potassium bromide in cases of arterial hypertension which are amenable to potassium chloride. *Can. Med. Assoc. J.* 18:281, 1928.
3. Berenson, G. S., Foster, T. A., Frank, G. C., Frevichs, R. R., Srinivasan, S. R., Voors, A. W., and Webber, L. S.: Cardiovascular disease risk factor variables at the preschool age. The Bogalusa Heart Study. *Circulation* 57:603, 1978.
4. Bulpitt, C., Shipley, M. J., and Semmence, A.: Blood pressure and plasma sodium and potassium. *Clin. Sci.* 61:85s, 1981.
5. Dahl, L. K., Heine, M., and Tassinari, L.: Effect of chronic excess salt ingestion. Role of genetic factors in both DOCA-salt and renal hypertension. *J. Exp. Med.* 118: 605, 1963.
6. Dahl, L. K., Leitl, G., and Heine, M.: Influence of dietary potassium and sodium/potassium molar ratios on the development of salt hypertension. *J. Exp. Med.* 136: 318, 1972.
7. Ganguli, M., Tobian, L., Iwai, J., and Johnson, M. A.: Potassium citrate feeding protects against nephron loss in severe sodium chloride hypertension in rats. *Clin. Sci.* 61:73s, 1981.
8. Garay, R. P., and Meyer, P.: A new test showing abnormal net Na+ and K+ refluxes in erythocytes of essential hypertensive patients. *Lancet* 1:349, 1979.
9. Grim, C. E., Luft, F. C., Miller, J. Z., Meneely, G. R., Battarbee, H. D., Hames, C. G., and Dahl, L. K.: Racial differences in blood pressure in Evans County, Georgia: Relationship to sodium and potassium intake and plasma renin activity. *J. Chron. Dis.* 33:87, 1980.
10. Hayduk, K., Krause, D. K., Kaufman, W., Huenges, R., Schillmoller, U., and Unbehaun, V.: Age-dependent changes of plasma renin concentration in humans. *Clin. Sci. Mol. Med.* 45:273s, 1973.
11. Hayes, C. P. Jr., McCleod, M. E., and Robinson, R. R.: An extrarenal mechanism for

the maintenance of K balance in severe chronic renal failure. *Trans. Assoc. Am. Physicians* 80:207, 1967.

12. Holly, J. M. P., Goodwin, F. J., Evans, S. J. W., Vandenberg, M. J., and Ledingham, J. M.: Reanalysis of data in two Lancet papers on the effect of dietary sodium and potassium on blood pressure. *Lancet* 2:1384, 1981.
13. Iimura, O., Kijima, T., Kikuchi, K., Miyama, A., Ando, T., Nakao, T., and Takigami, Y.: Studies on the hypotensive effect of high potassium intake in patients with essential hypertension. *Clin. Sci.* 61:77s, 1981.
14. Khaw, K. T., and Rose, G.: Population study of blood pressure and associated factors in St. Lucia, West Indies. *Int. J. Epidemiol.* 11:372, 1982.
15. Khaw, K. T., and Thorn, S.: Randomized double-blind cross-over trial of potassium on blood pressure in normal subjects. *Lancet* 2:1127, 1982.
16. Langford, H. G., and Watson, R. L.: Electrolytes and Hypertension. In *Epidemiology and Control of Hypertension,* edited by Paul, O., Miami, Symposium Specialists, 1975, pp. 119–128.
17. Linas, S. L., and Dickmann, D.: Mechanism of the decreased renal blood flow in the potassium-depleted conscious rat. *Kidney Int.* 21:757, 1982.
18. MacGregor, G. M., Smith, S. J., Markander, N. D., Banks, R. A., and Sagnella, G. A.: Moderate potassium supplementation in essential hypertension. *Lancet* 2:567, 1982.
19. McQuarrie, I., Thompson, W. H., and Anderson, J. A.: Effects of excessive ingestion of sodium and potassium salts on carbohydrate metabolism and blood pressure in diabetic children. *J. Nutr.* 11:77, 1936.
20. Meneely, G. R., and Ball, C. O. T.: Experimental epidemiology of chronic sodium chloride toxicity and the protective effect of potassium chloride. *Am. J. Med.* 25: 713, 1958.
21. Ueshima, H., Tanigaki, M., Iida, M., Shimamoto, T., Konishi, M., and Komachi, Y.: Hypertension, salt and potassium. *Lancet* 1:504, 1981.
22. Walker, W. G., Horvath, J. S., Moore, M. A., Whelton, P. K., and Russell, R. P.: Relation between plasma renin activity, angiotensin, aldosterone and blood pressure in mild untreated hypertension. *Circ. Res.* 38:470, 1976.
23. Walker, W. G., Whelton, P. K., Saito, H., Russell, R. P., and Hermann, J.: Relation between blood pressure, and renin, renin substrate, angiotensin II, aldosterone, urinary sodium and potassium in 574 subjects. *Hypertension* 1:287, 1979.

27

Relationship Between Potassium and Blood Pressure in General Population Samples

CHRISTOPHER J. BULPITT
London School of Hygiene and Tropical Medicine, London, England

Because hypertension is a common problem associated with such a high cardiovascular morbidity and mortality it is important to examine all potential causative factors. Studies on twins and investigations into the family history of patients with hypertension have conclusively shown that heredity is a determinant of blood pressure. However, the prevalence of hypertension varies within a given race according to environmental factors, for example: geographic location within a country (34), urban or rural location within the same region, and the socioeconomic status of the population. The prevalence of hypertension also varies more between countries than would be expected on the grounds of genetic differences alone. Langford and colleagues (20) have reviewed these findings and concluded that diet may explain these differences. The editor's summary of their review stated: "A very low sodium intake may prevent hypertension; a very high intake may directly cause hypertension." This hypothesis is supported by many animal experiments, but in humans there are other possible causes, and these include environmental temperature, poisoning from metals such as lead and cadmium, alcohol consumption, mental stress, and lack of exercise. In addition, the effect of diet may be mediated by a dietary component other than sodium.

Blood pressure is associated strongly with obesity, the relationship is independent of age, and weight reduction is accompanied by a fall in blood pressure in hypertensive subjects. These facts do not necessarily incriminate diet as a cause of hypertension since obesity indicates only an excess calorie intake over output over a period of time, and this balance is affected by exercise and metabolic rate. In addition, a subject with a genetic predisposition to obesity may also be prone to hypertension, which leads to a noncausal relationship. However, it is tempting to conclude that the relationship between obesity and hypertension supports a role for diet in producing hypertension. The dietary factors may not be total calorie consumption nor sodium intake. This chapter considers the experimental evidence implicating potassium and whether a lack of potassium can be causally related to the development of hypertension in the general population.

EXPERIMENTAL EVIDENCE LINKING POTASSIUM WITH HYPERTENSION

Hypertension can be induced by salt in certain strains of rats. Dahl et al. (4) selectively bred rats who were sensitive to salt and developed hypertension, and rats who were resistant and remained normotensive. These experiments showed the importance of both dietary and genetic factors in these animals, and it has been argued that the normotensive subject on a high-salt diet is the human equivalent of the "salt-resistant" rat.

Meneely and Ball (24) also reported that a high-potassium diet modified the increase in pressure in salt-sensitive rats, but most evidence suggests that potassium depletion decreases blood pressure in normal animals. Tannen (35) reviewed the literature and concluded that rats and dogs fed a diet low in potassium experienced a fall in blood pressure of between 10 and 20%. In hypertensive animals, a restriction in potassium intake lowers blood pressure (7,8,29) and prevents the rise that occurs with renal artery stenosis.

A trial of low-potassium diet in four hypertensive patients reported in 1953 revealed a fall in blood pressure of 15/8 mmHg with this treatment (26). Unfortunately, control patients were not studied and the effect could have been that of a placebo. There was also a fall in 24-hr urinary sodium excretion but this was thought to be due to sodium retention and not to any change in sodium intake. This experiment did not suggest a rise in pressure with a decrease in intake of potassium.

More recently Khaw and Thom supplemented the diets of normal medical students with 64 mmol slow-release potassium chloride daily and MacGregor et al. similarly gave these supplements to untreated hypertensive patients. The normal subjects experienced a fall in mean blood pressure of about 2% (19) and the hypertensive patients a fall of 4% (23). These trials were only short-term studies and it is not known whether these rather small effects would be maintained over several months or years. Holly and colleagues found a hypotensive effect from giving a 100-mmol potassium supplementation for 12 weeks to hypertensive patients on a low-salt diet (13). Iimura and his colleagues gave 175 mmol of potassium a day for 10 days, which reduced mean blood pressure by 8 mmHg (15).

On balance it would appear that if potassium intake is related to hypertension, a deficit in this cation is more likely to lead to hypertension than is an excess.

BLOOD PRESSURE AND POTASSIUM INTAKE IN DIFFERENT POPULATIONS

Isolated societies have been studied in many parts of the world. Several different races have been surveyed for the prevalence of hypertension and the results have been reviewed by Dahl and Love (5) and Gleibermann (11). The study of these isolated populations revealed a lack of both obese hypertensive persons and of subjects over the age of 60 years. Sodium consumption was low in these societies and blood pressure failed to rise with age. This may have been due to the paucity of salt in the diet, and it has therefore been suggested that a low sodium intake will prevent the development of hypertension in industrialized societies. This may be true, but it must be admitted that the diet of these isolated societies did not lead to a prolongation of life. These populations appeared to die from conditions unrelated to hypertension.

It must also be remembered that a low sodium intake is only one characteristic of these isolated societies. They may have a diet containing an excess of potassium, a low total calorie content, and without poisons such as cadmium and lead. Moreover, the subjects may take more exercise or suffer from gastrointestinal and other infections. In addition, isolated societies are popularly presumed not to be subject to psychological "stress."

Many unindustrialized societies who do not salt their food have a high intake of fruit and green vegetables and in such societies a high-potassium, low-sodium diet may be found. In such communities any "benefit" in terms of a low blood pressure may equally be ascribed to a high potassium intake or a low sodium consumption. In Western populations a person who eats heavily salted foods may or may not eat a large amount of potassium. However, a person of limited financial means may eat heavily salted foods such as bread and soup and yet consume little fruit or meat. A high salt intake will then be accompanied by a low consumption of potassium.

With cation excretion being used as a measure of intake, the level of blood pressure has been compared with sodium and potassium excretion in three studies using consistent methods to study different groups. One study compared blood pressure and electrolyte excretion in Belgian subjects with those of persons in two areas of South Korea (17); another studied blacks and whites in Evans County, Georgia (12), and one compared black girls with white girls in Jackson, Mississippi (21). In two of the three comparisons the populations with the greater intakes of sodium had the highest average blood pressures, but in all three studies those populations with the greatest intakes of potassium had the lowest blood pressures. These studies are not conclusive and cannot differentiate between the relative importance of sodium excess or potassium lack. However, the inverse relationship between blood pressure and potassium excretion was at least as good as the positive association between sodium excretion and pressure. In conclusion, studies in several populations generally support the concept that sodium increases blood pressure (11), but too few measurements of potassium intake have been made to allow any firm conclusion concerning the relationship between the intake of this cation and blood pressure between populations.

RELATIONSHIP BETWEEN POTASSIUM INTAKE AND BLOOD PRESSURE WITHIN A POPULATION

Three complex problems must be discussed before we evaluate the association between potassium consumption and blood pressure: the role of aldosterone, the interrelationship between potassium intake and other dietary elements, and the effects of stress.

Aldosterone

It has been suggested that patients with elevated blood pressure have an increased plasma level of aldosterone (9,10,22). Plasma potassium levels should therefore be decreased, and plasma sodium and urinary potassium levels increased in hypertensive persons. Walker and his colleagues have confirmed a significant positive correlation between plasma aldosterone and urinary potassium levels in their study (37). Ljungman (22) found a negative association between plasma aldosterone and the urinary Na/K ratio, but only in hypertensive patients. If the excessive secretion of aldosterone occurs intermittently, renal potassium excretion would be increased and sodium excretion decreased during this period. However, if there is a negative association between high blood pressure and both plasma and urinary potassium levels, then this combination of findings is more likely to result from a lack of potassium in the diet than from an excess of aldosterone in the blood. A high intake of potassium, not a low intake, increases plasma aldosterone (6,36).

Any positive relationship between plasma aldosterone and blood pressure may be due to an excess of renin (secondary hyperaldosteronism) and this could explain a low plasma potassium concentration in hypertensive patients, but not a low urinary potassium level.

Relationship Between Potassium Intake and Other Elements of the Diet

The dietary intake of potassium may be associated not only with sodium intake but also with the dietary intake of other substances such as calcium and fat. Any association between potassium intake and blood pressure could be due to these confounding variables. Serum calcium is positively related to high blood pressure (2,16) as is a high intake of fat (27).

Stress

It is also possible that a low plasma and urinary potassium level could be due not to diet but to other environmental factors such as stress. Figure 1 illustrates how stress could increase plasma catecholamines and lead to a fall in plasma and urinary potassium due to a

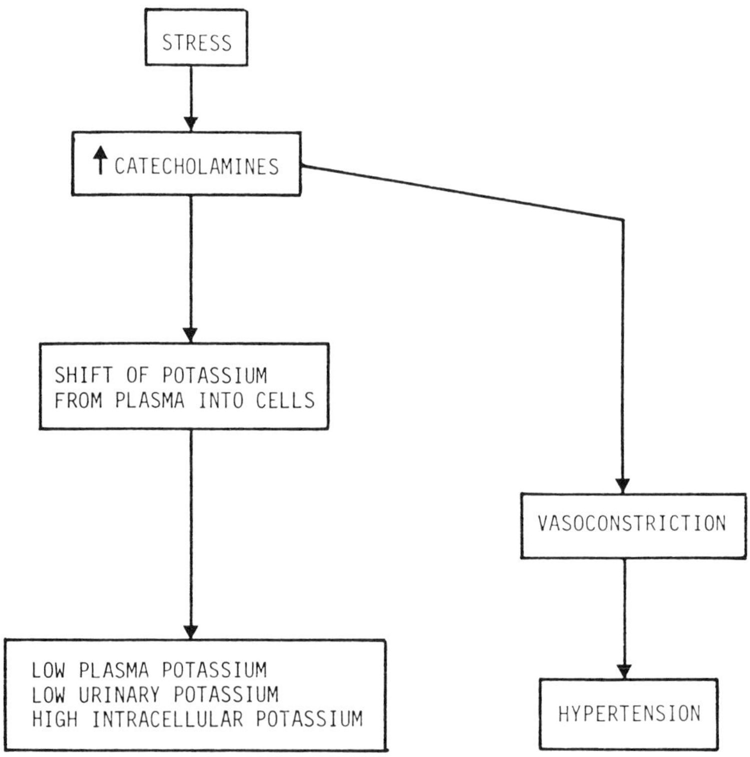

Figure 1 The mechanism whereby stress could produce a rise in blood pressure and a fall in both plasma and urinary potassium. (From Bulpitt, C. J.: Blood pressure and potassium consumption. In *The Epidemiology of Hypertension*, Vol. 6, Handbook of Hypertension, edited by Bulpitt, C. J., Amsterdam, New York, Oxford, Elsevier, 1985.

catecholamine-induced shift of potassium from plasma to the cells (25,28,31). The catecholamine pathway would produce a high intracellular potassium level, which might tend to lower pressure, but a high blood pressure will almost certainly result from direct vasoconstriction. Therefore it cannot be concluded that an association between a high blood pressure and a low concentration of potassium in the blood and urine at the same time is due to a diet deficient in potassium. Stress is obviously a potential confounding factor when one is relating casual blood pressure to the potassium concentration in plasma or urine collected at the same time. This may be less of a problem when blood pressure is related to a 24-hr measurement of urinary potassium collected on a different occasion.

Blood Pressure and Potassium Intake in the Same Population

Potassium intake may be assessed from a dietary history, urinary potassium excretion, and, although this is the subject of controversy, plasma potassium. It is doubtful how well plasma potassium is related to the dietary intake of this cation. Patients with accelerated or malignant hypertension usually have low concentrations of serum potassium due to

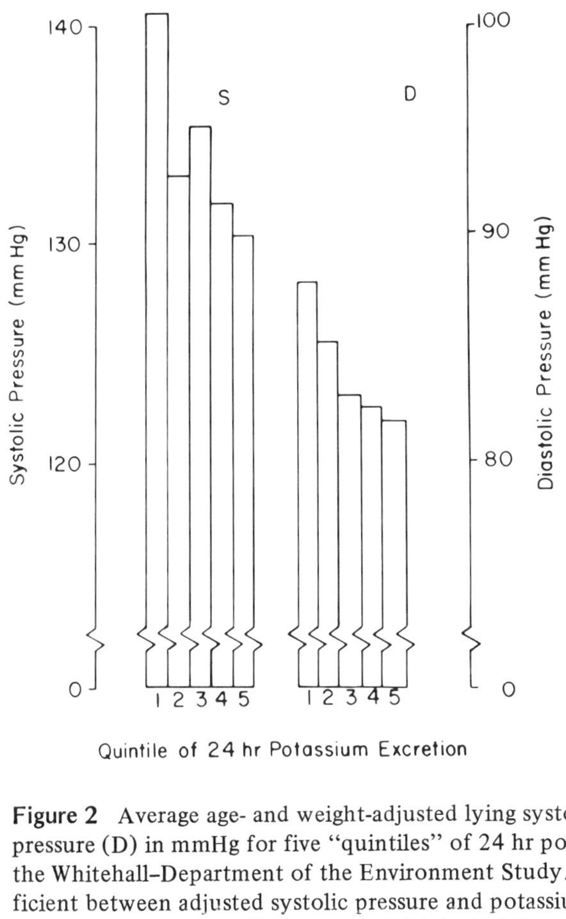

Figure 2 Average age- and weight-adjusted lying systolic blood pressure (S) and diastolic pressure (D) in mmHg for five "quintiles" of 24 hr potassium excretion for 452 men in the Whitehall–Department of the Environment Study. The first-order correlation coefficient between adjusted systolic pressure and potassium excretion was -0.17 ($p<0.001$) and for adjusted diastolic pressure -0.11 ($p<0.05$).

secondary hyperaldosteronism and patients with pyelonephritis also tend to have low levels of this ion in the serum. In both instances the disease process may lead to a loss of body potassium. However, it has been reported that in general populations, including very few subjects with these conditions, the lower the plasma potassium the higher the blood pressure (3,22,30).

It has also been shown that the lower the urinary potassium concentration the greater the blood pressure (18,37) and, most importantly, that the best indirect measure of dietary potassium intake, namely the 24-hr urinary excretion of this ion, is negatively related to systolic pressure in a random sample of men living in Belgium (33). This relationship was not found in women.

Recent studies of London civil servants have confirmed this finding in 452 men (1). Figure 2 shows the average systolic and diastolic pressure measured in the office (adjusted for age and body weight) according to five "quintiles" of 24-hr urinary potassium excretion estimated an average of 6 weeks later. The increase in average systolic and diastolic pressure with a low excretion of potassium is apparent. Figure 3, however, illustrates the results in 162 women: no such negative relationship was apparent between casual blood pressure and potassium excretion in these subjects.

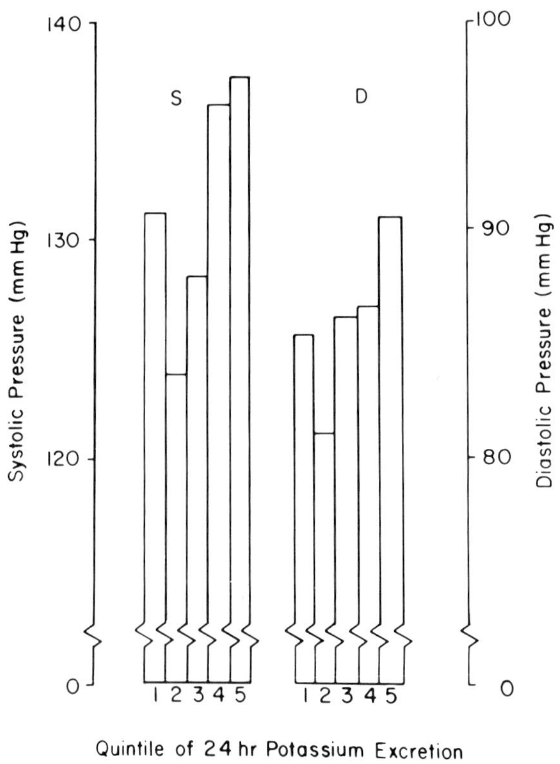

Figure 3 Average age- and weight-adjusted lying systolic blood pressure (S) and diastolic pressure (D) in mmHg for five "quintiles" of 24 hr potassium excretion for 162 women in the Whitehall–Department of the Environment Study. The first-order correlation coefficient between adjusted systolic pressure and potassium excretion was +0.20 ($p<0.05$) and for adjusted diastolic pressure +0.22 ($p<0.05$).

In men, it appears reasonable to accept the negative relationship between potassium excretion and both systolic and diastolic pressure. However, in women we must consider whether the failure to detect any such relationship is due to our having studied two few subjects or to a true difference between the sexes. The correlation coefficient for the association between systolic pressure and potassium excretion in women was +0.20 (95% confidence limits +0.02, +0.36), which leaves little chance of missing a *negative* association. For diastolic pressure the corresponding results were +0.22 (95% confidence limits +0.06, +0.38). Moreover the Belgian study also failed to find a negative association between 24-hr urinary potassium excretion and systolic blood pressure in 202 women. For systolic pressure (unadjusted for age or weight), the correlation coefficient between these variables was +0.07, which was not significant.

It is difficult to understand why, if potassium intake is an important causative factor in the genesis of hypertension, there should be a difference between the sexes. Average blood pressure in women tends not to reach that of men until after the age of 40 and any causative factor may be operative in men from an earlier age. There is also very indirect evidence that hormonal balance may influence the response of blood pressure to cation intake. In an extension of the Belgian study (32), blood pressure was positively related to sodium excretion only in women taking oral contraceptives. However, potassium excretion was not associated with blood pressure in women either taking or not taking oral contraceptives.

CONCLUSIONS

The recent study in London civil servants confirmed, in men, the negative association between blood pressure and both urinary and plasma potassium (1). Although these relationships may be explained by stress and partly accounted for by an increased secretion of aldosterone, it is unlikely that these mechanisms can explain the negative relationship in men between potassium excretion and the blood pressure measured weeks previously. The dietary intake of potassium appears to be decreased in male subjects with higher blood pressure, and potassium lack may be a causal factor in the genesis of male hypertension. It remains to be determined whether any such mechanisms operate in women.

REFERENCES

1. Bulpitt, C. J., Broughton, P. M. G., Markowe, H. L. J., Marmot, M. G., Rose, G. A., Semmence, A., and Shipley, M. J.: The relationship between potassium intake and blood pressure in London Civil Servants. The Whitehall–Department of Environment Study. *J. Chron. Dis.* (in press).
2. Bulpitt, C. J., Hodes, C., and Everitt, M. G.: The relationship between blood pressure and biochemical risk factors in a general population. *Br. J. Prev. Soc. Med.* 30:158–162, 1976.
3. Bulpitt, C. J., Shipley, M. J., and Semmence, A.: Blood pressure and plasma sodium and potassium. *Clin. Sci.* 61:85s–87s, 1981.
4. Dahl, L. K., Heine, M., and Tassinari, L.: Role of genetic factors in susceptibility to experimental hypertension due to chronic excess salt ingestion. *Nature* 194:480–482, 1962.
5. Dahl, L. K., and Love, R. A.: Evidence for relationship between sodium (chloride) intake and human essential hypertension. *Arch. Intern. Med.* 94:525–531, 1954.
6. Dluhy, R. G., Axelrod, L., Underwood, R. H., and Williams, G. H.: Studies of the

control of plasma aldosterone concentration in normal men. II Effect of the dietary potassium and acute potassium infusion. *J. Clin. Invest.* 51:1950–1957, 1972.
7. Fisher, E. R., and Funckes, A. J.: Effects of potassium deficiency on experimental renovascular hypertension. *Lab. Invest.* 16:539–549, 1967.
8. Friedman, M., Rosenman, R. H., and Freed, S. C.: Depressor effect of potassium deprivation on the blood pressure of hypertensive rats. *Am. J. Physiol.* 167:457–461, 1951.
9. Genest, J., Nowaczynski, W., Boucher, R., Kuchel, O., and Rojo-Ortega, J. M.: Aldosterone and renin in essential hypertension. *Can. Med. J.* 113:421–431, 1975.
10. Genest, J., Nowaczynski, W., Koiw, E., Sandor, T., and Biron, P.: Adrenocortical function in essential hypertension. In *Essential Hypertension. An International Symposium.* Edited by Bock, K. D., and Cottier, P. T., Berlin, Springer Verlag, 1960, p. 126.
11. Gleibermann, L.: Blood pressure and dietary salt in human populations. *Ecol. Food Nutr.* 2:143–156, 1973.
12. Grim, C. I., Luft, F. C., Miller, J. Z., Meneely, F. R., Battarbee, H. E., Hamies, C. G., and Dahl, L. K.: Racial differences in blood pressure in Evans County, Georgia: Relationship to sodium and potassium intake and plasma renin activity. *J. Chron. Dis.* 33:87–94, 1980.
13. Holly, J. M. P., Goodwin, F. J., Evans, S. J. W., Vandenburg, M. J., and Ledingham, J. M.: Re-analysis of data in two Lancet papers on the effect of dietary sodium and potassium on blood pressure. *Lancet* 2:1384–1386, 1981.
14. Hypertension Detection and Follow-up Program Co-operative Group: *Am. J. Epidemiol.* 106:351–361, 1977.
15. Iimura, O., Kijima, T., Kikuchi, K., Miyama, A., Ando, T., Nakao, T., and Takigami, Y.: Studies on the hypotensive effect of high potassium intake in patients with essential hypertension. *Clin. Sci.* 61 (suppl 7):77s–80s, 1981.
16. Kesteloot, H., and Geboers, J.: Calcium and blood pressure. *Lancet* 1:813–815, 1982.
17. Kesteloot, H., Park, B. C., Lee, C. S., Brems-Heyns, E., and Joossens, J. V.: A comparative study of blood pressure and sodium intake in Belgium and Korea. In *Epidemiology of Arterial Blood Pressure*, vol. 28, edited by Kesteloot, H., and Joossens, J. V., The Hague/Boston/London, Martinus Nijhoff, 1980, pp. 453–470.
18. Khaw, K. T., and Rose, G.: Population study of blood pressure and associated factors in St. Lucia, West Indies. *Int. J. Epidemiol.* 11:372–377, 1982.
19. Khaw, K. T., and Thom, S. Randomised double-blind cross over trial of potassium on blood pressure in normal subjects. *Lancet* 2:1127–1129, 1982.
20. Langford, H. G., Morino, T., and Watson, R. L.: Electrolyte intake in the treated and untreated hypertensive patients. In *Mild Hypertension Natural History and Management*, edited by Gross, F., and Strasser, T. Tunbridge Wells, Pitman Medical, 1979, pp. 139–146.
21. Langford, H. G., and Watson, R. L.: Electrolytes and hypertension. In *Epidemiology and Control of Hypertension*, edited by Paul, O., New York and London, Stratton Intercontinental Medical Book Corporation, 1975, p. 119.
22. Ljungman, S.: Renal function, sodium excretion and the renin-angiotensin-aldosterone system in relation to blood pressure. *Acta Med. Scand.* Suppl 663, 1982.
23. MacGregor, G. A., Smith, S. J., Markandu, N. D., Banks, R. A., and Sagnella, G. A.: Moderate potassium supplementation in essential hypertension. *Lancet* 2:567–570, 1983.
24. Meneely, G. R., and Ball, C. O. T.: Experimental epidemiology of chronic sodium chloride toxicity and the protective effect of potassium chloride. *Am. J. Med.* 25: 713–725, 1958.

25. Olsson, A. M., Persson, S., and Schoder, R.: Effects of terbutaline and isoproterenol on hyperkalemia in nephrectomized rabbits. *Scand. J. Urol. Nephrol.* 12:35-38, 1978.
26. Perera, G. A.: Depressor effects of potassium-deficient diets in hypertensive man. *J. Clin. Invest.* 32:633-636, 1953.
27. Puska, P., Iacono, J. M., Nissinen, A., Korhonen, J. H., Vartiainen, E., Pietinen, P., Dougherty, R., Leino, U., Mutanen, M., Moisio, S., and Huttenen, J.: Controlled, randomised trial of the effect of dietary fat on blood pressure. *Lancet* 1:1-5, 1983.
28. Rosa, R. M., Silva, P., Young, B., Landsberg, L., Brown, R. S., Rowe, J. W., and Epstein, F. H.: Adrenergic modulation of extrarenal potassium disposal. *N. Engl. J. Med.* 302:431-434, 1980.
29. Rosenman, R. H., Freed, S. C., St George, S., and Smith, M. K.: Effect of varying dietary potassium upon the blood pressure of hypertensive rats. *Am. J. Physiol.* 175: 386-388, 1953.
30. Sangal, A. K., and Beevers, D. G.: Serum calcium and blood pressure. *Lancet* 2:493, 1982.
31. Silva, P., Spokes, K., and Epstein, F. H.: Catecholamines and potassium homeostasis. *Kidney Int.* 12:544, 1977.
32. Staessen, J., Bulpitt, C. J., Fagard, R., Joossens, J. V., Lijnen, P., and Amery, A.: Contraceptive pill use, urinary sodium and blood pressure. A population study in two Belgian towns. *Acta Cardiol.* 39(1):55-64, 1984.
33. Staessen, J., Fagard, R., Lijnen, P., Amery, A., Bulpitt, C., and Joossens, J. V.: Salt and blood pressure in Belgium. *J. Epidemiol. Commun. Health* 35:256-261, 1981.
34. Takahashi, E., Sasaki, N., Takeda, J., and Ito, H.: The geographic distribution of cerebral hemorrhage and hypertension in Japan. *Hum. Biol.* 29:139-166, 1957.
35. Tannen, R. L.: Effects of potassium on blood pressure control. *Ann. Intern. Med.* 98 (Part 2):773-780, 1983.
36. Walker, W. G.: Relationships between sodium and potassium intake and blood pressure. In *Epidemiology of Arterial Blood Pressure*, edited by Kesteloot, H., and Joossen, J. V., The Hague/Boston/London, Martinus Nijhoff, 1980, p. 297.
37. Walker, W. G., Whelton, P. K., Saito, H., Russell, R. P., and Hermann, J.: Relation between blood pressure and renin, renin substrate, angiotensin II, aldosterone and urinary sodium and potassium in 574 ambulatory subjects. *Hypertension* 1:287-291, 1979.

28

Racial (Black/White) Differences in Blood Pressure in Children

GERALD S. BERENSON and GAIL C. FRANK
Louisiana State University Medical Center, New Orleans, Louisiana

Atherosclerosis and essential hypertension account for most of the cardiovascular deaths in the United States and in Western industrialized countries, and certain racial differences seem to influence the prevalence of these diseases (13). For example, coronary artery disease seems to be more common in young white males, while hypertension is more common in blacks, particularly in black females in whom the prevalence is two to three times greater than in whites. Hypertension is also a more severe disease in blacks. Although it is likely that major determinants of the pathogenesis of both atherosclerosis and hypertension are similar in both blacks and whites, observations of racial contrast provide clues to mechanisms contributing to the natural history of these diseases.

Epidemiological observations made over the past few years indicate that essential hypertension begins during childhood, and that precursors of this disease can be identified (22). Studies of general populations of children document the early onset of essential hypertension, and recent studies of blood pressure levels and other cardiovascular risk factor variables now allow us to identify in early life those persons at high risk of developing cardiovascular disease in adulthood.

The main purposes for exploring black-white contrasts in primary hypertension are that understanding differences may help to clarify mechanisms and pathogenesis of disease; and because these studies may guide development of more rational approaches to prevention. While both environmental and genetic factors are known to contribute to black-white differences, relatively little is known about the precise contribution made by the environmental or genetic factors in the general population. An environmental-genetic interaction undoubtedly occurs, influencing the course of essential hypertension and coronary artery disease over time. The strong familial relationship of hypertensive disease, and the impact of socioeconomic factors and diet are all known to influence essential hypertension greatly.

For over a decade extensive epidemiological studies in a number of populations of children have provided observations on cardiovascular risk factors and blood pressures in children (1). To complement the long-term studies of adults, the Bogalusa Heart Study has examined some 8,000 children in cross-sectional and longitudinal surveys for cardiovascular risk factor variables. Bogalusa is a semirural community of 22,000 individuals, one-third of whom are black and two-thirds white. Observations include measurements of height, weight, skinfold thickness, blood pressure levels, serum lipids and lipoproteins, cigarette smoking, Type A behavior, and results of nutrition studies. Methods for obtaining reproducible observations have been developed and special substudies have been conducted related to blood pressure and the role of sodium and potassium on blood pressure levels.

RACIAL DIFFERENCES IN THE GENERAL POPULATION

Based on several cross-sectional surveys (each includes approximately 4,000 children), several specific black-white differences were noted. White children and girls have greater skinfold thickness and tend to be fatter at similar heights and weights; these observations are also consistent with black children demonstrating a greater body density as measured by densitometric studies. Slightly higher blood pressure levels are detected in the black children, especially after age 12. This was particularly evident at the high percentiles for blood pressure in which a greater number of black children are found. Heart rates are slightly faster in white children. Serum total cholesterol levels are slightly higher in black children due to higher levels of α-lipoprotein cholesterol, while serum triglycerides and pre-β-lipoprotein cholesterol levels tend to be higher in white children. Fasting serum insulin levels are greater in black children, especially in young black girls who have a remarkably greater insulin response after a glucose load. These anthropometric and laboratory observations suggest that racial differences potentially influence the development of hypertension and cardiovascular disease beginning in early life. For example, body height and weight correlate closely with blood pressure levels, indicating a significant role of body mass in affecting levels in childhood (27). Body fatness and weight at an early age seem to correlate more closely with blood pressure levels in white children than in blacks. This relationship will likely change during the adolescent and young adult period when black girls begin to demonstrate a rapid onset of obesity.

NUTRITIONAL STUDIES

Extensive studies on infants and children explored dietary intakes of nutrients and electrolytes that might be related to cardiovascular disease (5). Figures 1 and 2 reflect Na^+ and K^+ intakes obtained from these studies. There are slight racial differences in dietary intake of electrolytes in the preschool age group, but because of difficulties in measurement and large variations of intake, these differences may not be significant. There is a progressive intake of both Na^+ and K^+, reaching childhood and young adult levels at age 3-4, with a suggestion of a slight increased intake in black children of preschool age. Reflecting total caloric intake and based on body size, a much greater relative intake of both Na^+ and K^+ is noted in infancy and in the preschool age group, reaching adult levels around age 13. The adult Na^+ intakes already considered excessive are considerably lower than that noted in infants and in young children. This circumstance may be important in preconditioning young children to hypertension later in life. Consequently, based on epidemiological studies, children are on high-Na^+ intake and relatively low-K^+ intake compared to optimal levels for prevention of hypertension. The flat curves noted in the distributions of blood pressure levels during infancy and early childhood, which are

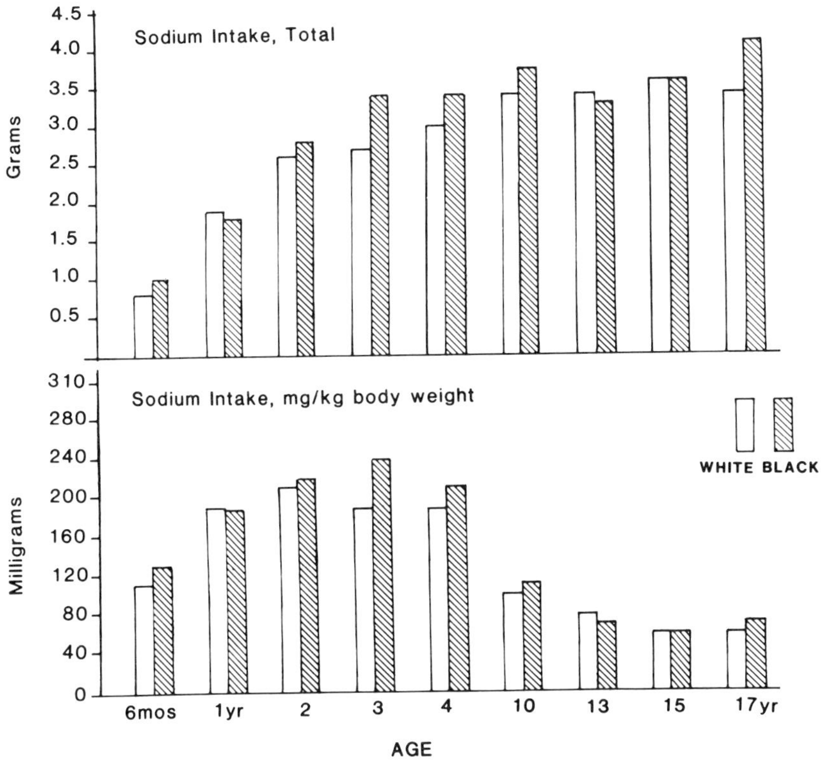

Figure 1 Na^+ intake of infants, children, and adolescents, aged 6 months to 17 years, obtained by 24-hr dietary recalls. The observations are expressed as actual amounts consumed and values based on body weight. The remarkable relatively high Na^+ intake during infancy reflects the relatively high caloric intake. (Bogalusa Heart Study.)

considered to be due to technical difficulties in measuring indirect pressure, may actually reflect the relatively high Na^+ intake during this period (25).

IN-DEPTH BLOOD PRESSURE STUDY

Findings

A special study was conducted on "normal" children selected from the general population at various levels of blood pressure. The purpose was to search for statistically meaningful factors that might distinguish between children at the high and the low end of the blood pressure distribution curve. Such studies in a biracial population may serve to document further the interaction of environmental and genetic factors influencing early hypertension. The general design of the study has been described (2,23). Two hundred and seventy-two children, selected at different levels of blood pressure with the

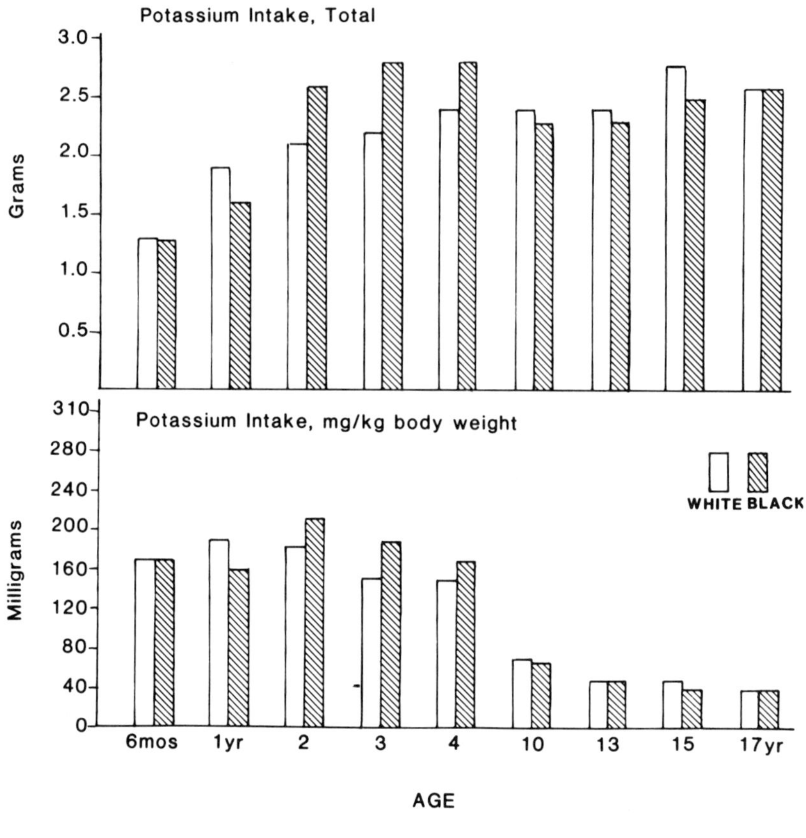

Figure 2 K^+ intake of young individuals, aged 6 months to 17 years, as shown in Figure 1. Interesting patterns emerge that suggest conditioning for hypertension in salt-responsive persons. Approximate adult levels relative to body size occur at 10–13 years of age, which are considerably different than during infancy. Even at that, the adult levels are considered excessive for Na^+ intake and meager for K^+ intake as ideal for prevention of hypertension. (Bogalusa Heart Study.)

extremes weighted, were studied extensively for a number of parameters that relate to hypertension. In addition to the examination to exclude secondary hypertension, several cardiovascular stresses on heart rate and blood pressure were also observed. Twenty-four-hour urine outputs were collected for electrolyte and creatinine excretion. Blood samples were obtained before and after an oral glucose load and blood was analyzed for multiple laboratory variables.

Consistent with cross-sectional observations, a greater percentage of body fat was found in white children, especially in those with high blood pressure. Serum dopamine-β-hydroxylase and renin values tended to be lower in black children, again especially in those with high blood pressure (Figure 3). One-hour plasma glucose levels were consider-

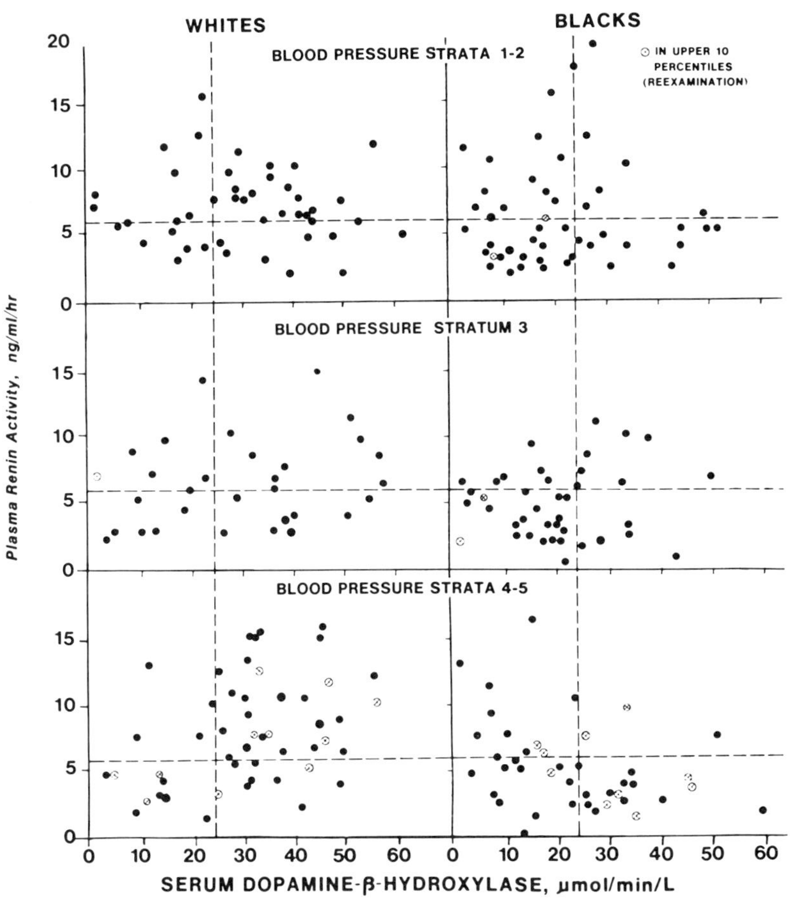

Figure 3 Scattergram of plasma renin activity by serum dopamine-β-hydroxylase, by race and by blood pressure stratum. Median values for the combined children are represented by dotted lines. The preponderance of children with combined high renin and high DβH, expected in the high-blood-pressure strata, is lacking among blacks. Children whose diastolic mercury sphygmomanometer pressure (4th phase) as measured during reexamination was in the upper 10% for age (7–15 years) and race group are marked with open circles. They conform to the above conclusions. (Bogalusa Heart Study, 1975–1976; from Ref. 23.)

Table 1 Electrolytes in Urine by Blood Pressure Stratum and Race (the Bogalusa Heart Study)

Electrolyte	Subject classification	Blood pressure stratum 1 (low)	2	3	4	5 (high)
				(Mean ± 2 SEM)		
Urine Na^+ (N=249)	Whites	86.5±17.7 (15)[a]	115.3±15.8 (31)	97.6±17.2 (31)	103.1±19.1 (30)	117.7±21.5 (18)
	Blacks	107.9±17.2 (11)	93.7±14.1 (33)	103.3±17.4 (37)	110.0±17.4 (34)	134.5±58.4 (9)
Urine K^+ (N=249)	Whites	33.2± 4.9 (15)	42.0± 5.6 (31)	34.2± 7.2 (31)	44.7±10.2 (30)	38.8± 6.8 (18)
	Blacks	24.8± 5.7 (11)	26.5± 4.2 (33)	27.4± 4.4 (37)	29.4± 5.0 (34)	29.8±11.6 (9)

[a]Sample size is given in parentheses.

ably higher in white children in the high-blood-pressure group. In the supine position, systolic blood pressure levels for black males in the high blood pressure group were considerably greater than those noted for the other black/white/gender groups. In contrast, heart rates in the high-blood-pressure group were significantly faster for white children. Reactivity to isometric hand grip stresses was greater in the black boys with high blood pressures (26).

A most intriguing observation of this study is related to urine electrolyte studies. The amount of Na^+ excreted in urine was very similar for the different blood pressure groups in both blacks and whites. However, black children in all blood pressure strata excreted considerably less K^+ in urine (Table 1) (2). This observation has been noted in other populations, and the phenomenon deserves further study. Their reduced excretion of K^+ is suggested to be related to diet, but since we do not find marked differences in dietary intakes in school-age children, diet may not explain the difference. Comparing the relationship of Na^+ to K^+ clearances in 24-hr urine samples from two different studies in Bogalusa and in Franklinton (24), we note that the correlation is much greater in black children (Figure 4).

The overall results of this study, from observation of a variety of parameters of the children stratified by high and low levels of blood pressure and showing the black-white differences, are summarized in Table 2.

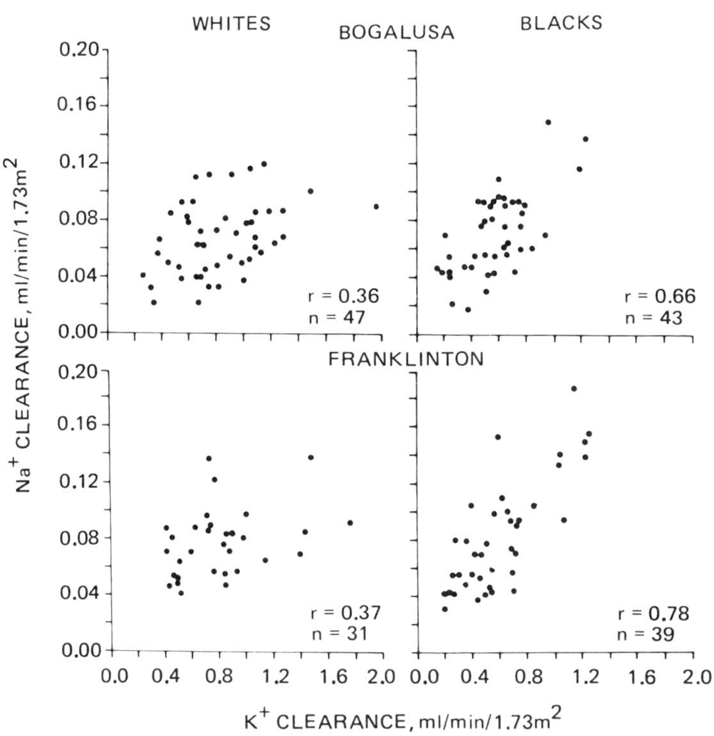

Figure 4 Relation of Na^+ and K^+ clearance for children age 7–18 years in upper decile of blood pressure, by race and community. Blacks tended to have stronger correlation of Na^+ with K^+ clearance than whites ($p < 0.01$ for untransformed data). (Bogalusa Heart Study, 1975–1980; from Ref. 24.)

Table 2 Racial Differences in Children's Blood Pressure

Higher values for characteristics noted in:	
All blood pressure strata	
Whites	Blacks
Percentage body fat	Blood pressure levels
Plasma renin activity	
Serum dopamine-β-hydroxylase (DβH)	
24-Hr urine K^+	
High-blood pressure strata	
Resting heart rate	Correlation 24-hr urine Na^+ and blood pressure
Renin activity and DβH	
1-Hr serum glucose	

Comments

Paffenbarger et al. (20), Kahn et al. (15), and Frohlich et al. (8) have found that heart rate is predictive of high blood pressure. Apparently this may be true for white children primarily and, as suggested by Julius and Conway (14), elevated recumbent heart rates in borderline hypertensive patients are associated with elevated cardiac output. The observations in children may be consistent with findings in more detailed studies that have been conducted on adults. The observation on low renin in black children is similar to that noted by Brunner et al. (4) in adult black hypertensive patients. These observations are now consistent with studies being conducted on racial differences in response to diuretic and other antihypertensive medication.

The differences in K^+ excretion are particularly interesting in view of the suggestions of Helmer (12) and Gleibermann (9) who propose an adaptive survival advantage for the genetic trait that would conserve body Na^+ in blacks by preventing hypernatremic collapse. Sodium losses could occur through sweating in persons in hot climates on a low-Na^+ diet that also tends to be very high in K^+. The possibility of an increased Na^+ sensitivity in the upper percentiles of blood pressure for black children in our high-Na^+ society certainly should be considered in any effort to prevent hypertension. The mechanisms for differences in K^+ excretion are not clear but certainly suggest adaptive mechanisms. Based on the observation of reduced urine K^+ excretion, additional studies were conducted.

POTASSIUM ADMINISTRATION TO NORMAL INDIVIDUALS

Methods

The above observations led to a special substudy on 13 normal persons to observe ambulatory Na^+/K^+ balance influenced by K^+ administration (24). The observations include dietary intake and total urine and stool excretions. After 3 days of baseline observations, each subject was given 80 mEq KCl daily in addition to his or her usual dietary intake. Potassium was administered orally in divided doses for 4 days. Twenty-four hour urine samples were collected and Na^+ and K^+ were measured in both urine and stools. The methods used have been described previously.

A simplified inventory method for quantitating dietary Na^+ and K^+ was developed to enable us to conduct a balance study on ambulatory persons (7). A method for monitoring

Table 3 Groups in Food Inventory Used to Quantitate Dietary Na^+, K^+, and Energy Intakes

Beverages	Fruits and juices
Bread and cereal	Milk and milk products
Fast foods	Home recipes
Fats, oils, and condiments	Snack items
Fish, meats, and poultry	Vegetables and soups

dietary Na^+, K^+, and energy was developed so that estimates of dietary intakes could be compared to urine and stool electrolyte measurements. Additional information included use of salt and the relationship of Na^+ to K^+ within the diet.

A food inventory included foods that the subjects were encouraged to consume during the study. This method provided ease of quantitation and reliability, heterogeneity of food preferences among participants, and accommodated the different energy requirements of participants. Participants were encouraged to repeat consumption of foods during the test period to simplify estimations of Na^+ and K^+.

The self-administered inventory consisted of 10 preselected food groups (Table 3). Each food group included 24–40 staple items, home-prepared recipes, and fast-food or vending-machine selections. Participants helped design the inventory by contributing names of foods most often purchased at work or brought from home. To improve selection and acceptance of foods on the inventory, restaurant and vending-machine items were included. Commonly consumed foods, additional condiments, and staple foods were added to increase validity of the tool. A total of 217 foods were selected and categorized into a 14-page food inventory; a partial list of one food group is given in Figure 5. The format allowed participants to "check" a column if the food was eaten, enter quantity consumed, and record ingredients or preparation procedures.

Participants received preweighed salt shakers to salt food as usual while quantifying topically applied salt. Total dietary Na^+ intake was calculated as the sum of Na^+ from the inventory plus Na^+ from the salt shaker.

Electrolyte and energy compositions of foods on the inventory were based on a computerized food composition table, the Extended Table of Nutrient Values (19), Pennington and Church handbook (21), and nutrition content values supplied by food companies. Recipes were selected that reflected "with salt added."

Effect of K^+ Administration on Electrolyte Balance

The mean daily dietary electrolyte (exclusive of supplemental K^+) and energy intakes for participants are outlined in Table 4. Figures 6 and 7 compare Na^+ and K^+ intakes and outputs for each day for all participants. Certain race and sex differences in the dietary components for this group of individuals were noted. White participants averaged 151 mEq Na^+, 70 mEq K^+, and 2,367 kcal/day. For black participants, mean intakes were 130 mEq Na^+, 50 mEq K^+, and 1,993 kcal/day. For the sexes combined, total energy ($p < 0.01$) and K^+ intakes ($p < 0.02$) were higher in whites than in blacks. For the races combined, Na^+ intakes ($p < 0.02$) and energy ($p < 0.10$) were higher in male than female participants. Based on caloric density, Na^+ intake was significantly higher for male than female participants ($p < 0.03$).

NAME ______________________ Page ___ of ___

ID ______________________ DATE ______________________

DAY ______________________

Food Item	Check if Eaten	Enter Amount Eaten	Comments	DO NOT WRITE IN THESE COLUMNS		
				Na^+	K^+	Kcal
FAST FOODS						
Burger King						
Cheeseburger						
French Fries						
Hamburger						
Vanilla Shake						
Whaler						
Whopper						
TACO BELL						
Bean Burrito						
Beef Burrito						
Taco						

Figure 5 A partial listing of the foods comprising the fast food groups, one of 10 subgroups in the Daily Food Inventory (Table 3). Participants entered the quantity and a description of each food eaten daily. A nutritionist then calculated the sodium, potassium, and energy content. (From Ref. 7.)

The overall Na^+/K^+ ratio of dietary intakes (1.4) was similar for whites (1.3) and blacks (1.5). Male patients had the same Na^+/K^+ ratio (1.8) whereas the Na^+/K^+ ratio for female white patients (1.0) was lower than that for female black subjects (1.4). The percentage of the daily Na^+ intake from the salt shaker for whites was 6%, 4% for males, and 10% for females. The total Na^+ intake from the shaker for blacks was 2%, 3%, for males and 2% for females. There is an obvious marked variability of intake and such studies need to be conducted on larger numbers of individuals.

Table 4 Daily Dietary Sodium, Potassium,[a] and Energy Intake of Participants, Food Inventory Study

		Sodium (mEq)		Potassium (mEq)		Energy (kcal)	
Group	n	Mean	Range	Mean	Range	Mean	Range
Whites	6	151	25–375	70	16–121	2367	551–4176
Male	3	190	55–375	74	16–121	2500	551–3781
Female	3	111	25–245	66	20–100	2235	880–4176
Blacks	7	130	1–263	50	15–101	1993	718–3302
Male	3	153	23–253	51	15–101	2220	947–3132
Female	4	112	1–263[b]	48	15–100	1823	718–3302

[a] K^+ supplement not included.
[b] One participant began a sodium-free diet on the last day of the study.

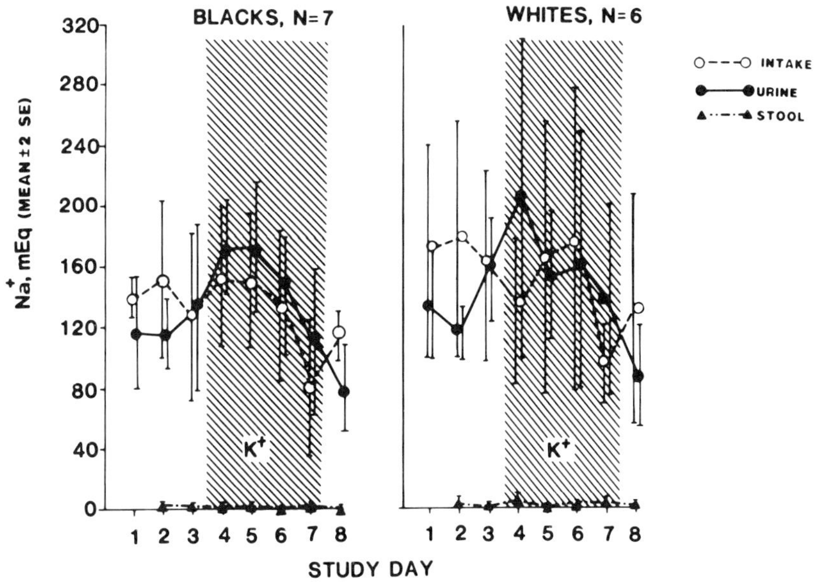

Figure 6 Daily 24-hr Na^+ in intake, urine, and stool (mEq, mean ± 2 SE) during K^+ administration, by race. A good matching of intake and output supports the validity of the measurement methods. Insensible loss was not measured, but was deduced from baseline observations during days 1–3. In blacks, a natriuresis following the K^+ medication onset is obvious ($p < 0.01$ by paired t test). In whites the natriuresis did not reach statistical significance. (From Ref. 24.)

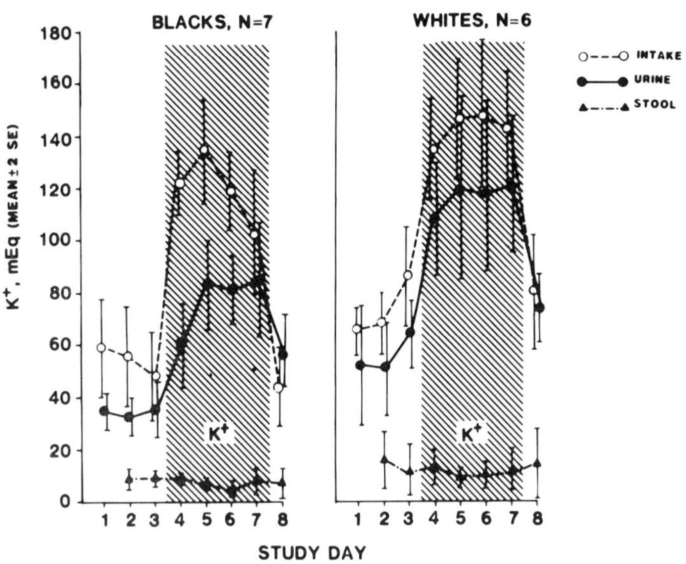

Figure 7 Daily 24-hr K^+ in intake, urine, and stool (mean ± 2 SE) during K^+ administration, by race. A close agreement between intake and output supports the validity of the measurement methods. Whites had higher K^+ excretion values than blacks during K^+ treatment ($p < 0.05$ by paired t test). This difference may have been caused in part by the higher dietary K^+ intake of the whites, and by the lag in K^+ excretion noted in the blacks. (From Ref. 24.)

Correlation coefficients among dietary components for both races showed higher correlations between Na^+ and energy intake than between K^+ and energy intake. Correlations are consistently positive and generally significant. The association between Na^+ and K^+/1,000 kcal was positive on some days and negative on others. Variations obviously occur based on the nature of foods and amount of exogenous NaCl consumed.

Administration of K^+ produced a marked natriuresis, especially in blacks. Blacks as a group also appeared to retain the additional K^+ for 24–48 hr. Increases of urine K^+ occurred in both whites and blacks, but a lag was noted in the blacks. The examination of stool electrolytes showed considerable interindividual variability for K^+ excretion with a relatively large amount of K^+ being excreted in the stool. Relatively small amounts of Na^+ are excreted and only slight differences were noted between whites and blacks; blacks had an insignificantly greater percentage of K^+ excretion.

Correlations between dietary Na^+ and K^+ intakes with urine and stool output were generally positive and higher for K^+ than for Na^+ for both races. An inverse relationship was noted on occasions for each component. There was a close parallel of K^+ intake and output each day, with intakes measuring 8 mEq higher for baseline days (range, 1–10 mEq/day). During the days of K^+ supplementation the differential between intake and output ranged from 10 to 40 mEq. During baseline days Na^+ intake was 20–40 mEq (about 22 mEq/day) higher than output; however, during K^+ supplementation an opposite trend in excretion was noted for Na^+. Output surpassed intake by as much as 40 mEq. By the second day of K^+ supplementation there was a close parallel between Na^+ in-

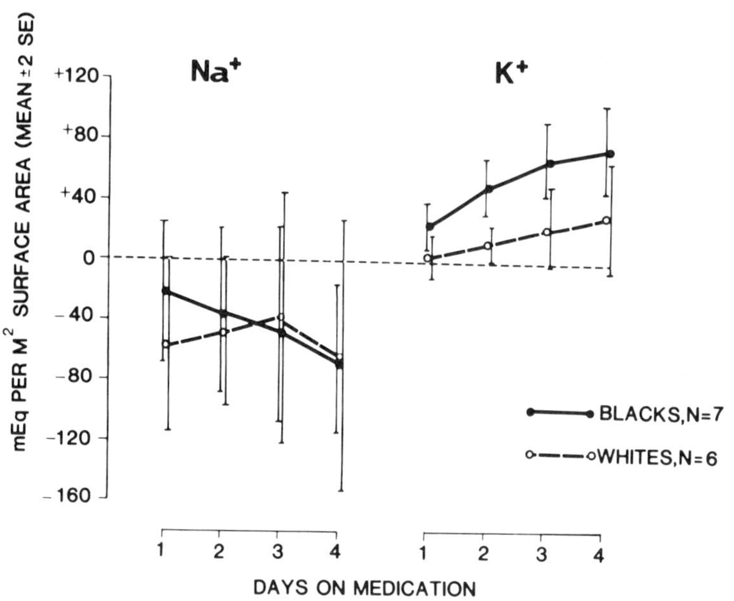

Figure 8 Cumulative dietary Na^+ and K^+ balance (mean ± 2 SE) during K^+ administration, by race. The mean baseline day values are used as zero. At the end of the K^+ administration, the cumulative Na^+ balance was different from zero for blacks ($p < 0.05$) but not for whites. The cumulative K^+ balance differed from zero for all medication days in blacks ($p < 0.05$–< 0.0001) but not in whites. (From Ref. 24.)

take and output for both races. A more consistent and continued natriuresis was noted in blacks.

The observations on stool electrolytes warrant further stool electrolyte studies along with observations of insensible losses. As might be expected, marked changes in plasma renin occurred during administration of K^+ with an indication that the responses might be greater in black men. These studies also showed that acute K^+ administration resulted in a decrease of blood pressure levels, particularly in blacks.

SUMMARY

The observations of racial contrasts related to blood pressure levels are consistent with mechanisms operating in the pathobiology of essential hypertension; however, they also document subtle changes occurring in early childhood that contribute to the development of essential hypertension in early life. Observations based on tracking and persistence of high or low blood pressure levels in childhood in a given person (16,29) and observations obtained from epidemiological studies over long periods (10,11) are consistent with the onset of essential hypertension in early life. Based on careful blood pressure measurements in children, coupled with family history, it is highly likely that young individuals destined to develop hypertensive disease in adulthood can be identified.

Increased body mass in the black children might enhance an increased blood volume and greater cardiac output, which could contribute to their higher blood pressure levels. Kidneys and other tissues of blacks may also have a decreased ability to handle Na^+, as suggested by Luft et al. (17,18). In our high-Na^+-consumption society, the slight aberration in electrolyte handling may be one of the mechanisms important in contributing to, or initiating, exaggerated hypertension in blacks. In contrast, observations on white children suggest the importance of other mechanisms. Their greater body fat and obesity, faster heart rates, higher blood sugars, high plasma renin and dopamine-β-hydroxylase values all indicate that greater neurohumoral factors may be operative in the onset of essential hypertension (22). These black-white contrasts provide several clues to the different mechanisms operating to produce essential hypertension, which is a complex disease process.

The observations also have bearing on prevention of hypertension. Although weight reduction and Na^+ restriction have been the basis of both primary prevention and nonpharmacological therapy, it appears from these observations that, at least in children, obesity has a greater influence on high blood pressure levels in whites and a lesser effect in blacks. Since an acceleration of obesity seems to occur in young black women (28), obesity may then begin to play a greater role in contributing to hypertension later in life in blacks. Because of a lesser response to antihypertensive medication by blacks, and a greater difficulty in dietary control of Na^+ intake, blacks likely require a more aggressive approach to hypertension prevention. In an intervention program on early hypertension, which used primary prevention approaches (6) and low-dosage medication (3), the response of blacks in general was less than that of the white children (Figure 9). The significant black-white differences described above emphasize the fact that multiple mechanisms contribute to hypertension. In the face of environmental factors in our culture that contribute to high Na^+ and excessive caloric intakes, a more aggressive approach to prevention of hypertension and obesity in blacks will be needed. The observations on K^+ suggest that the role of K^+ intake may be of even greater importance in control of hypertension in blacks.

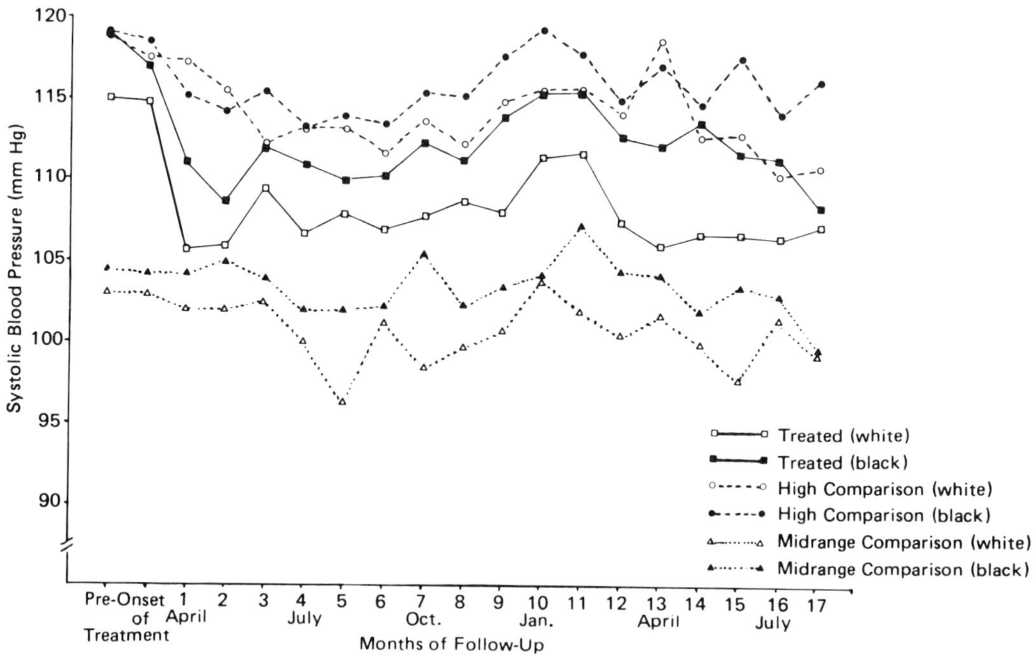

Figure 9 Systolic blood pressure levels in three groups of children over time, by race; observations extracted from an intervention study of children persisting with blood pressure levels at or above the 90th percentile (3). It might be noted that, although most children responded to treatment (here shown for a period of 17 months), the blacks did not respond as well as whites to a regimen of low-dosage medication (propranolol and chlorthalidone) and dietary and exercise management. (Franklinton Blood Pressure Study, 1979–1981.)

ACKNOWLEDGMENTS

This work was supported by funds from the National Heart, Lung and Blood Institute of the U.S. Public Health Service, Specialized Center of Research–Arteriosclerosis (SCOR-A), HL 15103.

The authors express appreciation to the SCOR-A staff in New Orleans and the Field Staff in Bogalusa for conducting the research. We also wish to recognize the major contributions to the above work by A.W. Voors, M.D., Dr. P.H. (deceased) and to Mr. E.R. Dalferes, Jr., for supervision of laboratory analyses. Finally, a special appreciation is expressed to the children of Bogalusa and Franklinton, without whom this work would not have been possible.

REFERENCES

1. Berenson, G. S., McMahan, C. A., Voors, A. W., Webber, L. S., Srinivasan, S. R., Frank, G. C., Foster, T. A., and Blonde, C. V.: *Cardiovascular Risk Factors in Children–The Early Natural History of Atherosclerosis and Essential Hypertension*, Oxford University Press, New York, 1980.
2. Berenson, G. S., Voors, A. W., Dalferes, E. R. Jr., Webber, L. S., and Shuler, S. E.:

Creatinine clearance, electrolytes, and plasma renin activity related to the blood pressure of white and black children–the Bogalusa Heart Study. *J. Lab. Clin. Med.* 93:535, 1979.

3. Berenson, G. S., Voors, A. W., Webber, L. S., Frank, G. C., Farris, R. P., Tobian, L., and Aristimuno, G. G.: A model of intervention for prevention of early essential hypertension in the 1980's. *Hypertension* 5:41, 1983.
4. Brunner, H. R., Sealey, J. E., and Laragh, J. H.: Renin subgroups in essential hypertension. Further analysis of their pathophysiological and epidemiological characteristics. *Circ. Res.* 33 (Suppl. 1):99, 1973.
5. Frank, G. C., Berenson, G. S., and Webber, L. S.: Dietary studies of infants and children. In *Promoting Adolescent Health: A Dialogue on Research and Practice*, edited by Coates, T., Petersen, A., and Perry, C., New York, Academic Press, 1982, p. 329.
6. Frank, G. C., Farris, R. P., Ditmarsen, P., Voors, A. W., and Berenson, G. S.: An approach to primary preventive treatment for children with high blood pressure. *J. Am. Coll. Nutr.* 1:357, 1982.
7. Frank, G. C., Voors, A. W., Berenson, G. S., and Webber, L. S.: A simplified inventory method for quantitating dietary sodium, potassium and energy. *Am. J. Clin. Nutr.* 38:474, 1983.
8. Frohlich, E. D., Tarazi, R. C., and Dustan, H. P.: Re-examination of the hemodynamics of hypertension. *Am. J. Med. Sci.* 257:9, 1969.
9. Gliebermann, L.: Blood pressure and dietary salt in human populations. *Ecol. Food Nutr.* 2:143, 1973.
10. Harlan, W. R., Oberman, A., Mitchell, R. E., and Graybiel, A.: A 30-year study of blood pressure in a white male cohort. In *Hypertension: Mechanisms and Management*, edited by Onesti, G., Kim, K. E., and Moyer, J. H., New York, Grune and Stratton, 1973, p. 85.
11. Heiss, G., Tyroler, H. A., and Hames, C.: Cholesterol tracking: prediction over time of serum cholesterol in Evans County. *Adv. Exp. Biol. Med.* 82:112, 1977.
12. Helmer, O. M.: In *Colloque Internationale, Les Concepts de Claude Bernard sur le Milieu Intérieur*, Paris, Masson, 1965, p. 115.
13. Hypertension Task Force, Report, Vol. I. General Summary and Recommendations. U.S. Department of Health, Education and Welfare, National Institutes of Health (NIH Publication No. 79-1623), September, 1978.
14. Julius, S., and Conway, J.: Hemodynamic studies in patients with borderline blood pressure elevation. *Circulation* 38:282, 1969.
15. Kahn, H. A., Medalie, J. H., Neufeld, H. N., Riss, E., and Goldbourt, U.: The incidence of hypertension and associated factors: The Israel Ischemic Heart Disease Study. *Am. Heart J.* 84:171, 1972.
16. Lauer, R. M., Clarke, W. R., and Beaglehole, R.: Level, trend, and variability of blood pressure during childhood: The Muscatine Study. *Circulation* 69:242, 1984.
17. Luft, F. C., Rankin, L. I., Bloch, R., Weyman, A. E., Willis, L. R., Murray, R. H., Grim, C. E., and Weinberger, M. H.: Cardiovascular and humoral responses to extremes of sodium intake in normal black and white men. *Circulation* 60:697, 1979.
18. Luft, F. C., and Weinberger, M. H.: Sodium intake and essential hypertension. *Hypertension* 4 (Suppl. III):14, 1982.
19. Moore, M. C., Goodloe, M. H., and Schilling, P. E.: *Extended Table of Nutrient Values*, New Orleans, LSU Medical Center, 1971.
20. Paffenbarger, R. S. Jr., Thorne, M. C., and Wing, A. L.: Chronic disease in former college students. 8. Characteristics in youth predisposing to hypertension in later years. *Am. J. Epidemiol.* 88:25, 1968.
21. Pennington, J. A., and Church, H. N. (eds.): *Bowes and Church's Food Values of Portions Commonly Used*, 13th ed., Philadelphia, J.B. Lippincott, 1980.

22. Voors, A. W., and Berenson, G. S.: Search for the determinants of the early onset of essential hypertension. In *Phasic Pressor Mechanisms: Hypertension in the Young and the Old*, edited by Onesti, G., and Eun Kim, K., New York, Grune and Stratton, 1981, p. 43.
23. Voors, A. W., Berenson, G. S., Dalferes, E. R., Webber, L. S., and Shuler, S. E.: Racial differences in blood pressure control. *Science* 204:1091, 1979.
24. Voors, A. W., Dalferes, E. R. Jr., Frank, G. C., Aristimuno, G. G., and Berenson, G. S.: Relation between ingested potassium and sodium balance in young blacks and whites. *Am. J. Clin. Nutr.* 37:583, 1983.
25. Voors, A. W., Webber, L. S., and Berenson, G. S.: Blood pressure of children, ages 2½–5½ years, in a total community–the Bogalusa Heart Study. *Am. J. Epidemiol.* 107:403, 1978.
26. Voors, A. W., Webber, L. S., and Berenson, G. S.: Racial contrasts in cardiovascular response tests for children from a total community. *Hypertension* 2:686, 1980.
27. Voors, A. W., Webber, L. S., Frerichs, R. R., and Berenson, G. S.: Body height and body mass as determinants of basal blood pressure in children–the Bogalusa Heart Study. *Am. J. Epidemiol.* 106:101, 1977.
28. Webber, L. S., Cresanta, J. L., Croft, J. B., Srinivasan, S. R., and Berenson, G. S.: Transitions of cardiovascular risk from adolescence to young adulthood–the Bogalusa Heart Study. II. Alterations in anthropometric, blood pressure and serum lipoprotein variables. *J. Chron. Dis.* (in press, 1985).
29. Webber, L. S., Cresanta, J. L., Voors, A. W., and Berenson, G. S.: Tracking of cardiovascular disease risk factor variables in school-age children. *J. Chron. Dis.* 36:647, 1983.

29

Sodium and Potassium Intake and High Blood Pressure

GRAHAM A. MacGREGOR
Charing Cross Hospital Medical School, London, England

Increasing epidemiological and experimental evidence in animals suggests that the ratio of sodium to potassium in the diet is an important determinant of blood pressure levels in both human communities and animal models of hypertension. This does not necessarily imply, however, that altering either sodium or potassium intake when high blood pressure is established will change the blood pressure. There are therefore two separate questions. First, does a high-sodium, low-potassium intake predispose towards the development of essential hypertension? Second, does lowering sodium intake or increasing potassium intake lower blood pressure when it is already raised?

Both sodium and potassium are vital cations, the major function of sodium being to regulate the extracellular fluid volume. For mammals living away from the sea, sodium or salt is difficult to obtain and there are several mechanisms in mammals designed to conserve sodium, both in the urine and sweat. Humans, quite recently in evolutionary terms, have developed the ability to obtain salt from both the sea and from mines and it was soon found that it could act as a preservative for food, which is of particular importance during the winter. Salt, therefore, became of great economic and religious importance in early civilizations. Most communities in the world are now eating between 100 and 400 mmol/day of sodium compared to the 5-10 mmol/day eaten by our ancestors during the last million or so years of evolution, and still in some communities where sodium chloride is not available (8). At the same time as this large increase in sodium intake, there has been a concomitant reduction in potassium intake. It has been estimated that potassium intake has fallen from a probable figure of 100-250 mmol/day to an average in most countries in the West of 30-80 mmol/day (8).

EVIDENCE FOR THE INFLUENCE OF SODIUM AND POTASSIUM ON BLOOD PRESSURE

Studies from different communities throughout the world have shown that differences in sodium and potassium intake appear to act as important determinants of the whole population's blood pressure levels (11). All of these studies have been criticized but epidemio-

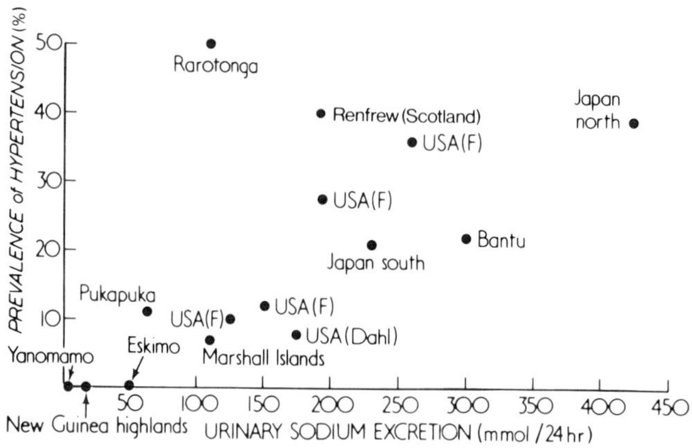

Figure 1 Relation between 24-hr urinary sodium excretion measured in different communities compared to the percentage of people in that community with high blood pressure [USA(F) taken from the Framingham data when grouped according to urinary sodium excretion].

logical evidence by its very nature can never prove a relationship. It is perhaps not surprising, given the genetic nature of essential hypertension, that there is no direct relationship within one community between salt intake and high blood pressure; this is seen only when different communities with different salt intakes are considered (Figure 1).

Some more recent studies in which potassium excretion has been measured suggest a direct relationship between potassium excretion or the sodium/potassium ratio in the urine, and blood pressure (34). None of these studies, however, will answer the vital question: does lowering sodium intake or increasing potassium intake prevent the development of essential hypertension in the Western world? Studies such as are beginning in Holland, in which babies are randomized to one of two different diets and are then followed up, may give us the answer but it will obviously take many years before definitive conclusions can be drawn. Nevertheless, after the first year in this study the babies who were consuming a low-sodium diet did have significant lower blood pressure values (13).

Recommendations, therefore, by various governmental health organizations in the West that the whole population should reduce sodium and increase potassium intake are based on circumstantial evidence. Further evidence may come if communities who are successful in decreasing sodium or increasing potassium in the diet are compared with communities that are less successful. Rose has made the important point that a small fall in blood pressure in the whole community would have the same benefit to the population as all of the current blood pressure treatment (29).

MECHANISM OF ACTION

There is general agreement that for sodium to be involved in high blood pressure, there must be some abnormality in the kidney's ability to excrete sodium. Initial ideas were that this abnormality would cause retention of sodium and water, increase cardiac output, and, by autoregulation, increase peripheral resistance. However, experimental evidence on the whole disagrees with this concept.

Several studies have demonstrated evidence of inhibition of the ouabain-sensitive component of the sodium pump in patients with essential hypertension (10) and that this inhibition of sodium transport is associated with a raised level of a sodium transport inhibitor in the plasma of patients with essential hypertension (12,20). Furthermore, cross-incubation studies in which normotensive white cells were incubated in hypertensive plasma showed that the hypertensive plasma produced the same abnormality in the normotensive white cells (i.e., inhibition of the ouabain-sensitive sodium pump) that occurred in their own white cells (27). Blaustein has suggested that this raised level of a circulating sodium transport inhibitor could, by slowing down sodium/calcium exchange across the arteriolar smooth-muscle cell wall, increase intracellular calcium concentration and thereby increase the sensitivity or tone of the smooth-muscle cell, giving rise eventually to an increase in peripheral resistance and the development of high blood pressure (5). Kidney cross-transplantation experiments in rats with inherited hypertension have demonstrated that the kidney carries the underlying message for the later development of high blood pressure (4,6,17) and it is likely, at least in the Dahl rat, that this abnormality of the kidney is a difficulty in excreting sodium. De Wardener and MacGregor therefore suggested that people who were going to develop essential hypertension might inherit a kidney that is less able to rid itself of sodium (9). With the high-sodium diet we eat, this would give a transient rise in blood volume, triggering the release of natriuretic hormones that would increase sodium excretion from the kidney, thereby restoring sodium balance to normal, however, this might be at the expense of causing an increase in peripheral resistance (Figure 2).

The protective effect of an increase in potassium intake on sodium-induced hypertension can be explained by potassium's well-known natriuretic effect and by its stimulating

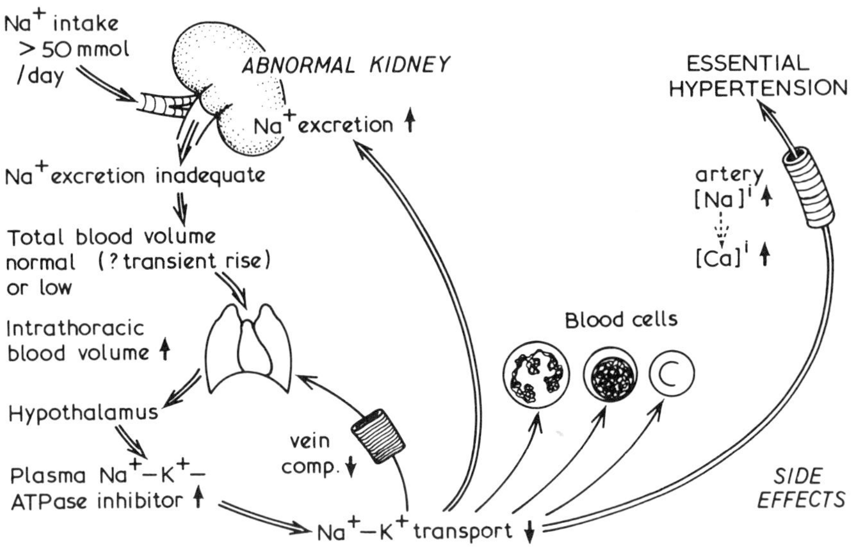

Figure 2 Sequence of events to explain a postulated inherited defect in the kidney's ability to excrete sodium, the observed rise in the concentration of a circulating sodium transport inhibitor, salt intake, and the rise in peripheral resistance in essential hypertension.

the sodium pump of either the smooth-muscle cell of the arteriole or the sympathetic neuronal junction. Potassium can oppose the effects of ouabain and therefore oppose the raised levels of a circulating inhibitor of Na^+-K^+-ATPase. While there is increasing evidence for a raised level of an inhibitor of sodium transport in the plasma of patients with high blood pressure, there is no direct evidence that this raised level causes the increase in peripheral resistance in essential hypertension.

DOES A LOWERED SALT INTAKE LOWER RAISED BLOOD PRESSURE?

Eighty years ago, Ambard and Beaujard showed that salt restriction lowered blood pressure (2). The fall in blood pressure was attributed to a reduction in chloride intake, mainly because these investigations could only measure chloride and not sodium. In the 1920s Allen and Sherill confirmed this finding in very careful studies (1). This work was largely ignored or forgotten until Kempner showed that a low-sodium, low-protein, high-potassium diet (using rice and fruit) had a pronounced blood-pressure-lowering effect in many patients with severe hypertension (18). Studies in the early 1950s, however, showed that in these patients who had severe and/or malignant hypertension, increasing sodium intake from approximately 10 mmol/day to 25 mmol/day caused the blood pressure to return towards the pretreatment levels (35). Based on this finding and also on the difficulty that patients had maintaining the very low sodium intakes and the advent of diuretics, sodium restriction was abandoned by most physicians. More recent studies have shown that more modest reduction in sodium intake does have a blood-pressure-lowering effect in patients with mild to moderate essential hypertension (24,26), although these studies have been criticized for their lack of proper controls, the fact that they were not double-blind, and for the methods of blood pressure measurement (30,32).

We therefore conducted a double-blind randomized cross-over study of the effect of modest restriction of dietary sodium intake alone on unselected patients with mild to moderate essential hypertension who were receiving no other treatment (21). Nineteen patients with mild to moderate essential hypertension who had been under observation by the Blood Pressure Unit for some months were instructed on how to cut their sodium intake by approximately half by not adding sodium chloride to food and by avoiding foods that were high in sodium. After 2 weeks of sodium restriction, they were entered into a double-blind, randomized cross-over study of Slow sodium tablets and matching placebos given for 1 month each. The number of Slow sodium tablets that each patient took was estimated to restore sodium intake back to the subject's usual intake. With sodium restriction alone, there was a significant fall in blood pressure but, more importantly, there was a rise in blood pressure from the end of the month in patients receiving Slow sodium tablets compared to those taking placebo, clearly demonstrating (Figure 3) that moderate sodium restriction does cause a fall in blood pressure. The percentage fall in blood pressure on the 4th week of placebo compared with the 4th week of Slow sodium was 6.1% (Figure 4), approximately equal to what has been seen in previous double-blind studies using either a diuretics or beta-blocker alone.

In our study, the patients who responded best to sodium restriction were those with the highest blood pressure; this confirmed what we had found in a more acute study of sodium restriction in which both normotensive and hypertensive subjects restricted

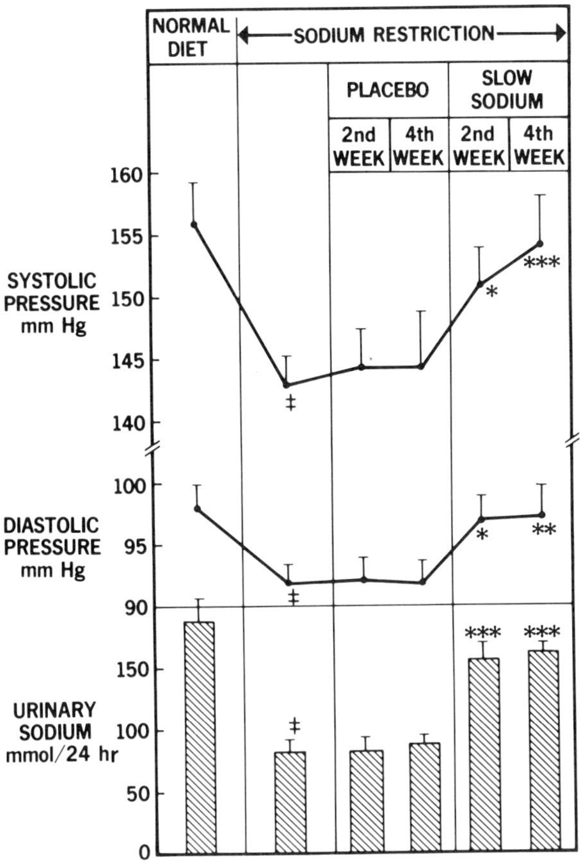

Figure 3 Average systolic and diastolic pressure and urinary sodium excretion in 19 patients (± SEM) with essential hypertension on their normal diet 2 weeks after restricting sodium intake, and at 2-weekly intervals during the randomized cross-over study of Slow sodium vs. placebo. Patients were not receiving any drug therapy. ***$p < 0.001$; **$p < 0.01$; *$p < 0.05$; comparing equivalent measurements on Slow sodium to placebo. ‡$p < 0.001$; comparing normal diet to 2 weeks of dietary sodium restriction. (From Ref. 23.)

sodium intake to 10 mmol/day for 5 days. In this study, the hypertensives but not the normotensives had a fall in blood pressure that was directly related to the height of the pretreatment blood pressure and inversely related to the activity of the renin-angiotensin system (25). This inverse relationship suggests that in essential hypertension the blunting of the response of the renin-angiotensin system to sodium restriction increases the fall in blood pressure that occurs with sodium restriction. This phenomenon is similar to that described for diuretics in which the hypotensive effect is greatest in those who respond to sodium depletion with the least rise in angiotensin II (22,33).

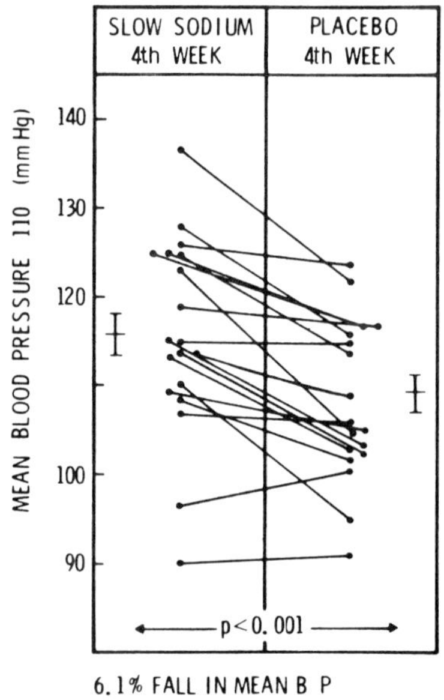

Figure 4 Fall in mean supine blood pressure in 19 (± SEM) patients during the fourth week of Slow sodium compared to the fourth week of placebo tablets. (From Ref. 23.)

DOES AN INCREASED POTASSIUM INTAKE LOWER RAISED BLOOD PRESSURE?

There is very little evidence of the effect of increasing potassium intake in patients with essential hypertension. One study in Japanese men with a high sodium intake and studied as inpatients did show a small decrease in blood pressure when potassium intake was doubled (15). In view of this finding, we conducted a double-blind study of the effect of increasing potassium chloride intake in patients with mild to moderate essential hypertension who were receiving no other treatment (23). As in the previous study, twenty-three patients were observed for some months and were then given 1 month of eight Slow K (64 mmol potassium chloride) which would approximately double their intake of potassium compared with identical matching placebos for 1 month in a 1-month double-blind randomized cross-over study. This study demonstrated that at least by the 4th week of Slow K supplementation, there was a small but significant fall in blood pressure in both systolic and diastolic pressure in the whole group (Figure 5).

A study by Holly et al. in which sodium intake was reduced and potassium intake increased in patients with essential hypertension also showed a fall in blood pressure, but this study did not differentiate between the effects of sodium restriction and those of potassium supplementation (14).

Evidence from animals suggests that the effect of potassium becomes more pronounced the higher the sodium intake (7) and the effect of potassium chloride supplementation may well be related to its natriuretic effect. A metabolic study in which we studied the effect of increasing potassium chloride intake demonstrated that potassium chloride supplementation did cause a natriuresis without an expected rise in renin (31). These findings, taken as a whole, suggest that the effect of potassium chloride may become less as sodium intake is restricted and it is likely that when patients restrict

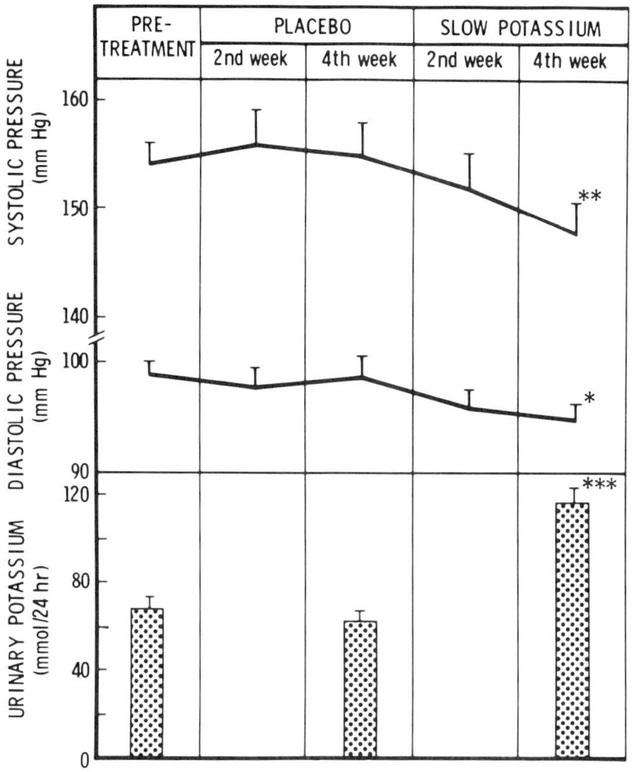

Figure 5 Average systolic and diastolic pressures and urinary potassium excretion in 23 patients (mean ± SEM) with essential hypertension before and during treatment with potassium chloride (8 Slow-K) and matching placebo. $*p < 0.05$; $**p < 0.025$; $***p < 0.001$; comparing equivalent measurements on Slow-K to placebo. (From Ref. 28.)

sodium intake, the effect of potassium chloride supplementation on blood pressure will be very small. From a practical point of view it is difficult to increase potassium chloride intake by 60 mmol/day. Studies that we have done using potassium salt substitutes have shown that many patients find them unacceptable and that even if they do accept them, the increase in potassium excretion is only 20–30 mmol/day.

It is relatively easy for patients to restrict sodium intake to approximately half of what they are now eating. Experience has shown that most patients can keep to this diet without problems and, indeed, many of them prefer their present diet and find high-salt foods unpleasant. This reduction in sodium intake does have a blood-pressure-lowering effect. Others have shown that this degree of sodium restriction is additive to blood-pressure-lowering drugs (3) and the effect of sodium restriction on blood pressure is greater, the higher the pretreatment blood pressure. It is not surprising that studies in which patients had normal blood pressure or pressure at the upper limit of normal have shown a less consistent fall in blood pressure with sodium restriction (28,36). Increasing potassium chloride intake is much more difficult but may be worthwhile if patients are unable to restrict their sodium intake. Chloride ions themselves have been shown to increase blood pressure in uninephrectomized DOCA-treated hypertensive rats (19) and chloride ions are known to inhibit directly renin release in humans (16). Clearly, more consideration should be given to the role of chloride ions in the regulation of extracellular volume and, thereby, blood pressure. No definitive conclusions can be drawn as to the blood-pressure-lowering effect of increasing potassium as a nonchloride salt, for example, by altering the diet through increasing fruit and vegetable intake. Increasing dietary potassium intake as a nonchloride salt may lower blood pressure when sodium intake is restricted. Such an increase in fruit and vegetable consumption would, in any case, help patients to comply with moderate sodium restriction. There may be other advantages to this type of diet, such as the higher fiber content and its lower saturated fat content, both of which have been claimed to lower blood pressure independent of reduction in sodium intake and may also be important in the long-term prevention of vascular disease.

REFERENCES

1. Allen, F. M., and Sherrill, J. W.: The treatment of arterial hypertension. *J. Metab. Res.* 2:429–545, 1922.
2. Ambard, L., and Beaujard, E.: Causes de l'hypertension arterielle. *Arch. Gen. Med.* 1:520–533, 1904.
3. Beard, T. C., Cooke, H. M., Gray, W. R., and Barge, R.: Randomised controlled trial of a no-added-sodium diet for mild hypertension. *Lancet* 2:455–458, 1982.
4. Bianchi, G., Fox, U., Di Francesco, G. F., Giovanetti, A. M., and Pagetti, D.: Blood pressure changes produced by kidney cross transplantation between spontaneously hypertensive rats and normotensive rats. *Clin. Sci. Mol. Med.* 47:435, 1974.
5. Blaustein, M. P.: Sodium ions, calcium ions, blood pressure regulation and hypertension: a reassessment and a hypothesis. *Am. J. Physiol.* 232 (Suppl 3):C-165, 1977.
6. Dahl, L. K., and Heine, M.: Primary role of renal homografts in setting chronic blood pressure levels in rats. *Circ. Res.* 36:692, 1975.
7. Dahl, L. K., Leith, G., and Heine, M.: Influence of dietary potassium and sodium/potassium molar ratios on the development of salt hypertension. *J. Exp. Med.* 136: 318–330, 1972.
8. Denton, D.: *The Hunger for Salt: An Anthropological, Physiological and Medical Analysis.* Berlin, Heidelberg, New York, Springer-Verlag, 1982.
9. de Wardener, H. E., and MacGregor, G. A.: The relation of a circulating sodium transport inhibitor (the natriuretic hormone?) to hypertension. *Medicine* 62(5):310–326, 1983.
10. Edmondson, R. P. S., Thomas, R. D., Hilton, P. J., Patrick, J., and Jones, N. F.: Abnormal leucocyte composition and sodium transport in essential hypertension. *Lancet* 1:1003, 1975.
11. Gleibermann, L.: Blood pressure and dietary salt in human populations. *Ecol. Food Nutr.* 2:143, 1973.
12. Hamlyn, J. M., Ringel, R., Schaeffer, J., Levinson, P. D., Hamilton, B. P., Avinoam Korwarski, A., and Blaustein, M. P.: A circulating inhibitor of (Na^+-K^+) ATPase associated with essential hypertension. *Nature* 300:650, 1982.
13. Hofman, A., Hazebroek, A., and Valkenburg, H. A.: A randomized trial of sodium intake and blood pressure in newborn infants. *JAMA* 250(3):370–373, 1983.
14. Holly, J. M. P., Goodwin, F. J., Evans, S. J. W., Vandenburg, M. J., and Ledingham, J. M.: Re-analysis of data in two Lancet papers on the effect of dietary sodium and potassium on blood pressure. *Lancet* 2:1384, 1981.
15. Iimura, O., Kijima, T., Kitchi, K., Kikuchi, K., Miyama, A., Amdo, T., Nakao, T., and Takigami, Y.: Studies on the hypotensive effect of high potassium intake in patients with essential hypertension. *Clin. Sci.* 61:77s, 1981.

16. Julian, B. A., Galla, J. H., Guthrie, G. P., and Kotchen, T. A.: Renin and aldosterone responses to short-term NaCl or $NaHCO_3$ loading in man. *Am. J. Physiol.* 241(4): 261-268, 1981.
17. Kawabe, K., Watanebe, T. X., Shiono, K., and Sokabe, H.: Influence of blood pressure on renal isografts between spontaneously hypertensive and normotensive rats utilizing the F_1 hybrids. *Jpn. Heart J.* 20:886, 1979.
18. Kempner, W.: Treatment of hypertensive vascular disease with rice diet. *Am. J. Med.* 4:545-577, 1948.
19. Kurtz, T. W., and Morris, R. C.: Dietary chloride as a determinant of "sodium-dependent" hypertension. *Science* 222:1139-1141, 1983.
20. MacGregor, G. A., Fenton, S., Alaghband-Zadeh, J., Markandu, N., Roulston, J. E., and de Wardener, H. E.: Evidence for a raised concentration of a circulating sodium transport inhibitor in essential hypertension. *Br. Med. J.* 283:1355, 1981.
21. MacGregor, G. A., Markandu, N. D., Best, F. E., Elder, D. M., Cam, J. M., Sagnella, G. A., and Squires, M.: Double-blind randomised crossover trial of moderate sodium restriction in essential hypertension. *Lancet* 1:351-355, 1982.
22. MacGregor, G. A., Markandu, N. D., Roulston, J. E., and Jones, B. E.: The antihypertensive action of spironolactone: The importance of the response of the renin-angiotensin system to the loss of sodium and water. *Aldosterone Antagonists in Clinical Medicine,* edited by Addison, G. M., Wirenfeldt, N., Corvol, P., et al., Amsterdam, Excerpta Medica, 1978, pp. 466-474.
23. MacGregor, G. A., Smith, S. J., Markandu, N. D., Banks, R. A., and Sagnella, G. A.: Moderate potassium supplementation in essential hypertension. *Lancet* 2:567, 1982.
24. Morgan, T., Gillies, A., Morgan, G., Adam, W., Wilson, M., and Carney, S.: Hypertension treated by salt restriction. *Lancet* 1:227-230, 1978.
25. Parfrey, P. S., Markandu, N. D., Roulston, J. E., Jones, B. E., Jones, J. C., and MacGregor, G. A.: Relation between arterial pressure, dietary sodium intake, and renin system in essential hypertension. *Br. Med. J.* 283:94-97, 1981.
26. Parijs, J., Joossens, J. V., Van der Linden, L., Verstreken, G., and Amery, A. K. P. C.: Moderate sodium restriction and diuretics in the treatment of hypertension. *Am. Heart J.* 85:22-34, 1973.
27. Poston, L., Sewell, R. B., Wilkinson, S. P., Richardson, P. J., Williams, R., Clarkson, E. M., MacGregor, G. A., and de Wardener, H. E.: Evidence for a circulating sodium transport inhibitor in essential hypertension. *Br. Med. J.* 282:847-849, 1981.
28. Richards, A. M., Nicholls, M. G., Espirer, E. A., Ikram, H., Maslowski, A. H., Hamilton, E. J., and Wells, J. E.: Blood pressure response to moderate sodium restriction and to potassium supplementation in mild essential hypertension. *Lancet* 1:757-761, 1984.
29. Rose, G.: Strategy of prevention: Lessons from cardiovascular disease. *Br. Med. J.* 282:1847-1851, 1981.
30. Simpson, F. O.: Salt and hypertension: A sceptical review of the evidence. *Clin. Sci.* 57:463s-480s, 1979.
31. Smith, S. J., Markandu, N. D., Sagnella, G. A., Poston, L., Hilton, P. J., and MacGregor, G. A.: Does potassium lower blood pressure by increasing sodium excretion? A metabolic study in patients with mild to moderate essential hypertension. *J. Hypertension* 1 (Suppl. 2):27-30, 1983.
32. Swales, J. D.: Dietary salt and hypertension. *Lancet* 1:1177-1179, 1980.
33. Vaughan, E. D., Carey, R. M., Peach, M. J., Ackerly, J. A., and Ayres, C. R.: The renin response to diuretic therapy: A limitation of anti-hypertensive potential. *Circ. Res.* 42:376-381, 1978.
34. Walker, W. G., Whelton, P. K., Saito, H., Russell, P. R., and Hermann, J.: Relation between blood pressure and renin, renin substrate, angiotensin II, aldosterone and urinary sodium and potassium in 574 ambulatory subjects. *Hypertension* 1:287, 1979.

35. Watkin, D. M., Froeb, H. F., Hatch, F. T., and Gutman, A. B.: Effects of diet in essential hypertension: II. Results with unmodified Kempner rice diet in fifty hospitalized patients. *Am. J. Med.* 9:441–493, 1950.
36. Watt, G. C. M., Edwards, C., Hart, J. T., Hart, M., Walton, P., and Roy, C. J. W.: Dietary sodium restriction of mild hypertension in general practice. *Br. Med. J.* 286:432–436, 1983.

30

Evidence for A Protective Effect of Potassium on Renal Function and Cerebral Arteries and Arterioles

LOUIS TOBIAN
University of Minnesota School of Medicine, Minneapolis, Minnesota

Primitive hunter-gatherers in remote corners of the world have very high intakes of potassium in the natural foods they eat (3). The males in these hunter-gatherer groups eat between 150 and 290 mEq K per day, whereas whites in the United States average 70 mEq/day and blacks average 40 mEq/day (6,8). Evidence indicates that men and women have eaten mainly unprocessed foods until about 10,000 years ago, and such a diet would have provided a high level of K. Evolutionary forces generally cause surviving species to adapt exceedingly well to their environments, including the foodstuffs in those environments (2). Thus during the long prehistoric period of primates, hominoids, and humans, evolutionary forces would have molded mankind to function well on this high K intake. The same general principles would apply to other mammals living in the wild and presumably eating the large amount of K in natural foods.

In a recent study we explored the possibility that adding K supplements to the diet might reduce the renal lesions in hypertensive, salt-fed Dahl S rats (5,10). They were fed a standard Purina chow with 4% added NaCl for 24 weeks. In the Dahl S rats this produced the expected hypertension (5) and the expected lesions in the tubules and arterioles of the kidney. In a number of these rats on the 4% high-salt intake, 1.36% K was added to the diet over the entire 24 weeks of the study, which did not lower the blood pressure whatsoever. However, the K supplements reduced renal tubular lesions in the renal cortex by 50%, in the outer medulla by 30%, and in the inner medulla by 44% (10). Thus without lowering the blood pressure, the addition of K provided a protective effect of major proportions against renal tubular lesions. Furthermore, in these same S rats fed a 4% high-salt diet, the hypertension had produced the expected 38% thickening of the walls of the renal arterioles. When K supplements were added to the diet (1.35% added K), the thickness of the arteriolar walls was reduced by 20–30% even though the blood pressure was not lowered (10).

We considered that if renal arteriolar lesions could be greatly lessened with K supplements, other hypertensive arterial lesions might also be favorably affected by extra dietary K. Stroke-prone SHR rats (SHRsp rats) develop cerebral arterial lesions quite readily, along with their severe hypertension; these lesions frequently lead to strokes from cerebral hemorrhage or from cerebral infarction. These SHRsp rats develop strokes more readily if there is extra NaCl in the diet and if they are fed a Japanese-type rather than an American-type rat chow. Dahl S rats also develop strokes quite readily on the same diet (11). These studies were done to determine whether supplements of K in the diet would protect SHRsp rats and Dahl S rats against death from strokes.

METHODS

Study I

Six-week old male SHRsp rats from our breeding colony were fed for 16 weeks a Japanese-type chow designed by Dr. J. Knapka of the NIH. This basic diet contains 0.75% K, and NaCl was added to the basic diet up to 4% to increase somewhat the likelihood of strokes. This basic diet was fed to 74 SHRsp rats in the study. Twenty-four of these rats received this basic diet alone without any added K. Twenty-five other SHRsp rats received this same basic diet with the addition of 1.36% K in the form of KCl. Twenty-five other SHRsp rats received this same basic diet plus 1.36% K in the form of K citrate. The K citrate was used in one of the diets because K in ordinary foodstuffs is rarely present as KCl. Blood pressures of all rats were measured after 6 weeks on the diets, using the microphonic method of Friedman and Freed (4) with gentle warming and without anesthesia.

Study II

The same basic type of feeding experiment was carried out with Dahl S rats (1). All the rats received the Japanese-type NIH chow supplemented with 4% NaCl between 3 and 5 weeks of age and up to 8% NaCl thereafter. These Dahl S rats were classified into three groups. The 33 Dahl S rats of group I received this basic diet without any added K. The 22 S rats of group II received this same basic diet with the addition of 1.36% K in the form of KCl. The 23 rats of group III received this same basic diet plus 1.36% K in the form of K citrate. The three diets were fed for 9 weeks. Blood pressures of all rats were measured after 6 weeks on the diets.

RESULTS

Study I

After 16 weeks of being fed the three Japanese-type diets with each diet containing 4% NaCl, 20 of the 24 SHRsp rats in the diet group with no added K had died of a stroke, an 83% mortality rate. During this same period, 49 of the 50 rats on the same diet but with the addition of 1.36% K, were still alive and showed no evidence of a nonfatal stroke. The two diets with K supplements had very similar effects on weight, blood pressure, and strokes, so the rats receiving these two types of K salts were combined into one group for comparison purposes. The results are striking: 83% of the rats on the diet with no added K died of a stroke while only 2% of the rats with the 1.36% added K died similarly. This 98% reduction in mortality rate is highly significant, with a p value less than 2×10^{-12} (7) (Figure 1).

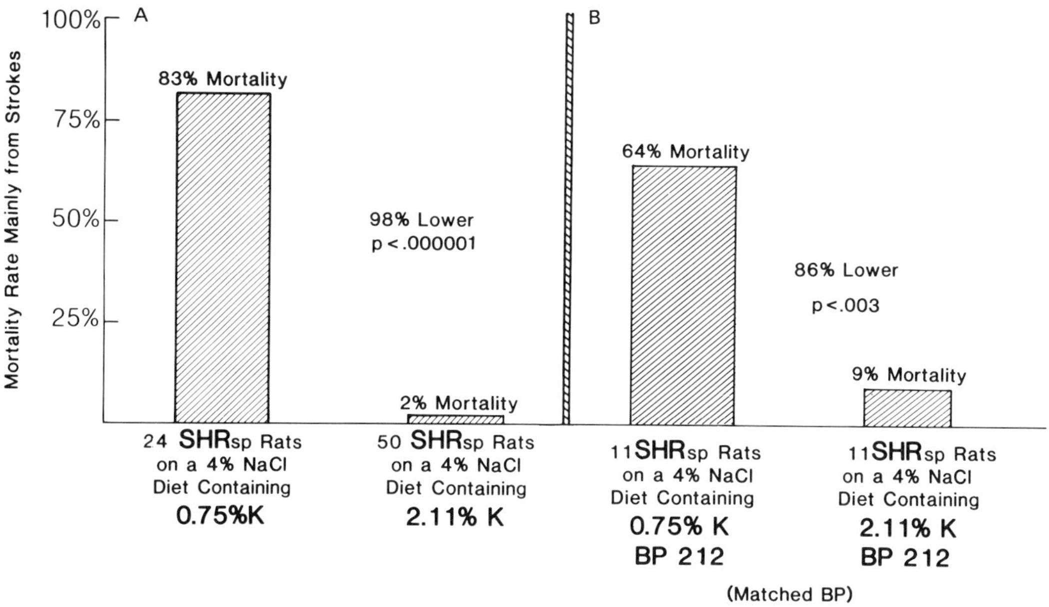

Figure 1 A, Mortality rates of hypertensive SHRsp rats on either normal or high dietary K intake. The actual final concentration of K in each diet is listed in the figure. B, Mortality rates of hypertensive SHRsp rats on either normal or high dietary K intake. The two groups being compared have virtually equal average systolic BP.

After 6 weeks on the diets, the blood pressure (BP) of the 20 surviving SHRsp rats on the diet with no added K averaged 233 mmHg. At this same time the average BP of the 50 rats on diets with 1.36% added K averaged 187 mmHg, a 46-mmHg decrease ($p < 0.0001$). Thus the K supplements significantly reduced BP in the SHRsp rats. This reduction in pressure would lessen the tension in the walls of the cerebral arteries and would therefore be expected to reduce the tendency to arterial lesions and strokes. This is undoubtedly one explanation for the remarkable protective effect of the K supplements.

However, the K supplements also appear to reduce the intrinsic susceptibility to cerebral artery lesions for a given level of hypertension. For instance, the 11 SHRsp rats with highest BP among the 50 rats in the K-supplemented groups and the 11 SHRsp rats with the lowest BP among the 20 rats with no added K had the same average systolic BP, 212 mmHg. Thus, these two groups had virtually the same average blood pressures of 212, yet the group of 11 K-supplemented rats had 1 death from stroke (9% mortality rate) while the group of 11 rats without K supplements had 7 deaths from strokes (64% mortality rate). In these two groups, very closely matched for blood pressure, the 86% decrease in mortality rate, 64% vs. 9% was significant, $p<0.003$ (Figure 1). This difference indicates that K supplementation in SHRsp rats is very effective for preventing stroke death, although blood pressure is almost identical in the two groups being compared. Postmortem urea analyses in skeletal muscle indicated that there were no deaths from uremia in either study I or II.

Study II

After 9 weeks of being fed the high-NaCl diets, 18 of 33 Dahl S rats on the diet with no K supplement had died, mainly from strokes (55% mortality rate); while only 2 of 45 Dahl S rats on the diets with 1.36% K supplements had died (4% mortality rate) (Figure 2). This 93% reduction in mortality rate, 55% vs. 4%, was significant, $p<10^{-6}$ (7).

Even though K-supplementation did not reduce the BP of Dahl S rats on a 4% NaCl diet in a previous study (10), it did effect a modest reduction in BP in the Dahl S rats in the present study. In the 33 rats of Group I (no added K) the systolic BP averaged 214.5 mmHg (SEM±4.1). In 22 rats of Group II (1.36% added K, as KCl), the BP averaged 198.5 (SEM±3.3). In the rats of Group III (1.36% added K, as K citrate), the BP averaged 202.7 (SEM±4.5). The Group II rats supplemented with KCl averaged 16 mmHg lower than Group I rats ($p<.005$). The Group III rats supplemented with K citrate averaged 12 mmHg lower than Group I ($p<.06$).

The modest reduction of BP in the K-supplemented groups could explain some of the lowered mortality rate in these groups. However, the 21 of 33 Dahl S rats with the lowest BP in the group with no K supplementation had the same average systolic BP as 39 of 45 Dahl S rats in the K-supplemented groups, 205 mmHg. In these two groups of Dahl S rats with very closely matched BP, the mortality rate was 38% (8 of 21) in the group with no K supplement vs 5% (2 of 39) in the groups with K supplementation (Figure 2). This 87% reduction in mortality rate was significant, $p<.001$ (7).

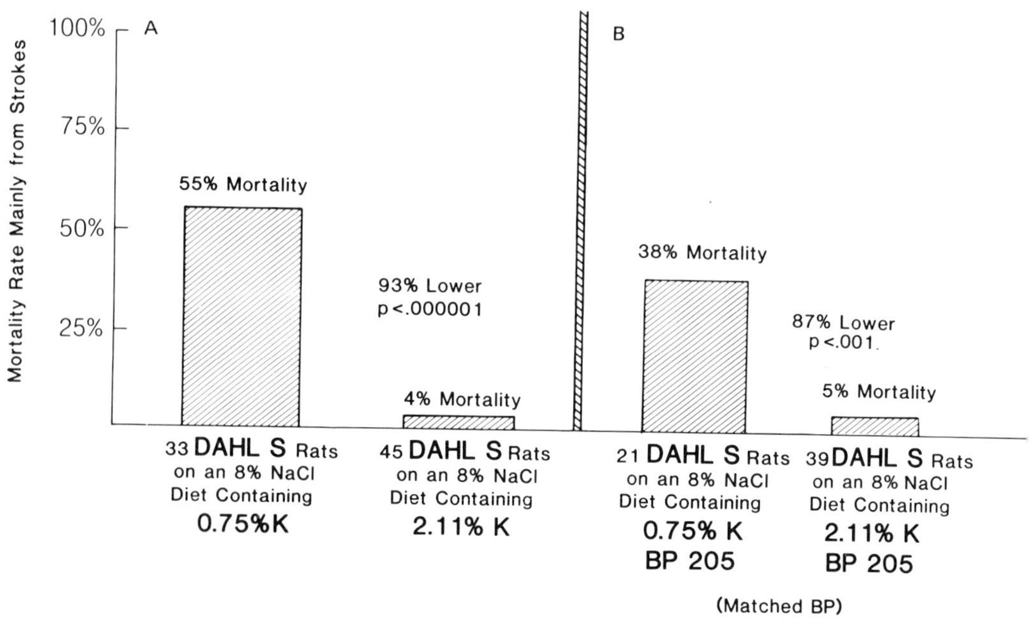

Figure 2 A, Mortality rates of hypertensive Dahl S rats on either normal or high dietary K intake. B, Mortality rates of hypertensive Dahl S rats on either normal or high dietary K intake. The two groups being compared have virtually the same average systolic BP.

COMMENTS

In both SHRsp and Dahl S rats, the addition of either KCl or K citrate strikingly reduced death from strokes. This marked reduction occurred even when BP was the same in the groups being compared. However, K supplements reduced BP considerably in SHRsp rats and modestly in Dahl S rats; and these reductions in BP undoubtedly contributed to the lower death rate from stroke.

The precise mechanism by which extra dietary K reduces stroke deaths is as yet elusive. It is worth considering that prehistoric humans and mammals had a very high K intake. The type of food processing that we take for granted results in a K intake among American whites that is only one-third that of a hunter-gatherer. Scottish people and American blacks have a daily K intake 80% lower than a hunter-gatherer. Thus, being "civilized" has greatly lowered our dietary K. American blacks have 18 times more hypertensive renal failure than whites (9) and also have a very significantly lower K intake than whites (6,8). People in Mississippi, Alabama, and Georgia have the highest death rate from strokes in the United States and also have the lowest K intake (6,8). Moreover, there would be no evolutionary adaptation to the modern low K diet because its bad effects on health mainly show up after the procreative years have ended. A return to the high K levels of prehistoric cuisine might very well diminish these high rates of stroke and hypertensive renal failure. As this study indicates, the added dietary K appears to retard the development of lesions in cerebral arteries exposed to high arterial pressure.

ACKNOWLEDGMENTS

I am greatly indebted to Drs. Michael Brody, Donald Heistad, Andrew Werber, and Richard Schaffer for invaluable help and advice for this study. This work was supported by grants from National Institutes of Health HL-17871 and The Cargill Foundation.

REFERENCES

1. Dahl, L. K., Heine, M., and Tassinari, L.: Effects of chronic salt ingestion: Evidence that genetic factors play an important role in susceptibility to experimental hypertension. *J. Exp. Med.* 115:1173–1190, 1962.
2. Darwin, C.: *On the Origin of Species* (a reprinting of the 1st edition). Cambridge, Harvard University Press, 1964.
3. Denton, D.: *The Hunger for Salt.* Berlin, Springer-Verlag, 1982, pp. 573–575.
4. Friedman, M., and Freed, S. C.: Microphonic manometer for indirect determination of systemic blood pressure in rats. *Proc. Soc. Exp. Biol. Med.* 70:670–672, 1949.
5. Ganguli, M. C., Tobian, L., Iwai, J., and Johnson, M. A.: Potassium citrate feeding protects against nephron loss in severe NaCl hypertension in rats. *Clin. Sci.* 61:73–75, 1981.
6. Grim, C. E., Luft, F. C., Miller, J. Z., Meneely, G. R., Battarbee, H. D., Hames, C. G., and Dahl, L. K.: Racial differences in blood pressure in Evans County, Georgia: Relationship to Na and K intake and plasma renin activity. *J. Chron. Dis.* 33:87–94, 1980.
7. Hill, A. B.: *A Short Textbook of Medical Statistics.* London, Hodder and Stoughton, 1977, pp. 118–126.
8. Langford, H. G.: Dietary potassium and hypertension: epidemiologic data. *Ann. Intern. Med.* 98(5, Suppl, Part 2):770–772, 1983.

9. Rostand, S. G., Kirk, K. H., Rutsky, E. A., and Pate, B. A.: Racial differences in the incidence of treatment for end-stage renal disease. *N. Engl. J. Med.* 306(21): 1276–1279, 1982.
10. Tobian, L., MacNeill, D., Johnson, M. A., Ganguli, M. C., and Iwai, J.: Potassium protects against lesions of the renal tubules, arteries and glomeruli and nephron loss in salt-loaded hypertensive Dahl S rats. *Hypertension* 6 (Suppl I):I-170–I-176, 1984.
11. Werber, A. H., Baumbach, G. L., Wagner, D. V., Mark, A. L., and Heistad, D. D.: Factors influencing stroke in Dahl salt sensitive rats. *Circulation* 68 (Suppl III):383, 1983 (abstract).

31

Can Black/White Differences in Blood Pressure and Hypertensive Mortality in the U.S. Be Explained by Differences in Potassium Intake?

HERBERT G. LANGFORD
University of Mississippi Medical Center, Jackson, Mississippi

There are major and consistent differences in blood pressure between blacks and whites in most parts of the United States. This chapter provides a logical dietary explanation for these black-white differences, and proposes that genetic factors are not necessarily involved.

FACTORS RELATED TO SOCIOECONOMIC STATUS AFFECT BLOOD PRESSURE IN BLACKS AND WHITES

We reported an observation from Robert Watson, based on a survey of the blood pressure of high school children of Jackson, Mississippi, and its surrounding county, Hinds. Urban children had lower blood pressures than rural children. In the city, the lower the socioeconomic status of the child's family, the higher the blood pressure. This effect was so marked that if black children from the upper third of the distribution of socioeconomic status of blacks were compared with rural white children, the usual black-white difference was abolished for girls and reversed for boys. Weight was not an adequate explanation for these observed differences (6).

Two more examples of the effect of social class and place of living on blood pressures of blacks and whites can be cited. The Hypertension Detection and Follow-up Program (HDFP) used years of education completed as a measure of socioeconomic status. In both blacks and whites, there was a clear stairstep relationship: with the higher the attained education, the lower the blood pressure. However, at each level of education, the blacks had higher blood pressures than whites (5). This information could be considered as evidence that a substantial residual racial effect was affecting blood pressure. However, a statewide survey of blood pressure in Connecticut found no difference between the blood pressures of blacks and whites (7). The examples I have quoted are open to various interpretations. However, it seems clear that there are major factors which affect blood pressure other than race, which are related to socioeconomic status and place of living. When the socioeconomic status is more or less equalized, or at least some crucial way of living equalized as seen in Connecticut, or when upper socioeconomic class blacks is compared with rural white, as in the example of Mississippi, the racial differences are abolished.

POTASSIUM INTAKE AS A TENABLE EXPLANATION

At least five nonracial explanations for the black-white differences can be advanced: emotional stress, sodium intake, potassium intake, calcium intake, and obesity. I will summarize evidence to suggest that differences in the potassium intake are a sufficient explanation for the observed blood pressure differences, but the evidence cannot exclude participation of other factors.

When Robert Watson and I noted the urban/rural and socioeconomic gradients of blood pressure, we were certain that differences in sodium intake explained the differences in blood pressure found in our population. We did not specifically look at a comparison of the social class differences in blood pressure and the social class differences in sodium intake. Instead, we wished to determine the correlation between sodium excretion and blood pressure in the total population group with enough observations to decrease the variability resulting from casual determinations of blood pressure and urinary excretion. We recruited 101 black girls between the ages of 19 and 21, whom we had previously identified in a school survey in Jackson, Mississippi, and in surrounding Hinds county. Each subject had her blood pressure measured daily for 8 days, and offered six sequential 24-hr urine specimens. To our dismay, there was no significant correlation between the mean blood pressure from the 24 determinations, and the mean sodium excretion, determined from the 6 days of collections. There was a suggestive negative correlation between potassium excretion and blood pressure. However, the correlation between Na/K excretion and blood pressure was found to be highly significant ($r=0.341$; $p=0.02$) (6).

This determination does not prove, of course, that the blood pressure differences between blacks and whites are dependent upon potassium.

One of our reports is the only one that I have found to date to document that blacks excreted more sodium than whites. However, both groups were excreting very little sodium. Black girls excreted 112 mEq Na/24 hr, the white girls 98 mEq Na/24 hours, which is a significant difference. However, the difference in potassium excretion was proportionally much larger, with the black girls excreting 28 mEq/24 hr, and the white girls excreting 36 mEq/24 hr. The urinary creatinine excretion was approximately the same: 1.1 g for both blacks and whites. Urinary Na/K ratio was 4:1 in the blacks, 2:9 in the whites. The difference was highly significant. The systolic blood pressure in the black girls was significantly higher than in the white girls (7).

A study comparing electrolyte excretion and intake in blacks and whites was performed in Evans County, Georgia. Evans County has been the site of studies in cardiovascular disease for several decades. A random sample of the biracial population was taken in 1961. Dietary electrolyte intake and excretion was estimated, with collection of simultaneous 24-hr urine samples and determination of dietary intake. The investigators paid the participants to save duplicate meals, which were then analyzed. Black men ate and excreted less sodium than the white men; white men had a dietary sodium intake of 186 ± 64 mEq/24 hr, black men had an estimated dietary sodium intake of 136 ± 14 mEq/24 hr, a significant difference ($p<0.05$).

Urinary sodium excretion was also significantly different: 160 ± 7.4 mEq/24 hr for the white men and 130 ± 10 mEq/24 hr for the black men ($p<0.05$). The dietary potassium was markedly lower in the black men than the white men (23±2.2 mEq/24 hr compared to 54±2.2 mEq/24 hr, $p<0.05$). The black men excreted 24 ± 2 mEq/24 hr potassium, compared to 40 ± 1.8 mEq/24 hr for the white men. Similar differences were found in the women. The blacks had significantly higher blood pressures than the whites.

This study is extremely important. Significantly less sodium, significantly less potassium, and significantly higher blood pressures marked the findings in the blacks. To use the most conservative interpretation of these data, they constitute strong evidence against a major role of sodium in the black-white blood pressure differences. Moreover, the data also provide a strong argument against the unlikely hypothesis of a difference in black/white, urine/stool partition of potassium excretion (4).

Further proof that the difference in urinary excretion of potassium by blacks and whites is given by the study of Frate et al. They determined the urinary excretion of potassium in blacks and whites in a rural county in Mississippi. Dr. Smoller estimated the sodium and potassium intake from computer-based analysis of dietary diaries. Blacks ingested 53.5 mEq potassium daily and excreted 28.1 mEq. Whites ingested 71.2 mEq potassium daily and excreted 39.1 mEq. These differences between blacks and whites were significant ($p<0.0001$). There was no significant difference in dietary sodium intake and urinary sodium excretion. The difference in potassium intake was not due to differences in protein intake, because this did not differ significantly between the two groups (3).

Cushman and Langford reported on the results from a Veterans Administration study of mild to moderate untreated hypertensive patients, 407 black men and 206 white men. Black hypertensive patients excreted slightly less sodium than white hypertensive patients. The difference was not significant. However, the difference in potassium excretion was statistically highly significant (40 vs. 78 mEq/24 hr, $p<0.001$). Although the study did not demonstrate a negative correlation between potassium excretion and blood pressure, it did demonstrate a significant positive correlation between urinary Na/K ratio and systolic blood pressure. There was a negative correlation between serum K and systolic blood pressure, but whether the serum K represents primarily a consequence of the amount of K taken is not clear (2).

A study that probably found a black-white difference in urinary excretion and blood pressure is that of Zinner and associates. They found that black children had significantly lower urinary kallikrein concentration than white children aged 5-18 years. Urinary potassium concentration was the most important predictor of urinary kallikrein concentration. Although Zinner's method of expressing the study's results makes it difficult to determine the mean urinary concentration by race, it appears that blacks were much more likely to have a low urinary potassium concentration than whites (8). Berenson and Frank's studies of young blacks and whites in Bogalusa, Louisiana, have demonstrated consistently higher blood pressures in young blacks, and lower potassium excretion. There was no significant difference in sodium excretion, and potassium excretion was consistently and significantly lower in blacks than in whites (28±2 mEq/24 hr vs. 39±4 mEq/24 hr, $p<0.0001$) (Chapter 27).

Not only in the United States are there black-white differences in blood pressure and electrolyte excretion. Barlow et al. compared urinary sodium and potassium excretion in normotensive South African blacks and whites (1). While the comparison was between normotensive blacks and whites, in South Africa, as in the United States, blacks have higher pressures. Their subjects were 30–50-year-old men with blood pressure <160/90 mmHg. Twenty-four-hour urine collections were obtained. Black male patients excreted 126.8 mEq urinary Na compared with 168 mEq urinary Na in whites, and they excreted 30.9 mEq urinary potassium vs. 59.3 mEq urinary potassium for male whites (1).

CAUSES OF LOW POTASSIUM INTAKE

The low potassium intake of blacks is probably a consequence of their geographic location and socioeconomic status. I have not given the evidence in this paper, and it is much less extensive than that for the black–white differences in potassium intake, but it is likely that Southern whites ingest much less potassium than Northern whites. Also, Southern whites are more likely to be hypertensive than Northern whites. As noted earlier, there was no black–white difference in blood pressure in Connecticut, suggesting that the phenomenon was concentrated more in the South, and especially in blacks in the South. The data from the Hanes survey showing that less potassium was eaten by individuals in the lower socioeconomic levels are another expression of this phenomenon.

One aspect of the problem is that, except during peak season, fresh fruits and vegetables are expensive. Therefore, it is reasonable to assume that poorer people will purchase and eat less of these sources of potassium than more affluent persons. However, I think there may be another important component. Root crops such as potatoes are an excellent source of potassium. Southerners eat fewer potatoes, and probably black Southerners eat less potatoes than white Southerners. The sweet potato is often considered a major part of the Southern diet, but it is actually more of a holiday food. Studies are urgently needed to determine the difference between the types of foods eaten by those who excrete a lot of potassium and those who eat and excrete little potassium. Until this research is done I do not see how we can arrange to alter potassium intake substantially.

REFERENCES

1. Barlow, R. J., Connell, M. A., Levendig, B. J., Gear, J. S. S., and Milne, F. J.: A comparative study of urinary sodium and potassium excretion in normotensive urban Black and White South African males. *South Afr. Med. J.* 62:939–941, 1982.
2. Cushman, W. C., and Langford, H. G.: Urinary electrolyte differences in black and white hypertensives. *Clin. Res.* 31(5):843-A, 1983.
3. Frate, D. E.: Personal communication.
4. Grim, C. E., Luft, F. C., Miller, J. Z., Luft, F. C., Christian, J. C.,and Weinberger, M. H.: Racial differences in blood pressure in Evans County, Georgia: Relationship to sodium and potassium intake and plasma renin activity. *J. Chron. Dis.* 33:87, 1980.
5. Hypertension Detection and Follow-up Program: Race, education and the prevalence of hypertension. *Am. J. Epidemiol.* 106:351, 1977.
6. Langford, H. G., and Watson, R. L.: Electrolytes and hypertension in epidemiology and control of hypertension. In *Epidemiology and Control of Hypertension,* edited by Paul, O., New York, Stratton, Intercontinental Medical Books, 1975, p. 119.
7. Watson, R. L., Langford, H. G., Abernethy, J., Barnes, T. Y., and Watson, M. J.: Urinary electrolytes, body weight and blood pressure, pooled cross-sectional results among four groups of adolescent females. *Hypertension* 2 (Suppl. 1):193, 1980.
8. Zinner, S. H., Margolius, H. S., Rosner, H. B., Keiser, H. R., and Kass, E. H.: Familial aggregation of urinary Kallifrien concentration in childhood: Relation to blood pressure, race and urinary electrolytes. *Am. J. Epidemiol.* 104:124, 1976.

32

The Role of Potassium Supplementation and Sodium Reduction in Controlling Blood Pressure in Hypertensive Men: The MSHT

RICHARD H. GRIMM, JR., PATRICIA J. ELMER,* JAMES D. NEATON
School of Public Health, University of Minnesota, Minneapolis, Minnesota

MARVIN S. SEGAL
Mt. Sinai Hospital and University of Minnesota, Minneapolis, Minnesota

RONALD J. PRINEAS
School of Public Health, University of Minnesota, Minneapolis, Minnesota

Results from the latest generation of clinical trials on hypertension have focused attention on improving current drug regimens with special emphasis on alternative and adjunctive treatments of hypertension. The problem of hypertension, when viewed over the long term, indicates that efforts should be continued to identify effective alternative and adjunctive therapies to antihypertensive drugs. Although currently the use of antihypertensive drugs appears safe and effective, the long-term effects are largely unknown. Some hypertensive patients cannot take drugs for a long period of time due to intolerance or other problems associated with the agents.

It has been suspected for several years that sodium and potassium intake and excretion play a major role in the development and treatment of hypertension. Epidemiological, clinical, and experimental investigations have shown that increased dietary sodium intake is associated with the development of hypertension, and that lowered sodium intake will lower blood pressure (1,3,5,8,10).

The role of potassium intake and excretion in the development and treatment of hypertension is less clear. Primitive cultures that have been studied have low sodium intakes and a low prevalence of hypertension. But these cultures also have higher dietary potassium intakes. It has been suggested that the ratio of sodium to potassium is perhaps one of the most important determinants of blood pressure (7).

**Current affiliation*: School of Public Health, University of Minnesota, and Minnesota Department of Health, Minneapolis, Minnesota

PURPOSE

Modest but significant lowering of blood pressure has been observed in recent small-scale clinical trials in which oral potassium was administered in daily doses ranging from 60 to 100 mEq (2,6,9,14) (the article cited in Ref. 9 was subsequently withdrawn). The purpose of the Mt. Sinai Hypertension Trial is to examine the ability of dietary sodium reduction with and without potassium supplementation to control blood pressure and reduce the need for antihypertensive medications. The study also addresses the ability of these electrolyte interventions to reduce the dosage and number of antihypertensive medications required to control blood pressure.

ELIGIBILITY CRITERIA

Men aged 45-69 years who have been taking antihypertensive drugs for at least 4 years and who have well-controlled blood pressures are eligible (diastolic blood pressure <95 mmHg at the second or third eligibility visit, and men with an average diastolic blood pressure <90 mmHg from the second and third eligibility visits combined). Participants with evidence of cardiovascular disease on physical examination or electrocardiogram are excluded. Men unwilling to modify their diet or whose conditions require potassium supplementation are also excluded.

DESIGN

The design of the study is shown in Figure 1.

Eligibility for participants in the MSHT is determined over four visits including a randomization visit (Figure 1). Initial eligibility is determined by reviewing records of prior studies to identify men who are hypertensive and likely to be on medication for at least 4 years. These men are telephoned and invited to attend an orientation visit (eligibility visit 1, EV01). The orientation visit is held in groups where the study's purpose, design, and requirements for participation are presented. Men who are interested in continuing to participate are invited to a second eligibility visit (EV02). This visit is 2-3

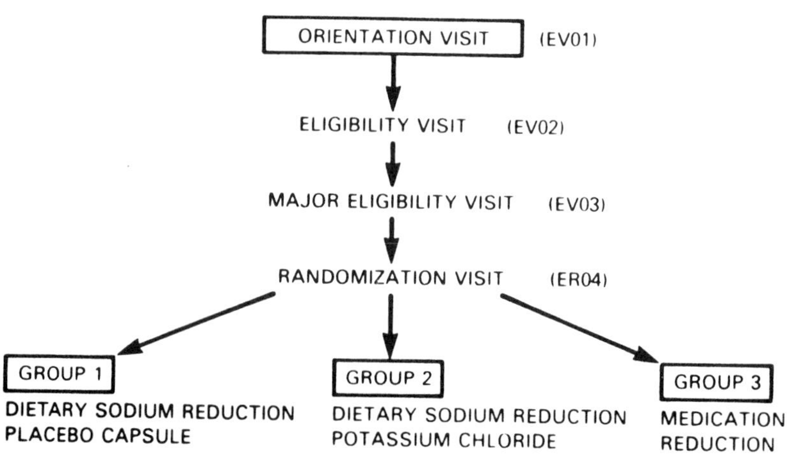

Figure 1 MSHT design.

weeks after the orientation visit and consists of a blood pressure measurement and a review of a self-administered medical history questionnaire. Men who meet basic eligibility requirements at this visit are scheduled for a third eligibility visit (EV03), the major eligibility visit. The third eligibility visit includes measurement of blood pressure, a physical examination, measurement of blood chemistries, urinalysis, complete blood count (CBC), and recording of an electrocardiogram. Participants at this visit are instructed on procedures for overnight and 24-hr urine collections and also on procedures for keeping 2-day food diaries. Men who remain eligible after the third eligibility visit are scheduled for a randomization visit (ER04) conducted 2 weeks after the third eligibility visit. At the randomization visit, the participants return their urine specimens and food diaries, blood chemistry determinations from the EV03 visit are reviewed, blood pressure is measured, and a sodium taste test is administered. Table 1 outlines the exclusions for the study determined at each eligibility visit.

Men eligible at ER04 are randomized to one of three treatment groups (Figure 2). Group 1 is advised on a dietary sodium reduction to $\leq$80 mEq/day and given placebo, 12 capsules a day. Group 2 is also advised on a dietary sodium reduction to $\leq$80 mEq/day and given supplemental potassium chloride (Micro-K) 96 mEq/day (12 capsules containing 8 mEq/capsule). Men in Groups 1 and 2 are instructed to take four capsules three times a day with meals. Subjects in both Groups 1 and 2 continue taking antihypertensive medication at this time. The men in Group 3 continue taking antihypertensive medications and their habits are not otherwise changed. Study conditions for Groups 1 and 2 are double-blind.

The dietary sodium goal for both Groups 1 and 2 is to reduce sodium excretion in the urine to less than or equal to 80 mEq (1,800 mg) sodium/24 hr. This level represents an average goal for men in Groups 1 and 2.

Table 1 Eligibility Visits and Exclusion Criteria

Visit	Exclusions
Visit 1 (EV01) Orientation	Age $<45>69$; duration of hypertension treatment ($\leq$4 years)
Visit 2 (EV02) Basic eligibility visit	Average DBP $>$95 mmHg
	History of significant renal disease
	Eats out more than five major meals/week
	Alcohol intake $>$four drinks/day
	Drugs: digitalis, nitroglycerine, antiarrhythmics, insulin, oral hypoglycemics
	Gross obesity $>$1.5 times ideal weight
	Refusal to participate in intervention
Visit 3 (EV03) Major eligibility visit	Average DBP $>$95 mmHg
	Average DBP at Visit 2 and Visit 3, $>$90 mmHg
	ECG abnormalities indicating past myocardial infarction
	Significant cardiovascular disease on physical examination
	Significant protinuria (2+ or greater)
	Significant hematuria (moderate or greater)
Visit 4 (ER04) Randomization	Serum creatinine $>$1.7 mg/dl
	Serum potassium $<$3.0 mEq/L
	Stool hemoccult positive (x2)
	Hematuria

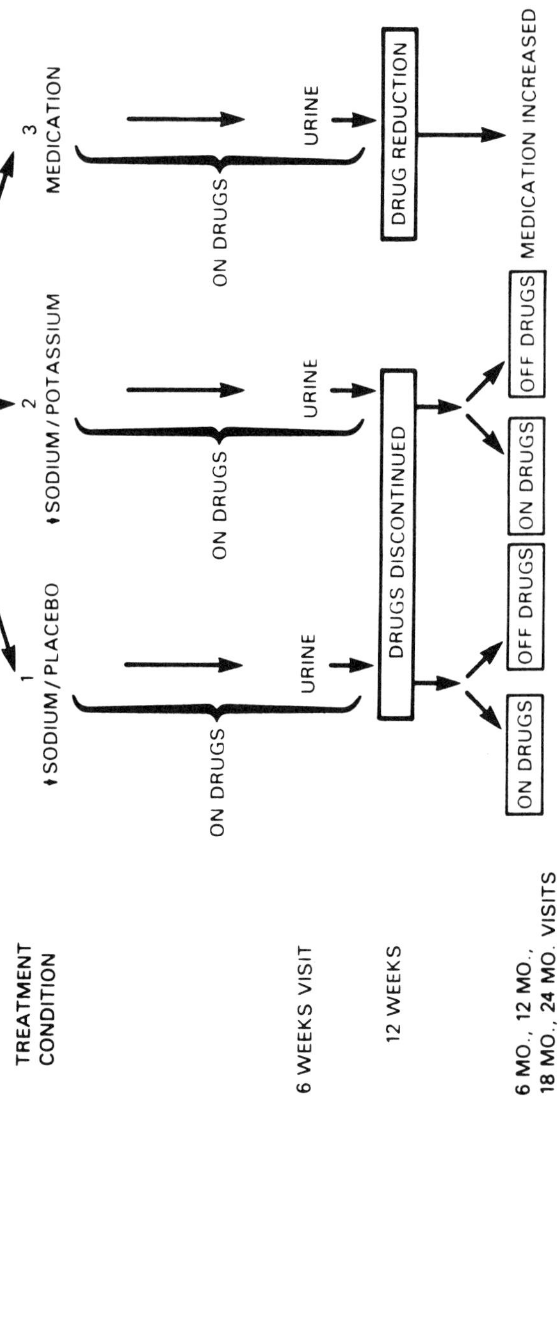

Figure 2 MSHT treatment timetable.

Twelve weeks after the subjects are randomized, antihypertensive medication is withdrawn from Groups 1 and 2. Men taking certain types of sympatholytic agents (i.e., beta blockers and methyldopa), have their dosages tapered and withdrawn over a 2-week period. After drug withdrawal, men in Groups 1 and 2 are seen at 2-3 week intervals for follow-up visits. If blood pressures remain under control after three consecutive visits, the subjects then enter a maintenance schedule (visits every 2 months).

The 75 men randomized to Group 3, the medication comparison group, continue with their regular antihypertensive drug regimen until the 12-week drug withdrawal visit, at which time their medication is reduced to the minimal dosage of diuretic (chlorthalidone 12.5 mg/day). Group 3 subjects are then evaluated on a regular basis and their dosages are increased when needed according to a standardized stepped-care protocol (Table 2) to a sufficient level with which to maintain diastolic blood pressure at less than or equal to 85 mmHg. Group 3 subjects are then seen at 2-month intervals unless blood pressures rise above goal, at which time they are seen more frequently so that their medication can be adjusted.

Table 2 Stepped-Care Regimen for Drug Reinstitution and Treatment

	Drug		Daily dosage (mg)
Step 1	Chlorthalidone		12.5
			25.0
			50.0
		or	
Step 2	Indapamide		2.5
		or	
	Hydrochlorothiazide		25
			50
	Reserpine		0.1
			0.25
		or	
	Propranolol		40
			80
			120
			160
		or	
	Methyldopa		500
			1000
			1500
			2000
Step 3	Hydralazine		25
			50
			75
			100
			150
			200

Table 3 Criteria for Reinstituting Antihypertensive Medication

Diastolic Pressure (mmHg)	
Monitoring visit	Recall visit
>115	immediate reinstitution of drugs
105–114	>95
95–104	>95 or 91–94 at two visits
91–94	91–94 at two visits

REINSTITUTION OF ANTIHYPERTENSIVE MEDICATIONS

Antihypertensive medication is reinstituted in Groups 1 and 2 according to a standard stepped-care protocol (Table 2). The specific drug and dosage used is listed in preferred order in Table 2. This treatment protocol is followed unless a specific contraindication exists at the time a drug is initiated or if a significant side effect develops. Criteria for reinstitution of antihypertensive medication are shown in Table 3. Any measurement of blood pressure greater than 90 mmHg at a regular follow-up visit will initiate a recall schedule. Visit intervals for recall visits are 3–4 weeks. Blood pressures taken at the recall visit determine if a participant's pressure is defined as uncontrolled and, if so, antihypertensive medication is then reinstituted.

END POINTS

The major end point of the study is a comparison of the proportion of participants from Groups 1 and 2 who require that antihypertensive medication be reinstated on visits (of record) conducted at 2-month intervals after randomization. Other end points include diastolic blood pressure changes and the proportion of participants at the various levels of medication (step and dosage).

Comparisons will also be made for the proportion of Group 1 and Group 2 subjects who have average diastolic blood pressures equal to or greater than 90 mmHg; mean levels, and distribution factors that reflect adverse or side effects associated with pharmacological treatment such as levels of serum potassium, uric acid, serum cholesterol, plasma lipoproteins, and plasma glucose; distribution of intervention variables which include sodium and potassium excretion; and dietary intakes. For these end points, comparisons will also be made across Groups 1, 2, and 3. Group 3 subjects, who continue on medication, provide a comparison group for adverse effects (biochemical and side effects), blood pressure change from standard care, and intervention results with respect to sodium and potassium.

MEASUREMENTS

Blood Pressure

Blood pressure is measured using a standard protocol by trained and certified observers using a standard sphygmomanometer, and a Hawkley random-zero sphygmomanometer. The random-zero device helps eliminate observer bias due to digit preference (11). Blood pressures are determined in the right arm using an adult-size cuff while the participant is seated after resting for at least 5 min. The initial reading is made with a standard mercury device followed by a second random-zero measure. The third measure is taken using the standard device and then a fourth random-zero measure is taken. The average of the second and fourth random-zero diastolic pressures forms the blood pressure measures that determine the major end point of the study. Blood pressure observers are certified according to the procedures of Rose and Prineas (12,13).

Urinalysis

Urine measures consist of one 24-hr and two timed-overnight collections for determination of sodium, potassium, and creatinine levels. Urine collections are done at the 6-week postrandomization visit, drug withdrawal visit, and subsequent "visit of record" every 6 months. Two-day food diaries are collected concurrently with urine specimens for determining dietary sodium, potassium, and other nutrients. Food records are kept by each participant and returned at the following visit. Men are given instructions on how to complete the records during the baseline period; ER04; 6- and 12-week; and 6-, 12-, 18-, and 24-month visits postrandomization. Food records returned to MSHT staff are reviewed and verified by staff nutritionists. They are then forwarded to a nutrition-coding center for processing and analysis.

Serum Chemical Values

A battery of chemical tests including measurement of electrolytes, creatinine, uric acid, and several other tests is performed using a multipanel SMA-C method. Blood values are measured at the major eligibility visit (EV03), the drug withdrawal visit, and then at 6-month visits of record.

Electrocardiogram

A standard 12-lead electrocardiogram is performed at the major eligibility visit and then at annual visits thereafter. Electrocardiograms are forwarded to the division of Epidemiology at the University of Minnesota for coding using the Minnesota Code (12).

Capsule Counts

When capsules are utilized, capsule counts of placebo/potassium antihypertensive medication are carried out in a standard fashion at 2-month visit intervals. Attempts are made to account for pills reported lost or destroyed.

INTERVENTION DESCRIPTION

The MSHT includes a major nutrition intervention–education component that helps participants in Groups 1 and 2 to reduce their dietary sodium intake to 80 mEq/day. After randomization, an intensive 12-week dietary sodium reduction phase begins. Participants undergo an initial nutrition assessment to determine their baseline sodium intake and eating patterns. Two-day food records are kept every 2 weeks for either individual nutrition counseling or group educational presentation.

The intervention trial is designed to make use of a variety of contact methods to enhance compliance and cost-effectiveness. The content of the intervention focuses on specific knowledge and behavioral areas. Family members are also included in all intervention activities to facilitate changes and to encourage participant support. Participants are provided with personal resource materials to be used at home and work: a Sodium Counter that provides information on sodium content of foods, a program guide, and a low-sodium cooking guide. Many of these materials will help the participants to self-monitor their dietary intake and to make appropriate food purchases and meal selections.

After the 12-week drug withdrawal visit, intervention visits occur at monthly intervals with similar formats as previously mentioned with special emphasis on solving individual problems, and maintaining low-sodium eating patterns.

RANDOMIZATION

At the fourth eligibility visit, participants are randomized to Group 1, 2, or 3. The randomization is stratified based on the current amount of antihypertensive medication used. Participants are included in stratum 1 if only a single antihypertensive agent (usually a diuretic) is prescribed. Stratum 2 is made up of participants taking two or more antihypertensive drugs.

The randomization is restricted to ensure approximate balance between Groups 1 and 2 and to approximate one-half as many patients in Group 3 within each stratum. This restriction is imposed by generating random permutations of the first 5 digits (1-5), or the first 10 digits (1-10) for each stratum. For a permutation of size 5, codes 1 and 2 are taken as Group 1, codes 3 and 4 as Group 2, and code 5 as Group 3. For a permutation of size 10, codes 1-4 correspond to Group 1, codes 5-8 to Group 2, and codes 9 and 10 to Group 3. For participants allocated to Groups 1 and 2, a unique four-digit bottle number is assigned by the Coordinating Center using a list provided by the company that supplies the potassium and placebo capsules. The first digit of the bottle number designates the participant's stratum.

The two randomization schedules, one each for stratum 1 and stratum 2, were prepared in advance. The actual treatment assignment (bottle number, or Group 3) is obtained by a designated clinic staff person who telephones the Coordinating Center. Before the assignment is issued, a prerandomization checklist is completed by the randomizer at the Coordinating Center to assure that the data are complete, and that participants not meeting eligibility criteria are excluded.

MAINTAINING THE DOUBLE BLIND

To reduce the likelihood of the clinical staff becoming aware of a participant's treatment assignment, serum and urine potassium measurements are sent only to the Coordinating Center, with the following exception: the clinic is informed only if serum potassium measurement is at high or low alert levels. if a participant's serum potassium level is <3.0 mEq/L or >6.0 mEq/L. For serum potassium readings of <3.2 mEq/L or >5.6 mEq/L, the participant is recalled for a repeat potassium measurement. As a precaution, the actual treatment assignment (KCl or placebo) for each participant is enclosed in a sealed envelope and stored at the clinical center. This envelope is opened only in the event of a severe illness or adverse reaction.

SAMPLE SIZE

To estimate the sample size for the proposed study, we assume that the major response variables for comparing Groups 1 and 2 are: (a) the proportion of participants who are prescribed antihypertensive medication, and (b) the difference in diastolic blood pressure change after 2 years of follow-up. The proportion of participants in Group 2 whom we estimated to have been prescribed antihypertensive medication after 2 years is 65%. We detected a 20% difference in the percentage of participants treated with antihypertensive drugs in Group 1 in relation to Group 2 by the 5% level of significance ($\alpha = 0.05$) for a two-sided alternative, and with a 90% probability ($1\text{-}\beta = 0.90$), leaving 128 participants required in each group. To allow for possible noncompliance with the assigned treatment, the sample size is increased by 15%, or 150 participants, in each group.

For the blood pressure change end point, it is considered important to detect a 4-mmHg difference in diastolic blood pressure. With 150 subjects in each group, the estimated power for detecting a 4-mmHg difference in diastolic blood pressure is 0.97 (we assumed the standard deviation for difference in blood pressure change to be 9.0 mmHg) when $\alpha = 0.05$ and a two-sided test is used.

The sample size required for Group 3 is determined so that a 4-mmHg difference between Group 1 or Group 2 and Group 3 could be detected with a power equal to 0.90 when $\alpha = 0.05$ (two-sided) test. We estimated a total of 75 subjects for Group 3 allowing for an approximately 15% noncompliance rate.

In summary, it is planned that a total of 375 participants will be recruited, 150 participants from each of Groups 1 and 2, and 75 participants from Group 3.

PLANNED DATA ANALYSIS

The proportion of subjects requiring antihypertensive treatment from Groups 1 and 2 will be compared at 6-month intervals using the 2x2 chi-square test. Since actual dates of medication withdrawal and reinstitution are available, the time for randomization to onset of treatment can be summarized using the life table methods of Kaplan and Meier (4). Blood pressure levels at 6-month intervals between treatment groups are compared using analysis of variance and covariance.

SUMMARY

Mt. Sinai Hypertension Trial is a major clinical trial designed to address the question of the role of potassium over and above dietary sodium reduction to control blood pressure in hypertensive men. By administering in double-blind fashion either placebo or potassium capsules, the trial will maximize the sodium/potassium excretion ratio in two groups of similar hypertensive men. After 12 weeks of sodium potassium/placebo intervention, participants will be withdrawn from their usual antihypertensive drugs and then evaluated at regular intervals. Antihypertensive medication is reinstituted if blood pressures rise to hypertensive levels. The trial will determine if potassium independently of sodium reduction aids in lowering blood pressure, and in reducing the number of participants requiring medication to reduce their blood pressure. The trial involves 375 men who will be evaluated for at least 2 years.

ACKNOWLEDGMENTS

This study is supported by a grant from the National Heart Lung and Blood Institute RO1-HL-29698-01 and the A.H. Robins Company. Dr. Grimm is an Established Investigator of the American Heart Association.

The authors wish to acknowledge Lorry Witte, R.N., Donna Rains-Clearman, R.D., Julie Levin, Sarah Taylor, R.D., M.P.H., Fran Galle, R.N., Linda Kiefer, R.D., M.P.H., and Mary Lemieux from our clinical staff; and also Kenneth Svendsen, Leslie Holland, Marie Hanson, Berit Aus, and Pat Stein from the coordinating center. Important contributions from these groups have made the study possible.

REFERENCES

1. Carney, S.: Sodium restriction and thiazide diuretics in the treatment of hypertension. *Med. J. Aust.* 1:803–807, 1975.
2. Holly, T. M. P., Evans, S. T. W., Goodwin, F. S., and Vandenberg, M. J.: Reanalysis of data in two Lancet papers on the effect of dietary sodium and potassium on blood pressure. *Lancet* 2:1384–1387, 1981.
3. Hunt, J. C.: Mild hypertension–appropriate diagnostic workup. *Ann. N.Y. Acad. Sci.* 304:373–380, 1978.
4. Kaplan, E. L., and Meier, P.: Non-parametric estimation from incomplete observers. *J. Am. Statist. Assoc.* 53:457–481, 1958.
5. Kempner, W.: Treatment of hypertensive vascular disease with rice diet. *Am. J. Med.* 4:545–577, 1948.
6. MacGregor, G. A., Markandu, N. D., Smith, S. J., Banks, R. A., and Sagnella, G. A.: Moderate potassium supplementation in essential hypertension. *Lancet* 2:567–570, 1982.
7. McNeely, G. R., and Battargee, H. D.: High sodium-low potassium environment and hypertension. *Am. J. Cardiol.* 38:768–785, 1976.
8. Morgan, T., Adam, W., Guillies, A., Wilson, M., Morgan, G., and Carney, S.: Hypertension treated by salt restriction. *Lancet* 1:227–230, 1978.
9. Parfrey, P. S., Wright, P., Goodwin, F. J., Vandenburg, M. J., Holly, J. M. P., Evans, S. J. W., and Ledingham, J. M.: Blood pressure and hormonal changes following alterations in dietary sodium and potassium in mild essential hypertension. *Lancet* 1:59–63, 1981.
10. Parijs, J., Joossens, J. V., Van der Linden, L., Verstreken, G., and Amery, A. K. P. C.: Moderate sodium restriction and diuretics in the treatment of hypertension. *Am. Heart J.* 85:22–34, 1973.
11. Prineas, R. J.: Blood pressure sounds: their measurement and meaning. Gamma Medical Products Corporation, 1978.
12. Prineas, R. J., Crow, R., and Blackburn, H.: *The Minnesota Code Manual of Electrocardiographic Findings*, Littleton, Massachusetts, John Wright-PSG, 1982.
13. Rose, G.: Standardization of observers and blood pressure measurement. *Lancet* 1:673, 1975.
14. Skrabal, F., Aubeck, J., Hortnagl, H., and Braunsteiner, H.: Effect of moderate salt restriction and high potassium intake on pressor hormones, responses to noradrenaline and baroreceptor function in man. *Clin. Sci.* 59:157s–160s, 1980.

33

Desirability of Changing Potassium Intake in the Community

GEOFFREY ROSE
London School of Hygiene and Tropical Medicine, London, England

Any recommendation for a general increase in potassium intake can be, at most, a matter of opinion: we do not know enough to be sure. This, however, does not necessarily preclude advice. For example, recommendations on a desirable intake of vitamins and of major nutrients are widely accepted, even though founded on very incomplete evidence. And in 1974 the U.S. National Academy of Sciences advised that healthy adults "need about 65 mmol (2.5 g) of potassium daily" (6).

We cannot hope for certainty in many public health issues; but we can draw up a balance sheet of supposed benefits, costs, and hazards, weight each item appropriately, and finally arrive at a best judgement. Disagreements must be expected, not only on the evidence itself but also on the relative importance of each item on the balance sheet.

WOULD AN INCREASED POTASSIUM INTAKE LOWER THE BLOOD PRESSURE OF POPULATIONS?

When the blood pressures of different populations are compared (Figure 1) the main difference is a shift affecting the whole distribution, to which the differences in the prevalence of hypertension are secondary phenomena. This means that the factors that determine these differences between populations operate on most individuals, not just on hypertensive subjects or other susceptible minority. Clearly, environmental factors can have powerful mass effects.

Variations in salt intake offer one possible explanation, and claims have been made (Table 1) for strong correlations and steep gradients when populations are compared. Unfortunately the data on which these claims rest are of poor or unknown quality; moreover, investigators have mostly concentrated exclusively on the sodium hypothesis and have failed to measure potassium intake and other key variables. Populations with a low-salt intake tend to have a high intake of potassium, and this might account for at least some of the effect attributed to sodium.

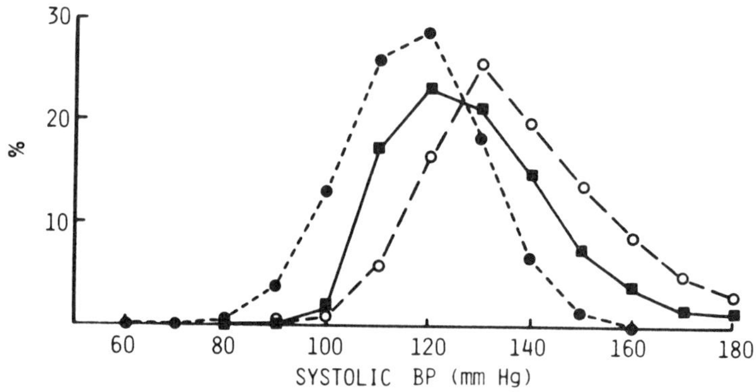

Figure 1 Distributions of systolic blood pressures of men aged 40–59: Kenyan nomads ●- - -●; London civil servants ■——■; Japanese railwaymen ○— —○.

These deficiencies in the data will be remedied in Intersalt, a new, prospectively planned international study which we are undertaking, under the auspices of the International Society and Federation of Cardiology and the World Health Organization. We shall obtain standardized measurements from about 30 populations on blood pressure, sodium and potassium intake, and other critical variables.

All the existing population data which link sodium intake with blood pressure might equally be interpreted as an effect of variations in the Na/K ratio, since any changes in the numerator necessarily also change the ratio. Thus the variation in mean blood pressure between populations could be due to variations in sodium intake or potassium intake or the Na/K intake ratio (or to something quite different). Within populations there is some evidence (3,5) that an individual's blood pressure may be related to potassium intake; and there are plausible mechanisms for a possible cause-and-effect relationship (9). Thus, taking the evidence as a whole it seems likely that an increase in potassium intake of the population would have *some* effect on its mean blood pressure, but this is not certain.

HOW LARGE MIGHT THE BENEFITS BE?

If potassium intake itself is a determinant of population blood pressures (whether directly or by influencing the Na/K ratio), no available data directly estimate the size of the effect. But if the Na/K ratio were the critical factor, then an indirect estimate can be made, based on the international data (Table 1). On this basis, and with typical Western

Table 1 Relation of Mean Blood Pressure to Supposed Sodium Intake in 27 Populations

	Slope (mmHg/mmol Na)	Correlation coefficient
Systolic	0.094	0.54
Diastolic	0.046	0.69

Source: Ref. 20.

electrolyte intake, a similar effect on mean blood pressure would be predicted from either a 25% reduction in intake of sodium or a one-third increase in potassium. This increase in potassium (from, say, 60 to 80 mmol daily) would correspond to a fall of 4 mmHg in mean systolic pressure, with a halving of the prevalence of hypertension.

Figure 2 shows the prevalence distribution of diastolic blood pressures (single reading, phase 4) in men aged 40-64 in the Whitehall Study (7), together with corresponding 10-year death rates. If the whole distribution were to be lowered by 4 mmHg, with corresponding falls in death rates, there would be a 25% reduction in the total deaths attributable to raised blood pressure.

Whether or not such a benefit would actually follow a reduction in mean blood pressure depends largely on whether the primary prevention of hypertension is more effective than treatment in reducing the risk of coronary heart disease. A major limitation of antihypertensive medication as a public health measure is its failure to control the coronary risk, since this is responsible for most of the excess deaths. The prospect of success in this respect for primary prevention seems much better, especially if control were to be instituted from childhood. If this hope were fulfilled, then a reduction in mean diastolic pressure of as little as 4 mmHg would probably reduce mortality by more than all the existing antihypertension medication.

This reasoning shows the potential public health importance of even a small reduction in pressure of the population as a whole. Unfortunately it involves two serious problems. First, a difference in mean pressure which could be very important may be too small to be demonstrable. Secondly, one encounters the "prevention paradox": *a preventive measure that brings much benefit to the population offers little to each individual* (8). If the population's mean blood pressure could be lowered there would be a small benefit to a lot of people, and the cumulative effect would be large; but each individual would expect to gain little. This reduces motivation, and it also underlines the necessity that any mass preventive measure must be safe.

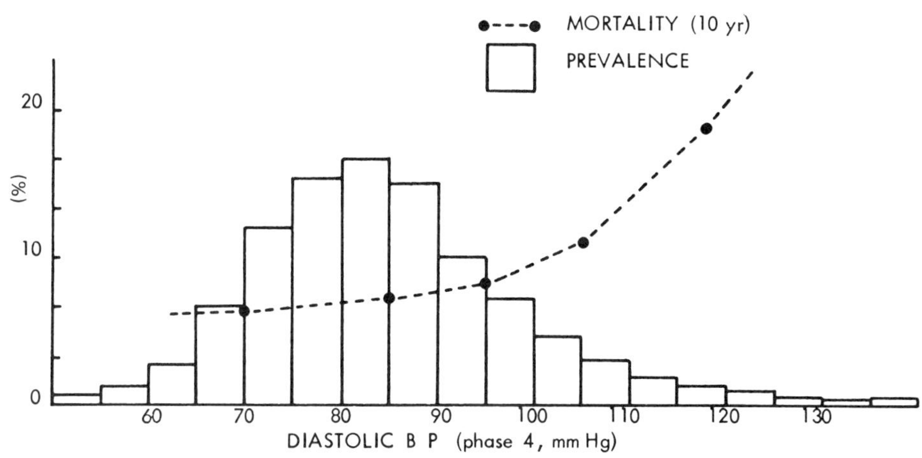

Figure 2 Distribution of diastolic (phase 4) blood pressure and corresponding 10-year mortality rates in men aged 40–64 in the Whitehall Study (7).

HOW COULD AVERAGE POTASSIUM INTAKE BE INCREASED?

The potassium contents of some common foods are shown in Table 2. The highest concentrations are in vegetables, especially potatoes. More than half of this is lost by boiling. All meats and fish, and most fruits, are also relatively rich sources. Cow's milk contains more than twice as much potassium as human milk.

A rather different picture emerges in Table 3, which shows where the population gets most of its potassium from. The main source is root vegetables; but milk comes second (because so much is consumed); and (at least in the United Kingdom) milk, meat, and eggs together account for one-third of the total potassium intake.

For an average individual, taking in perhaps 60 mmol potassium daily, a one-third increase would not be difficult to achieve. The cheapest way would be to add 120 g daily of baked potato, or a similar quantity of boiled potato plus other vegetables. For someone eating four slices of white bread daily, changing to wholemeal bread would yield an extra 16 mmol potassium. The rich man's preference might be to eat more fruit: 200 ml daily of orange juice yields about 10 mmol potassium.

Another cheap way of increasing potassium intake is by the use of a sodium-reduced, potassium-enriched salt substitute. About one-third of the sodium chloride can be replaced in this way without serious loss of palatability, particularly when the product is

Table 2 Potassium Content of Some Common Foods

Food	K content (mmol/100g)
Potatoes	
baked	17
boiled	8
Baked beans	9
Carrots	4
Peas	4
Cabbage	3
Stewed prunes	11
Bananas	9
Orange juice	5
Apples	3
Bread	
wholemeal	7
white	3
Cornflakes	3
Milk	
cow	4
human	2
Cheese: cheddar	3
Eggs	4

Source: Ref. 4.

Table 3 Main sources of potassium in British diet

	Average K/person per day	
Food	mmol	%
Root vegetables	11	27
Milk	8	19
Meat + eggs	5	13
Cereal products	4	11
Other vegetables	4	10
Fruits	3	6
Other	5	14
Total	40	100

Source: Ref. 1.

used in cooking. Replacing 3 g daily of common salt in this way would add an extra 13 mmol potassium, with a slightly augmented effect on the Na/K ratio due to the reduction in sodium.

In our studies of London civil servants we find that the 24-hr urinary excretion of potassium is about 50% greater among those in higher grades of employment compared to those in unskilled lower grades. Evidently a higher income, with its accompanying food preferences, leads to a higher potassium intake, apart from any motivation for health reasons.

SAFETY

The potassium intake of Western populations is probably much lower than that to which humans have become genetically adapted by evolutionary history. Thus an increase, by restoring "biological normality," carries an a priori expectation of safety. This is supported by the experience of vegetarian and other groups with higher intakes, who seem not to suffer harm.

Within the population, individuals with renal failure might be at risk; but they are identifiable and could be forewarned. Conversely, for the enormous numbers of people taking diuretic treatment, an increase in potassium intake could well be beneficial. On grounds of safety there seems no cause for concern.

WIDER IMPLICATIONS

Specialists tend to be interested only in the disease they are studying, but public health policy must consider the wider implications. The largest cardiovascular problem facing Western populations is coronary heart disease, and the main determinant of its high incidence is a dietary pattern conducive to a high serum cholesterol level. Such populations are therefore urged (10) to reduce their intake of fat, especially saturated fat, and to obtain a higher proportion of energy from vegetable sources. An increased intake of fiber is also encouraged. Such changes will increase the intake of potassium, because they encourage the consumption of cereal products, vegetables, and fruit.

Based on less strong but still suggestive evidence, an increased intake of fiber and complex carbohydrates is also being suggested as a possible means of preventing diverticulitis, colon cancer, and diabetes. Finally, the incidence of breast cancer correlates strongly with fat intake, and it might be reduced if the population chose to derive less energy from fat and more from carbohydrate.

CONCLUSION

Thus it seems from many points of view that a Western diet would be healthier if it derived a greater proportion of energy from cereal, vegetable, and fruit sources; such a diet happens also to be rich in potassium. If, then, current dietary advice is accepted, potassium intake will increase. It is possible, though in no way certain, that this could bring some lowering of average blood pressure as a bonus. It is highly likely that even a small reduction of this kind, shared by the population as a whole, would bring substantial cardiovascular benefits. No new policy decision is needed to move things in this direction.

The present evidence does not justify additional advice, aimed specifically at increasing the intake of potassium. However, such a policy is readily achieved by any individual who is so minded; it is safe, and it might be beneficial. The choice is a matter of personal preference.

REFERENCES

1. Bull, N. L., and Buss, D. H.: Contributions of foods to sodium intakes. *Proc. Nutr. Soc.* 39:31A, 1980.
2. Gleibermann, L.: Blood pressure and dietary salt in human populations. *Ecol. Food Nutr.* 2:143, 1973.
3. Khaw, K. T., and Rose, G.: Population study of blood pressure and associated factors in St. Lucia, West Indies. *Int. J. Epidemiol.* 11:372, 1983.
4. McCance, R. A., and Widdowson, E. M: *The Composition of Foods,* Medical Research Council Special Report Series No. 297, Her Majesty's Stationery Office, London, 1960.
5. MacGregor, G. A.: Dietary sodium and potassium intake and blood pressure. *Lancet* 1:750, 1983.
6. National Academy of Sciences: *Recommended Dietary Allowances,* 8th edition, National Academy of Sciences, Washington, D.C., 1974.
7. Reid, D. D., Hamilton, P. J. S., McCartney, P., Rose, G., Jarrett, R. J., and Keen, H.: Smoking and other risk factors for coronary heart disease in British civil servants. *Lancet* 2:979, 1976.
8. Rose, G.: Strategy of prevention: Lessons from cardiovascular disease. *Br. Med. J.* 282:1847, 1981.
9. Skrabal, F., Auböck, J., and Hörtnagl, H.: Low sodium/high potassium diet for prevention of hypertension: Probable mechanisms of action. *Lancet* 2:895, 1981.
10. World Health Organization: Prevention of Coronary Heart Disease: Report of a WHO Expert Committee. Technical Report Series 678, WHO, Geneva, 1982.

34

Feasibility of Changing Potassium Intake in the Community

KAY-TEE KHAW
University of California-San Diego, La Jolla, California

REASONS FOR CONSIDERING DIETARY POTASSIUM CHANGE IN THE COMMUNITY

Raised blood pressure is a major risk factor for cardiovascular disease, which is the leading cause of death in most countries. Medical treatment of patients with blood pressure levels above 160/105 undoubtedly lowers mortality and the benefits of drug treatment of subjects who have levels below this have also been demonstrated in some trials (12,53,61). However, the traditional approach of identifying and treating high-risk subjects has proved unsatisfactory for several reasons, as exemplified by the debate over treatment of individuals with "mild hypertension," that is, systolic blood pressure 140-160 mmHg, diastolic pressure 90-105 mmHg (3,36,39,41,54). Side effects of drugs in asymptomatic but hypertensive individuals are often not acceptable, compliance is poor, and costs are high (cost of treating the 20% of the U.S. population or 40 million people estimated to be "hypertensive" would exceed $1 billion annually). Additionally, because risk increases with every increment of blood pressure from the lowest level, approximately half the cardiovascular deaths attributable to raised blood pressure occur at levels below accepted treatment threshholds (44). Because of these problems, alternative strategies such as the lowering of risk factor distribution in the population as a whole by means other than drug treatment have been suggested (44).

Many dietary constituents have been implicated in the causes of high blood pressure. These include high saturated fat, protein, and alcohol intake and low magnesium, calcium, and fiber intake (4,10,13,27,28,45,45,50). Considerable epidemiologic, clinical, and experimental evidence exists for the role of high sodium intake, and, more recently for low potassium intake (7,8,18,22,29,31,37,40,47,52,56,57,59,62). Clinical trials have shown that potassium supplementation can lower blood pressure in hypertensives (14,29), and biologically plausible mechanisms for the effects of potassium on blood pressure control have been demonstrated (31,57). Populations with low mean blood pressures generally have high potassium and low sodium intakes and in populations with similar sodium intakes, mean blood pressure is lower in those with higher potassium intake (18,47).

Though correlation between sodium intake alone and blood pressure has been difficult to demonstrate within a population (49,58), several studies have reported positive and negative correlations with sodium/potassium ratio and potassium respectively, estimated from dietary intake or urinary samples (7,18,20,43,52,59). A continuing longitudinal rural-urban migration study in Kenya found that the increased blood pressures in urban migrants who had come from the rural area was significantly associated with higher urinary sodium/potassium ratio and lower urinary potassium (40). Ethnic, geographic, and socioeconomic differences in blood pressure patterns are also consistent with differences in potassium intake. The suggestion that sodium raises blood pressure only in those genetically susceptible has been used as an argument against any effort to achieve community reduction of sodium intake (23,49). Several lines of evidence suggest that potassium affects blood pressure not just in hypertensives but in the whole population. Two population-based studies (20,43) have reported significant negative correlation of individual blood pressure with dietary potassium intake estimated from 24 hr recall; in our study (23) this negative correlation in fact increased after excluding hypertensive subjects and those using antihypertensive medication. Though evidence from intervention trials is not conclusive (55), potassium supplementation has been reported to lower the blood pressure of normotensive subjects (22).

The "normal" mean daily potassium intake worldwide ranges from 20 to 200 mmol. In the United States the mean is approximately 60 mmol a day but there is wide socioeconomic as well as geographic variation (9,48). Even within a homogeneous, upper-middle-class white community in southern California the reported 24-hr intake ranged from 10 to 130 mmol (mean, 40 mmol) (23). The optimum level of dietary potassium intake is unknown but, at least in terms of blood pressure, a dietary increase might be expected to be beneficial and a twofold increase in the U.S. mean daily intake would still be within the range of "normal" human intake.

SOURCES OF DIETARY POTASSIUM

With the exception of the use of potassium salt substitute, potassium intake is nondiscretionary. In the typical "Western" diet approximately 50% of the dietary potassium intake is derived from vegetable and fruit sources, 25% from dairy sources, in particular milk, and 25% from other foods such as meat and cereal (10,23,48). Potassium is generally lost in food processing while sodium is added. Dietary intake can be increased by:

1. Potassium salt supplementation
    a. In tablet form
    b. As sodium chloride substitute in cooking and at table
    c. As sodium salt substitute in food processing
2. Decreasing loss in food processing
3. Increasing intake of potassium-rich foods.

The feasibility of each of these methods depends largely on acceptability in terms of taste and cost; desirability encompasses other questions such as the long-term effects. For high-risk, highly motivated individuals, such as those taking diuretics, all these methods may be considered; on a community basis the cost-benefit balance may be weighted differently.

Potassium supplementation in tablet form (usually 8 mmol each) can increase potassium intake sizably but is not realistic on a community basis (though not as impossible as might seem judging from the large proportion of people in the U.S. regularly taking vitamin supplements). Potassium salt substitutes are now widely available; use of this in place of sodium chloride could increase daily potassium intake by up to 100 mmol. Another alternative is the use of potassium salts in place of sodium salts in food processing.

There are, however, several major disadvantages to the use of potassium salts. Trials of their use in hypertensives, who might be expected to be more highly motivated than the general population, have reported that subjects found the taste unpalatable, though mixtures of potassium and sodium salts in, for example, a 1:1 molar proportion have been reported to be more acceptable (32). In food processing, sodium salts are used partially as food preservative and the effectiveness of potassium salts as a substitute food preservative is unknown. Additionally, a potassium salts are expensive—currently about ten times the cost of sodium salts—and widespread use would result in noticeably increased food costs.

Dietary potassium can also be increased by increasing the intake of potassium rich foods. Table 1 shows the potassium index of nutritional quality (INQ=mmol of potassium/100 kcal) for examples of selected food categories. Foods richest in potassium are vegetables and fruit. One average (100 g), serving of green vegetable or fruit has 5-15 mmol potassium (2). Increasing the average diet by two to three servings of these relatively low-calorie foods a day could be achieved without severely displacing other essential foods and compromising nutritional requirements. The palatibility of high fruit and vegetable intake is subject to individual preferences as well as cultural conditioning, but these foods are generally acceptable, given the wide range of possible choices. In a recent small trial, subjects preferred increasing potassium intake by eating fruit and vegetables to using potassium salt substitute (15). The relatively high cost of these foods in some urban environments may be a major difficulty, though this potentially could be overcome.

Food processing such as canning can reduce potassium content by half (Table 2); in a diet consisting largely of processed food, potassium could be increased by 50% by changing to the fresh equivalent. Food processing may be the only way of storing food safely in many communities and it may be preferable to lose potassium and overeat sodium than to suffer from malnutrition or food poisoning. With the increasingly widespread use of refrigeration and year-round availability of fresh food, processing may be less of a necessity than a convenience and reduction of processed food intake in these circumstances more feasible. Additionally, steaming or stir-frying food instead of prolonged boiling can reduce potassium loss.

Table 1 Index of Nutritional Quality (INQ) (mmol potassium/100 kcal)

Food type	Example	Kcal per 100g	Potassium (mmol/100g)	Sodium (mmol/100g)	INQ	Na/K ratio
Vegetable	celery	17	8.7	<0.1	51.1	<0.1
Fruit	orange	49	5.1	<0.1	10.4	<0.1
Milk	whole	66	3.7	2.3	5.6	0.6
Meat	beef	263	9.9	2.4	3.8	0.2
Cereal	macaroni	147	2.0	<0.1	1.4	<0.1
Fat	butter	716	0.6	0.3	<0.1	0.5

Source: Ref. 2.

Table 2 Effect of Processing on the Potassium and Sodium Content of Food

	Potassium (mmol/100g)	Sodium (mmol/100g)	Na/K ratio
Peas			
fresh cooked	8.1	0.1	0.1
frozen cooked	3.5	5.0	1.4
canned	2.5	23.6	9.4
Pork			
fresh cooked	5.5	1.3	0.2
bacon	1.4	10.9	7.8

Source: Ref. 2.

WHAT IS A FEASIBLE COMMUNITY CHANGE?

Several studies have increased potassium intake by up to 120 mmol a day using supplements or salt substitutes but these have generally been in motivated hypertensive or volunteer subjects (29,32,55). Although the mean potassium intake in Western countries could be doubled or even tripled with the use of potassium salt substitutes, this is probably not feasible in terms of acceptability of taste and cost, nor desirable in terms of unknown possible side effects. Though no large studies have specifically addressed dietary potassium intake, several substantial studies have achieved long-term reductions in saturated fat intake (11,13,33,34,53); a usual concomitant of such change is an increase in fruit and vegetable intake. In one trial, during the low-fat intervention period, the study group was found to have an increase in 24-hr potassium excretion of approximately 13 mmol (13). Though it could be argued that these trials are in highly motivated groups, the large differences and range of intake of dietary potassium between communities and even within one community suggest a wider potential for change. Further, unlike the difficulties of decreasing dietary sodium and fat, it is usually easier to add to a diet than to take away from it. A realistic community change might be to increase intake of fruit and vegetable by an extra serving of either at two meals (caloric value, on average, less than half an ounce of butter). Would a community change of this size be worth making in terms of the impact on blood pressure and cardiovascular disease?

ESTIMATED POTENTIAL BENEFIT

No randomized community trials of increased dietary potassium have yet been undertaken. Studies of potassium supplementation in hypertensives found that a 64-mmol daily increase in potassium intake reduced mean blood pressure by approximately 10% or 6–8 mmHg (29). These findings are consistent with population studies which have found the regression slopes of blood pressure on estimated dietary potassium intake to be approximately 1–2 mmHg decrease per 10 mmol increase in potassium (18,20). A mean community dietary increase of 10–20 mmol potassium achievable by an increase of two fruit or vegetable servings a day might be expected to result in a decrease in population mean of 2–4 mmHg. The population impact might be considerable. A change of this magnitude might be estimated to reduce ischemic heart disease deaths by up to 10% and stroke deaths by up to 20% (26). Rose has estimated that, given the problems of noncompliance and ineffective treatment, all the life-saving benefits of current antihypertensive treatment could be equalled by a downward shift of the whole blood pressure distribution in the population by a mere 2-3 mmHg (44). Some indirect observations agree with the idea that quite small population differences in blood pressure may be important; in both the United States and United Kingdom there has been a marked decrease in hypertension-associated deaths beginning before and not entirely attributable to widespread use of antihypertensive medications (24,38). Specific surveys have reported a secular decrease in mean blood pressures (8,21). There are many assumptions in such estimates of potential benefit from dietary change; however, one study has correlated geographic and socioeconomic differences in stroke mortality with fruit and vegetable intake that are consistent with such estimates (1).

POSSIBLE ADVERSE EFFECTS

Estimates of possible benefit have to be balanced by consideration of potential adverse effects. The clofibrate trial has shown us that apparent benefits of intervention on coronary heart disease can be counterbalanced by unexpected adverse effects (35,36). The potential adverse effects of mass measures on healthy individuals are a primary consideration. Even if increasing dietary potassium does lower blood pressure and lead to concomitant lowering of cardiovascular risk, are there any adverse effects of lowering blood pressure or increasing dietary potassium on the normotensive population?

Some cardiovascular risk factors such as serum cholesterol and obesity have been associated with U-shaped mortality curves (17,25,51). Though the increased mortality at lowest values has been ascribed to preexisting disease and selective mortality and not to a causal relationship, for example, between low serum cholesterol and mortality, this finding has led some to caution in recommending mass reduction of these risk factor levels. However, blood pressure shows no such U-shaped mortality curve. Several cohort studies have reported that blood pressure is a risk factor not only for cardiovascular but for cancer and other diseases (6,19,42). This finding was supported by the Hypertension Detection and Follow-Up Program, which, though not a randomized trial, found mortality from not only cardiovascular but also other causes to be reduced in the treatment group (12). Geographic correlations between hypertension-related mortality and cancer or other chronic disease mortality have also been reported (5). These studies indicate no adverse effects of lower blood pressure levels, even in "normotensives" and even suggest some possible beneficial effect.

No trials have been conducted of the effect of increased dietary potassium on mortality, as opposed to blood pressure. However, both case-control and observational studies have shown that diets high in potassium-rich foods such as vegetables are associated with lower incidence of, or mortality from, not only cardiovascular but also cancer and other diseases (16,30).

Potassium in the diet is linked with anions other than chloride or bicarbonate, the usual supplement form. Chloride has been suggested to have an additional effect to sodium in raising blood pressure (60). Gastrointestinal upset is a well-recognized short-term side effect of potassium chloride ingestion; long-term effects of potassium salt supplements that are not usual human dietary constituents are unknown.

CONCLUSIONS

Long-term trials are the oft-cited ideal but they are usually not feasible nor ethical, and dietary recommendations are made based on accumulation of opinion from imperfect evidence. When we are considering dietary potassium increase in the community, potassium salt supplementation is inadequately tested, less acceptable in taste and cost, and its long-term effects unknown. It cannot be recommended on a mass basis without further observation or trials. However, a moderate increase in dietary potassium can be achieved by a modest increase in fruit and vegetable intake, which is feasible in terms of acceptability and cost. This change would be well within the "normal" dietary human range. Available evidence from observational studies suggest no adverse effect and indeed, would indicate a beneficial effect not only on cardiovascular but also other chronic disease.

REFERENCES

1. Acheson, R. M., and Williams, D. R. R.: Does consumption of fruit and vegetables protect against stroke? *Lancet* 2:1191–1193, 1983.
2. Adams, C. F.: *Nutritive Value of American Foods in Common Units.* United States Department of Agriculture, 1975, p. 456.
3. Alderman, M. H.: High blood pressure: Do we really know whom to treat and how? *N Engl J Med* 296:753–754, 1977.
4. Anderson, J. W.: Plant fiber and blood pressure. *Ann. Intern. Med.* 98 (Part 2):842–845, 1983.
5. Armstrong, B., and Doll, R.: Environmental factors and cancer incidence and mortality in different countries with special reference to dietary practices. *Int J Cancer* 15:617–631, 1975.
6. Conti, S., Farchi, G., and Menotti, A.: Coronary risk factors and excess mortality from all causes and specific causes. *Int. J. Epidemiol.* 12:301–307, 1983.
7. Dai, W. S., Kuller, L. H., and Miller, G.: Arterial blood pressure and urinary electrolytes. *J. Chron. Dis.* 37:75–84, 1984.
8. Feinleib, M., Kannel, W. B., Garrison, R. J., McNamara, P. M., and Castelli, W. P.: The Framingham offspring study: Design and preliminary data. *Prev. Med.* 4:518–525, 1975.
9. Fregly, M. J.: Estimates of sodium and potassium intake. *Ann. Intern. Med.* 98 (Part 2):792–799, 1983.
10. Friedman, G. D., Klatsky, A. L., and Siegelaub, A. B.: Alcohol intake and hypertension. *Ann. Intern. Med.* 98 (Part 2):846–849, 1983.
11. Hjermann, I., Holme, I., Velve Byre, K., and Leren, P.: Effect of diet and smoking intervention on the incidence of coronary heart disease. *Lancet* 2:1303–1310, 1981.
12. Hypertension Detection and Follow-up Program Cooperative Group: Five year findings of the Hypertension Detection and Follow-up Program. *JAMA* 242:2562–2571, 1979.
13. Iacono, J. M., Puska, P., Dougherty, R. M., Pietinen, P., Vartianen, E., Leino, U., Mutanen, M., and Moisio, S.: Effect of dietary fat on blood pressure in a rural Finnish population. *Am. J. Clin. Nutr.* 38:860–869, 1983.
14. Iimura, O., Kijima, T., Kikuchi, K., Miyama, A., Ando, T., Nakao, T., and Takigami, Y.: Studies on the hypotensive effect of high potassium intake in patients with essential hypertension. *Clin. Sci.* 61:77s–80s, 1981.
15. Jeffery, R. W., Pirie, P. L., Elmer, P. J., Bjornson-Benson, W. M., Mullenbach, V. A., Kurth, C. L., and Johnson, S. L.: Low-sodium high-potassium diet: Feasibility and acceptability in a normotensive population. *Am. J. Public Health* 74:492–494, 1984.
16. Kahn, H. A., Phillips, R. L., Snowdon, D. A., and Choi, W.: Association between reported diet and all-cause mortality. *Am. J. Epidemiol.* 119:775–787, 1984.
17. Kannel, W. B., and Gordon, T.: The search for an optimum serum cholesterol. *Lancet* 2:374–375, 1982.

18. Khaw, K. T., and Rose, G.: Population study of blood pressure and associated factors in St. Lucia, West Indies. *Int J Epidemiol.* 11:372-377, 1982.
19. Khaw, K. T., and Barrett-Connor, E.: Systolic blood pressure and cancer mortality in an elderly population. *Am. J. Epidemiol.* 120:550-558, 1984.
20. Khaw, K. T., and Barrett-Connor, E.: Dietary potassium and blood pressure in a population study. *Am. J. Clin. Nutr.* 39:964-968, 1984.
21. Khaw, K. T., Barrett-Connor, E., and Suarez, L.: Seasonal and secular variation in blood pressure in man. *J. Cardiac. Rehab.* 4:440-444, 1984.
22. Khaw, K. T., and Thom, S.: Randomised double-blind crossover trial of potassium on blood pressure in normal subjects. *Lancet* 2:1127-1129, 1982.
23. Lancet editorial: Genetics, environment and hypertension. *Lancet* 1:681-682, 1983.
24. Lancet editorial: Why has stroke mortality declined? *Lancet* 1:1195-1196, 1983.
25. Lew, E. A., and Garfinkel, L.: Variations in mortality by weight among 750,000 men and women. *J. Chron. Dis.* 32:563-576, 1979.
26. Marmot, M. G.: Diet, hypertension and stroke. In *Nutrition and Health–A Perspective*, edited by Turner, M. R., Lancaster, MTP Press, 1982, pp. 243-254.
27. McCarron, D. A.: Calcium and magnesium nutrition in human hypertension. *Ann. Intern. Med.* 98 (Part 2):800-806.
28. McCarron, D. A., Stanton, J., Henry, H., and Morris, C.: Assessment of nutritional correlates of blood pressure. *Ann Intern. Med* 98 (Part 2):715-719, 1983.
29. MacGregor, G. A., Markandu, N. D., Smith, S. J., Banks, R. A., and Sagnella, G. A.: Moderate potassium supplementation in essential hypertension. *Lancet* 2:567-570, 1982.
30. McGee, D. L., Reed, D. M., Yano, K., Kagan, A., and Tillotson, J.: Ten year incidence of coronary heart disease in the Honolulu Heart Program. *Am. J. Epidemiol.* 119:667-675, 1984.
31. Meneely, G. R., and Battarbee, H. D.: High sodium-low potassium environment and hypertension. *Am. J. Cardiol.* 38:768-85, 1976.
32. Mickelson, O., Makdani, D., Gill, J. L., Frank, R. L.: Sodium and potassium and excretions of normal men consuming sodium chloride or a 1:1 mixture of sodium and potassium chlorides. *Am. J. Clin. Nutr.* 30:2033-2040, 1977.
33. Multiple Risk Factor Intervention Trial Research Group: Multiple Risk Factor Intervention Trial: Risk factor changes and mortality results. *JAMA* 248:1465-1477, 1982.
34. National Diet-Heart Study Research Group: The National Diet–Heart Study Final Report. *Circulation* 37 (suppl 1):1-428.
35. Oliver, M. F., Heady, J. A., Morris, J. N., and Cooper, J.: World Health Organization trial on primary prevention of ischaemic heart disease using clofibrate to lower cholesterol: Mortality follow-up. *Lancet* 2:379-385, 1980.
36. Oliver, M. F.: Risks of correcting the risks of coronary disease and stroke with drugs. *N. Engl. J. Med.* 306:297-298, 1983.
37. Ophir, O., Peer, G., Gilad, J., Blum, M., and Aviram, A.: Low blood pressure in vegetarians: The possible role of potassium. *Am. J. Clin. Nutr.* 37:755-762, 1983.
38. Ostfeld, A. M.: A review of stroke epidemiology. *Epidemiol. Rev* 2:136-152, 1980.
39. Pickering, T. G.: Treatment of mild hypertension and the reduction of cardiovascular mortality: the "of or by" dilemma. *JAMA* 249:399-400, 1983.
40. Poulter, N., Khaw, K. T., Hopwood, B. E. C., Mugambi, M., Peart, W. S., and Sever, P. S.: Salt and blood pressure in various populations. *J. Cardiovasc. Pharmacol.* 6 (Suppl 1):S197-S203, 1984.
41. Ram, C. V. S.: Should mild hypertension be treated? *Ann. Intern. Med.* 99:403-405, 1983.
42. Raynor, W. J., Shekelle, R. B., Rossof, A. H., Maliza, C., and Paul, O.: High blood

pressure and 17 year cancer mortality in the Western Electric Health Study. *Am. J. Epidemiol.* 113:371-377, 1981.

43. Reed, D., Yano, K., and McGee, D.: Diet and blood pressure among elderly Japanese males in Hawaii. *Cardiovascular epidemiology newsletter* no. 35, American Heart Association, January 1984, p. 50.
44. Rose, G.: Strategy of prevention. *Br. Med. J.* 282:1847-1851, 1981.
45. Rouse, I. L., Beilin, L. J., Armstrong, B. K., and Vandongen, R.: Blood pressure lowering effect of a vegetarian diet: Controlled trial in normotensive subjects. *Lancet* 1:5-10, 1983.
46. Salonen, J. T., Tuomilehto, J., and Tanskanen, A.: Relation of blood pressure to reported intake of salt, saturated fats and alcohol in healthy middle-aged population. *J. Epidemiol. Commun. Health* 37:32-37, 1983.
47. Sasaki, N.: High blood pressure and the salt intake of the Japanese. *Jpn. Heart J.* 3:313-324, 1982.
48. Shank, F. R.: Recent data on the amounts of sodium and potassium being consumed and future considerations for food labeling. In *Sodium and Potassium in foods and drugs,* edited by White, P. L., American Medical Association, Chicago, 1980.
49. Simpson, F. O.: Salt and hypertension: A sceptical review of the evidence. *Clin. Sci.* 57 (suppl 5):463s-480s, 1979.
50. Smith-Barbaro, P. A., and Pucak, G. J.: Dietary fat and blood pressure. *Ann. Intern. Med.* 98 (Part 2):828-831, 1983.
51. Sorlie, P., Gordon, T., and Kannel, W. B.: Body build and mortality. The Framingham study. *JAMA* 243:1828-1831, 1980.
52. Staessen, J., Bulpitt, C., Fagard, R., Joossens, J. V., Lijnen, P., and Amery, A.: Four urinary cations and blood pressure. A population study in two Belgian towns. *Am. J. Epidemiol.* 117:676-687, 1983.
53. Stamler, J., and Stamler, R.: Intervention for the prevention and control of hypertension and atherosclerotic diseases: United States and international experience. *Am. J. Med. Coronary and Hypertension symposium*, February 1984.
54. Stason, W. B., and Weinstein, M. C.: Allocation of resources to manage hypertension. *N. Engl. J. Med.* 296:732-739, 1977.
55. Treasure, J., and Ploth, D.: Role of dietary potassium in the treatment of hypertension. *Hypertension* 5:864-872, 1983.
56. Vital and Health Statistics: Dietary Intake and Cardiovascular risk factors, part 1. Blood pressure correlates: United States, 1971-1975. *DHHS Publication No. (PHS) 83-1676*, 1983.
57. Walker, W. G., Whelton, P. K., Saito, H., Russell, R. P., and Hermann, J.: Relation between blood pressure and renin, renin substrate, angiotensin II, aldosterone and urinary sodium and potassium in 574 ambulatory subjects. *Hypertension* 1:287-291, 1979.
58. Watt, G. C. M., and Foy, C. J. W.: Dietary sodium and arterial pressure: Problems of studies within a single population. *J. Epidemiol. Commun. Health* 36:197-201, 1982.
59. Watson, R. L., Langford, H. G., Abernethy, J., Barnes, T. Y., and Watson, M. J.: Urinary electrolytes, body weight and blood pressure. *Hypertension* 2 (suppl 1): 193-198, 1980.
60. Whitescarver, S. A., Ott, C. E., and Jackson, B. A.: Salt-sensitive hypertension: Contribution of chloride. *Science* 223:1430-1432, 1984.
61. W.H.O./I.S.H. Mild Hypertension Liaison Committee: Trials of the treatment of mild hypertension. *Lancet* 1:149-156, 1982.
62. Yamori, Y., Kihara, M., Nara, Y., Ohtaka, M., Horie, R., Tsunematsu, T., and Note, S.: Hypertension and diet: Multiple regression analysis in a Japanese farming community. *Lancet* 1:1204-1205, 1981.

TREATMENT OF HYPOKALEMIA

35

Approaches to the Correction of Diuretic-Induced Hypokalemia

TREFOR OWEN MORGAN
University of Melbourne, Melbourne, Victoria, Australia

Depression of plasma potassium and depletion of the body stores of potassium have a number of important metabolic consequences (5,8,13). In individual patients these have to be marked before serious side effects can be demonstrated. A large number of people with moderate falls in plasma potassium have alterations in frequency of ventricular ectopic beats (7,9), the importance of which was dismissed in the past and may be exaggerated at present. From the evidence that has accumulated, a fall in plasma potassium, even though the final value is in the normal range, is believed to cause an increased number of ectopic beats when the patient is stressed (9). In an individual it is difficult to show that ventricular ectopics have a bad prognostic significance. However, if plasma potassium is low, there is an increased number of serious ventricular arrhythmias if the person has a myocardial infarction (7,12,14). The situation is complicated by the finding that falls in magnesium aggravate the situation and also affect replenishment of potassium stores (3,4).

It should be emphasized that the risk caused by diuretic-induced hypokalemia is small but when lifetime therapy is being considered for mild hypertension this effect becomes important and may outweigh the gains to be achieved. Any step that would minimize this complication should be taken.

The results summarized in the present chapter have been reported in a number of studies (1,2,6,10,11,16).

EFFECT OF SODIUM RESTRICTION ON PLASMA POTASSIUM

This study was performed in 548 patients, many of whom were involved in other studies. Of these patients 416 received no drug treatment for hypertension at the time of the study (Table 1). Two hundred and thirty-five of these had never been treated for hypertension. Ninety-seven had been treated with a regimen including a diuretic and drugs, which had been stopped 4 weeks earlier, and 84 had been treated with a drug regimen that had not included a diuretic for 6 months. Their other antihypertensive drugs had been stopped 4 weeks before the study. In the remaining 132 patients conventional

Table 1 Patients Treated with Sodium Restriction According to Previous and Present Therapy

	Number	Male	Female
Never treated	235	212	23
Treatment ceased			
No diuretic 4 weeks	97	85	12
No diuretic > 6 months	84	76	8
Treated including diuretic	132	113	19
Total	548	486	62

Most of the patients were older: < 55 years = 59; 55–70 years = 441; > 70 years = 48.

therapy, which in all instances contained a thiazide diuretic, was continued throughout the study.

Three blood samples were taken over a 4-week period prior to the giving of dietary advice, which was to reduce their daily intake of sodium. The advice given, if followed strictly, would have increased K^+ intake by approximately 15 mmol/day. The aim of the dietary advice was to obtain a daily urinary Na^+ and K^+ excretion of approximately 70 mmol (Table 2). The compliance with dietary advice was checked by measurement of urinary electrolytes and three subsequent plasma samples were taken while patients were on their diet.

In all groups of patients, plasma K^+ during the reduced-sodium intake was higher than during the normal sodium intake (Table 3). The rise in plasma K^+ was greatest in the patients who had been on a diuretic that was discontinued 4 weeks earlier and part of this response was possibly due to the lower starting level and a "natural" replenishment of body stores. The rise in plasma K^+ overall was 0.28 mmol/L. This is a relatively small change but, when it is taken in conjunction with the use of low-dosage diuretics, at least 50% of the fall in plasma K^+ is reversed.

In a previous study (11) we had demonstrated that, when used in hypertension, diuretics had most of their antihypertensive effect at a dosage that did not cause total body potassium depletion or a significant incidence of hypokalemia ($K < 3.4$). The fall in plasma potassium was greatest after 2–4 weeks of therapy and rose towards normal levels after that time. The mean fall in plasma K^+ was 0.24 mmol/L.

Table 2 Urinary Electrolyte Excretion (mean ± SEM) Before and After Alteration of Diet

	Before	After
N (for samples)	1124	1518
Sodium (mmol/day)	186 ± 2	85 ± 1[a]
Potassium (mmol/day)	52 ± 1	61 ± 1[a]
Creatinine (mmol/day)	12.2 ± 0.1	12.3 ± .1
Na/K ratio	3.6	1.4[a]

[a] $p < 0.001$

Patients were requested to provide two or three urine collections before the diet intervention and after the intervention. Patients without urine collections were not included in the analysis.
N for patient = 548.

Table 3 Effect of Sodium Restriction on Plasma Potassium

	N	Plasma potassium (mmol/L; mean ± SEM)	
		Before	After
Never treated	235	3.91 ± 0.01	4.17 ± 0.01[a]
No diuretic 4 weeks	97	3.72 ± 0.02	4.14 ± 0.02[a]
No diuretic > 6 months	84	4.02 ± 0.02	4.19 ± 0.02[a]
On therapy	132	3.68 ± 0.02	3.95 ± 0.02[a]

[a] $p < 0.001$, paired "t" test.
N refers to number of patients. Three plasma samples were taken before and three after sodium restriction, thus N for samples is approximately three times greater.

In a study of a thiazide diuretics given to patients on a normal dietary intake of sodium compared with those subjected to a reduction of sodium intake to 70 mmol/day we have demonstrated that patients who responded to sodium restriction were those who had responded to diuretic therapy. Sodium intake had an effect on the response of individuals to thiazide diuretics. The fall in blood pressure with a thiazide diuretic was less in people on a low or a very high sodium intake (Table 4). The small fall in pressure in people on a low sodium intake may be because those who had responded to low sodium intake were not recruited to this study. In a separate study 12 people were given chlorothiazide 500 mg/day when on a sodium intake of <70 mmol/day, 70–150 mmol, or >150 mmol/day. The results are summarized in Table 5. The thiazide diuretic caused the greatest fall in blood pressure in people with a sodium intake between 70 and 150 mmol/day, but if patients were on a low sodium intake, diuretics had little or no incremental effect.

Thus we advocate the initial use of a reduced sodium intake to treat hypertension. If reduction of sodium intake to between 50 and 100 mmol/day does not control blood pressure adequately, a low-dosage thiazide diuretic can be added. This will allow control of blood pressure with minimal disturbance of plasma or total body K^+. It should be noted that there is still a fall in plasma K^+ and, depending on the distribution curve of the

Table 4 Effect of Chlorothiazide (500 mg daily) on Blood Pressure of People on Different Sodium Intakes

Urine Na^+ excretion (mmol/day)	N	Fall in supine diastolic blood pressure (mmHg)
<50	19	-1 ± 1
50–100	45	5 ± 1[a]
100–200	50	8 ± 1[a]
200–300	25	5 ± 2[b]
>300	12	3 ± 2

[a] $p < 0.001$
[b] $p < 0.05$
All patients were receiving no other antihypertensive drugs. Some patients had been placed on restricted sodium intake. People who had responded to a low-sodium diet were therefore not included in this study.

Table 5 Effect of Chlorothiazide (500 mg) on Mean Blood Pressure of Patients on Different Sodium Intake

	Supine blood pressure (mmHg)				
	No drug		Chlorothiazide		
Sodium intake	Systolic	Diastolic	Systolic	Diastolic	Δ Diastolic
<70 mmol	152	88	147	86	2
70–150 mmol	165[a]	97[a]	151[a]	87[b]	10[b]
>150 mmol	172[a]	102[a]	161[a,b]	96[a,b]	6[b]

N = 12, paired "t" test
[a]$p < 0.01$ compared to values in the column above
[b]$p < 0.01$ compared to control value

response, some individuals will be hypokalemic. Effects of thiazide diuretics on Mg^{2+} and H^+ will be reduced by the restricted sodium intake but not normalized. These statements refer to a sodium intake of between 50 and 100 mmol/day. At very low sodium intakes the situation may be different because of excess aldosterone stimulation.

EFFECT OF POTASSIUM-SPARING DIURETICS ON PLASMA POTASSIUM

A study was undertaken of the effect of diuretics on plasma and total body potassium and the means of restoring this to the normal range. Twelve male patients with essential hypertension entered a study in which their antihypertensive medication was kept constant apart from their diuretic therapy. Plasma and total body potassium (whole body counter) was measured on each regimen.

The following regimens were studied in a randomized order and each lasted for 2 months:

Hydrochlorothiazide: 100 mg (2 periods; I and II in Table 6)
Hydrochlorothiazide: 100 mg, Slow K 48 mmol
Hydrochlorothiazide: 100 mg, amiloride 10 mg
Hydrochlorothiazide: 100 mg; $KHCO_3$ 48 mmol
Placebo

Total body potassium expressed as g/kg body weight or as g did not alter significantly with any of the therapeutic regimens (Table 6). Plasma K^+ levels fell significantly with hydrochlorothiazide. The fall was reversed by the addition of amiloride and the value at the end of that period was not different from the value without a diuretic. $KHCO_3$ supplementation caused a further fall in plasma K^+. KCl given as Slow K did not elevate plasma K^+ but it was absorbed as measured by changes in urinary electrolyte excretion. Changes were noted in pH and plasma HCO_3. Amiloride corrected the pH and caused plasma HCO_3^- to return to normal values, while KCl had no significant effect. $KHCO_3$ caused the situation to worsen. In view of the absence of change in total body potassium we ascribe the major cause of the fall in plasma potassium to the alkalosis caused by diuretics. If this is correct it is not surprising that supplemental KCl had little effect,

Table 6 Effect of Diuretics, Amiloride, and Potassium Supplements on Plasma and Total Body Potassium Levels

	Plasma K^+ (mmol/L)	Total body K^+ (g/kg)
Placebo	4.23 ± 0.10	1.69 ± 0.04
Hydrochlorothiazide I	4.11[a] ± 0.11	1.76 ± 0.05
Hydrochlorothiazide II	4.07[a] ± 0.15	1.72 ± 0.07
Hydrochlorothiazide + $KHCO_3$	3.75[b]	1.64
Hydrochlorothiazide + KCl	4.11[a] ± 0.17	1.78 ± 0.08
Hydrochlorothiazide + amiloride	4.33 ± 0.14	1.71 ± 0.05

N = 12
[a]$p < 0.01$ compared with placebo and with hydrochlorothiazide + amiloride; these values are not significantly different from each other.
[b]N = 4 for this value.

as no potassium depletion is present. If higher dosages of diuretics are used, total body potassium depletion can be produced.

The combination of amiloride with a thiazide diuretic may prevent the fall in plasma K^+. It is appropriate to remember that amiloride by itself may cause hyperkalemia. In studies we have undertaken (Table 7) it can be observed that hypokalemia still occurred with combination therapy but less frequently than with a thiazide diuretic alone. When fixed combination therapy with a thiazide was used, hyperkalemia was uncommon. It must be noted that these results are likely to differ depending on the sodium and potassium intake of individuals and the general population.

Table 7 Frequency of Hyperkalemia (>5.0 mmol/L) and Hypokalemia (<3.4 mmol/L) in People Treated with Hydrochlorothiazide, Amiloride, or Moduretic

	N	Percentage of people: Hypokalemia	Percentage of people: Hyperkalemia
Control	200	1	0
Hydrochlorothiazide, 50 mg or chlorothiazide, 500 mg	200	15	0
Hydrochlorothiazide, 50 mg b.i.d. or chlorothiazide, 500 mg b.i.d.	50	20	0
Amiloride 5 mg	36	0	8
5 mg b.i.d.	20	0	20
Hydrochlorothiazide, 50 mg Amiloride, 5 mg	100	5	2
Hydrochlorothiazide, 50 mg b.i.d. Amiloride, 5 mg b.i.d.	35	9	0

Male patients being treated for hypertension with only a diuretic at time of study.

Table 8 Effect of Oral KCl on Plasma and Total Body Potassium in People Receiving Diuretics with Hypertension or Cardiac Failure

	N	Plasma K^+ (mmol/L)		Total body K^+ (g/kg)	
		Diuretic	Diuretic + KCl	Diuretic	Diuretic + KCl
Hypertension	16	4.0 ± 0.1	4.1 ± 0.2	1.72 ± 0.04	1.76 ± 0.06
Cardiac failure	10	3.5 ± 0.2	3.8[a] ± 0.1	1.41 ± 0.04	1.47[a] ± 0.03

Mean ± SEM
[a]$p < 0.05$ compared with before KCl therapy. Patients were all on hydrochlorothiazide 50 mg b.i.d. and were given 48 mmol/day KCl.

EFFECT OF POTASSIUM SUPPLEMENTATION ON PLASMA POTASSIUM

In acute experiments referred to above, we have found that supplementation with alkaline potassium salts did not correct any plasma or total body deficit and may make the situation worse in patients taking a diuretic. KCl supplementation had minimal effect in the studies we have undertaken when a low dosage of diuretic was being used to treat people with hypertension. However, in people with cardiac failure who have a total body potassium deficit, K^+ will correct the deficiency in part (Table 8), although, as shown by Dyckner (4), an associated magnesium depletion may need to be corrected first.

Potassium supplementation does not acutely (2-8 weeks) elevate plasma K^+, however, the plasma K^+ is higher in people eating a diet high in potassium. This may be a long-term effect or could be due to failure to correct magnesium depletion in the short-term studies.

EFFECT OF BETA-BLOCKING DRUGS ON PLASMA POTASSIUM

Elegant experiments by Struthers and Reid (15) have confirmed an older observation that continuous epinephrine infusions at concentrations achieved in stress cause a fall in plasma potassium. This fall is prevented by beta-blocking drugs. There may be differences in the protection offered by various beta-blocking drugs with the cardioselective drugs being less effective than others. In a number of studies, beta-blocking drugs have caused a rise in plasma potassium. We showed that alterations in plasma K^+ induced by chlorothiazide were reversed (Table 9) by timolol but there was no effect on plasma K^+ in

Table 9 Effect of Timolol on Plasma K^+ in People Receiving Hydrochlorothiazide or Hydrochlorothiazide + Amiloride

	N	Plasma K^+ (mmol/l)	
		No timolol	Timolol
Hydrochlorothiazide	30	3.74 ± 0.03	3.92 ± 0.04[a]
Hydrochlorothiazide + amiloride	26	3.82 ± 0.03	3.84 ± 0.04

Mean ± SEM
[a]$p < 0.01$ compared without Timolol. The other values are not significantly different.

people given amiloride and chlorothiazide (6). It is known that timolol suppresses plasma renin and thus it seemed logical to assume that this effect may work via a reduction in aldosterone secretion. However, the fall may be due to epinephrine outpouring due to stress associated with blood collection and that reduction of this effect due to beta-blocking drugs provides protection.

DISCUSSION AND CONCLUSION

Two situations merit discussion. In patients with hypokalemia with a total body deficit of potassium, potassium with or without magnesium must be given. This will occur when large dosages of diuretics are given to most people, particularly patients with fluid-retaining states who are receiving diuretics. Thus people with liver disease, nephrotic syndrome, cardiac failure, and Conn's syndrome often have a high circulating level of aldosterone and are potassium-depleted before a diuretic is given. It would appear reasonable to correct such potassium depletion before using a diuretic. In some circumstances it may be advisable to start with a potassium-sparing diuretic.

The more common situation is depression of plasma potassium without total body potassium deficit, which occurs most commonly in the treatment of hypertension. Except in people with Conn's syndrome or with severe hypertension with secondary hyperaldosteronism, K^+ deficit is uncommon prior to therapy. If low dosages of thiazide diuretics are used, total body potassium does not fall significantly and there is a small fall (about 0.3 mmol) in plasma K^+. The distribution of this fall means that certain individuals do become hypokalemic.

In people with hypertension I would suggest reducing sodium intake to between 50 and 70 mmol/day. If blood pressure is not controlled and the patient has reduced his or her Na^+ intake below 50 mmol/day as measured by urinary sodium excretion, then a thiazide diuretic has little additional effect and a beta-blocking drug should be used. If the patient has refused dietary advice or still has an intake above 50 mmol/day then a thiazide diuretic in modest dosages should be used. If plasma K^+ falls below 3.5 mmol/L or falls by 0.4 mmol or more, then amiloride should be added. A case can be made to use combined therapy of a thiazide and a potassium-sparing diuretic from the start. This will prevent the fall in Mg^{2+} and H^+ as well as the fall in K^+, which is probably an advantage. If a patient is on a thiazide diuretic and blood pressure is not controlled the addition of a beta-blocking drug may improve control and also return the K^+ level to normal. Potassium chloride supplements are of little use. They fail to correct the fall in K^+ and have no effect on the associated metabolic changes in Mg^+ and H^+. The real treatment is prevention. The need to prevent hypokalemia is now established. I believe that it is also important to prevent plasma potassium from falling; if you have hypertension and are thus likely to develop coronary artery disease you should maintain your plasma K^+ in the high normal range.

ACKNOWLEDGMENTS

These studies were supported by the National Health and Medical Research Council, the National Heart Foundation, and the Department of Veteran Affairs. The help of M. Hodgson, S. Waga, S. Carney, M. Wilson, A. Gillies, W. Adam, J. Myers, Bee Ho Teow, C. Nouson, A. Anderson, and other medical and nursing staff is acknowledged. The studies were performed at the Repatriation Hospital, Heidelberg, and the Royal Newcastle Hospital. Special thanks are given to the patients who cooperated in the studies.

REFERENCES

1. Carney, S., Gillies, A., and Morgan, T. O.: Optimal dose of a thiazide diuretic. *Med. J. Aust.* 2:692, 1976.
2. Carney, S., Morgan, T., Wilson, M., Matthews, G., and Roberts, R.: Sodium restriction and thiazide diuretics in the treatment of hypertension. *Med. J. Aust.* 1:803, 1975.
3. Dyckner, T.: Serum magnesium in acute myocardial infarction. Relation to arrhythmia. *Acta Med. Scand.* 207:59, 1980.
4. Dyckner, T., and Wester, P. O. Diuretic induced magnesium losses. Influence on potassium metabolism and on ventricular arrhythmias. *R. Soc. Med. Int. Congress Sympos. Series* 44:43, 1981.
5. Fisch, C.: Relation of electrolyte disturbance to cardiac arrhythmias. *Circulation* 47:408, 1973.
6. Gillies, A., Morgan, T., Morgan, G., and Wilson, M.: A simplified approach to the treatment of hypertension. *Med. J. Aust.* 2:593, 1977.
7. Holland, O. B., Nixon, J. V., and Von Kuhnert: Diuretic induced ventricular ectopic activity. *Am. J. Med.* 70:762, 1981.
8. Hollander, W., Jr., and Blythe, W. B.: Nephropathy of potassium depletion. In *Diseases of the Kidney*, edited by Strauss, M. B., and Welt, L. G., Boston, Little Brown, 1971, p. 933.
9. Hollifield, J. W., and Slatow, P. E.: Thiazide Diuretics, hypokalaemia and cardiac arrhythmias. *Acta Med. Scand. Suppl.* 647:67–74, 1981.
10. Morgan, T., and Myers, J.: Potassium maintenance, potassium supplements or potassium sparing agents. *Acta. Med. Scand. Suppl.* 647:117, 1981.
11. Morgan, T., and Myers, J.: The rationale of potassium conservation. *R. Soc. Med. Int. Congress Sympos. Series* 44:75, 1981.
12. Nordrehaug, J. E.: Serum potassium and arrhythmias in acute myocardial infarction. *R. Soc. Med. Int. Congress Sympos. Series* 44:83, 1981.
13. Schwartz, W. B., and Relman, A. S.: Metabolic and renal studies in chornic potassium depletion resulting from overuse of laxatives. *J. Clin. Invest.* 32:258, 1953.
14. Solomon, R. J., and Cole, A. G.: Importance of potassium in patients with acute myocardial infarction. *Acta Med. Scand. Suppl.* 647:87, 1981.
15. Struthers, A. D., Reid, J. L., McLean, K. and Rodger, J. C.: Adrenaline hypokalaemia and cardiac arrhythmias. Effect of beta adrenoreceptor antagonists. *Clin. Sci.* 62:1, 1982.
16. Whight, C., Morgan, T., Carney, S., et al.: Diuretics cardiac failure and potassium depletion. A rational approach. *Med. J. Aust.* 2:831, 1974.

36

Effectiveness and Tolerance of "Solid" vs. "Liquid" Potassium Replacement Therapy

DAVID Y. GRAHAM
Veterans Administration Medical Center and Baylor College of Medicine, Houston, Texas

Shortly after the introduction of the thiazide diuretics, it became evident that a modest percentage of patients receiving such drugs would develop potassium depletion. The pharmaceutical industry responded with the development of a number of potassium products that employed a variety of potassium salts and formulations. Because of the poor taste of potassium solutions, enteric-coated forms of potassium chloride and combinations of diuretics with enteric-coated potassium chloride were soon introduced.

POTASSIUM CHLORIDE-ASSOCIATED GASTROINTESTINAL INJURY

In 1964, Lindholmer and co-workers (39) reported four cases of nonspecific small bowel ulceration with stenosis. They also noted the possible association with use of enteric-coated potassium, often in combination with thiazides, in a total of 17 recent cases and called attention to the problem. The relatively frequent occurrence of a heretofore rare disease prompted a flurry of additional reports, along with studies in experimental animals that sought to elucidate the pathogenesis of small-bowel ulcers associated with enteric-coated potassium preparations (1,3,10,11,20,32,34,36,38,46,47,58,61). The typical lesion was a single circumferential, stenosing ulcer in the jejunum or ileum. The clinical presentation was nonspecific since the presence of the ulcer was often made known by complications which included hemorrhage, obstruction, and perforation of the small intestine. The disease was not limited to patients of either sex and involved those at any age, although most cases occurred in the older population, reflecting the fact that it was this group who was most likely to use potassium supplements. The risk of developing such a lesion associated with enteric-coated potassium was low (see below), even in the highest-risk group (30).

There was considerable difficulty in producing the intestinal lesions in experimental animals. Oral doses of 1,000 mg enteric-coated potassium chloride given twice daily to 6- and 8-week-old swine produced lesions, whereas doses from 500 to 2,000 mg twice daily for 5 days failed to produce ulcerations in the gastrointestinal tracts of dogs. Intestinal ulcerations were finally achieved in dogs by Boley et al. (10), who used sutures to suspend potassium chloride tablets within the intestine, thus restricting the area where the medication was dissolved and absorbed. In dogs, mucosal ulceration developed whenever potassium was absorbed in high concentration over a short segment of bowel.

Typical lesions were readily produced in monkeys (9,19), although a much higher dosage of potassium (approximately 14 times the human dosage on a mg/kg basis) had to be employed to produce ulcers consistently. In monkeys, investigators were able to detect tablets in various states of disintegration near lesions, suggesting that the ulceration was restricted to the area where the greatest amount of potassium chloride was released from the tablet. A dosage–response relationship was investigated: a 100-mg tablet of potassium chloride caused no lesions, hyperemia was seen with 250 mg, necrosis with 500 mg, and ulceration with 1,000 mg.

The role of tablet size was also investigated. Development of intestinal damage appeared to be related to the total amount of potassium administered, irrespective of whether the dosage was administered in one or more tablets. For example, lesions were produced equally well with a single 1,000-mg tablet, four 250-mg tablets, or ten 100-mg tablets (although the severity of the ulceration was reduced considerably in the presence of the 100 mg tablets).

The form in which potassium was given also had a significant effect on the development of intestinal lesions. For example, enteric-coated potassium produced lesions in the small intestine or colon, whereas tablets with short disintegration times and gradual-release tablets, which dissolved slowly but steadily, produced lesions located predominantly in the stomach or duodenum.

The pathogenesis of potassium-associated mucosal lesions remains unclear, although it has been definitely proven that lesions are directly related to the potassium as neither the thiazide diuretic nor the enteric coating alone caused histological changes. The current hypothesis for the genesis of intestinal lesions is that a high local concentration of potassium causes spasm of blood vessels, leading to hemostasis and subsequent infarction. Mucosal damage to the stomach and esophagus appears to be a form of direct corrosive injury. This hypothesis is bolstered by the observation of the formation of a painless oral ulcer in the mouth of a patient who sucked a wax-matrix potassium chloride preparation (41).

Intestinal damage prompted the withdrawal of enteric-coated potassium chloride preparations from the market. They were soon replaced by wax-matrix products that were designed to release the potassium slowly and continuously, thereby preventing the high concentrations of potassium that presumably produced mucosal damage. Young olive baboons were used to compare the effects of enteric-coated and wax-matrix dosage forms of potassium chloride (KCl–diuretic combinations) (40). Numerous lesions developed in the ileum and jejunum of animals exposed to enteric-coated potassium, whereas no lesions were observed in two baboons treated with the wax-matrix product. A second experiment with four baboons confirmed those findings, suggesting that the slow-release potassium chloride preparations did not cause mucosal injury. It subsequently became evident that the risk of small-bowel injury, although significantly reduced, was not entirely eliminated; several cases of stenosis and ulcer of the small intestine have been associated with the wax-matrix potassium forms in humans (25,26). The risk of small-bowel injury with wax-matrix potassium has been estimated at 1.59 cases per million patient years (about the same as the rate of spontaneous occurrence) compared with 441 cases per million patient years for the enteric-coated potassium products (30).

Gastric ulcers have been reported in several patients taking enteric-coated potassium. Jacob and Pringot (32) reported three cases in which there was reasonable evidence to support a causal relationship: no previous history of ulcer symptoms, close temporal relationship between symptoms and KCl administration, location of ulcer on posterior wall of antrum, and radiological features of acute ulcers. More recently, gastric ulcer has been reportedly associated with administration of wax-matrix potassium (43). The cause and effect of this latter association was less secure (the patient was also taking indomethacin). It may have occurred by chance, since gastric ulcers occur commonly in the age group of patients for whom potassium is most commonly prescribed. Acute gastric ulcers have also been observed in two of six young adult rhesus monkeys receiving a wax-matrix potassium preparation (23).

Recent clinical studies in which volunteers underwent gastroscopic evaluation following potassium administration suggested that wax-matrix forms of potassium might cause upper-gastrointestinal erosions and ulcers in humans (6,43,44,54). These observations have formed the basis for a major advertising campaign designed to promote multiple-unit dosage forms of potassium over the now-traditional single-unit wax-matrix solid dosage forms.

CONTROLLED-RELEASE MEDICATION

Controlled-release dosage forms can be classified into single-unit or multiple-unit dosage forms (21). The standard single-unit dose of potassium is the wax-matrix tablet. Multiple-unit dosage forms consist of many small depots or pellets, such as microencapsulated KCl crystals, contained within a capsule or tablet. The main theoretical difference between single-unit and multiple-unit dosage preparations is the difference in the rate of gastric emptying. Theoretically, the small drug depots in the multiple-unit dosage form will empty rapidly from the stomach and disperse throughout the gastrointestinal tract. In contrast, large single-unit dosage forms empty slowly from the stomach and much of the disintegration of tablets may occur within the stomach.

Postprandially, the stomach contents are sieved and particles >2 mm in diameter are emptied poorly (49). Thus, indigestible tablets and capsules are retained in the stomach in an attempt to grind them into smaller particles. The exception is the interdigestive period when gastric motility serves as a housekeeper to sweep undigested material from the stomach. Even during the interdigestive period, the emptying of tablets and particles large than 2 mm in diameter is a random process, and emptying can occur any time from minutes to several hours after ingestion.

If multiple-unit formulations were to disperse rapidly throughout the gastrointestinal tract, one would predict a relatively uniform absorption and a reproducible curve of plasma concentration of drug. Recent studies have suggested that the multiple dosage forms do not disperse widely but, instead, may move as a bolus through the gastrointestinal tract much like a liquid (8,21). The gelatin capsule may lodge within a gastric fold and release its material locally (12,27-29). The material may then become trapped by gastric mucus, allowing a large accumulation of drug (e.g., potassium), possibly causing acute gastric mucosal damage (12,27).

CLINICAL STUDIES OF POTASSIUM-ASSOCIATED GASTROINTESTINAL MUCOSAL INJURY

The description of gastric mucosal changes associated with solid dosage forms of potassium chloride prompted clinical studies in which a large number of subjects were enrolled. Most studies used a protocol similar to that initially described by the Tulane group and included an anticholinergic drug, glycopyrrolate (45). All studies required endoscopy to demonstrate that the esophagus, stomach, and duodenum were normal at the outset. Subjects then received 24-96 mEq potassium daily in divided doses. Drug administration usually lasted 1 week, although the relation to meals was not constant: In some instances, drugs were administered after fasting, whereas in other studies they were given with food. The effect of the drug on the gastrointestinal mucosa was evaluated by a second endoscopic procedure. Typically, study parameters included the presence of mucosal edema or erythema, mucosal erosions, or acute gastric ulcers. The methods of analysis varied, but the most common was to sum the scores from the three areas (esophagus, stomach, and duodenum) to achieve a final score that was used to compare the results between groups.

The endoscopic method of evaluating lesions may yield misleading information. Classically, the differentiation between mucosal erosions and acute ulcers is based on histological criteria. An erosion is an epithelial defect which does not penetrate the muscularis mucosae and heals spontaneously without scar formation (within 2-8 days). The differentiation between an ulcer and an erosion relates to whether the muscularis mucosa has been breached. Erosions are shallow circular or oval lesions, usually less than 0.5 cm in diameter, with sharply defined edges. Acute ulcers have the same general appearance and distribution as erosions, but are larger and penetrate through the muscularis mucosae. The base of an acute ulcer has little or no fibrosis, whereas chronic ulcers have underlying fibrous tissue. In these drug studies, we are forced to rely on the endoscopist's opinion and, endoscopically, it is impossible to differentiate a large erosion from a small ulcer. The distinction between ulcer and erosion is usually based upon size, which is often inaccurate. The impression of "depth" is also misleading because of the surrounding edema. It is likely that the number of ulcers is overestimated at the expense of an underestimation of erosions.

I have received published and unpublished data from investigators working in this field (4,6,44,45,50,54, see the section "Acknowledgments"), and I have been able to compile the results from the majority of the subjects. A number of different products have been evaluated, including wax-matrix products, microencapsulated potassium chloride products, liquid potassium chloride, and a number of experimental products, such as potassium chloride enclosed in an osmotic membrane. I will limit my analyses to gastric mucosal changes. Based on my experience with mucosal damage associated with antiinflammatory drugs, I have separated the endoscopic findings into two categories, erosions and acute ulcers. I have excluded "hyperemia and edema" because these are subtle, subjective findings of no known clinical significance. The data are presented as a total experience of the group; different experiments using the same dosage of potassium were combined.

I have summarized data from 16 studies in 5 centers, involving almost 600 subjects and using 8 different dosages of potassium (range, 24-96 mEq/day). It should be noted that only five studies have included a placebo-control group. I have classified the data into four groups: those using glycopyrrolate, those without glycopyrrolate, acute gastric ulcers, and gastric erosions. Although many comparisons could be made, I have restricted

Table 1 Frequency of Acute Gastric Ulcers Reported in Clinical Studies with Wax-Matrix and Microencapsulated KCl

Site	Wax-matrix	Microencapsulated	Total
Tulane	8/113	1/84	9/197
Hershey	1/27	2/56	3/83
Miami	1/24	0/24	1/48
Utah	0/60	0/30	0/90
Arizona	0/18	0/12	0/30
Totals	10/242	3/206	13/448

my analyses to commercial wax-matrix potassium chloride (single-unit dosage) and microencapsulated multiple-unit potassium formulations.

The study sites and the number of acute gastric ulcers reported are shown in Table 1, without regard to whether the subject was also receiving glycopyrrolate. Acute gastric ulcers occurred in 4% of those taking wax-matrix potassium and in 1.5% of those taking the multiple-unit form; a difference that is not statistically significant ($p = 0.08$, Fisher's exact test, two-tailed). It is of interest that five of the eight acute gastric ulcers reported with the use of wax-matrix potassium were reported from Tulane and the frequency of ulcer in their studies was significantly greater than that in the other studies combined ($p<0.05$). Further review of the data from which the summary table was derived (Tables 2-5; note that two centers found no acute gastric ulcers) shows that acute ulcers occurred in about 2.9% of those receiving either type of solid dosage form of potassium (Table 6).

Table 7 shows the summary data for the occurrence of gastric erosions in the study populations. Gastric erosions occurred more frequently in those taking wax-matrix potassium than in those receiving microencapsulated potassium formulations (26.4% vs. 9.7%, $p<0.01$). As noted before, erosions in the wax-matrix groups were overrepresented in the Tulane studies ($p<0.001$ compared to the remainder of the studies). The statistically significant difference between wax-matrix and microencapsulated potassium was not maintained when the data from the Tulane group were deleted (14.7% vs. 5.3%, respectively; $p>0.1$). The data from which Table 7 was derived are tabulated in Tables 8-15. As noted with acute gastric ulcer, glycopyrrolate seemed to accentuate the mucosal damage. There was no statistical difference between the frequencies of erosions when the results in subjects not receiving concomitant glycopyrrolate were compared (Table 16).

Table 2 Frequency of Acute Gastric Ulcer in Volunteers Receiving KCl in the Presence of Glycopyrrolate (Tulane)

	mEq KCl/day				
Product	96	72	24	Totals	%
Slow-K	2/6	1/15	2/24	5/45	11.1
Micro-K	0/6		1/24	1/30	3.3
Kaon-Cl liquid			0/15	0/15	0.0
Placebo			1/15	1/15	6.7

Table 3 Frequency of Acute Gastric Ulcer in Volunteers Receiving KCl in the Absence of Glycopyrrolate (Tulane)

	mEq KCl/day					
Product	96	80	40	24	Totals	%
Slow-K	0/12	1/15		2/30	3/68	4.4
Kaon-Cl tablets			0/11			
Micro-K	0/12		0/13	0/29	0/54	0.0
Placebo			0/11		0/11	0.0

Table 4 Frequency of Acute Gastric Ulcer in Volunteers Receiving KCl in the Presence of Glycopyrrolate (Hershey)

	mEq KCl				
Product	96	91	48	Totals	%
Slow-K	1/21		0/6	1/27	3.7
Micro-K	2/31			2/56	3.6
K-timekap[a]	0/25				
P-M KCl[b]		2/15		2/15	13.3
Kay-ciel elixir	0/15			0/15	0.0
Placebo	0/15			0/15	0.0

[a]Experimental microencapsulated product
[b]Experimental membrane-coated tablet

Table 5 Frequency of Acute Gastric Ulcer in Volunteers Receiving KCl in the Presence of Glycopyrrolate (Miami)

	mEq KCl			
Product	96	24	Totals	%
Slow-K	1/6	0/18	1/24	4.2
Micro-K	0/6	0/18	0/24	0.0

Table 6 Summary of Acute Gastric Ulcers in Clinical Trials

	Total		Minus Tulane results	
Drug	No. with	%	No. with	%
With glycopyrrolate				
Wax-matrix	7/138	5.1	2/93	2.1
Microencap	3/146	2.1	2/116	1.7
Liquid KCl	0/45	0.0	0/30	0.0
Placebo	1/45	2.2	0/30	0.0
Without glycopyrrolate				
Wax-matrix	3/104	2.9	0/36	0.0
Microencap	0/60	0.0	0/6	0.0
Placebo	0/25	0.0	0/14	0.0

Table 7 Frequency of Gastric Erosions in Clinical Studies with Wax-Matrix and Microencapsulated KCl

Site	Wax-matrix	Micro	Total
Tulane	45/113	9/84	54/197
Hershey	5/27	3/56	8/83
Miami	5/24	1/24	6/48
Salt Lake	5/60	4/30	9/90
Arizona	4/18	3/12	7/30
Totals	64/242	20/206	84/448

Table 8 Frequency of Gastric Erosions in Volunteers Receiving KCl in the Presence of Glycopyrrolate (Tulane)

	mEq KCl/day				
Product	96	72	24	Totals	%
Slow-K	5/6	7/15	11/24	23/45	51.1
Micro-K	0/6		0/24	0/30	0.0
Kaon-Cl liquid			0/15	0/15	0.0
Placebo			0/15	0/15	0.0

Table 9 Frequency of Gastric Erosions in Volunteers Receiving KCl in the Absence of Glycopyrrolate (Tulane)

	mEq KCl/day					
Product	96	80	40	24	Totals	%
Slow-K	5/12	1/15		12/30	22/68	32.3
Kaon-Cl tablets			4/11			
Micro-K	1/12		1/13	7/29	9/54	16.6
Placebo			2/11		2/11	18.2

Table 10 Frequency of Gastric Erosions in Volunteers Receiving KCl in the Presence of Glycopyrrolate (Hershey)

	mEq KCl				
Product	96	91	48	Totals	%
Slow-K	5/21		0/6	5/27	18.5
Micro-K	1/31			3/56	5.4
K-timekap[a]	2/25				
P-M KCl[b]		2/15		2/15	13.3
Kay-ciel elixir	0/15			0/15	0.0
Placebo	0/15			0/15	0.0

[a]Experimental microencapsulated product
[b]Experimental membrane-coated tablet

Table 11 Frequency of Gastric Erosions in Volunteers Receiving KCl in the Presence of Glycopyrrolate (Miami)

	mEq KCl			
Product	96	24	Totals	%
Slow-K	3/6	2/18	5/24	20.8
Micro-K	0/6	1/18	1/24	4.2

Table 12 Frequency of Gastric Erosions in Volunteers Receiving KCl in the Presence of Glycopyrrolate (Utah)

	mEq KCl			
Product	72	70	Totals	%
Slow-K	3/15		5/30	16.7
Exp-tab[a]		2/15		
Micro-K	2/15		4/30	13.3
Exp-cap[b]	2/15			
KCl liq[c]	0/15		0/15	0.0
Placebo	4/15		4/15	26.6

[a]Experimental wax-matrix tablet
[b]Experimental microencapsulated KCl
[c]Potassium chloride, in solution

Table 13 Frequency of Gastric Erosions in Volunteers Receiving KCl in the Absence of Glycopyrrolate (Utah)

	mEq KCl			
Product	60	30	Totals	%
K-tab[a]	0/15	2/15	2/30	6.7
Placebo	0/14		0/14	0.0

[a]Wax-matrix KCl

Table 14 Frequency of Gastric Erosions in Volunteers Receiving KCl in the Presence of Glycopyrrolate (Arizona)

	mEq KCl			
Product	96	48	Totals	%
Slow-K	2/6	2/6	4/12	33.3
Micro-K	2/6		2/6	33.3

Table 15 Frequency of Gastric Erosions in Volunteers Receiving KCl in the Absence of Glycopyrrolate (Arizona)

Product	mEq 48	Totals	%
Slow-K	0/6	0/6	0.0
Micro-K	1/6	1/6	16.7

The increased frequency with which acute gastric ulcer and gastric erosions were reported with wax-matrix potassium by the Tulane group deserves comment. Those investigators were forced to exclude a larger fraction of potential subjects because of endoscopic abnormalities found prior to drug administration (2). In fact, 37% of their subjects had abnormal endoscopic findings on screening examination, and 11 of 21 subjects with normal endoscopic examinations developed mucosal lesions following admission to the Clinical Research Unit (1 week of placebo therapy). One Tulane subject was reported to have developed an ulcer while receiving placebo. These observations suggest that the subjects studied by the Tulane group may have differed from those used in the other studies. It is not possible to identify with certainty a reason for this difference, such as type of subject (medical student vs. transient), type of diet (spicy New Orleans food), differences in diet or environment. Because the data from Tulane were possibly not representative, I chose to reanalyze the data after subtracting the results of the Tulane studies (Tables 6, 16). I believe this gives a more representative sample, and this thought is bolstered by knowledge of the results of another large study that I was not given permission to quote directly.

One of the problems with the above-mentioned clinical studies has been the frequent lack of placebo-controls or even liquid potassium chloride control groups. This is particularly important when evaluating the presence of minor findings such as hyperemia or edema. Another possible problem relates to the amount of potassium administered; the dosages used varied between 24 and 96 mEq potassium/day (the average dosage of potassium administered as Slow-K is about 20 mEq/day).

Table 16 Summary of Gastric Erosions in Clinical Trials

Drug	Total		Minus Tulane results	
	No. with	%	No. with	%
With glycopyrrolate				
Wax-matrix	42/138	30.4	19/93	20
Microencap	10/146	6.8	10/116	6
Liquid KCl	0/45	0.0	0/30	0
Placebo	4/45	8.8	4/30	13
Without glycopyrrolate				
Wax-matrix	24/104	23.1	2/50	4
Microencap	10/60	16.7	1/6	17
Placebo	2/25	8.0	0/14	0

The use of glycopyrrolate adds another important and confounding variable. Glycopyrrolate was employed to slow gastric emptying. In actuality, it was not necessary because large tablets depend on the housekeeping waves in the stomach for emptying and these waves occur only during the interdigestive period. Although I know of no evidence suggesting that glycopyrrolate is ulcerogenic, it may have influenced the results in unforeseen ways. For example, it may have altered gastric mucus secretion or produced other subtle changes that made a particular potassium preparation appear more injurious than it otherwise would be (a bias?). If so, one could speculate that it might have a similar permissive role with other drugs.

The finding of gastric ulcers has played a prominent role in the discussion of the importance of the published studies. Acute gastric ulcers exhibit a different course from chronic gastric ulcers: acute ulcers heal rapidly with or without therapy. Studies in experimental animals have shown that the ability of the gastric mucosa to heal after acute injury is phenonomenal. Similar rapid healing has been seen in humans after gastric biopsy or mucosal damage during surgery. The acute ulcers associated with potassium therapy have frequently been considered as chronic ulcers, which is very misleading. By and large the acute ulcers identified have been asymptomatic and would not have been identified, or even suspected, except for the involvement of the subjects in research involving gastroscopy. In one study performed in Utah, gastric erosions that occurred during potassium chloride therapy were followed prospectively and were observed to heal despite continued potassium administration.

I believe the accumulated data can be summarized as follows: Acute gastric ulceration may occur following the administration of either wax-matrix or microencapsulated potassium chloride. The frequency of ulcer formation is low and with coadministration of glycopyrrolate is in the range of 1-2%. Both wax-matrix and microencapsulated potassium preparations appear equivalent in this regard. The role that glycopyrrolate plays in accentuating injury is unknown and may be either permissive or active. Gastric erosions may occur with either type of drug formulation and the frequency is increased by glycopyrrolate. There does not seem to be a definite dosage-response relationship between the frequency of damage and the amount of potassium administered for either type of product. Potassium chloride when administered in solution form does not appear to damage the gastric mucosa. A large body of epidemiological data suggests that neither the acute ulcers nor the gastric erosions have clinical significance. The acute-injury-gastroscopy model seems to have little or no predictive value and the use of glycopyrrolate would not seem justified.

GASTRIC EMPTYING OF MICROENCAPSULATED POTASSIUM

At first look, it appears incongruous that the multiple-unit form of microencapsulated potassium chloride would cause gastric mucosal erosions and acute ulcers. The presence of such lesions implies a local high concentration of potassium and is not consistent with the hypothesis that widespread dispersal of the microcrystalline potassium occurs in vivo. Scintigraphic studies have shown that capsules frequently lodge between gastric folds and, after dissolving, release the drug which may remain localized due to gastric mucus (12,28, 29). Such localization has been associated with mucosal injury by drugs, such as pivampicillin, not commonly thought to damage mucous membranes (27).

We investigated the gastric emptying and distribution of microencapsulated potassium chloride following ingestion by normal volunteers (55). In our study, volunteers received 4 capsules (32 mEq) of Micro-K or placebo and then underwent endoscopy after 30, 60, or 120 min (on separate days). The material within the stomach was localized endoscopically and was quantitatively removed for analysis. The placebo dispersed widely throughout the stomach whereas the microencapsulated potassium tended to remain in large clumps in the distal stomach. Clumps of crystals were also adherent to the gastric mucosa, held in place by gastric mucus. The lack of widespread dispersal of the microencapsulated potassium chloride obviates the theoretical advantages associated with the use of multiple-unit dosage form medication and explains how, on occasion, such a form may cause acute gastric mucosal injury, including acute ulcer.

DRUG-INDUCED GASTROINTESTINAL MUCOSAL INJURY

Gastrointestinal mucosal irritants can be classified into those in which mucosal irritation is an intrinsic property of the substance and those in which injury occurs as a random event. The second category includes substances that are intrinsically not irritating, but during the use of which an untoward event mediates a formulation–mucosal interaction (such as when a capsule of pivampicillin lodges between gastric folds).

Aspirin is a good example of a drug with intrinsic ability to damage the gastric mucosa. Mucosal irritation in the form of submucosal hemorrhages or erosions is seen in most patients following acute oral administration of aspirin. Continued administration of aspirin is associated with mucosal adaptation that results in healing of existing lesions and resistance to the development of additional lesions (24). Continued administration of the irritating agent is required for gastric mucosal adaptation to remain in effect. Thus, it seems unlikely that drugs that cause random and infrequent injury (e.g., potassium) would promote mucosal adaptation. For example, aspirin administration is associated with an increase in fecal blood loss as measured by studies using radiochromium-labeled red blood cells. In contrast, neither wax-matrix nor microencapsulated potassium chloride produced an increase in fecal blood loss in normal volunteers (14,52,56).

DRUG-INDUCED ESOPHAGEAL INJURY

A wide variety of drugs has been shown to cause esophageal injury following retention in the esophagus. The initial report of caustic esophageal injury appeared in 1970 and by 1983 more than 220 cases had been described (13,17,35). Esophageal injury has been reported with 26 different types of pills; antibiotics and the anticholinergic, emepronium bromide, accounted for most of the cases (35). Potassium chloride, ferrous sulfate, quinidine, and nonsteroidal antiinflammatory compounds are also included on the list. Sixteen cases of esophageal injury involving wax-matrix potassium chloride tablets have been reported (35,42,51); many of those patients had preexisting esophageal compression due to left atrial enlargement (42) or adhesions following thoracic surgery. The risk is low (estimated at 1.9 cases per million patient years), but it would seem prudent not to prescribe solid dosage forms of potassium to patients known to have problems of esophageal emptying. That such a wide variety of drugs are able to cause corrosive injury in the esophagus suggests that they may also cause gastric mucosal injury, but this has never been evaluated.

Whether one chooses a wax-matrix or a microencapsulated form of potassium, it is important to be aware of the problems associated with the manner in which tablets and capsules are administered. Either tablets or capsules may remain trapped in the esophagus for an extended time after ingestion. Fisher et al. (22), in an elegant study, used scintigraphic techniques to investigate the best approach to administering solid dosage medication. It was found that the best technique began with a sip of water followed by ingestion of the medication, followed by additional water. Sitting or standing was preferable to a supine position. The preliminary sip of water was apparently critical to help ensure that the tablet or capsule would be cleared from the esophagus following ingestion.

COMPARISON OF SOLID DOSAGE FORMS OF POTASSIUM CHLORIDE

Is it possible to estimate what difference, if any, might exist between potassium solid-dosage formulations? It is difficult to interpret data obtained from studies, in volunteers, lasting only 1 or 2 weeks, and it is impossible to project those results to many thousands of patients who take such drugs daily. Current evidence suggests that there is no major difference between solid dosage forms of potassium. If they do differ at all, it is by less than an order of magnitude. Current data suggest that both types of solid dosage forms of potassium chloride are safe, but not as safe as the liquid forms of potassium chloride. The observed very low level of risk must be balanced against the benefits gained from such a dosage form of potassium.

The frequency of stenosing small bowel ulcer with solid-dosage potassium is similar to the spontaneous rate (i.e., that not associated with potassium therapy). Esophageal injury has been associated with wax-matrix potassium chloride in those patients with delayed esophageal emptying. The experience with microencapsulated potassium is still too small to allow us to identify whether the risk will be reduced compared with wax-matrix dosage forms. Nevertheless, neither type of product should be prescribed to patients with known problems of esophageal emptying. There is still no evidence to suggest that either solid dosage form of potassium causes clinically important injury to the stomach or duodenum. In fact, when evidence of such injury has been looked for, it has not been found (5) and it has not been possible to demonstrate an increased frequency of ulcer complications (bleeding, obstruction, or perforation), or chronic gastric or duodenal ulcer production in patients receiving solid dosage forms of potassium chloride. If such an untoward event were discovered with wax-matrix products, I predict that the same event would also be present with the microencapsulated preparations.

RECOMMENDATIONS FOR ADMINISTRATION OF POTASSIUM CHLORIDE

What is the best method for administering these preparations? Potassium chloride has advantages over many other drugs in that where the potassium is released is not critical; it will be absorbed whether it is released in the stomach, small intestine, or, probably, the colon. Bioavailability studies with the wax-matrix and microencapsulated potassium preparations demonstrated that, in all instances, the potassium was highly bioavailable (7,14-16,18,33,37,48,53,57).

I recommend that potassium preparations be administered after meals, despite slowing of gastric emptying. This takes advantage of the large postprandial gastric volume and enhanced gastric motility. During this time, the tablet or capsule could move freely from place to place, thereby reducing high local concentrations of potassium.

Although potassium chloride in solution is not palatable, it is clear, from looking at studies of patient compliance, that patients take the potassium that is prescribed (31). One must assume that the majority of patients are able to discover a method of taking the potassium that is palatable for them; for example, in a mix with fruit juice to disguise the taste. The large number of patients who receive solid dosage forms of potassium suggests that the decision that liquid potassium is too unpalatable must often be made by the physician and that patients are not given the opportunity to learn to use liquid potassium dosage forms.

I recommend, first, that when a decision is made to administer potassium, that decisions be reconsidered. It has become increasingly clear that the prescription of potassium is often a reflex action and not the result of a risk/benefit calculation. If, after reconsideration, the decision is remade to administer potassium, then one should begin with potassium chloride in solution. Patients should be instructed that there may be a period of adjustment and that they should explore various combinations in order to achieve a palatable product. I recommend a solid-dosage form only if the patient is unable or unwilling to take the liquid dosage form. Solid-dosage form products should not be prescribed to patients with disorders of intestinal transit, including disorders affecting emptying of the esophagus, stomach, and small intestine. I see no major difference between the wax-matrix and microencapsulated products. Cost and patients' preference for tablets or capsules should probably be the major factors in deciding which form of solid-dosage potassium to prescribe.

ACKNOWLEDGMENTS

The author gratefully acknowledges the cooperation given to him by investigators from medical schools throughout the country who were willing to share their raw data, both published and unpublished. In particular, I would like to thank Drs. K. Akdamar, A. Ertan, and J. Ryan from Tulane, D. Ernest from the University of Arizona, J. Barkin from the University of Miami, and K. Tolman from the University of Utah.

REFERENCES

1. Abbruzzese, A. A., and Gooding, C. A.: Reversible small-bowel obstruction. Withdrawal of hydrochlorothiazide potassium chloride therapy. *JAMA* 192:111–112, 1965.
2. Akdamar, K., Ertan, A., Agrawal, N. M., McMahon, G., Ryan, J., Kedia, S., and Burk, J.: Upper gastrointestinal endoscopy in normal asymptomatic volunteers. *Am. J. Gastroenterol.* 78:670, 1983.
3. Allen, A. C., Boley, S. J., Schultz, L. and Schwartz, S.: Potassium-induced lesions of the small bowel. II. Pathology and pathogenesis. *JAMA* 193:85–90, 1965.
4. Alsop, W. R., Moore, J. G., Rollins, D. E., and Tolman, K. G.: The effects of five potassium chloride preparations on the upper gastrointestinal mucosa in healthy subjects receiving glycopyrrolate. *J. Clin. Pharmacol.* 24:208–212, 1984.
5. Aselton, P. J., and Hershel, J.: Short-term follow-up study of wax-matrix potassium chloride in relation to gastrointestinal bleeding. *Lancet* 1:184, 1983.
6. Barkin, J. S., Harary, A. M., Shamblen, C.E., and Lasseter, K. C.: Potassium chloride and gastrointestinal injury. *Ann. Intern. Med.* 98:129–276, 1983.

7. Barlow, C. G.: Release of potassium chloride from tablets. *J. Pharm. Pharmacol.* 17:822–824, 1965.
8. Bechgaard, H., and Nielsen, G. H.: Controlled-release multiple-units and single-unit doses. A literature review. *Drug Dev. Indust. Pharm.* 4:53–67, 1978.
9. Bokelman, C., Bagdon, W., Zwickey, R. E., and Mattis, P. A.: Ulcerogenic effect of potassium chloride on the gastrointestinal tract of the monkey. *Fed. Proc.* 24:715, 1965.
10. Boley, S. J., Schultz, L., Krieger, H., Schwartz, S., Elguezabal, A., and Allen, A. C.: Experimental evaluation of thiazides and potassium as a cause of small-bowel ulcer. *JAMA* 192:93–98, 1965.
11. Boley, S. J., Allen, A. C., Schultz, L., and Schwartz, S.: Potassium-induced lesions of the small bowel. *JAMA* 193:81–84, 1965.
12. Casey, D. L., Beihn, R. M., Digenis, G. A., and Shambhu, M. B.: Method for monitoring hard gelatin capsule disintegration times in humans using external scintigraphy. *J. Pharm. Sci.* 65:1412–1413, 1976.
13. Collins, F. J., Matthews, H. R., Baker, S. E., and Strakova, J. M.: Drug-induced oesophageal injury. *Br. Med. J.* 1:1673–1676, 1979.
14. Cordano, A., Vitale, J. J., Gunther, B. J., Velez, H., and Franco, T.: Controlled-release potassium chloride: Effectiveness in the repair of an experimentally-induced potassium depletion and effects on fecal blood loss. *Curr. Ther. Res.* 20:156–163, 1976.
15. Cordano, A., Vitale, J. J., Hamby, R., Velez, H., and Franco, T.: A new controlled-release oral potassium supplement: An extended study on safety and efficacy. *Clin. Ther.* 2:263–270, 1979.
16. Cordano, A., Winter, L., Elliott, D. L., Ali, N., Carter, T. N., and Bazo, A.: Acceptance, safety, and efficacy of Klotrix. A controlled-release potassium supplement: A long-term study. *Curr. Ther. Res.* 26:471–477, 1979.
17. Creteur, V., Laufer, I., Kressel, H. Y., Caroline, D. F., Goren, R. A., Evers, K. A., Glick, S. N., and Gatenby, R. A.: Drug-induced esophagitis detected by double-contrast radiography. *Radiology* 147:365–368, 1983.
18. Dickerson, J., Bressler, R., Gelderman, G. A., Cohn, J. B., and Goldstein, J. A.: Bioavailability, efficacy, safety and acceptance of Klotrix. A slow-release potassium chloride supplement. *Curr. Ther. Res.* 28:340–354, 1980.
19. Diener, R. M., Shoffstall, D. H., and Earl, A. E.: Production of potassium-induced gastrointestinal lesions in monkeys. *Toxicol. Appl. Pharmacol.* 7:746–755, 1965.
20. Emerson, D. N.: Potassium therapy and gastrointestinal lesions. *J. Indiana State Med. Assoc.* 63:228–232, 1970.
21. Fara, J. W.: Gastrointestinal transit of solid dosage forms. Drug Delivery Systems: Proceedings of an International Conference. *Pharm. Tech.* 1983.
22. Fisher, R. S., Malmud, L. S., Applegate, G., Rock, E., and Lorber, S. H.: Effect of bolus composition on esophageal transit: Concise communication. *J. Nucl. Med.* 23:878–882, 1982.
23. Goble, F. C., Lillis, W. G., Bladridge, J., Jacob, J. T., and Casorso, D. R.: Evaluation of intestinal ulcerogenesis potential of potassium chloride solid dosage forms. *Curr. Ther. Res.* 27:40–54, 1980.
24. Graham, D. Y., Smith, J. L., and Dobbs, S. M.: Gastric adaptation occurs with aspirin administration in man. *Dig. Dis. Sci.* 28:1–6, 1983.
25. Heffernan, S. J., Fogarty, O., and Murphy, J. J.: Stenosing ulcers of the small intestine associated with slow release potassium tablets. *J. Irish Med. Assoc.* 68:366–368, 1975.
26. Heffernan, S. J., and Murphy, J. J.: Ulceration of small intestine and slow-release potassium tablets. *Br. Med. J.* 2:746, 1975.

27. Hey, H., Matzen, P., Andersen, J. T., Didriksen, E., and Nielsen, B.: A gastroscopic and pharmacological study of the disintegration time and absorption of pivampicillin capsules and tablets. *Br. J. Clin. Pharmacol.* 8:237–242, 1979.
28. Hunter, E., Fell, J. T., Calvert, R. T., and Sharma, H.: 'In vivo' disintegration of hard gelatin capsules in fasting and non-fasting subjects. *Int. J. Pharm.* 4:175–183, 1980.
29. Hunter, E., Fell, J. T., and Sharma, H.: The gastric emptying of pellets contained in hard gelatin capsules. *Drug Dev. Indust. Pharm.* 8:751–757, 1982.
30. Hutcheon: Benefit-risk factors associated with supplemental potassium therapy. *J. Clin. Pharmacol.* 16:85–87, 1976.
31. Inui, T. S., Carter, W. B., Pecoraro, R. E., Pearlman, R. A., and Dohan, J. J.: Variations in patient compliance with common long-term drugs. *Med. Care* 18:986–993, 1980.
32. Jacobs, E., and Pringto, J.: Gastric ulcers due to the intake of potassium chloride. *Am. J. Dig. Dis.* 18:289–294, 1973.
33. Jouhar, A. J., Garnett, E. S., and Wallington, J. S.: Potassium absorption—a comparison of in vitro and in vivo studies. *J. Pharm. Sci.* 57:617–620, 1968.
34. Karacadag, S.: Effects of potassium chloride and chlorothiazide on gastric secretion and gastric mucosa in dogs. *Am. J. Gastroenterol.* 52:495–499, 1969.
35. Kikendall, J. W., Friedman, A. C., Oyewole, M. A., Fleischer, D., and Johnson, L. F.: Pill-induced esophageal injury. Case reports and review of the medical literature. *Dig. Dis. Sci.* 28:174–182, 1983.
36. Lawrason, F. D., Alpert, E., Mohr, F. L., and McMahon, F. G.: Ulcerative-obstructive lesions of the small intestine. *JAMA* 191:105–108, 1965.
37. Levene, D. L.: The absorption of potassium chloride—liquid vs. tablet. *C.M.A. Journal* 108:1480–1481, 1973.
38. Levowitz, B. S., Boley, S. J., Agrawal, G. P., Glotfelty, E., Kamil, N., and Allen, A. C.: Vascular basis of the potassium ulcer and its reversal by magnesium ion. *Surg. Forum* 18:315–317, 1967.
39. Lindholmer, B., Nyman, E., and Raf, L.: Nonspecific stenosing ulceration of the small bowel. A preliminary report. *Acta Chir. Scand.* xx:xx–xx, 19xx.
40. Lister, R. E.: Potassium chloride and intestinal ulceration. *Lancet* 2:794–795, 1965.
41. McAvoy, B. R.: Mouth ulceration and slow-release potassium tablets. *Br. Med. J.* 4:164–165, 1974.
42. McCall, A. J.: Slow-K ulceration of oesophagus with aneurysmal left atrium. *Br. Med. J.* 3:230–231, 1976.
43. McMahon, F. G., and Akdamar, K.: Gastric ulceration after "Slow-K." *N. Engl. J. Med.* 295:733–734, 1976.
44. McMahon, F. G., Ryan, J. R., Akdamar, K., and Ertan, A.: Effect of potassium chloride supplements on upper gastrointestinal mucosa. *J. Clin. Pharmacol. Ther.* 35:852–855, 1984.
45. McMahon, F. G., Ryan, J. R., Akdamar, K., and Ertan, A.: Upper gastrointestinal lesions after potassium chloride supplements: A controlled clinical trial. *Lancet* 2:1059–1060, 1982.
46. Morganstern, L., Freilich, M., and Panish, J. F.: The circumferential small-bowel ulcer. Clinical aspects in 17 patients. *JAMA* 191:101–104, 1965.
47. Myers, R. N., Brown, C. E., and Deaver, J. M.: In vivo effect of potassium on small bowel. *Ann. Surg.* 166:693–703, 1967.
48. Nordin, B. E. C., and Wilkinson, R.: Potassium supplements. *Br. Med. J.* 1:433, 1970.
49. Park, H. M., Chernish, S. M., Rosenek, B. D., Brunelle, R. L., Hargrove, B., and Wellman, H. N.: Gastric emptying of enteric-coated tablets. *Dig. Dis. Sci.* 29:207–212, 1984.

50. Patterson, D. J., Weinstein, G. S., and Jeffries, G. H.: Endoscopic comparison of solid and liquid potassium chloride supplements. *Lancet* 2:1077–1078, 1983.
51. Pemberton, J.: Oesophageal obstruction and ulceration caused by oral potassium therapy. *Br. Heart J.* 32:267–268, 1970.
52. Rider, J. A., Manner, R. J., and Swader, J. I.: Potassium chloride preparations and fecal blood loss. A parallel study with a 10% solution and a non-enteric-coated waxy-matrix tablet. *JAMA* 231:836–837, 1975.
53. Ryan, J. R.: A multicenter trial of microencapsulated potassium chloride. *Curr. Ther. Res.* 29:838–848, 1981.
54. Ryan, J. R., McMahon, F. G., Akdamar, K., Ertan, A., and Agrawal, N.: Mucosal irritant potential of a potassium-sparing diuretic and of wax-matrix potassium chloride. *Clin. Pharmacol. Ther.* 35:90–93, 1984.
55. Smith, J. L., Hurley, M. E., Jones, R. D., and Graham, D. Y.: Endoscopic evaluation of gastric emptying of drugs: How microencapsulated KCl (Micro-K Extencaps) can cause gastric mucosal damage. *Gastrointest Endosc.* 30:153, 1984.
56. Tannen, R. L., and Cordano, A.: Pharmacokinetics and effects on fecal blood loss of a controlled release potassium chloride tablet. *J. Pharmacol. Exp. Ther.* 204:240–246, 1978.
57. Tarpley, E. L., and Cordano, A.: Evaluation of efficacy, safety and patient acceptance of the controlled-release potassium chloride oral supplement, Klotrix. *Curr. Ther. Res.* 21:282–288, 1977.
58. Teicher, I., Arlen, M., Muehlbauer, M., and Allen, A. C.: The clinical-pathological spectrum of primary ulcers of the small intestine. *Surg. Gynecol. Obstet.* 116:196–202, 1963.
59. Treasure, T.: Ulceration of small intestine and slow-release potassium tablets. *Br. Med. J.* 3:302, 1975.
60. Watson, M. R., and Mark, J. B. D.: Ulceration of the small intestine. Relation to enteric-coated potassium. *Am. J. Surg.* 112:421–425, 1966.
61. Wilson, I. H., Cooley, N. V., and Luibel, F. J.: Nonspecific stenosing small bowel ulcers. *Am. J. Gastroenterol.* 50:449–455, 1968.

TREATMENT OF HYPERKALEMIA

37

The Treatment of Hyperkalemia

ROBERT C. MAY and WILLIAM E. MITCH
Harvard Medical School and Brigham and Women's Hospital, Boston, Massachusetts

Recent data reported by the Boston Collaborative Drug Surveillance Program highlight aspects of current potassium (K) therapy (63). Of 16,048 consecutive hospitalized patients, 4,921 (31%) were treated with potassium chloride; the prevalence of its use varied from 17 to 53% among the hospitals participating in the study. Adverse reactions attributed to K occurred in 283 or nearly 6% of those being treated. Hyperkalemia was the most frequent adverse reaction, occurring in 179 patients, or 3.6%, of those treated with K. This was not trivial hyperkalemia; the average peak serum level was 6 mEq/L and was judged to have contributed to the death of 7 patients while threatening the lives of 21 other patients. The incidence of iatrogenic hyperkalemia was highest in patients older than 50 years or with azotemia and in those receiving K-sparing diuretics or a combination of oral and intravenous K. This report is especially distressing since 87% of patients receiving K were being treated solely to prevent the development of hypokalemia; nearly half of all treated patients were given K intravenously. The incidence of adverse effects resulting from K supplements in ambulatory patients is unknown.

An awareness of these data has prompted some authors to question the practice of prescribing K prophylactically for patients receiving diuretics (47). Besides this caveat, an increasing number of commonly used drugs impair normal defenses against hyperkalemia and increase the risks of prophylactic K therapy. Drugs that affect K homeostasis include not only the K-sparing diuretics, but also angiotensin-converting enzyme inhibitors, beta-adrenoreceptor antagonists, and the nonsteroidal, antiinflammatory agents (42,45,89,90). Because of the increasing age of patients, the higher prevalence of azotemia and diabetes in the population, and the increasing use of these drugs, we predict that hyperkalemia will constitute an increasing problem unless prophylactic prescribing of K is curtailed.

DEFENSES AGAINST HYPERKALEMIA

A brief overview of the partition and disposal of K is necessary for understanding therapeutic approaches to hyperkalemia. Both carcass analysis (34) and determination of the body content of the naturally occurring isotope, ^{40}K (75), indicate that there is 55–65 mEq K/kg of fat-free weight in normal adults. Since the concentration of serum or extracellular K is tightly regulated between 3.5 and 5 mEq/L (85), it follows that extracellular K represents only about 2% of total K stores. In fact, the amount of K in extracellular fluid of a 70-kg human might well be less than the amount prescribed for prophylactic therapy each day. To prevent K intoxication, the body must dispose of K loads effectively to minimize changes in the concentration ratio of extra- to intracellular K. At the same time, K balance must be regulated precisely (75) in the face of sporadic K loading, as occurs with meals or with exercise and trauma. Disposal of an acute K load involves poorly understood interactions between insulin, aldosterone, and catecholamines (7,18), while K balance is largely regulated by aldosterone (12,22,70). During K adaptation, the activity of NaK-ATPase in kidneys and colon changes, leading to an increase in K excretion (24,33,82).

Several defenses are activated simultaneously to prevent serious hyperkalemia when foods rich in K, such as fruits and meats, are eaten. High-carbohydrate foods (especially fruit juices) and protein-rich foods stimulate osmoreceptors in the duodenum and activate gastric hormonal responses, thereby slowing gastric emptying. This delays transit of the K-enriched meal into the small intestine which is the most important site of K absorption (61). During absorption of food, insulin and catecholamines are secreted and, by shifting K into cells, blunt the rise in plasma K (7,16,17,99). Besides cellular redistribution, another defense against hyperkalemia after a meal is the increasing renal elimination of K. Approximately 2-½ hr after a meal containing protein, the glomerular filtration rate of normal subjects increases (8). This response could increase K excretion either by raising distal tubular flow or by modifying the constituents of distal tubular fluid (38,41). In addition, a rise in serum K of only 0.1 mEq/L is sufficient to stimulate aldosterone release, further augmenting K secretion in the distal nephron (52). Within 6 hours, these renal responses account for excretion of about 50% of an oral or I.V. K load in normal subjects (19,40). It is important to note that except for aldosterone, these defenses do not depend upon the K content of the meal nor do they act specifically to regulate extracellular K concentration. Consequently, an oral dose of K chloride or another K salt is unlikely to activate them.

Disposal of an endogenous K load (e.g., accompanying trauma or exercise) differs from disposal of an oral K load. A rise in plasma K occurring after the sudden release of K from tissue must be damped immediately; renal K excretion rises too slowly to accomplish this. Since plasma insulin is usually low during stress or exercise (96), it cannot account for the increase in K uptake by tissues in these conditions. However, stress and exercise do stimulate catecholamine release (96) and both norepinephrine and epinephrine promote active K transport into skeletal muscle, presumably by an adenylate-cyclase-dependent activation of NaK-ATPase (16). Since there is almost instantaneous activation of NaK-ATPase by catecholamines, sympathetic nervous system is the most rapid defense against sudden shifts in serum K. Experimentally, an infusion of sufficient epinephrine into humans to produce a physiological increase in plasma epinephrine blunts the increase in serum K caused by a concomitant infusion of K (19,77,83). Although catecholamine infusion is not suitable for treating most cases of hyperkalemia because of its effects in cardiac excitability, salbutamol inhalation has been used successfully to treat patients with familial hyperkalemic periodic paralysis (94). On the other hand, beta-adrenergic blockade with propranolol interferes with disposal of a K load in humans (77), rats (83), and cats (65). The importance of this is highlighted by the observation that serum K usually rises when propranolol is used to treat hypertensive persons (90). Preliminary evidence also suggests that the ability to dispose of K generated during exercise is blunted by propranolol (13). Besides causing a release of catecholamines, stress also stimulates aldosterone secretion by promoting ACTH release from the pituitary (57) and by stimulating renin release (80). These latter responses increase K excretion and reestablish steady-state levels of plasma K. Thus, the sympathetic nervous system is ideally suited for disposing of an endogenous K load because of the following characteristics: (a) catecholamines directly stimulate uptake of K into skeletal muscle, the major repository of K; (b) the rapidity of catecholamine turnover (serum half-life 2 min [62]) prevents the development of serious hypokalemia; (c) the effectiveness is not dependent upon augmenting K excretion. Experimental studies indicate that administration of exogenous K does not by itself stimulate the sympathetic nervous system (77,83); the food, tissue damage, and other factors evoke a response from the sympathetic nervous system.

CLINICAL MANIFESTATIONS

Most reviews stress that patients with hyperkalemia complain of muscle fatigue (69); more serious problems include respiratory failure and quadriplegia (10). Most commonly, however, the physician is alerted to impending K intoxication by serum electrolyte values, rather than symptoms (63). Although prolonged application of a tourniquet or hemolysis can produce a false increase in serum K, whenever serum K is reported to be high, an electrocardiographic reading should be obtained immediately.

The most commonly occurring adverse reaction due to hyperkalemia is the development of abnormalities in conduction of cardiac impulses. At a plasma K level of 6-7 mEq/L, "tenting" of T waves may occur due to an increase in the K conductance of cardiac membranes which accelerates repolarization of the membrane. Tenting of T waves is invariably found when plasma K rises to 8-9 mEq/L (26). Other EKG findings include variable shortening of the PR interval and a value of only 0.15-0.18 seconds for the difference between the QT and QRS intervals (88). At a plasma K above 8 mEq/L, atrial conduction is generally impaired, causing a reduced amplitude of the P wave and a prolonged PR interval (26). When plasma K rises above 9 mEq/L, there is a sharp increase in the duration of the QRS and the H-Q intervals in both animals (26) and humans (4), which suggests progressively impaired conduction. At this stage, the QRS morphology may resemble a bundle branch block (4). In the rare circumstance when plasma K has been documented to exceed 10 mEq/L, atrioventricular conduction stops and a junctional rhythm may ensue (26). As the effects of hyperkalemia worsen, conduction through the Purkinje's fibers and ventricular muscle either ceases or variable blocks in conduction arise resulting in "circus rhythms" and, ultimately, ventricular fibrillation.

TREATMENT

The strategy for treating hyperkalemia is heavily influenced by the urgency of the clinical condition. When hyperkalemia is mild and unaccompanied by impairment of cardiac or skeletal muscles, investigation of the cause of hyperkalemia can be initiated while K stores are reduced by dietary or other means. Our discussion will focus on the therapy of life-threatening hyperkalemia. Therapeutic options may be categorized as: (a) methods for improving cardiac conduction, including intravenous administration of $CaCl_2$, hypertonic sodium, and placement of a cardiac pacemaker; (b) systemic alkalinization with sodium bicarbonate; (c) injection of insulin to increase tissue uptake of K; and (d) extrarenal removal of K using cation exchange resins or dialysis. Diuretics also have been used to treat hyperkalemia but the response usually is too slow and inadequate to be relied on in life-threatening conditions.

Calcium

As noted above, the most frequent life-threatening complication of hyperkalemia is abnormal conduction of cardiac impulses. Since the resting membrane potential of the specialized Purkinje's conducting tissues depends on the intra-/extracellular concentration gradient for K (53), and since the K concentration within cells remains virtually constant even in hyperkalemia (25), it follows that hyperkalemia causes the resting membrane potential to become less negative. This affects cardiac conduction because conduction velocity is determined by phase 0 depolarization mediated by the voltage- and time-dependent sodium gate (53). A less negative, resting membrane potential decreases the availability of sodium channels that can respond to an action potential. Consequently, a high serum K is always associated with poor cardiac conduction. It has been known since 1883 that calcium can reverse the effects of hyperkalemia on the cardiac membrane (76). Injection into dogs of KCl alone or a mixture of KCl and $CaCl_2$ revealed that a higher plasma K was tolerated without fatal cardiac effects in dogs also receiving $CaCl_2$ (97). Using isolated Purkinje's fibers, Weidmann showed that calcium has a "membrane-stabilizing effect" (95); at any resting membrane potential, fibers bathed in 10.4 mmol calcium had a greater rate of rise in voltage upon depolarization than fibers bathed in solutions containing 2.6 mmol calcium. More recent studies have demonstrated that a high calcium concentration also reduces the rectifying current, thereby delaying repolarization in cardiac tissue; this effect would counteract the accelerated repolarization caused by hyperkalemia (56).

Several studies document the benefits of I.V. calcium in the treatment of hyperkalemia. Merrill et al. treated K intoxication in 11 patients with acute renal failure (69). Of the five patients treated with calcium salts, three experienced an improvement in cardiac conduction. Meroney and Herndon summarized their experience with soldiers who developed acute renal failure in the Korean War (68). They reported that intravenous calcium provided an immediate, albeit transient, improvement in cardiac conduction in hyperkalemic patients. When they observed a poor response to calcium therapy, it invariably meant that plasma K was still rising. In vitro studies have suggested that the benefits of calcium are directly related to the concentration of ionized calcium. The temporary nature of the beneficial effect of calcium on cardiac conduction is almost certainly related to the fact that the increase in ionized calcium is not sustained, especially in patients with high serum phosphate levels (68). For this reason, several authors have recommended that large dosages of calcium be administered. Meroney and Herndon infused 10 g of a 10% calcium gluconate solution over 4 hr (68) and obtained satisfactory results, but others (15) have reported that a 10-g dose of $CaCl_2$ can raise serum calcium to values as high as 16 mg/dl. The benefits of intravenous calcium are immediate (15) which is fortunate because infusion of an excessive amount of calcium can be avoided simply by monitoring the electrocardiogram. This will tend to reduce the frequency of adverse effects of calcium infusions including hypercalcemia and soft-tissue calcification (15,93). It should be noted that much of the data from animal and in vitro experiments resulted from the use of very high calcium concentrations: 20–40 mg/dl. Such levels would be extremely dangerous to humans and probably are unnecessary for counteracting the effects of hyperkalemia, although clinical studies have not established a clear relationship between changes in cardiac conduction and either the rate of calcium administration or the calcium salt infused. Because of the immediate effect of calcium in improving the conduction abnormalities, it frequently is the first measure used.

Hypertonic Sodium

Besides calcium, infusion of hypertonic sodium solutions also can immediately reverse the abnormal cardiac conduction caused by hyperkalemia (31,37). This method can be especially useful in patients with acute renal failure and hyperkalemia who develop hyponatremia and acidosis, which can further depress the slowed cardiac conduction. One of the patients reported by Merrill et al. improved as his hyponatremia was corrected despite the persistence of hyperkalemia (69). Therapeutic regimens of hypertonic sodium chloride vary in the total amount of sodium given, the rate of infusion, and the percentage of sodium chloride in the infusate. A typical regimen is 100 ml of 3 or 5% sodium chloride infused over 1-3 hr (31,37). As with calcium, hypertonic sodium increases the maximum velocity of the action potential in isolated ventricular muscle strips or Purkinje's cells (3). Slowed conduction in cardiac tissue incubated in a high-K bath has been reversed by increasing the sodium concentration of the bath (3). In contrast to calcium, however, infusion of hypertonic sodium chloride leads to a considerable increase in the extracellular volume; infusion of 200 cc of 5% sodium chloride would expand the extracellular volume by almost 1 L. Besides this adverse effect, a large amount of hypertonic sodium chloride might aggravate an accompanying acidosis. For these reasons, hypertonic sodium has mainly been given as sodium bicarbonate.

Bicarbonate

Since the report of Fenn and Cobb (29), it has been known that acidosis is associated with net flux of K from skeletal muscle into extracellular fluid while the development of alkalosis is associated with uptake of K into skeletal muscle. However, this hydrogen-K exchange does not adequately explain the complex interrelationship between plasma K and changes in blood pH. On the basis of only nine studies of five patients with different illnesses who were undergoing different therapies directed at modifying their blood pH, the notion has been promulgated that for every 0.1 unit change in pH, an inverse change in serum K of 0.6 mEq/L occurs (11). Although this relationship was generally confirmed in another study of 79 chronically ill patients with acid-base disorders, plasma K varied far less in patients who had respiratory acidosis or alkalosis than in those with metabolic acid-base disorders (64). Moreover, in both studies, there was a large degree of individual variation in the response of plasma K to changes in acid-base status. In a study designed to unravel the pathophysiology of the relationship between K and hydrogen ion in dogs, Simmons and Avelone (84) found that an isohydric change in blood bicarbonate did not cause plasma K to rise or fall; this finding supported the concept that a change in blood pH, rather than bicarbonate, determines the cellular partitioning of K. When the pH of humans with acute respiratory failure was raised without bicarbonate being changed, their plasma K fell prior to any significant change in K excretion or blood bicarbonate (58). Thus, a rise or fall in blood pH clearly can change plasma K acutely, but the degree of the change in plasma K cannot be predicted reliably because of a high degree of individual variability.

More recent studies have uncovered additional complexities in the relationship between acid–base changes and the cellular partitioning of K. In contrast to earlier studies (84), Kim and Brown reported that inducing isohydric changes in the blood bicarbonate of dogs was associated with an inverse change in plasma K (59). Fraley and Adler have confirmed in rats (35) and in humans (36) that an isohydric change in the blood bicarbonate is associated with an inverse change in plasma K concentration that does not depend on K excretion. Thus, it seems that a rise or fall in blood bicarbonate can affect the cellular partitioning of K independently of changes in pH. In addition to changing cellular partition of K, bicarbonate infusion also could lower plasma K by promoting a kaliuresis (67). Besides pH and bicarbonate, the nature of the acid load also can affect the change in plasma K that occurs in response to an acid load. Infusion of a strong mineral acid (e.g., NH_4Cl or HCl) caused a dramatic rise in plasma K concentration of dogs while there was a negligible change in plasma K when an organic acid (e.g., lactate, methylmalonate) was infused, even though both solutions produced a comparable degree of acidosis and reduction in blood bicarbonate (72,73). It should be emphasized that infusion of hypertonic sodium chloride or mannitol (66,71) causes plasma K to rise, in contrast to the fall in plasma K that occurs with infusion of hypertonic sodium bicarbonate (71).

The decision to treat hyperkalemia with bicarbonate and the rate of its infusion depend upon several factors. Acidotic patients with subnormal plasma bicarbonate levels experience a marked change in pH and blood bicarbonate and, hence, the greatest change in plasma K concentration when infused with sodium bicarbonate. In contrast, patients with a normal pH and bicarbonate who are volume-expanded should be treated with another regimen since they experience little benefit from sodium bicarbonate therapy. The osmolality of the sodium bicarbonate solution used and the rate of administration depend upon: (a) the degree of impairment in cardiac conduction and hence the urgency of therapy; (b) the presence of hyponatremia; and (c) the cardiovascular capacity to accommodate the extra sodium. An immediate benefit is generally achieved when hypertonic sodium bicarbonate is infused rapidly because of the cardiac membrane effects of a hypertonic sodium infusion. The benefit derived from raising blood pH and bicarbonate does not become apparent for 30 min.

Insulin

Experimentally, the perfused pancreas or cultured islet cell preparations release insulin in response to K (44,55) and infusion of K into dogs or humans stimulates insulin secretion (23,50,51,74,79). However, the quantity of insulin released or the rise in plasma insulin in these studies was small, and the effect was achieved only at very high concentrations of K. In fact, when the plasma K of humans was increased <3 mEq/L by infusing K, there was no significant increase in plasma insulin (23,77,87). On the other hand, an increase in plasma insulin reliably reduces the concentration of K in plasma and this effect occurs independently of glucose removal from plasma (2). Insulin promotes active transport of K into tissues by a poorly understood mechanism(s) involving hyperpolarization of the cell membrane (54,100). From experiments using incubated skeletal muscle (17) and from in vivo studies across human forearms (2,32) and the splanchic bed (1), it is clear that skeletal muscle and liver are major sites of insulin-mediated K uptake. Insulin also affects "steady-state" regulation of plasma K; K tolerance is markedly impaired in diabetic anephric subjects (86) and in normal subjects infused with somatostatin which suppresses insulin secretion (21).

In order to use insulin properly in the treatment of hyperkalemia, several aspects of insulin pharmacokinetics should be understood. The rate of insulin-stimulated K uptake is maximal when the plasma level of insulin exceeds 500 μU/ml (20). This concentration of insulin will decrease plasma K at a rate of ∿ 1 mEq/L per hr. There is essentially no lag period after beginning the infusion of insulin and the onset of the decrease in plasma K caused by uptake of K into tissues (20,46,92). Moreover, when plasma insulin is held constant, plasma K falls linearly with respect to time (20). Following intravenous injection, both porcine and human insulin disappear from plasma with a $t_{1/2}$ varying between 3.8 min for human monocomponent insulin (92) and 5-8 min for porcine insulin (39,92). The best estimate of the volume of distribution of monocomponent human insulin in healthy, young adult subjects who are within 10% of their ideal body weight is 16% of body weight (range, 12-18%) (92).

Guerra and Kitabchi compared the effects of different routes of insulin administration on the fall in plasma K (46). When 0.1 U/kg was given subcutaneously or intramuscularly, plasma insulin increased to 40.6 μU/mo and 51.5 μU/l, respectively, but plasma K did not decrease significantly. When the same dosage was given intravenously, plasma insulin increased sharply and plasma K decreased 27.5%. Since the goal of insulin therapy is to lower plasma K, we conclude that insulin should be given intravenously. This regimen is necessary because the decrease in plasma K is proportional to the increase in plasma insulin (20) and intravenous administration will achieve the highest plasma level of insulin in the shortest period of time. Maximal levels of plasma insulin after subcutaneous or intramuscular injection are too low and the time to achieve peak plasma insulin is too variable (39,46) for emergency therapy.

As noted, the maximal potassium-lowering effects of insulin occur at a plasma insulin level of ∿ 500 μU/ml (20). The dosage of insulin that can achieve this concentration can be calculated from the volume of distribution (16% weight) and t ½ (∿ 6 min) of porcine insulin using a monoexponential, single-compartment model for insulin kinetics. Thus, a loading dose of 0.08 U/kg and a constant infusion of 0.00924 U/kg per min (approximately 0.5 U/kg per hr) should increase plasma insulin to a steady concentration of 500 μU/ml. Other regimens are less desirable. For example, it would be necessary to inject 2.6 U/kg every 30 min to maintain plasma insulin above 500 μU/ml because of the short half-life of intravenously administered insulin. The metabolic consequences of such large dosages of insulin are unclear and we recommend that insulin be given as a constant infusion. Even though glucose is not required for the K-lowering effect of insulin (2), it will be necessary to infuse glucose with this regimen to prevent hypoglycemia. The rate of glucose uptake is dependent upon plasma insulin; the peak glucose disappearance rate occurs when plasma insulin exceeds 300-500 μU/ml and is approximately 10 mg/kg per min or 600 mg/kg per hr (20). Consequently, about 600 mg/kg or 3 cc/kg per hr of D20 will be required to prevent hypoglycemia. Obviously, blood glucose must be monitored to prevent hypoglycemia as well as hyperglycemia which, by causing hypertonicity, could aggravate hyperkalemia (66).

Cation Exchange Resins

These therapies for hyperkalemia either cause only a transient shift in K from the extra- to intracellular space or counteract (e.g., calcium infusion) the cardiac effects of hyperkalemia. Consequently, treatment of hyperkalemia also must include a regimen that reduces K stores. Most commonly, hyperkalemic patients also have renal insufficiency so that a method for promoting extrarenal K elimination, such as gastrointestinal loss or dialysis, is necessary. Regarding gastrointestinal elimination, K primarily is transported across colonic epithelia by a passive mechanism linked to active sodium reabsorption (61). Potassium also is secreted in the colon by an energy-requiring process which tends to maintain a large K concentration gradient between colonic fluid and plasma (61). Studies in humans (78) and rats (60) suggest that when K in colonic fluid rises to 30-50 mEq/L, net K secretion ceases. The high K gradient in colonic fluid decreases in diarrheal states (14) thereby reducing the factor that normally limits passive net K loss. Consequently, K losses rise in patients with diarrhea. Besides intestinal transit time, other factors that increase colonic K loss include: (a) a high aldosterone level (5); (b) a low-sodium diet (49); (c) a high plasma K (49); (d) increased colonic NaK-ATPase activity and a more negative transluminal potential difference caused by adaptation to a high K intake (49); and (e) renal insufficiency, possibly through stimulation of NaK-ATPase activity (6,33,48,70). To augment gastrointestinal K losses, a cation exchange resin such as Kayexalate, the sodium salt of a sulfonic polystyrene resin, can be administered. This resin not only increases the amount of sodium presented to the colon, which tends to maintain the transcolonic potential, it also binds K. Kayexalate has a theoretical binding capacity of 3.4 mEq K/g resin (27) but when given orally, it binds only 0.7-1.7 mEq K/g resin (30,81). The difference between the theoretical and clinical efficacy is related to the binding of other cations. Potassium exchanges with sodium because it is bound about 50% more avidly than sodium (43); multivalent cations (e.g., calcium, magnesium) have a much higher affinity for the resin. Other cations, such as ammonium, also can compete with K and account in part for the lower capacity of the resin when it is given orally (43). For these reasons, Kayexalate should not be given with phosphate binders containing aluminum or antacids such as magnesium hydroxide or calcium carbonate. Frequently, Kayexalate is given with a cathartic to avoid constipation and to ensure elimination of the bound K. The usual dosage of Kayexalate is 10-20 g mixed with 100-200 cc water and given orally as a slurry. This dosage may be repeated several times daily and if constipation develops, an oral osmotic cathartic, such as sorbital or mannitol, can be added. Kayexalate also has been given as a retention enema, but available evidence suggests that it is less effective when given by this route, even when the retention time is prolonged to 18 hr (27).

Dialysis

The efficacy of hemodialysis in the treatment of hyperkalemia in patients with renal failure was emphasized by Merrill et al. (69). When plasma K increases rapidly, as in patients with rhabdomyolysis and acute renal failure, for those with impaired GI motility or with congestive heart failure and inability to tolerate the sodium load associated with Kayexalate, dialysis is the best method for controlling hyperkalemia. With hollow-fiber dialyzers, the clearance of K is essentially equal to urea (98), though this can be manipulated by varying the concentration of K in the dialysate. When dialysate K is zero, K clearance at a blood flow of 200 ml/min would be approximately 150 cc/min or 9 L/hr. This could clear K from the extracellular volume of a 70-kg human in approximately 1-½ hr. The greatest decrease in plasma K occurs in the first 2 hr of dialysis. Thereafter, plasma K levels reach a plateau, so that during the remainder of the dialysis all K removed represents a loss of tissue K stores (91). This explains the findings of Feig et al. who noted that, after a 3-hr dialysis against a K-free dialysate, the average amount of K removed was correlated with the predialysis plasma K and was proportional to body weight (28). In their studies, total K losses amounted to 1.22 mEq/kg. After dialysis,

Table 1 Regimens for Treating Hyperkalemia

Treatment	Dosage	Onset	Comment
Calcium	$\leqslant$ 100 ml of 10% Cagluconate or $CaCl_2$ I.V. over 1–4 hr	Immediately	Effectiveness is transient especially in hyperphosphatemic patients
Sodium bicarbonate	>50 ml of 7.4% solution	Immediately	Effect of hypertonic Na occurs immediately while that of HCO_3 requires $\geqslant$ 30 min
Insulin	0.5 U/kg per hr I.V. drip	∿30 min	I.V. glucose required to prevent hypoglycemia
Cation-exchange/Resin (Kayexalate)	10–15 g in 100–200 ml H_2O given P.O.	$\geqslant$2 hr	Effectiveness depends on elimination
Hemodialysis	–	Within 30 min of beginning dialysis	Effectiveness dependent upon availability; variable rise in serum K after dialysis

plasma K rises progressively for at least 5 hr. At 5 hr, the percentage decrease in plasma K was found to be greatest in those patients who had the highest initial values of plasma K (28). In contrast to hemodialysis, peritoneal dialysis is considerably less efficient in removing K; K clearances are only 17-22 ml/min, even when the dialysate dextrose was varied from 1.5 to 7% (9). In considering dialytic removal of K, it must be remembered that it takes 1-2 hr before either peritoneal or hemodialysis can be started. Thus, other methods (Table 1) are necessary to defend against the toxic effects of hyperkalemia. Rational treatment of hyperkalemia, therefore, depends upon knowledge of the time that will elapse before the regimen can reduce plasma K or reverse the effects of hyperkalemia and knowledge of the duration of effectiveness of different regimens.

ACKNOWLEDGMENTS

Supported in part by a National Research Service Award (AM 07131) and an RCDA (AM 00750) from the National Institutes of Health. We thank Paula Dolan for expert editorial assistance.

REFERENCES

1. Alvestrand, A., Wahren, J., Smith, D., and DeFronzo, R. A.: Insulin-mediated potassium uptake is abnormal in uremic and healthy subjects. *Am. J. Physiol.* 246: E174–E180, 1984.
2. Andres, R., Baltzan, M. A., Cader, G., and Zierler, K. L.: Effect of insulin on carbohydrate metabolism and on potassium in the forearm of man. *J. Clin. Invest.* 41: 108–115, 1962.
3. Ballantyne, F., Davis, L. D., and Reynolds, E. W.: Cellular basis for reversal of hyperkalemic electrocardiographic changes by sodium. *Am. J. Physiol.* 229:935–940, 1975.
4. Bashour, T., Hsu, I., Gorfinkel, H. J., Wickramespkavan, R., and Rios, J. C.: Atrioventricular and intraventricular conduction in hyperkalemia. *Am. J. Cardiol.* 35: 199–203, 1975.
5. Bastl, C. P., Binder, H. J., and Hayslett, J. P.: Role of glucocorticoids and aldosterone in maintenance of colonic cation transport. *Am. J. Physiol.* 238:F181–F186, 1980.
6. Bastl, C., Hayslett, J. P., and Binder, H. J.: Increased large intestinal secretion of potassium in renal insufficiency. *Kidney Int.* 12:9–16, 1977.
7. Bia, M. J., and DeFronzo, R. A.: Extrarenal potassium homeostasis. *Am. J. Physiol.* 240:F257–F268, 1981.
8. Bosch, J. P., Saccaggi, A., Laner, A., Ronco, C., Belledonne, M., and Glabman, S.: Renal functional reserve in humans. *Am. J. Med.* 75:943–950, 1983.
9. Brown, S. T., Ahearn, D. J., and Nolph, K. D.: Potassium removal with peritoneal dialysis. *Kidney Int.* 4:67–69, 1973.
10. Bull, A. M., Carter, A. B., and Loew, K. G.: Hyperpotassaemic paralysis. *Lancet* 2:60–61, 1953.
11. Burnell, J. M., Villamil, M. F., Uyeno, B. T., and Scribner, B. H.: The effect in humans of extracellular pH change on the relationship between serum potassium concentration and intracellular potassium. *J. Clin. Invest.* 35:935–939, 1956.
12. Cannon, P. J., Ames, R. P., and Laragh, J. H.: Relation between potassium balance and aldosterone secretion in normal subjects and in patients with hypertensive or renal tubular disease. *J. Clin. Invest.* 45:865–878, 1966.

13. Carlsson, E., Fellenius, E., Lundborg, P., and Svensson, L.: Beta-adrenoceptor blockers, plasma potassium, and exercise. *Lancet* 2:424–425, 1978.
14. Carpenter, C. C. J.: The pathophysiology of secretory diarrheas. *Med. Clin. North Am.* 66:597–610, 1982.
15. Chamberlain, M. J.: Emergency treatment of hyperkalemia. *Lancet* 1:464–467, 1964.
16. Clausen, T., and Flatman, J. A.: The effect of catecholamines on Na-K transport and membrane potential in rat soleus muscle. *J. Physiol.* 270:383–414, 1977.
17. Clausen, T., and Hansen, O.: Active Na-K transport and the rate of ouabain binding. The effect of insulin and other stimuli on skeletal muscle and adipocytes. *J. Physiol.* 270:415–430, 1977.
18. Cox, M., Sterns, R. H., Singer, I.: The defense against hyperkalemia: The roles of insulin and aldosterone. *N. Engl. J. Med.* 299:525–532, 1978.
19. DeFronzo, R. A., Bia, M., and Birkhead, G.: Epinephrine and potassium homeostasis. *Kidney Int.* 20:83–91, 1981.
20. DeFronzo, R. A., Felig, P., Ferrannini, E., and Wahren, J.: Effects of graded doses of insulin on splanchnic and peripheral potassium metabolism in man. *Am. J. Physiol.* 238:E421–E427, 1980.
21. DeFronzo, R. A., Sherwin, R. S., Dillingham, M., Hendler, R., Tamborlane, W. V., and Felig, P.: Influence of basal insulin and glucagon secretion on potassium and sodium administration. *J. Clin. Invest.* 61:472–479, 1978.
22. Dluhy, R. G., Axelrod, L., Underwood, R. H., and Williams, G. H.: Studies of the control of plasma aldosterone concentration in normal man. *J. Clin. Invest.* 51:1950–1957, 1972.
23. Dluhy, R. G., Axelrod, L., and Williams, G. H.: Serum immunoreactive insulin and growth hormone response to potassium infusion in normal man. *J. Appl. Physiol.* 33:22–26, 1972.
24. Doucet, A., and Katz, A. I.: Renal potassium adaptation: NaK-ATPase activity along the nephron after chronic potassium loading. *Am. J. Physiol.* 238:F380–F386, 1980.
25. Drescher, A. N., Talbot, N. B., Meara, P. A., Terry, M., and Crawford, J. D.: A study of the effects of excessive potassium intake upon body potassium stores. *J. Clin. Invest.* 37:1316–1321, 1958.
26. Ettinger, P. O., Regan, T. J., and Oldewurtel, H. A.: Hyperkalemia, cardiac conduction and the electrocardiogram: A review. *Am. Heart J.* 88:360–371, 1974.
27. Evans, B. M., Milne, M. D., Hughes Jones, N. C., and Yellowlees, H.: Ion-exchange resins in the treatment of anuria. *Lancet* 2:791–795, 1953.
28. Feig, P. U., Shook, A., and Sterns, R. H.: Effect of potassium removal during hemodialysis on the plasma potassium concentration. *Nephron* 27:25–30, 1981.
29. Fenn, W. O., and Cobb, D. M.: The potassium equilibrium in muscle. *J. Gen. Physiol.* 17:629–645, 1934.
30. Field, H., Swell, L., Flick, D. F., and Dailey, R. E.: Cation uptake by exchange resin in vitro and the colon as a sodium-conserving organ. *Circulation* 9:32–37, 1954.
31. Finch, C. A., Sawyer, C. G., and Flynn, J. M.: Clinical syndrome of potassium intoxication. *Am. J. Med.* 1:337–352, 1946.
32. Fineberg, S. E., and Merimee, T. J.: Effects of comparative perfusions of equimolar, single component insulin and proinsulin in the human forearm. *Diabetes* 22:676–686, 1973.
33. Fisher, K. A., Binder, H. J., and Hayslett, J. P.: Potassium secretion by colonic mucosal cells after potassium adaptation. *Am. J. Physiol.* 231:987–994, 1976.
34. Forbes, G. B., and Lewis, A. M.: Total sodium, potassium, and chloride in adult man. *J. Clin. Invest.* 35:596–600, 1956.

35. Fraley, D. S., and Adler, S.: Isohydric regulation of plasma potassium by bicarbonate in the rat. *Kidney Int.* 9:333–343, 1976.
36. Fraley, D. S., and Adler, S.: Correction of hyperkalemia by bicarbonate despite constant blood pH. *Kidney Int.* 12:354–360, 1977.
37. Garcia-Palmieri, M. R.: Reversal of hyperkalemic cardiotoxicity with hypertonic saline. *Am. Heart J.* 64:483–488, 1962.
38. Giebisch, G., and Stanton, B.: Potassium transport in the nephron. *Annu. Rev. Physiol.* 41:241–256, 1979.
39. Ginsberg, S., Block, M. B., Mako, M. E., and Rubenstein, A. H.: Serum insulin levels following administration of exogenous insulin. *J. Clin. Endocrinol. Metab.* 36:1175–1179, 1973.
40. Gonick, H. C., Kleeman, C. R., Rubini, M. E., and Maxwell, M. H.: Functional impairment in chronic renal disease. III. Studies of potassium excretion. *Am. J. Med. Sci.* 261:281–290, 1971.
41. Good, D. W., and Wright, F. S.: Luminal influences on potassium secretion: sodium concentration and fluid flow rate. *Am. J. Physiol.* 236:F192–F205, 1979.
42. Greenblatt, D. J., and Koch-Weser, J.: Adverse reactions to spironolactone. *JAMA* 225:40–43, 1973.
43. Greenman, L., Peters, J. H., Mateer, F. M., and Danowski, T. S.: Probable clinical utility of cation exchange resins. *J. Clin. Invest.* 30:1027–1031, 1951.
44. Grodsky, G. M., and Bennett, L. L.: Cation requirements for insulin secretion in the isolated perfused pancreas. *Diabetes* 15:910–913, 1966.
45. Grossman, A., Echland, D., Price, P., and Edwards, C. R. W.: Captopril: Reversible renal failure with severe hyperkalemia. *Lancet* 1:712, 1980.
46. Guerra, S. M. O., and Kitabchi, A. E.: Comparison of the effectiveness of various routes of insulin injection: Insulin levels and glucose response in normal subjects. *J. Clin. Endocrinol. Metab.* 42:869–874, 1976.
47. Harrington, J. T., Isner, J. M., and Kassirer, J. P.: Our national obsession with potassium. *Am. J. Med.* 73:155–159, 1982.
48. Hayes, C. P., McLeod, M. E., and Robinson, R. R.: An extrarenal mechanism for the maintenance of potassium balance in severe chronic renal failure. *Trans. Am. Assoc. Physiol.* 58:207–216, 1967.
49. Hayslett, J. P., Myketey, N., Binder, H. J., and Aronson, P. S.: Mechanism of increased potassium secretion in potassium loading and sodium deprivation. *Am. J. Physiol.* 239:F378–F382, 1980.
50. Hiatt, N., Davidson, M. B., and Bonorris, G.: The effect of potassium chloride infusion on insulin secretion in vivo. *Horm. Metab. Res.* 4:64–68, 1972.
51. Hiatt, N., Morgenstern, L., Davidson, M. B., Bonorris, G., and Miller, A.: Role of insulin in the transfer of infused potassium to tissue. *Horm. Metab. Res.* 5:84–88, 1973.
52. Himathongkam, T., Dluhy, R. G., and Williams, G. H.: Potassium–Aldosterone–renin interrelationships. *J. Clin. Endocrinol. Metab.* 41:153–159, 1975.
53. Hoffman, B. F., Rosen, M. R., and Wit, A. L.: Electrophysiology and pharmacology of cardiac arrythmias. VII. Cardiac effects of quinidine and procaineamide. *Am. Heart J.* 90:117–122, 1975.
54. Hougen, T. J., Hopkins, B. E., and Smith, T. W.: Insulin effects on monovalent cation transport and Na-K-ATPase activity. *Am. J. Physiol.* 234:C59–C63, 1978.
55. Howell, S. L., and Taylor, K. W.: Potassium ions and the secretion of insulin by islets of Langerhans incubated in vitro. *Biochem. J.* 198:17–24, 1968.
56. Kass, R. S., and Tsien, R. W.: Multiple effects of calcium antagonists on plateau currents in cardiac Purkinje fibers. *J. Gen. Physiol.* 66:169–192, 1975.
57. Kem, D. C., Gomez-Sanchez, C., Kramer, N. J., Holland, O. B., and Higgins, J. R.:

Plasma aldosterone and renin activity response to ACTH infusion in dexamethasone-suppressed normal and sodium-depleted man. *J. Clin. Endocrinol. Metab.* 40:116-124, 1975.

58. Kilburn, K. H.: Movements of potassium during acute respiratory acidosis and recovery. *J. Appl. Physiol.* 21:679-684, 1965.
59. Kim, W. G., and Brown, E. B.: Potassium transfer with constant extracellular pH. *J. Lab. Clin. Med.* 71:678-685, 1968.
60. Kliger, A. S., Binder, H. J., Bastl, C., and Hayslett, J. P.: Demonstration of active potassium transport in the mammalian colon. *J. Clin. Invest.* 67:1189-1196, 1981.
61. Krejs, G. J., and Fordtran, J. S.: Physiology and pathophysiology of ion and water movement in the human intestine. In *Gastrointestinal Disease*, 2nd ed, edited by Fordtran, J. S., and Sleisenger, M. H., Philadelphia, W. B. Saunders, 1978, pp. 297-313.
62. Lake, C. R., Ziegler, M. G., and Kopin, I. J.: Use of plasma norepinephrine for evaluation of sympathetic neuronal function in man. *Life Sci.* 18:1315-1326, 1976.
63. Lawson, D. H.: Adverse reactions to potassium chloride. *Q. J. Med.* 43:433-439, 1974.
64. Leibman, J., and Edelman, I. S.: Interrelationships of plasma potassium concentration, plasma sodium concentration, arterial pH and total exchangeable potassium. *J. Clin. Invest.* 38:2176-2188, 1959.
65. Lockwood, R. H., and Lum, B. K. B.: Effects of adrenergic agonists and antagonists on potassium metabolism. *J. Pharmcol. Exp. Ther.* 189:119-129, 1974.
66. Makoff, D. D., DaSilva, J. A., and Rosenbaum, B. J.: On the mechanism of hyperkalemia due to hyperosmotic expansion with saline or mannitol. *Clin. Sci.* 41:383-393, 1971.
67. Malnic, G., DeMello Aires, M., and Giebisch, G.: Potassium transport across renal distal tubules during acid-base disturbances. *Am. J. Physiol.* 221:1192-1208, 1971.
68. Meroney, W. H., and Herndon, R. F.: The management of acute renal insufficiency. *JAMA* 155:877-885, 1954.
69. Merrill, J. P., Levine, H. D., Somerville, W., and Smith, S.: Clinical recognition and treatment of acute potassium intoxication. *Ann. Intern. Med.* 33:797-830, 1950.
70. Mitch, W. E., and Wilcox, C. S.: Disorders of body fluids, sodium, and potassium in chronic renal failure. *Am. J. Med.* 72:536-550, 1982.
71. Moreno, M., Murphy, C., and Goldsmith, C.: Increase in serum potassium resulting from the administration of hypertonic mannitol and other solutions. *J. Lab. Clin. Med.* 73:291-298, 1969.
72. Oster, J. R., Perez, G. O., Castro, A., and Vaamonde, C. A.: Plasma potassium response to acute metabolic acidosis induced by mineral and nonmineral acids. *Min. Elect. Metab.* 4:28-36, 1980.
73. Oster, J. R., Perez, G. O., and Vaamonde, C. A.: Relationship between blood pH and potassium and phosphorus during acute metabolic acidosis. *Am. J. Physiol.* 235: F345-F351, 1978.
74. Pettit, G. W., Vick, R. C., and Swander, A. M.: Plasma K^+ and insulin: Changes during KCl infusion in normal and nephrectomized dogs. *Am. J. Physiol.* 228:107-109, 1975.
75. Pierson, R. N., Lin, D. H. Y., and Phillips, R. A.: Total-body potassium in health: Effects of age, sex, height, and fat. *Am. J. Physiol.* 226:206-212, 1974.
76. Ringer, S.: A further contribution regarding the influence of the deficient constituents of the blood on the concentration of the heart. *J. Physiol.* 4:29-42, 1883.
77. Rosa, R. M., Silva, P., Young, J. B., Landsberg, L., Brown, R. S., Rowe, J. W., and Epstein, F. H.: Adrenergic modulation of extrarenal potassium disposal. *N. Engl. J. Med.* 302:431-434, 1980.

78. Salas-Coll, C. A., Kermode, J. C., and Edmonds, C. J.: Potassium transport across the distal colon in man. *Clin. Sci.* 51:287–296, 1976.
79. Santeusanio, F., Faloona, G. R., Knochel, J. P., and Unger, R. H.: Evidence for a role of endogenous insulin and glucagon in the regulation of potassium homeostasis. *J. Lab. Clin. Med.* 81:809–817, 1973.
80. Sassard, J., Vincent, M., Annat, G., and Bizollon, C. A.: A kinetic study of plasma renin and aldosterone during changes of posture in man. *J. Clin. Endocrinol. Metab.* 42:20-27, 1976.
81. Scherr, L., Ogder, D. A., Mead, A. W., Spritz, N., and Rubin, A. L.: Management of hyperkalemia with a cation-exchange resin. *N. Engl. J. Med.* 264:115–119, 1961.
82. Silva, P., Hayslett, J. P., and Epstein, F. H.: The role of Na-K-ATPase in potassium adaptation. *J. Clin. Invest.* 52:2665–2671, 1973.
83. Silva, P., and Spokes, K.: Sympathetic system in potassium homeostasis. *Am. J. Physiol.* 241:F151–F155, 1981.
84. Simmons, D. H., and Avedon, M.: Acid–base alterations and plasma potassium concentration. *Am. J. Physiol.* 197:319–326, 1959.
85. Sterns, R. H., Cox, M., Feig, P. U., and Singer, I.: Internal potassium balance and the control of the plasma potassium concentration. *Medicine* 60:339–354, 1981.
86. Sterns, R. H., Feig, P. U., Pring, M., Guzzo, J., and Singer, I.: Disposition of intravenous potassium in anuric man: A kinetic analysis. *Kidney Int.* 15:651–660, 1979.
87. Sterns, R. H., Guzzo, J., and Feig, P. U.: The disposition of intravenous potassium in normal man: The role of insulin. *Clin. Sci.* 61:23–28, 1981.
88. Surawicz, B., Chlebus, H., and Mazzoleni, A.: Hemodynamic and electrocardiographic effects of hyperpotassemia. Differences in response to slow and rapid increases in concentration of plasma K. *Am. Heart J.* 73:647–664, 1967.
89. Tan, S. Y., Shapiro, R., Franco, R., Stockard, H., and Mulrow, P. J.: Indomethacin-induced prostaglandin inhibition with hyperkalemia. *Ann. Intern. Med.* 90:783–785, 1979.
90. Traub, Y. M., Rabinor, M., Rosenfeld, J. B., and Treuherz, S.: Elevation of serum potassium during beta blockade: Absence of relationship to the renin-aldosterone system. *J. Clin. Pharmacol. Ther.* 28:765–767, 1980.
91. Tu, W. H., Blair, G. O., and Schloerb, P. R.: Removal of excess body potassium by hemodialysis. *Am. J. Physiol.* 199:671–676, 1960.
92. Turner, R. C., Grayburn, J. A., Newman, G. B., and Nabarro, J. D. H.: Measurement of the insulin delivery rate in man. *J. Clin. Endocrinol.* 33:279–286, 1971.
93. Wallach, S., Bellavia, J. V., Schorr, J., and Schaffer, A.: Tissue distribution of electrolytes, ^{47}Ca and ^{28}Mg in experimental hyper- and hypoparathyroidism. *Endocrinology* 78:16–28, 1966.
94. Wang, P., and Clausen, T.: The treatment of attacks in hyperkalemic familial periodic paralysis by inhalation of salbutamol. *Lancet* 1:221–223, 1976.
95. Weidmann, S.: Effects of calcium ions and local anaesthetics on electrical properties of Purkinje fibers. *J. Physiol.* 129:568–582, 1955.
96. Winder, W. W., Hickson, R. C., Hagberg, J. M., Ehsani, A. A., and McLane, J. A.: Training-induced changes in hormonal and metabolic responses to submaximal exercise. *J. Appl. Physiol.* 46:766–771, 1979.
97. Winkler, A. W., Hoff, H. E., and Smith, P. K.: Factors affecting the toxicity of potassium. *Am. J. Physiol.* 124:430–437, 1938.
98. Wolf, A. V., Rump, D. G., Kiley, J. E., and Currie, G. D.: Artificial kidney function: Kinetics of hemodialysis. *J. Clin. Invest.* 30:1062–1074, 1951.
99. Young, J. B., and Landsberg, L.: Stimulation of the sympathetic nervous system during sucrose feeding. *Nature* 269:615–617, 1977.
100. Zierler, K., and Rogns, E.: Insulin does not hyperpolarize rat muscle by means of a ouabain-inhibitable process. *Am. J. Physiol.* 241:C145–C149, 1981.

38

Drug Interactions Causing Hyperkalemia

RICHARD L. TANNEN
University of Michigan Medical School, Ann Arbor, Michigan

Potassium concentration in plasma is dictated both by factors that regulate the distribution of potassium between the intracellular and extracellular compartments and by those that determine renal excretion, and thereby total body potassium stores. Hyperkalemia can result from a disturbance in either of these two critical regulatory systems. Because of the multiple mechanisms that defend against hyperkalemia, abnormalities in more than one regulatory system are usually required to provoke life-threatening hyperkalemia. Nevertheless, it is critical for the clinician to be aware of all potential hyperkalemia-inducing mechanisms in order to diagnose the cause of mild hyperkalemic states and to anticipate and thereby prevent severe hyperkalemia. For this reason it is especially important to be aware of all the therapeutic agents that have the propensity to interfere with normal potassium regulation.

This chapter will consider all drug-induced hyperkalemic syndromes and, where understood, the underlying mechanisms. As might be anticipated a broad subdivision can be made into (a) hyperkalemia resulting from interference with the mechanisms for distribution between the cell and the extracellular fluid, and (b) hyperkalemia resulting from agents that interfere with the normal renal potassium excretory mechanisms.

HYPERKALEMIA SECONDARY TO ALTERED DISTRIBUTION OF POTASSIUM BETWEEN THE INTRA- AND EXTRACELLULAR COMPARTMENTS

The intracellular potassium concentration is approximately 150 mEq/L, resulting in an intracellular to extracellular ratio (Ki/Ke) of about 30:1.

The potassium content of cells is regulated by an energy-dependent uptake mechanism and by a passive leak process, whereby potassium exits from the intracellular compartment.

Uptake of potassium by the cells is driven by the Na-K pump catalyzed by the enzyme Na-K-ATPase, which utilizes the energy of ATP to transport potassium into the cell against the cell's electrochemical gradient in exchange for countertransport of sodium into the extracellular fluid. The chemical gradient (Ki/Ke) for potassium exit from the cell exceeds the electrical gradient (cell-interior-negative), thereby promoting passive leak of potassium from the intracellular compartment, a process that is also regulated by the permeability characteristic of the membrane. Under steady-state conditions, the pump-leak processes are equivalent and stable intracellular potassium concentrations and a normal Ki/Ke are maintained. Drugs can produce hyperkalemia by impeding the activity of the Na-K pump, increasing the K^+ permeability of the membrane, or modifying the passive forces favoring K leak from the cells. Examples of hyperkalemia produced by all of these mechanisms are detailed on Table 1.

Beta-Adrenergic Blockers

Beta-adrenergic agonists promote cellular K^+ uptake by a direct effect on the Na-K pump, an action mediated by the B_2 system (7,12,53,58). Recent studies have clearly demonstrated that the nonselective beta-blocking agent propranolol heightens and prolongs the hyperkalemia induced in normal human volunteers by potassium infusions (15,48).

An analysis of the effects of therapy with beta blockers in several large groups of patients suggests that plasma potassium concentration is increased, but that the increment is quite modest (0.1-0.2 mEq/L) (4,30,44,45,62). The increase appears to be attributable predominantly to an alteration in potassium distribution rather than an increase in total body potassium stores secondary to the effects of beta blockade on the renin-aldosterone system (62). Although life-threatening hyperkalemia has not been reported, it should be noted that exercise-induced hyperkalemia is heightened and prolonged during beta blockade, similarly to the response to an exogenous potassium load (11).

Hence it should be appreciated that therapy with beta-blocking drugs has the potential to accentuate hyperkalemia, and might pose a risk to patients with other mechanisms of disordered K^+ regulation. When such agents are needed under such conditions, it would seem prudent to use selective beta_1 blockers.

Alpha-Adrenergic Agonists

The alpha-adrenergic nervous system affects potassium redistribution in exactly the opposite fashion to the beta-adrenergic system (4). Epinephrine, which has both alpha- and beta-adrenergic properties, results in hyperkalemia of several minutes' duration, but its beta-adrenergic properties subsequently become dominant and the major effect is a sustained decrease in plasma potassium levels. The pure alpha agonist, phenylephrine, heightens and prolongs the rise in plasma K^+ in response to either a KCl infusion or to

Table 1 Hyperkalemia Secondary to Redistribution

Drug	Mechanism
Beta-adrenergic blockers (propranolol)	↓Na-K pump
Alpha-adrenergic agonists	?
Digitalis	↓Na-K pump
Succinylcholine	↑membrane permeability
Arginine HCl	?
Mannitol (hyperosmolality)	$\uparrow K_i/K_e$

exercise and these effects are abolished by the alpha-adrenergic antagonist, phentolamine (56,66,67). The hyperkalemic effect of alpha agonists results, in part, from accentuated hepatic potassium release; however, an effect on potassium uptake by muscle also seems highly probable (29).

Digitalis

Cardiac glycosides are specific inhibitors of the Na-K pump and represent one of the important experimental probes for dissecting the role of the Na-K ATPase in physiological and pathophysiological conditions. Therapeutics amounts of these agents perturb the Ki/Ke ratio minimally, but appear to result in a slight decrease in intracellular K^+ concentration rather than in hyperkalemia (19). However, severe digitalis poisoning commonly results in overt hyperkalemia (54,55).

Succinylcholine

The muscle relaxant succinylcholine results in a prolonged increase in the potassium permeability of muscle cells (7,55). In normal subjects this can be associated with an increase in plasma potassium concentration of approximately 0.5 mEq/L. However use of this muscle-depolarizing agent can pose a significant risk for the development of hyperkalemia in patients with increased body K^+ stores who are under anesthesia. The risk for development of hyperkalemia also appears to be accentuated in patients with burns or with underlying neuromuscular diseases (8,26,47).

Arginine HCl

The infusion of cationic amino acids, including both arginine HCl and lysine HCl, can result in profound hyperkalemia (10,16,27,38,39). Presumably the positively charged amino acids displace intracellular potassium; however, the precise transport mechanism whereby this occurs has not been delineated. In normal humans the average maximal increase in potassium with a 30-g arginine infusion ranges from 0.5-1.0 mEq/L (27). As with other hyperkalemic stimuli, the risk for substantial hyperkalemia is greatest in patients with other derangements in potassium regulation, especially those with diabetes mellitus or impaired renal function.

Mannitol (Hyperosmolality)

Hyperosmolality, produced by an infusion of mannitol, or more commonly clinically by hyperglycemia in insulin-deficient patients, increases plasma potassium concentration (2,23,24,35,36,41,42,59). The mechanism relates to the shift of water from the intracellular to extracellular fluid compartment. The attendant cellular dehydration will increase the ratio of Ki/Ke and promote potassium exit from the cell, although solvent drag as water exits from the cell could also play a role.

The increase in plasma potassium concentration with mannitol-induced hypertonicity averages approximately 0.6 mEq/L for each 10 mOsm/kg H_2O increase in osmolality (41).

HYPERKALEMIA SECONDARY TO IMPAIRED RENAL POTASSIUM EXCRETION

Potassium excretion by the kidney is primarily dictated by a secretory process localized to the distal nephron, and largely by segments comprising the collecting duct system. A normal capacity to excrete potassium requires a functionally operative distal nephron, an appropriate delivery of sodium and fluid to the distal nephron K^+ secretory sites, and an intact regulatory system for production of aldosterone, the hormonal modulator of collecting-duct K^+ secretion. In addition, a normal K^+ excretory capacity obviously requires a normal number of intact, functional nephron units, usually reflected clinically by the glomerular filtration rate. Abnormalities in any of these components of the K^+ excretory system lead to impaired renal regulation. Overt hyperkalemia, except with extreme renal failure, is frequently not evident until more than one component of the system is disordered.

Drug-induced hyperkalemia can result from agents that cause hypoaldosteronism and those which directly impede K^+ secretion by acting on the renal tubule itself. Interference with normal aldosterone production has been described at virtually every step of the renin–angiotensin–aldosterone axis. The specific drugs implicated and their site of action are outlined in Table 2.

Drug-Induced Hypoaldosteronism

Prostaglandin Synthetase Inhibitors (Indomethacin)

Since the original reports in 1979, a variety of publications have documented that indomethacin, as well as other prostaglandin synthetase inhibitors, can produce clinically significant hyperkalemia (6,21,25,31-34,60). Many of the patients reported with this complication have had glomerulonephritis (31-34,60); however, patients with arthritis of various types (rheumatoid, gout, meningococcal) some of whom did not have evidence of underlying renal disease, have also developed hyperkalemia during therapy with indomethacin (6,21,25).

Prostaglandins, specifically PGE_2 and PGI_2 (prostacyclin), are known stimulators of renin secretion. In most reports indomethacin-induced hyperkalemia has been accompanied by a decrease in renin and aldosterone levels, along with a reduction in urinary potassium excretion (6,21,25,32-34,60). Thus it appears that protoglandin synthetase inhibition can result in hypoaldosteronism mediated through prostaglandin-related inhibition of renin secretion. Hence prostaglandin synthetase inhibitors seem capable of producing a drug-induced form of the syndrome of hyporeninemic hypoaldosteronism.

Table 2 Hyperkalemia Secondary to Hypoaldosteronism

Drug	Mechanism
Prostaglandin synthetase inhibitors (indomethacin)	↓PRA
Angiotensin-converting enzyme inhibitor (captopril)	↓A_{II}
Heparin	↓Aldosterone biosynthesis
Cyclosporine	↓PRA (?) tubular effect

In addition to producing hypoaldosteronism, prostaglandin synthetase inhibition can also decrease the glomerular filtration rate (GFR) and diminish sodium delivery to the distal nephron, especially in patients with diminished actual or effective extracellular fluid volume. These effects might also play a role in impeding K^+ excretion and provoking hyperkalemia (21,33,60).

Based on the change in plasma K^+ in response to an acute KCl infusion in a single patient, it has been suggested that indomethacin may interfere with the cellular uptake of potassium (34). Since prostaglandin synthetase inhibition can impair pancreatic insulin release, drug-mediated insulin deficiency has been suggested as a potential mechanism. However, neither the possibility of a defect in cellular K^+ uptake nor its putative underlying mechanism has undergone rigorous examination.

Angiotensin-Converting Enzyme Inhibitor (Captopril)

A variety of studies have documented an increase in serum potassium levels in patients with either hypertension or congestive heart failure, who are treated with captopril (3,17, 37,40,43,61,64). Patients with reduced renal function and those receiving potassium supplements are at risk for the development of serious hyperkalemia (17,40,61,64).

Captopril-mediated hyperkalemia results from the drug-induced decline in aldosterone levels. Since its predominant pharmacological effect is inhibition of angiotensin-converting enzyme, angiotensin II levels are decreased with a resultant decrease in aldosterone (3,64, 68). In contrast to the syndrome of hyporeninemic hypoaldosteronism (SHH); however, PRA is increased during therapy with captorpil.

Heparin

Despite its widespread use, only a few cases of heparin-induced hyperkalemia have been reported (46,68). However, in a recent study of hospitalized patients, it was estimated that 8% of the patients who receive heparin develop hyperkalemia (50).

The mechanism appears to relate to a direct effect of heparin on the adrenal gland to produce hypoaldosteronism (46,49). A recent study in normal human volunteers showed that aldosterone production is depressed substantially with dosages of heparin as low as 10,000 units/day (51). Studies both in animals and in humans have demonstrated reduction in the width of the zona glomerulosa with heparin administration (46,68). The findings of slightly reduced levels of corticosterone along with subnormal levels of 18-hydroxycorticosterone and aldosterone suggest that heparin may impair aldosterone biosynthesis by inhibition of the enzyme 18-hydroxylase (46).

Cyclosporine

Hyperkalemia has recently been described in renal and cardiac transplant recipients treated with the newly released immunosuppressive agent, cyclosporine (1,18,22). In the most detailed report, the majority of hyperkalemic renal transplant recipients appeared to have low renin and aldosterone levels, suggesting that cyclosporine might cause a drug-induced form of hyporeninemic hypoaldosteronism. However low PRA levels have not been a uniform finding, the drug does not cause renin suppression in animals, and it has known toxic effects on the renal tubule (1,22,52). In view of these observations, the possibility that cyclosporine inhibits K^+ secretion by a direct effect on the renal tubule cannot be discounted. Further studies are clearly needed to elucidate the mechanism of cyclosporine-induced hyperkalemia.

Table 3 Potassium-Sparing Diuretics

Drug	Mechanism
Spironolactone	Aldosterone receptor antagonist
Triamterene	?
Amiloride	Na channel blocker and Na/H exchange inhibitor

Potassium-Sparing Diuretics

Several drugs, which fall under the broad classification of potassium-sparing diuretics, directly interact with the cortical collecting duct to impede potassium secretion. These agents, listed in Table 3, are all also mildly natriuretic. Therapy with this class of drugs represents one of the major causes of hyperkalemia (50).

Spironolactone

This drug is an aldosterone antagonist. It competes with the mineralocorticoid for its receptor and thereby blocks the mineralocorticoid effect on the distal tubule as well as in other aldosterone-responsive tissues (14). Hyperkalemia results, as it does with low circulating levels of aldosterone, and is likely to be accentuated by similar factors.

Triamterene

This diuretic inhibits K^+ secretion by an aldosterone-independent action that has not been precisely delineated.

Amiloride

This diuretic also impairs K^+ secretion by an aldosterone-independent action. While it is a specific inhibitor of the Na–H exchanger in a variety of cells, its effect on K^+ secretion at distal nephron sites relates primarily to blockade of the luminal sodium channel with a concurrent reduction in transtubular voltage (5). The reduced transtubular potential difference impedes both potassium and hydrogen ion secretion.

As might be anticipated, patients with impaired renal function, those receiving concurrent potassium supplements, and patients with other defects in their K^+ regulatory system, especially diabetics, are more prone to develop hyperkalemia during therapy with K^+-sparing diuretics. All of these settings should be viewed as contraindications to the use of these drugs. However, it is important to be aware that significant hyperkalemia can occur in the presence of normal glomerular filtration rates and even when diuretics that promote K^+ wastage are ingested simultaneously with K^+-sparing agents (13,20,50,63,65).

SUMMARY

This chapter has reviewed the currently identified drug interactions that can result in hyperkalemia. In terms of their mechanism of action, they fall into two broad categories: (a) drug-induced hyperkalemia due to a redistribution of K^+ from the intracellular to extracellular compartment, and (b) drug-induced impairment of renal potassium excretion. It is important for the clinician to be aware of all these drug-induced defects in K^+ homeostasis to avoid precipitating severe hyperkalemia in patients already predisposed because of existing abnormalities in their K^+ regulatory defenses. Furthermore it should be appreciated that combinations of drugs that impair K^+ regulation significantly increase the risks of serious hyperkalemia.

REFERENCES

1. Adu, D., Turney, J., Michael, J., and McMaster, P.: Hyperkalaemia in cyclosporin-treated renal allograft recipients. *Lancet* 2:370–372, 1966.
2. Ammon, R. A., May, W. S., and Nightingale, S. D.: Glucose-induced hyperkalemia with normal aldosterone levels. *Ann. Intern. Med.* 89:349–351, 1978.
3. Atlas, S. A., Case, D. B., Sealey, J. E., Laragh, J. H., and McKinstry, D. N.: Interruption of the renin-angiotensin system in hypertensive patients by captopril induces sustained reduction in aldosterone secretion, potassium retention and natriuresis. *Hypertension* 1:274–280, 1979.
4. Bauer, J. H.: Effects of propranolol therapy on renal function and body fluid composition. *Arch. Intern. Med.* 143:927, 1983.
5. Benos, D. J.: Amiloride: A molecular probe of sodium transport in tissues and cells. *Am. J. Physiol.* 242:C131–C145, 1982.
6. Beroniade, V., Corneille, L., and Haraoui, B.: Indomethacin-induced inhibition of prostaglandin with hyperkalemia. *Ann. Intern. Med.* 90:499–500, 1979.
7. Bourke, D. L., and Rosenberg, M.: Changes in total serum Ca^{++}, Na^+, and K^+ with administration of succinylcholine. *Anesthesiology* 49:361–363, 1978.
8. Brooke, M. M., Donovon, W. H., and Stolov, W. C.: Paraplegia: Succinylcholine-induced hyperkalemia and cardiac arrest. *Arch. Phys. Med. Rehabil.* 59:306–309, 1978.
9. Brown, M. J., Brown, D. C., and Murphy, M. B.: Hypokalemia from beta$_2$-receptor stimulation by circulating epinephrine. *N. Engl. J. Med.* 309:1414–1419, 1983.
10. Buchinsky, D. A., and Gennari, F. J.; Life-threatening hyperkalemia induced by arginine. *Ann. Intern. Med.* 89:632–634, 1983.
11. Carlsson, E., Fellenius, E., Lundborg, P., and Svensson, L.: Beta-adrenoceptor blockers, plasma-potassium, and exercise. *Lancet* 2:424–425, 1978.
12. Clausen, T., and Flatman, J. A.: Beta$_2$-adrenoceptors mediate the stimulating effect of adrenaline on active electrogenic Na-K-transport in rat soleus muscle. *Br. J. Pharmacol.* 68:749–755, 1980.
13. Cohen, A. B.: Hyperkalemic effect of triamterene. *Ann. Intern. Med.* 65:651–527, 1966.
14. Corvol, P., Claire, M., Oblin, M. E., Geering, K., and Rossier, B.: Mechanism of the antimineralocorticoid effects of spironolactones. *Kidney Int.* 20:1–6, 1981.
15. DeFronzo, R. A., Bia, M., and Birkhead, G.: Epinephrine and potassium homeostasis. *Kidney Int.* 20:83-91, 1981.
16. Dickerman, H. W., and Walker, W. G.: Effect of cationic amino acid infusion on potassium metabolism in vivo. *Am. J. Physiol.* 206:403–408, 1964.
17. Dzau, V. J., Colucci, W. S., Williams, G. H., Curfman, G., Meggs, L., and Hollenberg, N. K.: Sustained effectiveness of converting-enzyme inhibition in patients with severe congestive heart failure. *N. Engl. J. Med.* 302:1373–1379, 1980.
18. Egel, J., Thompson, M. E., Hardesty, R. L., Griffith, B. P., Bahnson, H. T., Bernstein, R. L., and Puschett, J. B.: Renal failure in heart transplant patients receiving cyclosporine. *Transplant. Proc. 15* (Suppl. 1):2706–2707, 1983.
19. Ericsson, F., Carlmark, B., Jogestrand, T., and Sundqvist, K.: Effect of digoxin upon intracellular potassium in man. *Scand. J. Clin. Lab. Invest.* 41:457–463, 1981.
20. Feinfeld, D. A., and Carvounis, C. P.: Fatal hyperkalemia and hyperchloremic

acidosis. Association with spironolactone in the absence of renal impairment. *JAMA* 240:1516, 1978.

21. Findling, W., Beckstrom, D., Rawsthorne, L., Kozin, and Itskovitz, M.: Indomethacine-induced hyperkalemia in three patients with gouty arthritis. *JAMA* 244:1127–1128, 1980.
22. Foley, R. J., Van Buren, C. T., Hammer, R., and Weinmann, E. J.: Cyclosporine-associated hyperkalemia. *Transplant. Proc.* 15 (Suppl. 1):2726–2729, 1983.
23. Goldfarb, S., Cox, M., Singer, I., and Goldberg, M.: Acute hyperkalemia induced by hyperglycemia: hormonal mechanisms. *Ann. Intern. Med.* 84:426–432, 1976.
24. Goldfarb, S., Strunk, B., Singer, I., and Goldberg, M.: Paradoxical glucose-induced hyperkalemia. Combined aldosterone–insulin deficiency. *Am. J. Med.* 59:744–749, 1975.
25. Goldszer, R. C., Coodley, E. L., Rosner, M. J., Simons, W. M., and Schwartz, A. B.: Hyperkalemia associated with indomethacin. *Arch. Intern. Med.* 141:802–804, 1981.
26. Gravlee, G. P.: Succinylcholine-induced hyperkalemia in a patient with Parkinson's disease. *Anesth. Analg.* 59:444–446, 1980.
27. Hertz, P., and Richardson, J. A.: Arginine-induced hyperkalemia in renal failure patients. *Arch. Intern. Med.* 130:778–780, 1972.
28. Ho-Yen, D. O., and Pennington, C. R.: Pseudohyperkalemia and infectious mononucleosis. *Postgrad. Med. J.* 56:435–436, 1980.
29. Jauchem, J. R., and Vick, R. L.: Phenyleprine-induced hyperkalemia: Role of the liver. *Proc. Soc. Exp. Biol. Med.* 162:207–210, 1979.
30. Karlberg, B. E., Kagedal, B., Tegler, L., Tolagen, K., and Bergman, B.: Controlled treatment of primary hypertension with propranolol and spironolactone. A cross-over study with special reference to initial plasma renin activity. *Am. J. Cardiol.* 37:642–649, 1976.
31. Kimberly, R. P., Bowden, R. E., Keiser, H. R., and Plotz, P. H.: Reduction of renal function by newer nonsteroidal anti-inflammatory drugs. *Am. J. Med.* 64:804–807, 1978.
32. Kutyrina, I. N., Androsova, S. O., and Tareyera, I. E.: Indomethacin-induced hyporeninemic hypoaldosteronism. *Lancet* 1:785, 1979.
33. Kutyrina, I. M., Androsova, S. O., Warshavskii, V. A., and Tareyeva, I. E.: Effects of indomethacin on the renal function and renin-aldosterone system in chronic glomerulonephritis. *Nephron* 32:244–248, 1982.
34. MacCarthy, E. P., Frost, G. W., and Stokes, G. S.: Indomethacin-induced hyperkalemia. *Med. J. Aust.* 1:550, 1979.
35. Makoff, D. L., Sa Silva, J. A., and Rosenbaum, B. J.: On the mechanism of hyperkalemia due to hyperosmotic expansion with saline or mannitol. *Clin. Sci.* 41:383–393, 1971.
36. Makoff, D. L., Da Silva, J. A., Rosenbaum, B. J., Levy, S. E., and Maxwell, M. E.: Hypertonic expansions: Acid–base and electrolyte changes. *Am. J. Physiol.* 218:1201–1207, 1970.
37. Maslowski, A. H., Ikram, H., Nicholls, M., Espiner, E. E., Turner, J. G.: Hemodynamic, hormonal, and electrolyte responses to captopril in resistant heart failure. *Lancet* 1:71–74, 1981.
38. Massara, F., Caliero, E., Bisbocci, D., Passarino, G., Carta, Q., and Molinatti, G. M.: The risk of pronounced hyperkalaemia after arginine infusion in the diabetic subject. *Diabete Metab.* 7:149–153, 1981.
39. Massara, F., Martelli, S., Cagliero, E., Camanni, F., and Molinatti, G. M.: The hypophosphatemic and hyperkalemic effect of arginine in man. *J. Endocrinol. Invest.* 3:177–180, 1979.

40. Matson, J. R., Norby, L. H., and Robillard, J. E.: Interaction of minoxidil and captopril in the treatment of refractory hypertension. *Am. J. Dis. Child.* 135:256–258, 1981.
41. Moreno, M., Murphy, C., and Goldsmith, C.: Increase in serum potassium resulting from the administration of hypertonic mannitol and other solutions. *J. Lab. Clin. Med.* 73:291–298, 1969.
42. Nicolis, G. L., Kahn, T., Sanchez, A., and Gabrilove, J. L.: Glucose-induced hyperkalemia in diabetic subjects. *Arch. Intern. Med.* 141:49–53, 1981.
43. Nicholls, M. G., Espiner, E. A., Ikram, H., Maslowski, A. H., Lyn, S., and Scandrett, M. S. Angiotensin II is more potent than potassium in regulating aldosterone in cardiac failure: evidence during captopril therapy. *J. Clin. Endocrinol. Metab.* 52: 1253–1256, 1981.
44. Pedersen, G., Pedersen, A., and Pedersen, E. G.: Effect of propranolol on total exchangeable body potassium and total exchangeable body sodium in essential hypertension. *Scand. J. Clin. Lab. Invest.* 39:167–170, 1979.
45. Pedersen, E. B., and Kornerup, H. J.: Relationship between plasma aldosterone concentration and plasma potassium in patients with essential hypertension during alprenolol treatment. *Acta Med. Scand.* 200:263–267, 1976.
46. Phelps, K. R., Oh, M. S., and Carroll, H. J.: Heparin-induced hyperkalemia: report of a case. *Nephron* 25:254–258, 1980.
47. Rao, T. L. K., and Shanmugam, M.: Succinylcholine administration—another contraindication? *Anesth. Analg.* 58:61–62, 1979.
48. Rosa, R. M., Silva, P., Young, J. B., Landsberg, L., Brown, R. S., Rowe, J. W., and Epstein, J. H.: Adrenergic modulation of extrarenal potassium disposal. *N. Engl. J. Med.* 302:431–434, 1980.
49. Schlatmann, R. J. A. F. M., Jansen, A. P., Prenen, H., Van der Korst, J. D., and Majoor, C. L. H.: The nutriuretic and aldosterone-suppressive action of heparin and some polysulfated polysaccharides. *J. Clin. Endocrinol. Metab.* 24:35–47, 1964.
50. Shemer, J., Modan, M., Ezra, D., and Cabili, S.: Incidence of hyperkalemia in hospitalized patients. *Isr. J. Med. Sci.* 19:659–661, 1983.
51. Sherman, R. A., and Ruddy, M. C.: Suppression of aldosterone (A) production by low dose heparin (H). *Abstr. Am. Soc. Nephrol.* 16:39A, 1983.
52. Siegel, H., Ryffel, B., Petric, H., Shoemaker, P., Muller, A., Donatsch, P., and Mitash, P.: Cyclosporine, the renin-angiotensin-aldosterone system, and renal adverse reactions. *Transplant. Proc. 15* (Suppl. 1):2719–2725, 1983.
53. Silva, P., and Spokes, K.: Sympathetic system in potassium homeostasis. *Am. J. Physiol.* 241:F151–155, 1981.
54. Smith, T. W., Butler, V. P. Jr., Haber, E., Fozzard, H., Marcus, F. I., Brenner, W. F., Schulman, I. C., and Phillips, A.: Treatment of life-threatening digitalis intoxication with digoxin-specific Fab antibody fragments. *N. Engl. J. Med.* 307:1357–1362, 1982.
55. Sterns, R. H., Fieg, P. U., and Singer, I.: Internal potassium balance and the control of the plasma potassium concentration. *Medicine* 60:339–354, 1981.
56. Sterns, R. H., Izzo, J. L. Jr., Thomas, D., Turgeon, K.: Control of the plasma (K^+) in hyperkalemia. Role of α and β adrenoreceptors. *Clin. Res.* 32:457A, 1984.
57. Stewart, G. W., Corrall, R. J. M., Fyffe, J. A., Stockdill, G., and Strong, J. A. Familial pseudohyperkalemia: A new syndrome. *Lancet* 2:175–177, 1979.
58. Struthers, A. D., Reid, J. L., Whitesmith, R., and Rodger, J. C.: The effects of cardioselective and non-selective β-adrenoceptor blockade on the hypokalemic and cardiovascular responses to adrenomedullary hormones in man. *Clin. Sci.* 65:143–147, 1982.
59. Sunderlin, F. S., Jr., Anderson, G. H. Jr., Streeten, H. P., and Blumenthal, S. A.:

The renin–angiotensin–aldosterone system in diabetic patients with hyperkalemia. *Diabetes* 30:335–340, 1981.

60. Tan, S. Y., Shapiro, R., Franco, R., Stockard, H., and Mulrow, P. J.: Indomethacin-induced prostaglandin inhibition with hyperkalemia. *Ann. Intern. Med.* 90:783–785, 1979.
61. Textor, S. C., Bravo, E. L., Fouad, F. M., and Tarazi, R. C.: Hyperkalemia in azotemic patients during angiotensin-converting enzyme inhibition and aldosterone reduction with captopril. *Am. J. Med.* 73:719–725, 1982.
62. Traub, Y. M., Rabinov, M., Rosenfeld, J. B., and Treuherz, S.: Elevation of serum potassium during beta blockade: Absence of relationship to the renin–aldosterone system. *Clin. Pharmacol. Ther.* 28:765–768, 1980.
63. Wan, H. H., and Lye, M. D. W.: Moduretic-induced metabolic acidosis and hyperkalemia. *Postgrad. Med. J.* 56:348–350, 1980.
64. Warren, S. E., and O'Connor, D. T.: Hyperkalemia resulting from captopril administration. *JAMA* 244:2551–2552, 1980.
65. Whiting, G. F. M., Mclaran, C. J., and Bochner, F.: Severe hyperkalemia with moduretic. *Med. J. Aust.* 1:409, 1979.
66. Williams, M. E., Rosa, R. M., Gervino, E. V., Silva, P., Brown, R. S., and Epstein, F. H.: Alpha-adrenergic modulation of potassium homeostasis. *Clin. Res.* 32:460A, 1984.
67. Williams, M. E., Spokes, K., and Silva, P.: Alpha-adrenergic agents impair extrarenal potassium disposal. *Clin. Res.* 32:536A, 1984.
68. Wilson, I. D., and Goetz, F. C.: Selective hypoaldosteronism after prolonged heparin administration. *Am. J. Med.* 36:635–640, 1964.

CONTINUING CONTROVERSIES

39

Are Physicians Obsessed with the Treatment of Hypokalemia?

JOHN T. HARRINGTON
New England Medical Center Hospital and Tufts University School of Medicine, Boston, Massachusetts

BACKGROUND

I have been involved in the controversy regarding the appropriateness of routine potassium supplementation in hypertensive patients receiving diuretics since the late 1970s. At that time, Kassirer and I reviewed the literature on the effect of diuretics on potassium metabolism for a symposium on potassium in *Kidney International* (8). When I began that analysis, I shared the same bias that most nephrologists of my generation had at the time: that virtually all patients receiving diuretic therapy required additional potassium, usually given as an organic potassium salt and not as potassium chloride.

This review was written before the current controversy regarding the *possible* predisposition to serious arrhythmias in hypokalemic patients. We concluded then that "Neither potassium-sparing diuretics nor potassium supplementation should be given routinely . . . to the nonedematous patient treated with diuretics." That conclusion was based on the following data, that are still valid and important as background to today's argument regarding arrhythmias.

1. Most nonedematous patients receiving thiazide diuretics have a decline in serum potassium concentration, ranging from 0.3 to 1.2 mEq/L. Values less than 3.0 mEq/L are unusual and occur in less than 5% of patients. The majority of patients receiving diuretics have serum potassium concentrations between 3.3 and 3.7 mEq/L.
2. Total body potassium content is either not different from control or less than 200 mEq below control in the vast majority of nonedematous patients receiving thiazides. Such a reduction in body potassium content, if it exists at all, is at the threshold of sensitivity of the radioisotope techniques used.
3. Standard therapy with oral potassium supplements often is inadequate and ineffective in restoring serum potassium levels to normal. In one representative study, a substantial minority of patients remained hypokalemic despite receiving up to 100 of potassium/day (20).
4. Finally, the risks, albeit small (such as hyperkalemia and small-bowel ulcerations), recently raised even with the wax matrix preparations (13)) and costs of the proposed treatment (both psychic and dollar costs) are rarely included in the cost-benefit equation.

PRESCRIPTIONS FOR POTASSIUM

You ask if I feel that U.S. physicians are obsessed with the need to treat hypokalemia. (I might add that this title was adapted from the title of our recent editorial, which I will discuss shortly, but you should know that the title was assigned to me by the Brothers Whelton!) Let me give you some facts regarding potassium prescribing and you decide if we are obsessed with (or even possessed by) prescribing potassium. The number of prescriptions for oral potassium supplements increased approximately 25%/year during the years 1976–1980. The cost of potassium replacement and potassium-sparing diuretics now approaches $250 million per year. CIBA, manufacturer of Slow-K, the most widely prescribed potassium chloride capsule, has a classic full-page ad, which states that "if pennies were Slow-K, patients are up to $9,361,240." CIBA states in the same ad that between 1975 and 1981, 7.3 million patients were treated with Slow-K and in 1982 alone an additional 2 million patients were treated. Since both the proponents of and the skeptics about routine potassium supplementation therapy agree that the potassium ingested daily is quantitatively excreted daily in the urine, I must reluctantly conclude that we are "poisoning" the ground water of the United States with recycled potassium.

FREQUENCY OF ARRHYTHMIA

Round II of the hypokalemia debate was summarized in an editorial that Drs. Kassirer, Isner, and I wrote in 1982 (6). In that paper, we reviewed the frequency of arrhythmia in hypokalemic patients in the best 17 studies then available. Table 1 of that 1982 paper details the problems in design in those studies. Using a number of different criteria we made the following conclusions.

1. Adequate documentation of the *temporal relationship* between serum potassium measurements and arrhythmias was available in only 4 of the 17 studies.
2. In only 1 of the 17 studies were other potential causes of arrhythmias excluded, such as digitalis. Since our editorial, Ruskin et al. have pointed out that quinidine has the ability to provoke arrhythmias in a small, but significant, subset of patients (19). Few of the retrospective studies of arrhythmias associated with hypokalemia provide information regarding the utilization of such "antiarrhythmic" drugs.
3. In the three studies that did demonstrate a reduction in ventricular ectopic activity after serum potassium was restored to normal, multiple 24-hr recordings (pre- and postcorrection) were not obtained.
4. No fatality from diuretic-induced hypokalemia was documented.
5. In regard to arrhythmias in patients who were hypokalemic and experienced acute myocardial infarction:
    a. There were problems of lack of documentation of timing between the arrhythmia and the measurement of serum potassium.
    b. The fact that many resuscitative measures commonly employed (e.g., administration of glucose and insulin, bicarbonate and epinephrine), can lower serum potassium levels was not taken into account.

Before returning to more recent data, I'd like to point out again, as I have in the past (6), that we must consider factors that predispose to hyperkalemia and the risks of hyperkalemia as well as the risks of hypokalemia. Table 1 lists several factors that are known to predispose to hyperkalemia, including advancing age, impaired renal function, diabetes,

Table 1 Factors that Predispose to Hyperkalemia

Age
Impaired renal function
Diabetes
Hypoaldosteronism
Catabolism
High potassium intake
Certain drugs

hypoaldosteronism, catabolism, high potassium intake, and the ingestion of a number of drugs. Table 2 lists the drugs in common use that predispose to hyperkalemia, including potassium supplements, salt substitutes (some of which are pure potassium chloride), potassium-sparing diuretics, indomethacin, captopril, heparin, and beta-adrenergic blocking agents.

The risks of potassium treatment in inpatients have been reviewed by The Boston Collaborative Drug Surveillance Program (9). I stress that these are *inpatient* data; good data on the relative risk of hyperkalemia in the outpatient setting are not available. In that inpatient study, 16,000 consecutive patients in 12 hospitals across the world were studied prospectively. Forty-nine hundred received potassium chloride; in 87%, KCl was given for *prophylaxis* and not for *treatment* of established hypokalemia. Nineteen hundred and ten patients received oral potassium supplements only. Hyperkalemia occurred in 176 such treated patients. Life-threatening reactions occurred in 10 and 7 patients died from hyperkalemia. The risk of hyperkalemia from oral potassium treatment in this setting is therefore approximately 1:100; the risk of death is approximately 1:250. The relative risk of death from chloramphenicol is 1:20,000–50,000. The same Boston Collaborative Drug Surveillance Program compiled similar information regarding spironolactone, the classic potassium-sparing diuretic, and found a 9% incidence of hyperkalemia (5).

Since our 1982 editorial (6), a number of studies have reexplored the issue of arrhythmias in diuretic-treated hypokalemic patients. Five of these studies have shown no increased incidence of arrhythmias in hypokalemic patients. Papademetriou et al. (18)

Table 2 Drugs that Predispose to Hyperkalemia

Potassium supplements
chloride
acetate, bicarbonate, and citrate (triplex)
gluconate
Salt substitutes
Potassium-sparing diuretics
spironolactone
triamterene
amiloride
Indomethacin
Captopril
Heparin
Beta-adrenergic blocking agents

showed that correction of hypokalemic did not significantly alter the occurrence of ventricular ectopy in 16 patients with uncomplicated hypertension and diuretic-induced hypokalemia (see Chapter 21).

The Medical Research Council Working Party reported their analysis on the relationship between ventricular ectopy and thiazide treatment (14). Ninety-one patients with mild hypertension, randomly assigned to receive thiazide diuretics with potassium supplements, thiazide diuretics without potassium supplements, or placebo therapy satisfactorily completed 24-hr EKG monitoring before and after 9-10 weeks of treatment. Analysis of the data revealed no significant increase in ventricular ectopy in any group. Dr. Paul Whelton, involved in some aspects of this study, reviews his interpretation of these data in Chapter 20. Two abstracts also have been published recently, one by Caralis et al. (11) and one by Lief et al. (10) demonstrating that their patients with uncomplicated hypertension did not experience any change in ventricular ectopy following diuretic-induced hypokalemia.

In the fifth and finaly study, Drs. John Madias, Nicolaos Madias, and Harry Gavras from Mt. Sinai School of Medicine, Tufts University School of Medicine, and the Boston University School of Medicine, respectively, intensively studied twenty patients with uncomplicated hypertension (11). Ambulatory EKG monitoring (using two-channel recorders), before and after 1 month of therapy with hydrochlorothiazide, was carried out. Serum potassium levels were 4.4 ± 0.09 mEq/L pretreatment and 3.0 ± 0.06 mEq/L after 4 weeks of hydrochlorothiazide. Sixteen patients with no arrhythmias prior to therapy did not develop arrhythmias as a result of diuretic-induced hypokalemia of 1 month's duration. In the four patients with low-grade ventricular ectopy prior to therapy, there was no progress to higher grades of ventricular ectopy. The reasons for the conflicting results between these five studies and the study by Holland and his colleagues (7) are not clear.

OTHER CAUSES OF HYPOKALEMIA

Before concluding with some preliminary information from studies the Renal Lab at New England Medical Center is carrying out in collaboration with Dr. Jeremy Ruskin and his colleagues in the Electrophysiological Laboratory at the Massachusetts General Hospital, let me briefly comment on the *genesis* of hypokalemia in the patient with acute myocardial infarction. We need to ask how much of the hypokalemia seen in the patient with acute myocardial infarction is actually due to chronic diuretic use and how much has a different pathogenesis.

In only a minority of such patients is the hypokalemia related to the use of diuretics. If you go back to the literature, an interesting observation is buried there. Daniell reported in 1971 that of five hypokalemic patients with acute myocardial infarction who had suffered arrhythmias, only one of the five had, in fact, been treated with diuretics (2). Second, Nordrehaug (17) looked at 1,035 patients with acute myocardial infarctions who had serum potassium measured and electrocardiographs done. There were 918 normokalemic patients and only 117 hypokalemic patients; thus, we are already down to only 11% of all patients with acute myocardial infarction being at increased risk because of hypokalemia. Nordrehaug noted that ventricular fibrillation and ventricular tachycardia were seen in 156 of the 918 normokalemic patients (17%) compared with 34 of 117 hypokalemic patients (29%). Data are given only for the 19 (of the 34) patients with ventricular fibrillation; and only 6 of these 19 patients had *diuretic*-induced hypokalemia.

Therefore, the data say that only 6 of 1,035 patients with acute myocardial infarction had ventricular fibrillation related to *diuretic-induced* hypokalemia. Nordrehaug himself says on page 175 of Supplement 647 of *Acta Medica Scandinavia* (1981) he did not know if the serum potassium measurements were obtained before or after glucose infusion! Such problems abound in the literature.

Dyckner examined 450 patients with acute myocardial infarctions who were admitted to a coronary care unit (3). Serum potassium levels were measured in 444; 15% were hypokalemic, which figure is in substantial accord with the 11% found by Nordrehaug. Of the hypokalemic patients, only 43% had been receiving diuretics. Thus, only 28 of the entire group of 444 patients with myocardial infarction had diuretic-induced hypokalemia. Dyckner could find no significant differences in the instance of ventricular ectopy and ventricular tachycardia in the first day in the coronary care unit between patients with and without hypokalemia.

In 1982 Morgan and Young analyzed patients admitted to hospital for a variety of disorders (16). Few had serum potassium levels less than 2.8 mEq/L; the incidence of such levels was 1.9%. In only 20 of the 70 hypokalemic patients were facts available regarding diuretic therapy, but in these 20 patients, only 5 had been treated with diuretics before admission to hospital. Plasma potassium returned to normal in 4 days even without treatment and the authors concluded that oral potassium did not help in replenishing the serum potassium. In an earlier article in the *British Medical Journal* in 1980, Morgan concluded that "the overall effect of diuretics on the frequency of hypokalemia was therefore small and the surprising finding was the high frequency of hypokalemia which was not due to diuretics and which could be regarded as acute hypokalemia" (15).

Finally, Thompson and Cobb have studied hypokalemia in patients who had been resuscitated from out-of-hospital ventricular fibrillation (21). They noted that the mean serum potassium level was substantially lower in resuscitated than in control patients, but that after resuscitation mean serum potassium was not significantly different in patients who had been taking diuretics and patients who had not. The genesis of this acute non-diuretic-associated hypokalemia in the patient with an acute myocardial infarction who has not been resuscitated is not totally clear, but acute catecholamine release probably plays a substantial role.

CURRENT STUDIES

Let me end by briefly reviewing studies we are carrying out in collaboration with Dr. Jeremy Ruskin and his associates at the Massachusetts General Hospital (4,12). Graded degress of potassium depletion and hypokalemia were produced in approximately 10-kg dogs in our laboratory and quantitative balance studies performed. Electrophysiological studies then were performed at the Massachusetts General Hospital, before and after production of acute myocardial infarction by standard techniques. Mild to moderate degrees of hypokalemia (plasma [K^+] 2.9 mEq/L; mean negative K^+ balance of 28 mEq) did not alter the ease of induction of ventricular fibrillation in the absence of ischemia, whereas profound hypokalemia did (plasma [K^+] 2.6 mEq/L; negative K^+ balance of 55 mEq). Ventricular tachycardia could not be induced in any dog. Even in the presence of acute ischemia (transmural, anteroapical myocardial infarction), mild hypokalemia and K^+ depletion did not increase the ease of inducing ventricular fibrillation. However, profound hypokalemia and moderate to severe K^+ depletion (plasma K^+ 2.6 mEq/L; mean negative

K^+ balance of 55 mEq) did significantly increase the risk of electrically induced ventricular fibrillation but not sustained ventricular tachycardia.

Given all this information, I would certainly consider administering potassium to any hypokalemic patient admitted with an acute myocardial infarction. But for long-term prophylaxis, I would prefer administering one aspirin a day rather than one Slow-K tablet per day. I remain skeptical about the efficacy of reducing the risk of myocardial infarction by mass treatment of our hypertensive population with potassium or K-sparing agents. Only a small fraction of patients with acute myocardial infarctions are hypokalemic and, in fact, most are hypokalemic from reasons other than diuretics. Treatment of acute myocardial infarction is still the obligation of the cardiologist and not the nephrologist.

REFERENCES

1. Carolis, P., Perez-Stable, E., Materson, B., and Rozanski, J.: Ventricular ectopy and diuretic-induced hypokalemia in hypertensive patients. *Clin. Res.* 29:832A, 1981 (abstr).
2. Daniell, H. W.: Arrhythmias in hypokalemia (letter). *N. Engl. J. Med.* 284:385, 1971.
3. Dyckner, T., Helmers, C., Lundman, T., and Webster, P. O.: Initial serum potassium level in relation to early complications and prognosis in patients with acute myocardial infarction. *Acta Med. Scand.* 197:207–210, 1975.
4. Garan, H., McGovern, B., McCauley, J., Yano, K., Ruskin, J. N., Madais, N., and Harrington, J. T.: Prior potassium depletion predisposes the heart to inducible ventricular fibrillation after myocardial infarction (abstr). American Heart Association's 57th Scientific Session, November, 1984.
5. Greenblatt, D. J., and Koch-Weser, J.: Adverse reactions to spironolactone. *JAMA* 225:40–43, 1973.
6. Harrington, J. T., Isner, J. M., and Kassirer, J. P.: Our national obsession with potassium. *Am. J. Med.* 73:155–159, 1982.
7. Holland, D. B., Nixon, J. V., and Huhnert, L. K.: Diuretic-induced ventricular ectopic activity. *Am. J. Med.* 70:762–768, 1981.
8. Kassirer, J. P., and Harrington, J. T.: Diuretics and potassium metabolism. A reassessment of the need, effectiveness and safety of potassium therapy. *Kidney Int.* 11: 505–515, 1977.
9. Lawson, D. H.: Adverse reactions to potassium chloride. *Q. J. Med.* 43:433–440, 1974.
10. Lief, P. D., Belizon, I., Matos, J., and Bank, N.: Diuretic-induced hypokalemia does not cause ventricular ectopy in uncomplicated essential hypertension. *Proc. Am. Soc. Nephrol.* 16:66A, 1983 (abstr).
11. Madias, J. E., Madias, N. E., and Gavras, H. P.: Evidence for the nonarrhythmogenecity of diuretic-induced hypokalemia in patients with uncomplicated hypertension. *Arch. Intern. Med.* xx:xx–xx, 198x.
12. McGovern, B., Madias, N., Ruskin, J. N., Bodvarsson, M., Canzanello, V., Harrington, J. T., and Garan, H.: Isolated graded depletion of body potassium and ventricular fibrillation (abstr). American Heart Association's 57th Scientific Sessions, November, 1984.
13. McMahon, F. G., Ryan, R. J., Akdamar, K., and Ertan, A.: Upper gastrointestinal lesions after potassium chloride supplements: A controlled clinical trial. *Lancet* 2: 1059–1061, 1982.
14. Medical Research Council Working Party on Mild to Moderate Hypertension:

Ventricular extrasystoles during thiazide treatment. Substudy of MRC mild hypertension trial. *Br. Med. J.* 287:1249–1253, 1983.

15. Morgan, D. B.: Hypokalemia and diuretics. In *Arrhythmias and Myocardial Infarction: The Role of Potassium.* Royal Society of Medicine International Congress and Symposium Series, Number 44. London, Academic Press, and the Royal Society of Medicine.
16. Morgan, D. B., and Young, R. M.: Acute transient hypokalaemia: New interpretation of a common event. *Lancet* 2:751–752, 1982.
17. Nordrehaug, J. E.: Malignant arrhythmias in relation to serum potassium values in patients with an acute myocardial infarction. *Acta Med. Scand.* (S)647:101–107, 1981.
18. Papademetriou, V., Fletcher, R., Khatri, I. M., and Freis, E. D.: Diuretic-induced hypokalemia in uncomplicated systemic hypertension: Effects of plasma potassium correction on cardiac arrhythmias. *Am. J. Cardiol.* 52:1017–1022, 1983.
19. Ruskin, J. N., McGovern, B., Garan, H., DiMarco, J. P., and Kelly, E.: Antiarrhythmic drugs: A possible cause of out-of-hospital cardiac arrest. *N. Engl. J. Med.* 309: 1302–1306, 1983.
20. Schwartz, A. B., and Swartz, C. D.: Dosage of potassium chloride elixir to correct thiazide-induced hypokalemia. *JAMA* 230:702–704, 1974.
21. Thompson, R. G., and Cobb, L. A.: Hypokalemia after resuscitation from out-of-hospital ventricular fibrillation. *JAMA* 248:2860–2863, 1982.

40

Are Physicians Undertreating Hypokalemia?

PHILIP A. POOLE-WILSON
The Cardiothoracic Institute and National Heart Hospital, London, England

The question of whether physicians should consider prophylactic measures to avoid hypokalemia when prescribing diuretics for the treatment of mild hypertension in otherwise healthy persons has been the subject of debate for more than 25 years. Controversy (1, 17,30,38,39,41) has reappeared because of new evidence regarding the effectiveness of treatment for mild hypertension (20,22); several reports on the putative link between arrhythmias, hypokalemia, and thiazide diuretic therapy (18,19,30,36); and a better understanding of the underlying physiology (3,7,43). The emphasis in the debate appears to be different in the United States and in the United Kingdom. In the United States it seems that physicians already take note of the possible dangers of thiazide-induced hypokalemia although some, such as Harrington et al. (17), are arguing against that policy. In the United Kingdom the position is almost the reverse. The British National Formulary for 1980 (5) stated "The majority of patients taking diuretics for hypertension or heart failure do not require potassium replacement therapy." This opinion has been challenged (38,39,41) and it has been argued that such a nihilistic approach is not appropriate in the face of more recent evidence. A small change in attitude has occurred. The National Formulary for 1984 (6) states "Potassium supplements are seldom necessary but plasma potassium concentration should be measured regularly. Potassium-sparing diuretics are usually not necessary in the routine treatment of hypertension unless hypokalaemia develops." The three essential facets of the argument are that hypokalemia can cause arrhythmias, that hypokalemia occurs with thiazide diuretics, and that some arrhythmias occurring in patients prescribed thiazide diuretics can be attributed to hypokalemia.

DOES HYPOKALEMIA CAUSE ARRHYTHMIAS?

The evidence that hypokalemia causes arrhythmias comes from both animal experiments and observations in patients (44). The experimental scientist has known for many years that if isolated hearts are perfused with solutions containing a low concentration of potassium, arrhythmias are frequent (10); it has become common practice to increase the potassium concentration in the perfusate to 5 mmol/L or above to avoid arrhythmias.

Numerous reports in the literature claim to show an association between hypokalemia and arrhythmias in patients. These have been reviewed by Harrington et al. (17) who put forward several criticisms of the published data: that often no firm temporal relationship has been established between the potassium concentration and the observed ventricular ectopic activity, that 24-hr recordings before and after potassium repletion have not been obtained so that some responses may be due to spontaneous variation in ventricular ectopic activity, that alternative causes for ventricular ectopic activity have not always been excluded, and finally that many of the patients were suffering from an acute myocardial infarction. Though all these criticisms have some validity they do not appear to me to have sufficient weight to counter the enormous body of evidence suggesting a direct association between hypokalemia and arrhythmias in humans.

In this context perhaps the most important evidence is the common observation that when an arrhythmia occurs in the presence of hypokalemia in patients soon after cardiac surgery or during acute myocardial infarction, the arrhythmia usually responds almost immediately to restoration of a normal plasma potassium concentration. It has for many years been common medical practice to measure the plasma potassium concentration when such arrhythmias occur and to take the necessary therapeutic action (44).

In patients with acute myocardial infarction, evidence linking hypokalemia to arrhythmias has been obtained (35). That hypokalemia is common in patients with myocardial infarction is not a new observation. It is tempting but probably erroneous to suggest that there is a direct and simple link between hypokalemia and the onset of the arrhythmia. During an acute myocardial infarction, urinary and plasma catecholamine levels increase and a rise of catecholamines is known to bring about a reduction in the plasma potassium due to a beta-2-stimulated uptake of potassium by skeletal muscle (4,7,43). Some patients, possibly those with larger myocardial infarctions, will have a greater sympathetic response and hence a lower plasma potassium level. These patients maybe more likely to sustain lethal arrhythmias. Thus, a relationship between the plasma potassium and arrhythmias in the context of acute myocardial infarction may exist merely because both are more common in patients with a substantial sympathetic response. The arrhythmia may be caused by increased sympathetic drive, hypokalemia, or many other factors. Though evidence is only just becoming available, it would be predicted from this argument that the plasma potassium level during a myocardial infarction would fall in relation to the rise of catecholamines in the plasma and subsequently return to normal. I would not, however, deny that hypokalemia is a factor in the initiation of arrhythmias during myocardial infarction. The extracellular potassium in ischemic muscle rapidly attains high concentrations, up to 10 mmol/L. If, in adjacent normally perfused tissue, the plasma potassium is falling due to a release of catecholamines, then large differences in resting membrane potential will exist between almost adjacent cells. Such heterogeneity within the myocardium is likely to lead to the generation of arrhythmias either on an ectopic basis or as a result of a reentry circuit. Another important consideration is that the plasma potassium level can rise and fall from moment to moment. After exercise the plasma potassium increases rapidly, and on cessation of exercise may fall by up to 2 mmol/L over a period of 1 min (25). After prolonged exercise, the plasma potassium level is reduced (8). A rapidly varying extracellular potassium concentration in normal myocardium adjacent to ischemic myocardium with a high extracellular potassium concentration will promote electrical instability. Two reports suggest that a high proportion of patients dying suddenly in the community have previously been hypokalemic (27,42).

The known electrophysiological effects of hypokalemia can account for the observed increased incidence of arrhythmias. A fall in the extracellular plasma concentration to 3 mmol/L causes the resting membrane potential of cardiac muscle to become more negative as would be predicted from the Nernst equation for the potassium equilibrium potential. Below 3.0 mmol/L, however, the membrane potential becomes less negative rather than the expected more negative, possibly due to an effect on the potassium conductance of the cell membrane (34). Hypokalemia of a mild degree also increases diastolic depolarization, increases the duration of the action potential and the refractory period, and increases the conduction velocity. The increased rate of diastolic depolarization in normal cells is such that despite any increased difference between the resting membrane potential and the threshold potential, the threshold voltage is reached sooner and an ectopic beat can be initiated. These effects may be more pronounced in diseased myocardial cells. Diastolic depolarization is usually absent in myocardial cells but can occur in the presence of ischemia. Such effects of a low extracellular potassium concentration are likely to cause arrhythmias as a result of both ectopic foci and reentry pathways. Two additional factors are (a) that the effect of hypokalemia on the action potential may not be homogeneous throughout the heart, and (b) that arrhythmias may be related not just to the mean value of plasma potassium but to the rate of change of plasma potassium. In the presence of hypokalemia larger transient changes of potassium in response to everyday activities such as exercise may occur.

DO THIAZIDE DIURETICS CAUSE HYPOKALEMIA?

Morgan and Davidson (32) reviewed the literature on the occurrence of hypokalemia in patients taking diuretics. The incidence appears to depend on patients' age and sex, the type of diuretic prescribed (loop or thiazide diuretic), and on the condition being treated (hypertension or heart failure). The incidence will also depend on the definition of hypokalemia and the validity of the method for obtaining blood and measuring the potassium concentration. The serum potassium level is known to be approximately 0.1 mmol/L higher than the plasma potassium concentration because of some degree of hemolysis of red cells. Since plasma or serum potassium levels can change rapidly, single measurements may not reflect the true mean resting value unless care is taken to avoid stress, venous occlusion, and muscle activity at the moment of venipuncture. Nevertheless, Morgan and Davidson (32) reported that in patients with hypertension treated with thiazides, 50% had a plasma potassium level below 3.5 mmol/L and in 7% it was below 3.0 mmol/L. In patients with heart failure given frusemide the figures are 5% and 0.2%, respectively. Such a prevalence may appear high to many physicians but the results have been confirmed by the Medical Research Council (MRC) study in the United Kingdom (31), in which the mean potassium concentration fell by 0.5 mmol/L from 4.1 to 3.6 mmol/L over a 3-year period. I would suggest that such a high prevalence of hypokalemia is not seen by many physicians because prophylactic measures have been taken to avoid hypokalemia. It has been claimed in a study of 53 patients that the metabolic consequences of diuretics have been exaggerated, but that study did use potassium supplementation (2).

If diuretics are known to induce hypokalemia and hypokalemia is known to be associated with arrhythmias, it is reasonable to ask how it was that physicians were advised that it was safe to prescribe thiazide diuretics without any form of potassium therapy. This advice arose from evidence in the mid-1970s showing that the total body potassium was altered either not at all or only to a minor degree (9,17,46). This is now known to be a fallacious argument because it supposes that the initiation of arrhythmias is a consequence of changes in the intracellular potassium concentration presumably of heart muscle or of conducting tissue in the heart. Many studies have shown that if gross potassium loss is induced by either diuretics or diet the plasma potassium concentration and the amount of potassium in skeletal muscle will fall but the amount of potassium in cardiac muscle remains unchanged (37,45). The reason appears to be that in cardiac muscle loss of potassium induces an increase in sodium pump sites (45). Diuretics in therapeutic concentrations have no effect on potassium exchange in heart muscle (40). Furthermore it can easily be deduced from the Nernst equation that a small change in the plasma potassium of, perhaps, 1 mmol/L has major electrophysiological effects on cardiac muscle, whereas a similar change in the intracellular plasma concentration has a negligible effect. For these reasons the measurement of total body potassium is almost irrelevant to the development of cardiac arrhythmias. Total body potassium may be important in other symptoms such as muscle weakness, tiredness, and effects on the central nervous system of hypokalemia. With regard to the heart, however, the plasma potassium is the key factor and is undoubtedly reduced by thiazide diuretics.

DO THIAZIDE DIURETICS CAUSE ARRHYTHMIAS AS A CONSEQUENCE OF HYPOKALEMIA?

To design an experiment in humans which would demonstrate that thiazide or loop diuretics caused hypokalemia and that the hypokalemia caused arrhythmias is almost impossible. Nevertheless recent evidence has established some associations. Two groups (18,19) have attempted to measure arrhythmias during exercise or by monitoring of the electrocardiogram over 24 hr in hypertensive patients before and after treatment with thiazide diuretics. Both studies demonstrated that ventricular arrhythmias were increased in incidence when the patients were hypokalemic. A third study (36) using 24-hr ambulatory monitoring of the electrocardiogram has also been published and was unable to confirm a significant association between hypokalemia and spontaneous ventricular ectopic activity. The numbers of patients in these studies were small (21, 38, and 16, respectively) and it is not always clear from what population the patients originated. In the third study (36) 14 of 16 patients were black. Beta-blockers were given as concurrent therapy in four patients and other drugs in five patients. A beta-blocker may suppress arrhythmias in the presence of hypokalemia.

The Medical Research Council has recently reported on the incidence of ventricular extrasystoles obtained by monitoring of the electrocardiogram in 324 patients who were taking part in the MRC mild hypertension trial (30). Included in the study were patients who had been on treatment for some time and new entrants to the study. The results did show that the serum potassium was related to extrasystolic counts when all patients were considered, that those on long-term thiazide diuretics had an increased incidence of ventricular ectopic beats, and that those on thiazides had an increased incidence of complex arrhythmias. Correlations were not found with the decrement in serum potassium and correlations in some small selected subgroups were also absent. The trial also showed a correlation between uric acid and arrhythmias which probably demonstrates only that the patients were taking the tablets since uric acid itself is not arrhythmic in the short term. The association of arrhythmias with plasma potassium was a good as that with plasma uric acid. The serum potassium level was only measured once in relation to the period of monitoring and no account was taken of the time of day or the relation to meals.

The authors of this trial concluded "The explanation of the association between thiazide treatment and ventricular extrasystolic activity therefore remains uncertain." What is not clear from this trial, however, is what the authors originally expected to find. Many factors contribute to the initiation of arrhythmias and thiazides are known to alter not only the serum potassium but also the magnesium concentration (11,19). If hypokalemia were an important cause of ventricular arrhythmias, I would have anticipated results almost identical to those reported by the Medical Research Council and would argue that this study provides strong evidence that diuretic-induced hypokalemia is linked to arrhythmias. It is impressive that the correlation between plasma potassium and arrhythmias was as good as that for uric acid, a presumed marker of the biological activity of the drug. Further support for this hypothesis comes from the MRFIT study (33) and from the Oslo study (24), although in the latter the number of patients was small. In the MRFIT study one reason put forward for the negative results of risk factor intervention was that patients with initial electrocardiographic abnormalities who were treated with thiazide diuretics had an increased incidence of sudden death.

CONCLUSION

Incontrovertible evidence that thiazide diuretics induce hypokalemia and thereby bring about an increased incidence of lethal arrhythmias will never be obtained. The reason is simple. If 1 million patients were treated with thiazide diuretics alone, half would have a plasma potassium level below 3.5 mmol/l and 70,000 would have a plasma potassium level below 3.0 mmol/l. If life-threatening arrhythmias occurred in 1:1,000 of those with a potassium level below 3.5 mmol/l and 1:250 of those with a potassium level below 3.0 mmol/L, then 780 patients would die annually. This represents 1:1,300 patients per annum. Thus the possibility exists that the small benefit of treating patients with mild hypertension (20,22) might be offset by the complications of thiazide diuretics. It is of note that the benefit of treating mild hypertension has been reported as between 1:400 and 1:1,000 patients treated per year (20,22). A trial to detect an effect of this size would need to include almost 500,000 patients and is unlikely ever to be undertaken. The assumptions in this calculation are not unreasonable since Greenblatt et al. (14) showed that in 2,397 patients in hospital receiving frusemide, 3.6% had hypokalemia and three had cardiac arrhythmias. Lowe et al. (26) obtained similar results. Five patients of 2,580 had a plasma potassium level below 2.5 mmol/L and three patients were considered to have life-threatening arrhythmias. Thus, in severely hypokalemic patients the incidence of life-threatening arrhythmias may be between 15% and 3%, well above the figure of 1:250 used in my calculation.

Physicians will have to make a judgement upon the basis of available evidence. I would argue that we should take more account of the potential risks of hypokalemia when assessing patients for treatment with thiazide diuretics and that physicians should prescribe the prophylactic treatment most appropriate for any individual patient. An important consideration in this regard is that any prophylactic treatment should not be more dangerous than the risk of hypokalemia. Several reports of problems with the use of potassium chloride or potassium-sparing diuretics (14,15,21,23,26,29) have been published but physicians are more selective today in choosing patients prescribed such

Table 1 Clinical Approach to Prevention and/or Treatment of Diuretic-Induced Hypokalemia

Low dosages of thiazides
Early identification of hypokalemic patients
Dietary modification
Potassium supplements
Combined thiazide and beta-blocker therapy
Combined thiazide and angiotensin-converting enzyme inhibitor therapy
Potassium-sparing diuretics

treatment. In the European trial of hypertension in the elderly (12) a potassium-sparing diuretic was used and the plasma potassium level was shown to remain almost constant over a 4-year period without any complications. Earlier reports of the dangers of using prophylactic measures to prevent hypokalemia I believe to have been exaggerated because of inappropriate prescribing.

Many options are available to the physician to avoid hypokalemia, some of which are shown in Table 1. Perhaps the easiest method is to prescribe a low dosage of thiazide diuretics, since this brings about the same fall of blood pressure as a higher dosage but is less likely to induce hypokalemia. Treatment with thiazides can have unforeseen costs (28). Another possibility is to increase the dietary intake of potassium. The average British diet contains 64 mmol potassium/24 hr. To bring about a substantial increase would require a large change in national habits. A fall in sodium intake may be as important or more important than an increase in potassium intake. Diets high in potassium tend to be expensive. The combination of a diuretic with a beta blocker (13) does reduce the incidence of hypokalemia as does the combination of a diuretic with angiotensin-converting enzyme inhibitors (16). A different approach is to measure the plasma or serum potassium level regularly and treat only those patients in whom hypokalemia develops. Such a policy requires close observation of patients and will increase costs. Potassium supplements have been used but are not entirely without complications (21,23, 29). Finally there is the possibility of using potassium-sparing diuretics.

In my opinion there is an overwhelming case for the fact that hypokalemia does cause arrhythmias in humans and that thiazide diuretics are associated with hypokalemia and an increased incidence of arrhythmias. With such evidence available it is prudent for physicians to take active measures to avoid hypokalemia in patients being prescribed thiazide diuretics.

REFERENCES

1. Beeley, L.: When do patients on diuretics need potassium replacement. *Adverse Drug Reaction Bulletin* 84:304–307, 1980.
2. Berglund, G., and Andersson, O.: Beta-blockers or diuretic in hypertension; A six year follow-up of blood pressure and metabolic side-effects. *Lancet* 1:744–747, 1981.
3. Bia, M. J., and Defronzo, R. A.: Extrarenal potassium homeostasis. *Am. J. Physiol.* 240:F257–68, 1981.
4. Brewer, G., Larson, P. S., and Schroeder, A. R.: On the effect of epinephrine on blood potassium. *Am. J. Physiol.* 126:708–712, 1939.
5. British National Formulary: 1981, page 67.

6. British National Formulary: 1984, page 83.
7. Brown, M. J., Brown, D. C., and Murphy, M. B.: Beta 2-receptor stimulation by circulating epinephrine causes prolonged hypokalemia. *N. Engl. J. Med.* 309:1414–19, 1983.
8. Corea, L., Bentivoglio, M., and Verdecchia, P.: Plasma potassium during exercise. *Lancet* II:1292, 1981.
9. Dargie, H. J., Boddy, K., Kennedy, A. C., King, P. C., Read, P. R., and Ward, D. M.: Total body potassium in long-term frusemide therapy: Is potassium supplementation necessary? *Br. Med. J.* 4:316–319, 1974.
10. Daugherty, A., Mohamed, O. Y., and Woodward, B.: Effects of potassium on coronary artery ligation induced ventricular arrhythmias in the isolated rat heart. *J. Physiol.* 340:66P, 1983.
11. Dyckner, T., and Wester, P. O.: In *Arrhythmias and Myocardial Infarction. The Role of Potassium,* edited by Wood, C. and Somerville, W., Royal Society of Medicine, International Congress and Symposium series. 44:43–46, 1981.
12. Fourth Interim Report of the European Working Party on High Blood Pressure in Elderly: Antihypertensive therapy in patients above age 60 years. *Clin. Sci. Mol. Med.* 55:2635–2705, 1978.
13. Gotzen, R., and Hiemstra, S.: Total body and serum potassium during treatment with atenolol in combination with chlorthalidone. *J. Int. Med. Res.* 9:292–294, 1981.
14. Greenblatt, D. J., Duhme, D. W., Allen, M. D., and Koch-Weser, J.: Clinical toxicity of frusemide in hospitalised patients. *Am. Heart J.* 94:6–13, 1977.
15. Green Blatt, D. J., and Koch-Weser, J.: Adverse reactions to spironolactone. *JAMA* 225:40–43, 1973.
16. Griffing, G. T., Sindler, B. H., Aurecchia, S. A., and Melby, J. C.: Reversal of diuretic-induced secondary hyperaldosteronism and hypokalaemia by enalapril (MK-421), a new angiotensin-converting enzyme inhibitor. *Metabolism* 32:711–716, 1983.
17. Harrington, J. T., Isner, J. M., and Kassirer, J. P.: Our national obsession with potassium. *Am. J. Med.* 73:155–59, 1982.
18. Holland, O. B., Nixon, J. V., and Kuhnert, L.: Diuretic-induced ventricular ectopic activity. *Am. J. Med.* 70(4):762–768, 1981.
19. Hollifield, J. W., and Slaton, P. E.: Cardiac arrhythmias associated with diuretic induced hypokalaemia and hypomagnesaemia. *Royal Society of Medicine, International Congress and Symposium.* Arrhythmias and Myocardial Infarction. The role of potassium. 44:17–24, 1981.
20. Five year findings of the Hypertension Detection and Follow-up Program: 1. Reduction in mortality of persons with high blood pressure, including mild hypertension. 11. Mortality by race sex and age. *J. of Am. Med. Association.*
21. Kassirer, J. P., and Harrington, J. T.: Diuretics and potassium metabolism: a reassessment of the need, effectiveness and safety of potassium therapy. *Kidney Int.* 11:505–515, 1977.
22. *Lancet*: Australian therapeutic trial in mild hypertension. 1:1261–1267, 1980.
23. Lawson, D. H.: Adverse reactions to potassium chloride. *Q. J. Med.* 43:433–440, 1974.
24. Leren, P., Helgeland, A., Hjermann, I., and Holme, I.: MRFIT and the Oslo study. *JAMA* 249:893–894, 1983.
25. Lim, M., Linton, R. A. F., Wolfee, C. B., and Band, D. M.: Arterialolol, exercise and plasma potassium. *Lancet* 2:591, 1981.
26. Lowe, J., Gray, J., Henry, D. A., and Lawson, D. H.: Adverse reactions to frusemide in hospital inpatients. *Br. Med. J.* 2:360–362, 1979.

27. Lown, B., Calvert, A. F., Armington, R., and Ryan, M.: Monitoring for serious arrhythmias and high risk of sudden death. *Circulation* Suppl II, 52:189–198, 1975.
28. McCarron, D. A.: Diuretic therapy for mild hypertension: The "real" cost of treatment. *Am. J. Cardiol.* 53:9A–11A, 1984.
29. McMahon, F. G., Ryan, J. R., Akdamar, K., and Ertan, A.: Upper gastrointestinal lesions after potassium chloride supplements: a controlled clinical trial. *Lancet* 2: 1059–1061, 1982.
30. Medical Research Council Working Party on Mild to Moderate Hypertension: Ventricular extrasystoles during thiazide treatment: Substudy of MRC mild hypertension trial. *Br. Med. J.* 287:1249–53, 1983.
31. Medical Research Council Working Party on Mild to Moderate Hypertension: Adverse reactions to bendrofluazide and propranolol for the treatment of mild hypertension. *Lancet* 2:539–543, 1981.
32. Morgan, D. B., and Davidson, C.: Hypokalaemia and diuretics: an analysis of publications. *Br. Med. J.* 1:905–908, 1980.
33. Multiple Risk Factor Intervention Trial Research Group: Multiple risk factor intervention trial. Risk factor changes and mortality results. *JAMA* 248:1465–1477, 1982.
34. Noble, D.: *The Initiation of the Heart Beat.* Oxford, Clarendon Press, 1979.
35. Nordrehaug, J. E., and Von der Lippe, G.: Hypokalaemia and ventricular fibrillation in acute myocardial infarction. *Br. Heart J.* 50:525–529, 1983.
36. Papademetriou, V., Fletcher, R., Khatri, I. M., and Freis, E. D.: Diuretic-induced hypokalaemia in uncomplicated systemic hypertension: Effect of plasma potassium correction on cardiac arrhythmias. *Am. J. Cardiol.* 52:1017–1022, 1983.
37. Poole-Wilson, P. A.: The myocardial cell membrane: the effect of diuretics. Royal Society of Medicine International Congress and Symposium Series. 44:9–16, 1981.
38. Poole-Wilson, P. A.: Hypokalaemia induced by thiazide diuretics in the treatment of hypertension: a cause for concern not nihilism. *Postgrad. Med. J.* Suppl III, 59:137–139, 1983.
39. Poole-Wilson, P. A.: Ventricular extrasystoles during thiazide treatment. *Br. Med. J.* 2:1798–1799, 1984.
40. Poole-Wilson, P. A., Cobbe, S. M., and Fry, C. H.: Acute effects of diuretics on potassium exchange, mechanical function and the action potential in rabbit myocardium. *Clin. Sci. Mol. Med.* 55:555–559, 1978.
41. Poole-Wilson, P. A., and Webb, S. C.: Hypokalaemia: Is it a wolf in sheep's clothing. *Internat. Med.* Suppl 4:4–6, 1983.
42. Salerno, D. M., Asinger, R. W., Mikell, F. L., Ruiz, E., and Hodges, M.: Hypokalaemia in out of hospital cardiac arrest. *Am. J. Cardiol.* 49:929–1982.
43. Struthers, A. D., Whitesmith, R., and Reid, J. L.: Prior thiazide diuretic treatment increases adrenaline-induced hypokalaemia. *Lancet* 1:1358–60, 1983.
44. Surawicz, B.: Role of electrolytes in etiology and management of cardiac arrhythmias. *Prog. Cardiovasc. Dis.* 8:364–386, 1966.
45. Ward, J. P. T., and Cameron, I. R.: Adaptation of the cardiac muscle sodium pump to chronic potassium deficiency. *Cardiovasc. Res.* 18:257–263, 1984.
46. Wilkinson, P. R., Issler, H., Hesp, R., and Raftery, E. B.: Total body and serum potassium during prolonged thiazide therapy for essential hypertension. *Lancet* 1:759–762, 1975.

41

First-Step Therapy of Essential Hypertension: The Advantages of Initial Diuretic Treatment

RAY W. GIFFORD, JR.
The Cleveland Clinic Foundation, Cleveland, Ohio

Contrary to the experience in some other countries, notably the United Kingdom and Scandinavia, physicians in the United States continue to prescribe diuretics preferentially as initial therapy in the stepped-care approach to the management of hypertension.

This is more than habit or tradition. Diuretics have most of the attributes of the ideal step-one drug (Table 1). In addition, their long-term hemodynamic effect is to reduce total peripheral vascular resistance without changing cardiac output, thereby correcting the usual abnormality seen in patients with essential hypertension, namely increased total peripheral vascular resistance with normal or reduced cardiac output.

The direct vasodilators hydralazine and minoxidil are not appropriate drugs to use for step one because without a sympathetic inhibiting drug in the regimen they induce reflex tachycardia and palpitations and without a diuretic in the regimen they cause considerable fluid retention.

Although it may be presumptuous to speculate on the cause of essential hypertension, experimental and epidemiological data strongly implicate a role for sodium in many cases (6,16,22,23). Before effective antihypertensive drugs were developed, extremely-low-sodium diets were shown to have a hypotensive effect. There is a direct relationship between average dietary sodium intake and the prevalence of hypertension in population groups (6,16). For any given inflow pressure, isolated perfused kidneys from Dahl salt-sensitive ("S") rats excrete sodium more slowly than isolated, perfused kidneys from Dahl-resistant ("R") rats, even before hypertension develops in the "S" rats (22). In addition, administration of a diuretic along with the high-sodium chow will prevent development of hypertension in "S" rats (23). Conceivably, therefore, oral diuretics may be more specific than any of the other antihypertensive agents, at least for patients whose hypertension seems to be sodium-dependent.

Table 1 Relative Merits of Antihypertensive Drugs for Step 1

Drugs	Efficacy as mono-therapy	Desirable hemo-dynamic effect	Low side effect profile	No pseudo-resistance	Long duration of action	Easy titration	Augments action of other drugs	Inexpensive	Safety	Few contra-indications	Total score
Diuretic	3	3	3	3	3	3	3	3	2	3	29
Beta blocker	3	0[a]	3	3	3	1[b]	2	1	2	1	19
Converting enzyme inhibitor	3	3	2	3	3[c]	2	2	0	2	2	22
Central alpha agonist	2	3	1	1	1[d]	1	1	1	3	3	17
Prazosin	2	3	2	2	1	0	2	1	3	3	19
Reserpine	2	2	1	1	3	3	2	3	2	2	21
Guanethidine/guanadrel	2	2	1	1	3[f]	1	2	2	2	2	18
Hydralazine	1	2	0	0	1	1	2	3	1	2	13
Minoxidil	3	2	0	0	1	1	2	2	2	2	15
Calcium entry blockers	2	3	2	?	0	1	2	1	2	2	15

0, Does not have this attribute; 1, little of this attribute; 2, some of this attribute; 3, much of this attribute.
[a]Pindolol is exception.
[b]Atenolol is exception.
[c]Captopril is short-acting; enalapril can be given once daily.
[d]Exception is transdermal clonidine which can be given once a week.
[e]Methyldopa can cause hepatotoxicity and hemolytic anemia.
[f]Guanadrel must be given twice daily.

MONOTHERAPY

Efficacy as monotherapy is an important consideration in selecting a step-one agent. Diuretics administered alone have been shown to normalize blood pressure in up to 50% of patients with mild hypertension and in the VA study 65% of patients treated with diuretic alone had diastolic blood pressure <90 mmHg at the end of 58 weeks (24). Diuretics and beta blockers were equally effective in controlling mild hypertension in the study conducted by Berglund and Andersson (2), while in the double-blind VA study, hydrochlorothiazide was more effective than propranolol as monotherapy at the end of the 58-week trial.

The converting-enzyme inhibitor captopril was shown to be effective as monotherapy in relatively small dosages in another VA trial (25). Other antihypertensive agents have not been subjected to large-scale well-controlled clinical trials over a long period of time. It is a clinical impression, however, borne out by short-term trials, that most agents are effective as monotherapy but most have other disadvantages as step-one drugs (Table 1).

SIDE EFFECTS

It is obvious that the ideal step-one drug must not only be effective as monotherapy but must also have a low side effect profile so that most patients can tolerate it for years. Diuretics are as well tolerated by patients as are any of the alternatives and better than most. In the placebo-controlled double-blind study being conducted by the Medical Research Council (MRC) in the United Kingdom, 17.1% of men and 12.8% of the women discontinued bendrofluazide because of side effects compared to 15.5% of men and 18% of women who discontinued propranolol because of side effects (19). Sexual dysfunction in men was the main reason that men seemed to tolerate the diuretic less well than women did (Table 2).

Table 2 Prevalence of Symptoms at 12 Weeks

	Percentage of 1130 Men			Percentage of 958 Women		
Complaint	Bendro-fluazide	Propranolol	Placebo	Bendro-fluazide	Propranolol	Placebo
Dizziness	13.7[a]	6.9	5.9	25.3[b]	18.1	16.8
Muscle pain	13.5	15.7	14.6	25.2	21.6	22.5
Slowed walking	2.6	7.9	6.6	10.0	12.6[b]	6.2
Exertional dyspnea	16.1	19.4	14.0	20.9	18.4	21.0
Headaches	19.6	21.9	27.1	31.9[b]	33.1	42.4
Cold/numb digits	8.4	14.2	11.5	18.8	18.3	16.3
Paresthesia	11.6	14.7	14.7	28.9[b]	19.7	18.4
Dry mouth	13.7	11.2	7.7	26.6	18.8	21.3
Blocked or runny nose	13.7	23.2[a]	12.5	11.5	20.1	19.2
Vomiting/nausea	3.9	7.9[b]	3.2	13.4	6.3	8.2
Impotence	16.2[b]	13.8	8.9	–	–	–

Based on results of questionnaire.
[a]p <0.01.
[b]p <0.05.
Significance levels refer to prevalence rates for each active drug separately compared with those for all control patients. The figures do not indicate comparisons between the two active drugs.
Source: Ref. 19.

PSEUDORESISTANCE

It has long been recognized that nondiuretic antihypertensive drugs, especially direct vasodilators and some adrenergic inhibitors tend to cause subtle sodium and water retention that eventually leads to a loss of these agents' hypotensive effectiveness (3-5). This is not usually manifested by overt edema or abrupt weight gain and may take months to become apparent. This has been described with reserpine, guanethidine, methyldopa, hydralazine, and the ganglion-blocking agents. It is not true pharmacological resistance, but a reflection of volume expansion and is readily prevented or treated by including a diuretic in the regimen; hence it is called "pseudoresistance." Claims have been made that the newer centrally acting $alpha_2$ agonists (clonidine and guanabenz) and the $alpha_1$ receptor blocking drug prazosin do not lead to fluid retention but long-term studies have not been carried out to confirm this.

Obviously the ideal step-one drug should not cause pseudoresistance. Diuretics are the only antihypertensive drugs which by their action to reduce plasma and extracellular volume could not possibly lead to pseudoresistance but can also prevent it when other agents are added to the regimen. Beta blockers and converting-enzyme inhibitors, because they reduce the level of angiotensin II and hence of aldosterone, are not likely to lead to fluid retention. There has not been enough experience with calcium slow channel entry blockers to know whether they will cause fluid retention when administered as monotherapy for hypertension, but edema is a well-known side effect of nifedipine.

DURATION OF ACTION

The ideal step-one drug should have a duration of action long enough to permit one dose a day which enhances compliance. Long-acting diuretics have this desirable quality, but so do some of the other agents including long-acting beta blockers, reserpine, and guanethidine.

EASE OF TITRATION

A rather flat dosage-response curve is a desirable feature of a step-one drug to eliminate the inconvenience and expense of multiple office visits to titrate the dosage to an effective level. It is becoming apparent that the initial dosage of a diuretic should be 25 mg of hydrochlorothiazide or its equivalent in other diuretics and the maximal dosage, except in unusual cases should be the equivalent of 50 mg hydrochlorothiazide. Only atenolol and reserpine share this dosage-response relationship with diuretics.

Some drugs, such as prazosin, clonidine, guanabenz, guanethidine, guanadrel, and beta blockers other than atenolol can require four or more steps in dosage titration.

AUGMENTATION OF ACTION OF OTHER ANTIHYPERTENSIVE AGENTS

Diuretics enhance the action of all other classes of antipressor drugs, thus permitting smaller dosages and consequently fewer side effects when a step-two agent is required. The effect is at least additive and in some cases seems to be synergistic. Consequently, most authorities agree with the 1984 Report of the Joint National Committee which advocates that a diuretic be added as step two if it is not used in step one (21). While combinations of most classes of nondiuretic antihypertensive agents have additive effects, few combinations are as effective as when a diuretic is included, and some may even be antagonistic. For instance, there is evidence that the combination of prazosin and clonidine may not have any additional antihypertensive effect over either drug alone (12); pargyline and methyldopa may cause hyperexcitability. The combination of guanethidine or reserpine with pargyline can cause a hypertensive crisis. The hypertensive crisis associated with sudden clonidine withdrawal may be worse when a beta blocker is in the regimen (1). Isolated reports suggest that combinations of propranolol with methyldopa may result in a paradoxical pressor response (15). If this does occur, it is rare because this combination has been used successfully by many physicians. The combination of nifedipine and prazosin has led to severe hypotension in some cases (13). Beta blockers probably should not be used in the same regimen with either verapamil or diltiazem, because their negative effects on conduction and inotropism are additive.

CONTRAINDICATIONS

The ideal step-one drug should not be contraindicated in a large number of hypertensive patients. There are few contraindications to the use of an oral diuretic. Diuretics can be given with appropriate care to diabetics and patients with gout. On the other hand, beta blockers are contraindicated for patients with asthma, more than second-degree heart block, congestive heart failure, and are relatively contraindicated for patients with chronic occlusive arterial disease and insulin-dependent diabetes.

EXPENSE

The ideal step-one drug should be relatively inexpensive because antihypertensive therapy is a lifelong need. Only reserpine and hydralazine are less expensive than diuretics.

SAFETY

The metabolic effects of diuretics have been a source of concern with regard to their long-term efficacy. This has been highlighted by the results of the Multiple Risk Factor Intervention Trial (MRFIT) which reported more deaths, many of them sudden, in the special intervention (SI) group than in the usual care (UC) group of men with hypertension and abnormal findings on resting electrocardiograms (14). Although men in both groups were treated with diuretics, the dosage was higher in SI than UC group. While the difference (36 vs. 21 deaths) was not statistically significant, the specter of an adverse effect of the diuretic has been raised and must be considered. Other aberrations make this finding suspect. Men who had abnormal stress electrocardiograms before entering the study had a lower mortality rate in SI than UC. In UC, hypertensive men who had abnormal resting electrocardiograms had a lower mortality rate than hypertensive men who had normal resting electrocardiograms, a finding that is contrary to all previous experience in long-term follow-up studies.

Potassium

Hypokalemia is a frequent occurrence in patients treated with thiazide diuretics. Diuretic-induced hypokalemia has been associated with ventricular irritability manifested by increased ectopy on Holter monitor recordings (10), and after exercise (11), although Papademetriou et al. could not confirm this (17). Nevertheless, it has been difficult to detect any serious adverse clinical consequences of this, unless the higher death rate in the SI subgroup of MRFIT discussed above reflects the hypokalemic effects of the diuretics. Consequently, many have disregarded asymptomatic, diuretic-induced hypokalemia rather than make the regimen complicated and expensive by adding potassium chloride supplements or a potassium-retaining diuretic.

It is still not clear that every hypertensive patient who is going to be treated with a thiazide diuretic needs supplementary potassium chloride or a potassium-sparing diuretic from the outset, especially now that lower dosages of diuretic are being prescribed. The indications for maintaining the serum potassium at or restoring it to normal levels are given in Table 3. In general, patients who have or have had evidence of ventricular irritability, including frequent ectopy, or who have conditions which would make the ventricle susceptible to irritability (e.g., digitalis therapy, remote infarct, left ventricular hypertrophy on electrocardiogram) should have their serum potassium level maintained at normal concentrations during treatment with a thiazide diuretic.

The simplest and surest way to do this is to prescribe a combination tablet that contains both the thiazide and the potassium-sparing diuretic. This ensures compliance, because the patient cannot take the potassium-losing diuretic without also taking the potassium-retaining diuretic.

Potassium chloride supplements, whether elixirs, matrix tablets, or the microencapsulated preparations, are just as expensive as the potassium-retaining diuretics if adequate dosages are prescribed. Many physicians fail to recognize that it often takes 60-100 mEq or more of potassium chloride daily in addition to usual dietary intake to keep serum potassium levels normal during thiazide therapy. This is not easily achieved with the tablets containing 8 or 10 mEq each and the elixirs are often so unpalatable that patients will not take them. Compliance, therefore, is a problem.

It is unrealistic to expect that dietary manipulation can provide enough potassium to prevent or correct thiazide-induced hypokalemia. There is for instance, approximately 1 mEq of potassium in 2.5 cm of banana. If 60-100 mEq additional potassium are often required, the caloric load that must be consumed in potassium-rich foods to get the requisite amount of potassium is highly undesirable for most hypertensive patients (Table 4).

Ram et al. have shown that thiazide-induced kaliuresis was diminished when patients were placed on a low-sodium diet (18). Dietary sodium restriction is a more rational maneuver than dietary potassium supplementation. Most hypertensive patients should be

Table 3 Indications For K^+ Supplementation or Addition of K^+-Sparing Diuretic For Patients Taking Thiazide-Type Diuretics

Concomitant digitalis therapy
Frequent ventricular ectopy
History of tachyarrhythmias
Abnormal resting ECG (especially LVH)
Symptomatic hypokalemia
Serum $K^+ < 3.0$ mEq/L without symptoms
Before general anesthesia
During episodes of nausea, vomiting, diarrhea, anorexia

Table 4 Potassium and Caloric Values of Selected Foods

Food	K^+ (mEq)	Calories	Cal/mEq K^+
1 orange (medium)	7.4	66	8.9
Orange juice (225 g fresh)	12.7	111	8.7
1 banana	11.3	101	8.9
1 grapefruit (whole)	6.8	80	11.8
1 potato, baked (7–10-cm diam)	19.4	139	7.2
1 tomato, raw (small)	5.7	20	3.5
Tomato juice (225 g)	13.9	48	3.5
Honeydew melon (1/4 of 12-cm diam)	6.4	33	5.2
Cantaloupe (1 medium)	7.7	36	4.7
Grapefruit juice (225 g canned unsweetened)	9.2	75	8.1
Nectarine (1 medium)	3.8	32	8.4

on a low-sodium diet. The less sodium that reaches the distal tubule of the kidney, the less the sodium-potassium exchange at this site and hence the less potassium lost in the urine. Because of the vagaries of compliance with dietary sodium restriction, however, one cannot rely absolutely on dietary sodium restriction to keep the serum potassium at normal levels during thiazide therapy.

Finally, it must be emphasized that deaths from drug-induced hyperkalemia have been much easier to document than deaths from diuretic-induced hypokalemia (9). In addition, potassium-sparing diuretics should not be prescribed for patients with renal insufficiency and should not be prescribed in conjunction with supplements of potassium chloride or with converting-enzyme inhibitors that can elevate serum potassium (20). Elderly patients, particularly diabetics, who have hyporeninemic hypoaldosteronism are very susceptible to hyperkalemia when given supplements of potassium chloride or a potassium-sparing diuretic.

Glucose Metabolism

Thiazide diuretics sometimes impair glucose tolerance. Frequently this is only apparent when glucose tolerance tests are administered, because fasting blood glucose levels are usually not affected. In the study by Berglund and Andersson (2), the blood glucose level 1 hr after a glucose load was lower after 6 years of diuretic or propranolol therapy than it was initially. Propranolol has been shown to impair glucose tolerance after 1 or 2 years of treatment. The long-term implications of this with regard to coronary and cerebral vascular risk are unknown. Most diabetics can tolerate a thiazide diuretic with little or no perceptive change in the control of their diabetes.

Urate Metabolism

Thiazide diuretics increase serum urate levels so consistently that this measure is often used as a marker of compliance. In the absence of clinical gout, hyperuricemia is a weak risk factor at most for coronary disease and in the Framingham study it was not considered

Table 5 Effect of Diuretics on Serum Cholesterol and Triglyceride Levels

	Cholesterol (mg/dl)			Triglycerides (mg/dl)		
Reference	N	C	Rx	N	C	Rx
VA Coop Study (24)						
10-wk trial	343	224	231[a]	343	184	220
58-wk trial	167	226	223	170	187	184
Berglund and Andersson (2)						
1 yr	53	267	263		142	142
6 yr	49	267	255	49	142	151
MRC Trial (19) 3 yr						
Men	256	246	247		–	–
Women	229	262	265		–	–
VA-NHLBI Feasibility Trial[b]						
1 yr	302	203	213	297	152	167

[a] $p < 0.001$.
[b] *JAMA* 244:1691, 1980.
C, control; Rx, during treatment.

to be a risk factor at all (8). Only a very few patients with thiazide-induced hyperuricemia ever develop gout de novo, although thiazides will certainly exacerbate preexisting gout. In the absence of clinical gout, there is seldom justification for treating thiazide-induced hyperuricemia. Thiazide diuretics actually reduce urate excretion in the urine and therefore are not likely to cause urate stones.

Serum Lipids

Many short-term studies have shown that thiazide diuretics increase concentrations of serum triglyceride and cholesterol (7). While there is much debate regarding triglycerides as a risk factor for coronary disease and stroke, hypercholesterolemia is clearly a major

Table 6 Effect of Propranolol on Serum Cholesterol and Triglyceride Levels

	Cholesterol (mg/dl)			Triglycerides (mg/dl)		
Reference	N	C	Rx	N	C	Rx
VA Coop Study (24)						
10-wk trial	340	221	217[a]	340	160	191[c]
58-wk trial	121	223	231[b]	118	167	209[a]
Berglund and Andersson (2)						
1 yr	53	271	263	53	142	177
6 yr	49	271	255	49	142	159
MRC Trial (19) (3 yrs)						
Men	239	241	238		–	–
Women	218	260	256		–	–

[a] $p < 0.01$.
[b] $p < 0.02$.
[c] $p < 0.001$.
C, control; Rx, during treatment.

risk factor. Concern that thiazide treatment of hypertension may replace one risk factor with another is understandable. However, most long-term studies (1 year or more) have failed to show any effect of thiazide treatment on serum cholesterol or triglycerides (Table 5). Propranolol, on the other hand, seems to have a more lasting effect on serum cholesterol and triglycerides (Table 6).

COMMENTS

With the exception of metabolic side effects the thiazide diuretics fulfill all the criteria for the ideal step-one drug (Table 1). They are inexpensive, convenient, well-tolerated, and correct the hemodynamic abnormality most frequently seen in essential hypertension: increased total peripheral vascular resistance.

A closer look at the metabolic side effects reveals that the lipid changes are usually transient, hypokalemia can be corrected or prevented very easily with the addition of a potassium-sparing diuretic when indicated, asymptomatic hyperuricemia can be ignored, and the effect on glucose tolerance is usually minimal and not often reflected by an increase in fasting blood glucose. Moreover, since most of the metabolic side effects of diuretics are dosage-related, the widespread use of smaller dosages, as recommended in the 1984 Joint National Committee Report (21), should also reduce the frequency and severity of metabolic side effects.

This is not to say that a thiazide-type diuretic is indicated as step-one for every hypertensive patient. There are times when a beta blocker is a more appropriate step-one drug (Table 7). Converting-enzyme inhibitors and calcium slow channel blocking drugs also have many of the attributes of an ideal step-one drug and may be used in this role if further experience confirms their efficacy.

Not all the attributes shown in Table 1 are equally important. Obviously, efficacy as monotherapy and safety are the foremost considerations because absence of either one of these qualities would make a drug unacceptable even though other attributes were present.

It is my practice to initiate therapy with an oral diuretic providing there is no contraindication to its use and no special indication for using a beta blocker. If a nondiuretic antihypertensive agent is used as step one it is appropriate to introduce a diuretic as step two if needed.

Every controlled clinical trial that has shown a reduction in cardiovascular mortality and morbidity from treating hypertension has used a diuretic as step one. Moreover, in this country, where a diuretic is prescribed as step one by more than 90% of physicians, there has been a 25% decline in mortality from coronary disease and a 45% decline in mortality from stroke in the past 10 years.

Table 7 Special Indications for Step-One Treatment

Special Indications for Diuretics as Step One	Special Indications for Beta-Blockers as Step One
Elderly patients	Young patients
Black patients	Hyperkinetic circulation
Congestive heart failure	Symptomatic coronary disease
Contraindications to beta-blockers (intermittent claudication, asthma, heart block)	Past myocardial infarction
	Gout
	Migraine

REFERENCES

1. Bailey, R. R., and Neale, T. J.: Rapid clonidine withdrawal with blood pressure overshoot exaggerated by beta blockade. *Br. Med. J.* 1:942–43, 1976.
2. Berglund, G., and Andersson, O.: Beta-blockers or diuretics in hypertension? A six year follow-up of blood pressure and metabolic side effects. *Lancet* 1:744–747, 1981.
3. Dustan, H. P., Tarazi, R. C., and Bravo, E. L.: False tolerance to antihypertensive agents. In *Systemic Effects of Antihypertensive Drugs,* edited by Sambhi, M. P., New York, Stratton Intercontinental Medical Book Corporation, 1976, pp. 51–68.
4. Dustan, H. P., Tarazi, R. C., and Bravo, E. L.: Dependence of arterial pressure on intravascular volume in treated hypertensive patients. *N. Engl. J. Med.* 286:861–866, 1972.
5. Finnerty, F. Jr., Davidov, M., Mroczek, W. J., and Gavrilovich, L.: Influence of extra-cellular fluid volume on response to antihypertensive drugs. *Circ. Res.* 26–27: (Suppl I):71–80, 1970.
6. Freis, E. D.: Salt, volume and prevention of hypertension. *Circulation* 53:589–595, 1976.
7. Grimm, R. H., Leon, A. S., Hunninghake, D. B., Lenz, K., Hannan, P., and Blackburn, H.: Effects of thiazide diuretics on plasma lipids and lipoproteins in mildly hypertensive patients. A double-blind trial. *Ann. Intern. Med.* 94:7–11, 1981.
8. Hall, A. P.: Correlations among hyperuricemia, hypercholesterolemia, coronary disease and hypertension. *Arthritis Rheum.* 8:846, 1965.
9. Harrington, J. T., Isner, J. M., and Kassirer, J. P.: Our national obsession with potassium. *Am. J. Med.* 73:155–159, 1982.
10. Holland, O. B., Nixon, J. B., and Kuhnert, L.: Diuretic-induced ventricular ectopic activity. *Am. J. Med.* 70:762–768, 1981.
11. Hollifield, J. W., and Slaton, P. E.: Thiazide diuretics, hypokalemia and cardiac arrhythmias. *Acta Med. Scand.* (Suppl)647:67–73, 1981.
12. Hubbell, F. A., Weber, M. A., Drayer, J. I. M., and Rose, D. E.: Combined central and peripheral sympathetic blockade: Absence of additive antihypertensive effects. *Am. J. Med. Sci.* 285:18–26, 1983.
13. Jee, L. D., and Opie, L. H.: Acute hypotensive response to nifedipine added to prazosin in treatment of hypertension. *Br. Med. J.* 287:1514, 1983.
14. Multiple Risk Factor Intervention Trial Research Group: Multiple Risk Factor Intervention Trial. Risk factor changes and mortality results. *JAMA* 248:1465–1477, 1982.
15. Nies, A. S., and Shand, D. G.: Hypertensive response to propranolol in a patient treated with methyldopa—a proposed mechanism. *Clin. Pharmacol. Ther.* 14:823–826, 1973.
16. Page, L.: Hypertension and atherosclerosis in primitive and acculturating societies. In *Hypertension Update: Mechanisms, Epidemiology, Evaluation, Management.* Editorial Board of Dialogues in Hypertension. Bloomfield, NJ, Health Learning Systems, Inc., 1980, pp. 1–12.
17. Papademetriou, P., Fletcher, R., Khatri, I. M., and Freis, E. D.: Diuretic-induced hypokalemia in uncomplicated systemic hypertension: Effect of plasma potassium correction on cardiac arrhythmia. *Am. J. Cardiol.* 52:1017–1022, 1983.
18. Ram, C. V., Garrett, B. N., and Kaplan, N. M.: Moderate sodium restriction and various diuretics in the treatment of hypertension. Effects of potassium wastage and blood pressure control. *Arch. Intern. Med.* 141:1015–1019, 1981.
19. Report of Medical Research Council Working Party on Mild to Moderate Hypertension: Adverse reaction to bendrofluazide and propranolol for the treatment of mild hypertension. *Lancet* 2:539–543, 1981.

20. Texter, S. C., Bravo, E. L., Fouad, F. M., and Tarazi, R. C.: Hyperkalemia in azotemic patients during angiotensin-converting enzyme inhibition and aldosterone reduction with captopril. *Am. J. Med.* 73:719–725, 1982.
21. The 1984 Report of the Joint National Committee on Hypertension: Detection, Evaluation and Treatment of High Blood Pressure. *Arch. Intern. Med.* 144:1045–1057, 1984.
22. Tobian, L., Lange, J., Azar, S., Iwai, J., Koop, D., Coffee, K., and Johnson, M.: Reduction of natriuretic capacity and renin release in isolated, blood-perfused kidneys of Dahl hypertension-prone rats. *Circ. Res.* 43:I-92–I-98, 1978.
23. Tobian, L., Lange, J., Iwai, J., Hiller, K., Johnson, M., and Goossens, P.: Prevention with thiazide of NaCl-induced hypertension in "S" rats. Evidence for Na-retaining humoral agent in "S" rats. *Hypertension* 1:316–323, 1979.
24. Veterans Administration Cooperative Study Group on Antihypertensive Agents: Comparison of propranolol and hydrochlorothiazide for the initial treatment of hypertension. II: Results of long-term therapy. *JAMA* 248:2004–2011, 1982.
25. VA Cooperative Study Group on Antihypertensive Agents: Low-dose captopril for the treatment of mild to moderate hypertension. I. Results of a 14 week trial. *Arch. Intern. Med.* 144:1947–1953, 1984.

42

Nondiuretic as First-Step Drug Therapy for Hypertension

B. N. C. PRICHARD
School of Medicine, University College London, and University College Hospital, London, England

CORNELIUS J. CRONIN*
University College London, London, England

Diuretics have long been regarded as first-choice drugs for the treatment of hypertension. They can frequently be used alone to control the blood pressure in milder degrees of hypertension, and they are also very valuable in combination (230). They are relatively cheap, since once-daily dosage can be achieved (80). However, cheapness of the drug should not obscure consideration of the cost of complications of long-term diuretic therapy (163). They remain nevertheless a useful class of drugs (138) provided proper care is given to monitoring safety. McCarron (163) considered clonidine and prazosin as useful alternatives. Clonidine has a relatively high incidence of side effects including the occurrence of withdrawal hypertension and we would not regard it as a first-choice agent for hypertension (230). It is possible to use many drugs as first-choice alternatives to diuretics. In mild hypertension a low-dosage potent, or better-termed, efficacious, antihypertensive will suffice (230). In some parts of the world, beta-adrenergic blocking drugs have become first-choice antihypertensives, and are more frequently used than diuretics. A useful alternative is labetalol, a beta-blocking drug that also possesses alpha-blocking properties. More recently, calcium antagonists have come to be considered as possible first-choice drugs.

BETA-ADRENOCEPTOR BLOCKING DRUGS

The use of beta-adrenoceptor blocking drugs in hypertension was first described with pronethalol (218). Pronethalol was withdrawn because of its tumor-producing action in mice (205) but the use of propranolol in hypertension was reported later the same year (226).

The beta-adrenoceptor blocking drugs may be classified according to various associated properties, such as those which are nonselective and those which have a selective action on the beta-receptors, and further classified into those also possessing alpha-receptor blocking properties. They may be classified into various groups according to the presence or absence of intrinsic sympathomimetic activity and membrane activity (81,221) (Table 1). These various associated properties result in a number of differing pharmacodynamic effects (230).

Table 1 Classification of Beta-Adrenoceptor Blocking Drugs[a]

		Partial Agonist Effect (Intrinsic Sympathomimetic Effect)	Membrane Stabilizing Effect (Quinidine-Like Effect)
Division I: Nonselective ($beta_1$ + $beta_2$) block			
Group I	Oxprenolol	+	+
	Alprenolol		
	Penbutolol		
Group II	Propranolol	–	+
Group III	Pindolol	+	–
	Carteolol		
Group IV	Sotalol	–	–
	Timolol		
	Nadolol		
Division II: Cardioselective block ($beta_1$)			
Group I	Acebutolol	+	+
Group III	Practolol	+	–
Group IV	Atenolol	–	–
	Metoprolol		
Division III: Nonselective block + alpha block			
Group II	Labetalol	–	+
Division IV: Cardioselective block + alpha block			
No example yet available			

[a]All these drugs have been shown to lower the blood pressure.

The use of beta-blocking drugs in hypertension represents their principal therapeutic application and drugs with all the permutations of associated properties have been found effective.

Hemodynamic Effects

The proper assessment of beta blockade (164) requires a measure of the inhibition of endogenous sympathetic activity. The greater the level of endogenous sympathetic activity, the more sensitive is the test for beta blockade. The supine resting heart rate is the result of a low sympathetic tone, vagal tone predominating, while on standing there is a modest increase in sympathetic tone. Even these low levels of sympathetic activity are sufficient for us to demonstrate a dosage–response relationship with a beta antagonist that does not possess partial agonist activity (229). However, as levels of exercise are increased up until maximum, there is an increased discrimination for beta blockade (164).

Intravenous propranolol reduces heart rate and cardiac output; peripheral resistance increases; and thus there is little effect on resting blood pressure (255,286). The cardiac output and heart rate are reduced to a similar degree after acute and long-term drug administration (95,273) but usually only after prolonged administration does blood pressure fall and peripheral resistance decline (2,110,273). Other beta-blocking drugs that do not possess partial agonist activity (PAA) show similar results: sotalol (267), nadolol (279), and timolol (74,86).

At rest, a beta-blocking agent with PAA results in less of a fall in resting heart rate than those not having this property (3,142,164,231,268,277). At modest levels of exercise, heart rates may be similar for drugs with and without PAA, but at high levels of exercise drugs with PAA, at maximum dosage, produce less of a reduction of exercise tachycardia (47,164,165). Exercise tachycardia with a beta-blocking drug without PAA is a result of vagal deinhibition, whereas the possession of partial agonist activity supplies some modest sympathetic stimulus to increase heart rate further. This difference between drugs with and without PAA may only be seen at maximum blocking dosage, and dosages below maximum may not demonstrate this difference.

Alteration of heart rate after the administration of beta-blocking drugs usually parallels alterations in cardiac output (96). There is evidence that these drugs which possess PAA when given at low levels of sympathetic activity (e.g., rest), result in less of a reduction in cardiac output; examples include pindolol (268,290), practolol (171,268, 277), and oxprenolol (104,277). In association with the absence of a decline in cardiac output with beta-blocking drugs with partial agonist activity, such as pindolol (290), peripheral resistance does not increase, as is the case with drugs without this property, but may, indeed, fall. In spite of some suggestions to the contrary (96), it appears that non-PAA cardioselective drugs produce a similar fall in cardiac output to non-PAA nonselective agents (171,287).

The dual action of alpha- and beta-adrenoceptor inhibition (e.g., labetalol) produces different responses from those of beta blockade alone. Blood pressure is reduced acutely after oral or intravenous administration (240). Cardiac output at rest shows little change after administration of labetalol (75,141,179). At high levels of exercise there is some reduction of cardiac output (75) but changes in patients with ischemic disease have been found to be less than after propranolol (257).

Nonselective Beta-Blocking Drugs (Division 1)

Group I

These drugs have both membrane-stabilizing action and PAA. A double-blind study of oxprenolol showed that it was similar to propranolol, practolol, tolamolol, and metoprolol in antihypertensive effectiveness (62). The similarity remained when oxprenolol was compared with propranolol in combination with a diuretic (93). Many other studies have confirmed the effect of oxprenolol in hypertension (13,87,152,177,283,295), an efficacy that has also been demonstrated with 24-hr monitoring of blood pressure (183). Alprenolol is an effective antihypertensive drug (28,92,117,186,197,281); as is a further example of this group, penbutolol (45,120,160). More recently, a further nonselective beta-adrenergic blocking drug with membrane-stabilizing activity and partial agonist effect, indendolol, has been found to lower the blood pressure (252).

Group II

These beta-blocking agents have membrane activity but no intrinsic sympathomimetic action. Studies with propranolol demonstrated the value of beta-receptor blocking agents in hypertension (91,136,226-228,292,315). Propranolol was found to give similar overall control of blood pressure to that obtained with bethanidine, guanethidine, and methyldopa (228,232,235,315). In earlier studies propranolol was given three or four times a day but twice- (112), or even once-daily (310) administration is often effective. More recently, a slow-release form of propranolol has been developed (162) which may be given once daily for treatment of hypertension (84).

Group III

The members of this group have partial agonist activity but no significant membrane activity. Pindolol is the most potent beta-adrenoceptor blocker in general use. It is effective in the treatment of hypertension (79,185,297) and is similar in efficacy to propranolol (148) and other beta-blocking drugs (117). Likewise Gonasun (101) reported that pindolol was similar in its level of blood pressure control to propranolol, hydrochlorothiazide, methyldopa, and chlorthalidone. Similarly, Doyle (72) found pindolol (7.5 mg twice daily) gave similar control of the blood pressure to the calcium antagonist verapamil in patients with mild and moderate hypertension. Pindolol may be given once daily (310). Carteolol is a recently described member of this group that is highly potent, has an exceptionally long duration of action (265), and has been found effective in double-blind trials in hypertension (248).

Group IV

Beta-adrenoceptor blocking drugs of this group have no intrinsic sympathomimetic effect or significant membrane activity. Sotalol has been found to be as effective an antihypertensive drug as propranolol (31); it appears to have the same efficacy as methyldopa (223) and can be given once daily (172). Timolol is also effective (7,39,48,156,158,186) and in mild hypertension most effect was seen with 20 mg daily, with only a marginal further effect being achieved with a dosage of 60 mg/day (258). In a double-blind factorial trial (49) there was an additive effect with timolol (10 mg three times daily) and hydrochlorothiazide (50 mg once daily). Another member of this group, nadolol, which has a half-life of about 24 hr and a prolonged duration of action, has been shown to be effective in the treatment of hypertension (73,119,304). There has been some suggestion that, in contrast to other beta-blocking drugs, nadolol may increase renal flow (123,279), but other work does not support this (189,201).

Cardioselective Beta-Adrenergic Blocking Drugs (Division II)

Group I

These drugs possess intrinsic sympathomimetic activity (ISA) and membrane activity. Acebutolol has been found effective in the treatment of hypertension (115,154). Once-daily administration of acebutolol appears as effective as when given twice daily (199).

Group III

These drugs have intrinsic sympathomimetic action but no membrane action. The first in this group was practolol which has an antihypertensive effect (152,234) but it is no longer used as an antihypertensive because it produces serious adverse reactions involving the eye and skin and a sclerosing peritonitis.

Group IV

These drugs have neither ISA nor membrane activity. Atenolol is an effective antihypertensive drug (71,114,159,251,316). Intraarterial monitoring of blood pressure for 24 hr confirms that atenolol can be given once daily (84). In a variable dosage, comparative study of atenolol with oxprenolol, propranolol, and pindolol, the control of the blood pressure was similar, but the diastolic pressures on atenolol were lower during isometric (hand grip) exercise and mental arithmetic (296). It appears similar in efficacy to methyldopa (145, 168). Metoprolol lowers blood pressure (29,30,62,109) and it appears as effective as methyldopa in treating mild and moderate high blood pressure. A sustained-release preparation of metoprolol gave similar control of blood pressure at 24 hr as at 2 hr post-dose, but exercising systolic blood pressure and heart rate tended to be higher at 24 hr after administration (51). Betaxolol is a recently described drug of this group (98), which has been found effective in the treatment of mild and moderate hypertension (246).

BETA-RECEPTOR BLOCKING DRUGS IN COMBINATION WITH OTHER DRUGS

Diuretics

When one is treating more resistant cases, beta-adrenoceptor blocking drugs have been combined with diuretics since the earliest studies. Approximately equal numbers of patients were found to need a diuretic in addition to propranolol as with previous therapy with the then-generally used "potent" (i.e., efficacious) drugs, methyldopa and adrenergic neurone inhibitors (228,235). Beta-blocking drugs, besides exerting an additive antihypertensive effect (188), may also partially antagonize the hypokalemic effect of diuretics (48). The sum of the individual falls of blood pressure may not be as great as that seen when the beta-adrenergic blocking drug or the diuretic is given alone (23). In a recent study, 12.5 mg hydrochlorothiazide was found as effective as larger dosages when combined with acebutolol 400 mg (166).

Vasodilating Drugs

Vasodilators used alone in the treatment of hypertension often cause an unacceptable tachycardia (1,247), which is undesirable in patients with ischemic heart disease. Sodium and fluid retention and side effects such as headaches, nervousness, and gastrointestinal disturbances may also occur (97,139). Beta-adrenergic blocking agents inhibit the vasodilator-induced tachycardia and the increases of plasma renin activity which may be important in the combined antihypertensive regimen (216). Lower dosages of vasodilators may be used and better blood pressure control is achieved. The dosages should also be large enough to inhibit the reflex sympathetic activity caused by the vasodilator (4,57,70, 88,102,112,128,214,217,247,256,283,284,303,305,314).

Drugs Inhibiting the Innervation of the Alpha Receptor

Prazosin has been used in combination with beta blockade (139,176,263). Stokes et al. (264) reported a series of 171 patients treated by the $alpha_1$-blocking drug prazosin in combination with various beta-blocking drugs. Labetalol, which has alpha- and beta-receptor blocking activity, has become established in the treatment of hypertension (see below). The combination of beta-adrenergic blocking drugs such as propranolol with either methyldopa or a sympathetic inhibitor such as bethanidine has at least an additive effect or even a potentiating action, but there is a tendency for some postural and exercise hypotension which propranolol alone does not induce (64,220). Similar additive effects are seen with oxprenolol and guanethidine (207) and atenolol and methyldopa (300, 309).

POSSIBLE MODES OF ACTION

Beta-adrenoceptor blocking drugs lower the blood pressure as a result of their beta-receptor blocking action. There is a fall of blood pressure regardless of associated properties, and the membrane-active non-beta-blocking isomers are without antihypertensive effect (225,294). A number of attempts have been made to explain the hypotensive effect of beta-adrenergic blocking drugs, including a direct action on the central nervous system, adrenergic neurone blocking, antirenin activity, increase of vasodilator prostaglandins, effects secondary to reduced cardiac output, and resetting of baroreceptors secondary to reduced pressor peaks to various pressor stimuli from the reduction in cardiac activity consequent to beta blockade. However, the exact mode of action remains unclear (230). In some patients one of the many effects may be of overriding importance. Antirenin effect may be important in certain cases at low dosage, but other mechanisms may be involved at higher dosage levels (124).

ROLE IN HYPERTENSION

Beta-adrenoceptor blocking drugs have now become widely accepted as first-choice drugs for hypertension. Care should be taken in selecting patients for treatment. These drugs should be avoided in patients with heart failure as such patients are crucially dependent on sympathetic drive (230) and in patients with asthma, as they are sensitive to inhibition of adrenergic drive to bronchial smooth muscle; even cardioselective drugs are liable to cause significant increase in airway obstruction (66). Beta-blocking drugs are also likely to increase heart block and worsen Raynaud's phenomenon (99,175). It does not seem to be possible to predict reliably which patients will respond successully to beta-adrenergic blocking drugs. Bühler et al. (41,42) have suggested that renin levels are important; perhaps the basis for the suggestion that older patients respond less in that renin concentrations fall with age (42,43) but others have not found quite such a clear relationship (10,37,124,153,187). It has also been observed that beta-adrenoceptor sensitivity, as shown by a reduced response to isoprenaline, declines with age (68,291). However, it appears that beta-blocking drugs are effective and useful in the elderly (201,302) and some physicians consider them specifically indicated (9). There is no clear correlation between initial cardiac output and response to beta-blocking drugs (34,113,273) or age, in contrast to the findings of Bühler et al. (42), or blood volume (34,113). The measurement of peripheral resistance, urinary epinephrine and norepinephrine (113,178) aldosterone (113), and heart rate response to isoprenaline (113,258) has no value in predicting response to beta-blocking drugs. Distler et al. (69), however, found a correlation between the ratio of exercise to resting plasma norepinephrine and a good response to atenolol.

Value in Hypertension

Besides being able to be widely used, beta-blocking drugs have several special features; they lower the blood pressure to a similar degree regardless of the physiological circumstances; they probably have a cardioprotective effect; and finally in a given patient there may be a coexistent indication for treatment with a beta-blocking drug.

Response to Physiological Stimuli in Patients Treated with Beta-Blocking Drugs

When the blood pressure has been lowered by beta-blocking drugs, there is neither postural nor exercise hypotension (228,232,233,235). Peripheral resistance increases on standing, as might be expected, since innervation of the alpha-constrictor receptor is intact (233). Other evidence of normally functioning innervation of the alpha receptor is afforded by studying environmental temperature. A rise from 7° to 30° increases postural and exercise hypotension in patients treated with sympathetic neurone inhibitory drugs such as bethanidine and guanethidine. This is probably because of uncompensated vasodilation in skin blood vessels, whereas after propranolol the response of blood pressure to posture and exercise, when environmental temperature was increased, remained unchanged (232).

Cardioprotective and Vasculoprotective Effect

There is evidence that the long-term administration of beta-adrenergic blocking drugs may exert a cardioprotective effect. There are several mechanisms by which this may occur (222). A reduction of myocardial oxygen consumption may be of prime importance, possibly improved delivery of oxygen, better distribution of coronary flow, and enhanced substrate utilization may also contribute. A reduction in platelet adhesion may possibly inhibit actual coronary occlusion from taking place. Beta-blocking drugs, in addition to reducing heart rate and blood pressure, also reduce the rate of rise of systolic blood pressure, and therefore the force of the systolic pressure wave. This represents a reduction of vascular stress. The beta-adrenergic blocking drugs reduce the tachycardia, thus the oxygen consumption, and arrhythmias of everyday stress besides those of exercise. This reduced tachycardia has been documented in pilots undergoing simulated flights (77), in public speakers (270), racing car drivers (269), automobile drivers (275) and car or aircraft passengers (276).

If there is a reduction in cardiac necrosis, there should be less likelihood of pump failure (173) which is likely to occur when 40% or more of the left ventricle is involved (8,204). Notwithstanding the well-known propensity of beta-blocking drugs to precipitate heart failure in susceptible subjects (219), ischemic patients taking beta-blocking drugs do not appear to have a higher incidence of heart failure than those not taking these drugs (85).

Experimental studies in animals suggest that infarct size is reduced by beta-blocking drugs (140,174,238). Likewise, studies in humans after acute myocardial infarction suggest that beta-blocking drugs reduce the extent of the infarct, provided these drugs are administered promptly. This has been shown with postinfarct ST segment mapping (213), monitoring of cardiac enzyme changes (132,215,313), R wave changes (313), and chest pain (12); all parameters showed improvement after beta blockade. Overall trials of beta-blocking drugs postinfarction indicate that the drugs produce benefit (18,108,146,242, 285), although like all drugs, there is a benefit–risk ratio (38). A number of the studies can be criticized on methodological grounds (82,107) and there have been some negative results (19,306). But numerous reports now indicate that beta-blocking drugs are effective in reducing the recurrence rate of myocardial infarction (6,33,116,122,131,191,198, 278,307). This evidence and that for an effect in acute myocardial infarction suggests a cardioprotective effect in high-risk patients following myocardial infarction. There is also some evidence that propranolol-treated patients with hypertension may have a lower incidence of myocardial infarction than those not given beta-blocking drugs (262). In a further uncontrolled but larger study, Beevers et al. (26) found fewer heart attacks and also strokes in hypertensive patients treated with beta-adrenergic blocking drugs compared to those in whom similar blood pressure control was achieved with other antihypertensive drugs.

Coexistent Disease

Beta-blocking drugs are widely used. A number of conditions well-treated by beta-blocking drugs not infrequently coexist with hypertension, such as angina pectoris, migraine, or anxiety with somatic features (230).

COMBINATION OF BETA AND ALPHA BLOCKADE

Labetalol, at present the only drug with beta- and alpha-receptor blocking properties to be widely available (240), has been extensively evaluated in patients with hypertension (13,21,35,75,100,111,135,196,224,271,298). Studies of severe hypertension indicate that labetalol is a powerful drug (60,118,144,308). Double-blind trials of labetalol vs. placebo have confirmed the former's antihypertensive effect (35,46,89,134,147). There is no evidence of tolerance developing with long-term administration in studies of up to 6 years (236), 5 years (135), and an average of 57 months (298).

Unlike beta-adrenergic blocking drugs that do not possess alpha-blocking activity, acute labetalol controls the blood pressure of severely hypertensive patients (5,40,53,58, 130,149,206,241,282), in pheochromocytoma (20,137,239,243,245,271), and hypertensive reactions in clonidine withdrawal (127,243,244) as well as acting as an adjunct to produce hypotensive anesthesia (169). Several of the studies employed large-bolus injections of labetalol; this results in occasional excessive falls of blood pressure, possibly with concurrent symptoms (282). The use of repeated small-bolus injections or graded infusions can give smooth and rapid control of blood pressure. Overall, the parenteral use of labetalol appears safe; no neurological or cardiological sequelae were seen in a total of 70 severely hypertensive patients (54). Labetalol has been used in single oral doses to control blood pressure (94,254).

Intraarterial monitoring in mild hypertension confirmed a rapid fall of blood pressure after 200 mg oral labetalol. The greatest fall was seen by 1 hr, with a smaller further fall by 2 hr (63).

Medroxalol

This drug possesses both beta- and alpha-blocking properties, but additionally appears to have a vasodilator effect mediated by $beta_2$-adrenergic stimulation (55,56). Its beta- and alpha-blocking properties have been confirmed in humans (129) and it is an effective drug for the treatment of hypertension (249).

Beta-Adrenergic Blocking Vasodilator Drugs

Several drugs have recently been evaluated that possess beta-blocking as well as vasodilator activity. Prizidolol (161) has been extensively evaluated but has been withdrawn because of animal toxicity. Bucindolol (67,170), carvedilol (181,293), and other similar drugs are at present in an early stage of evaluation.

Mode of Action of Labetalol

Although the mechanism of action remains a matter for debate, it is well established that beta-adrenoceptor blocking drugs lower the blood pressure (see above). Alpha-receptor blocking drugs have long been demonstrated to reduce peripheral resistance and thus lower the blood pressure. The possession by labetalol, at present the only such drug generally available, of both beta- and alpha-receptor blocking properties (240) represents an additional mode of action to lower the blood pressure. In accordance with the well-established antihypertensive effect of chronic administration of beta-blocking drugs, it seems likely that the beta blocking component becomes relatively more important with more prolonged use. Weidmann et al. (301) have noted a 17% increase in blood volume with 6 weeks' oral labetalol; this will reduce the hypotensive effect of the initial alpha blockade. Hunyor et al. (126) and Rasmussen and Nielson (237) also found that labetalol increased blood volume, in contrast to propranolol. Additionally, Semplicini et al. (253) observed an inhibition of the alpha pressor response to phenylephrine with acute labetalol, as had been previously shown (240), which declined over 6 months of treatment, whereas the shift in the isoprenaline dosage-response curve was unchanged. Likewise, whereas the acute administration of labetalol is associated with an inhibition of the pressor responses to norepinephrine (240), it has been suggested that with 4 and 12 weeks' administration the response to norepinephrine is no longer inhibited but is indeed enhanced (317).

CALCIUM ANTAGONISTS

Calcium is central in its importance in cell membrane excitation and contraction of vascular smooth muscle and cardiac muscle. The transmembrane passage of calcium ions is an integral part of the genesis of the action potential of automatic and conduction tissue in the heart. Antagonism of calcium transport by calcium antagonist drugs has lead to their application in an increasing spectrum of cardiovascular disease, including angina pectoris, arrhythmias, and hypertension (36,61,202,209,266).

There are important pharmacological differences between the various antagonists (83, 121,180,209,288). Nifedipine is more effective in inhibiting slow-channel transport in smooth muscle cells, and has little effect on pacemaker activity or AV conduction tissue (289). Nifedipine inhibits slow calcium transport into cardiac muscle and therefore is a cardiodepressant in isolated tissue preparations. However, in the intact animal reflex changes induced by the peripheral vasodilation mask the direct cardiodepressant effect (133). Diltiazem is approximately equal in its effects on cardiac and smooth muscle cells (193). Verapamil has relatively less effect on smooth muscle cells (194) and has a preferential effect on the AV node.

In addition to drugs that act principally by inhibiting slow inward calcium currents, other drugs possess this action (e.g., aminophylline), but it is secondary to predominantly phosphodiesterase inhibition. Many local anesthetics (quinidine, procainamide, lignocaine), although they interfere primarily with fast sodium current, also inhibit slow calcium currents (184). Finally, other drugs owe at least part of their vasodilator action to calcium antagonism: nitroglycerine, inorganic nitrates, morphine (194).

Hemodynamics and Mode of Action

Vasodilators have been classified by Tarazi et al. (274) into those which produce little or no venodilation, such as hydralazine, minoxidil, or diazoxide, and those similar to the nitrates and prazosin which effect significant venodilation. The first group is associated with increased venous return, a rise in cardiopulmonary blood volume, and an increase in heart rate and cardiac output; in the second group this cardiac stimulation may not occur.

Calcium antagonists relax arterial smooth muscle, and peripheral resistance falls. This, coupled with the increase in venous capacity and fall in venous return, results in a fall of blood pressure.

Verapamil, and similar drugs, have a significant direct negative chronotropic and inotropic effect. This prevents the rise in heart rate and cardiac output that might otherwise occur. Studies with verapamil have suggested that heart rate and cardiac output do not change (17,90). Some investigators have found a fall in heart rate and cardiac output from verapamil or similar drugs, for example, after intravenous administration of gallopamil (D600) (150,151). Nifedipine has only a little calcium antagonist inhibitory effect on the sinus node and this is balanced by reflex sympathetic stimulation consequent to the peripheral vasodilation, thus heart rate and cardiac output show little change, with possibly a slight increase after acute administration (22,106,200). Chronic treatment has not been found to be associated with an increase in heart rate (167). Evidence of overall cardiac stimulation has been found with drugs similar to nifedipine, such as nitrendipine (151).

Use in Hypertension: Results

Many studies have shown that the acute administration of nifedipine produces a rapid fall of blood pressure (15,16,25,32,105,200,210,212,280). Bertel et al. (32) demonstrated the value of oral nifedipine 10 or 20 mg in 25 patients with hypertensive crises, in whom blood pressure fell from an average of 221/126 to 152/89 mmHg. Others have confirmed the value of nifedipine in lowering the blood pressure in patients with severe hypertension

(78,272). Continuous oral administration has demonstrated the effectiveness of nifedipine in the control of hypertension (16,24,76,190,210). These findings have been confirmed with studies using continuous intraarterial recording of blood pressure (125,167). Hornung et al. (125) used the delayed-release tablets of nifedipine (up to 60 mg twice daily) which give lower peak levels but more prolonged plasma levels than the previously used capsules.

Verapamil had been shown to lower the blood pressure when given intravenously (27); this has been confirmed (208). Only more recently has its useful effect in chronic oral treatment been demonstrated (11,72,155,182), and also shown with a slow-release formulation (250). The antihypertensive effect of verapamil has also been confirmed by studies using intraarterial monitoring (103).

Diltiazem also lowers the blood pressure in hypertensive patients (312) as do other newer calcium antagonists that have been assessed, such as nitrendipine (44) and tiapamil (50).

As might be expected from the increased reflex sympathetic activity to the heart, the combination of nifedipine with beta-adrenoceptor blockade, from propranolol (15,311), atenolol (203,299), or several different drugs (211), results in an additional fall in blood pressure. The combination of nifedipine and methyldopa has also been found to be additive in effect (106). Similarly, nifedipine added to a combination of a diuretic plus a beta-blocking drug is useful in patients with more resistant hypertension (65,192,260).

Role in Treatment of Hypertension

Side effects are not uncommon with calcium antagonists (143) and some series have shown relatively high dropout rates (14-22%), from nifedipine (76,124,212). Levels as high as 31% were reported in one series in which nifedipine was used in combination with propranolol (311), while others, in contrast, have had no dropouts in studies of nifedipine alone (125). Side effects associated with vasodilation (headache and flushing) are more common with nifedipine than verapamil, with rates for diltiazem probably between the two (143). Postural hypotension is rare but it was responsible for the withdrawal of 1 patient in the series of 15 reported by Murphy et al. (192) when nifedipine was added to atenolol and bendrofluazide. Ankle edema occurs in 0.6% of patients treated with nifedipine, possibly the result of increased capillary permeability; such edema is resistant to treatment with diuretics (143). Palpitations, presumably secondary to vasodilation are not uncommon with nifedipine (200), but are rare with verapamil. Significant negative inotropic effects and consequent depression of left ventricular function, dyspnea, and pulmonary edema may occur in patients with poor cardiac reserve who are treated with verapamil; it is rare with nifedipine (143). Constipation is quite frequent (12-42%) in patients receiving verapamil, in contrast to nifedipine with the use of which the gastrointestinal side effect is usually diarrhea (143).

Calcium antagonists can be used as first-line treatment in patients for whom beta-adrenoceptor blocking drugs are contraindicated. In patients with poor left ventricular function or bradyarrhythmias, nifedipine may be given. Likewise, in asthmatic patients, in contrast to beta-blocking drugs, calcium antagonists do not increase airway obstruction. There has been a report that nifedipine reduces exercise-induced asthma (52). Similarly, attacks of Raynaud's phenomenon are lessened after nifedipine (261).

There have not been any secondary prevention studies with calcium antagonists to assess whether they have a cardioprotective effect. However, there is evidence from animals that calcium antagonists have a protective effect in experimental ischemia, inhibiting the ischemic rise in cytosolic calcium (195). Coronary spasms may be a cause of sudden death and they are inhibited by calcium antagonists (14,157). Nifedipine also inhibits platelet aggregation (59). Finally, verapamil and similar drugs have a significant anti-arrhythmic action (259).

CONCLUSION

Overall, provided the specific contraindications associated with beta-adrenoceptor blockade are observed, these drugs are the first choice in the treatment of hypertension. They have become very widely used. They can be administered in all grades of hypertension and they do not cause postural falls in pressure. They have a cardioprotective action, and they may additionally be indicated because of coexistent diseases. Calcium antagonists are a more recently introduced group of vasodilators that may also have a cardioprotective effect, although evidence is at present based only on experimental results. These drugs are becoming more frequently used as first-choice agents for hypertension.

ACKNOWLEDGMENTS

We would like to express our appreciation to Miss C.F. Knights, S.R.N., Mrs. J. Raeburn, B.Sc., and Mrs. L. White, S.R.N. for their assistance in the preparation of the manuscript.

REFERENCES

1. Ablad, B.: A study of the mechanism of the haemodynamic effects of hydralazine in man. *Acta Phamacol. Toxicol.* 20 (Suppl. 1):1–53, 1963.
2. Ablad, B., Ljung, B., and Sannerstedt, R.: Haemodynamic effects of -adrenoceptor blockers in hypertension. *Drugs* 11 (Suppl. 1):127–134, 1976.
3. Aellig, W. H.: Clinical Pharmacology of β-adrenoceptor blocking drugs possessing partial agonist activity with special reference to pindolol. *J. Cardiovasc. Pharmacol.* 5:S16–S20, 1983.
4. Aenishanslin, W., Pestalozzi-Kerpei, J., Dubach, U. C., Imhof, P. R., and Turri, M.: Antihypertensive therapy with adrenergic beta-receptor blockers and vasodilators. *Eur. J. Clin. Pharmacol.* 4:177–181, 1972.
5. Agabiti-Rosei, E., Alicandri, C. L., Beschi, M., Castellano, M., Fariello, R., Montini, E., Muiesan, M. L., Romanelli, G., and Muiesan, G.: The acute and chronic hypotensive effect of labetalol and the relationship with pretreatment plasma noradrenaline levels. *Br. J. Clin. Pharmacol.* 3 (Suppl. 1):87s–92s, 1982.
6. Ahlmark, G., Saetre, H., and Korsgren, M.: Reduction of sudden deaths after myocardial infarction. *Lancet* 2:1563, 1974.
7. Alcocer, L., Aspe, J., and Gomez, E. A.: Anti-hypertensive effect of timolol, a new beta-blocking agent (double-blind study). *J. Int. Med. Res.* 3:1–9, 1975.
8. Alonso, D. R., Scheidt, S., Post, M., and Killip, L.: Pathophysiology of cardiogenic shock. Quantification of myocardial necrosis: clinical, pathologic and electrocardiographic correlations. *Correlation* 48:588–596, 1973.
9. Amery, A.: High blood pressure above age 60. In *Clinical Hypertension and Hypotension*, edited by Brunner, H. R., and Gavras, H., New York, Marcel Dekker, Inc., 1982, pp. 327–150.
10. Amery, A., Billiet, L., Boel, A., Fagard, R., Reybrouck, T., and Willems, J.: Mechanism of hypotensive effect during beta dreenergic blockade in hypertensive patients. Haemodynamic and renin response to a new cardio-selective agent: Tenormin or ICI 66082. *Am. Heart J.* 91:634–642, 1976.

11. Anavekar, S. N., Barter, C., Adam, W. R., and Doyle, A. E.: A double-blind comparison of verapamil and labetalol in hypertensive paients with coexisting chronic obstructive airways disease. *J. Cardiovasc. Pharmacol.* 4:5374–5377, 1982.
12. Andersen, M. P., Bechsgaard, P., Frederiksen, J., Hansen, D. A., Jurgensen, H. J., Nielsen, B., Pedersen, F., Pedersen-Bjergaard, O., and Rasmussen, S. L.: Effect of alprenalol on mortality among patients with definite or suspected acute myocardial infarction. *Lancet* 2:865–868, 1979.
13. Andersson, O., Berglund, G., and Hansson, L.: Anti-hypertensive action, time of onset and effects on carbohydrate metabolism of labetalol. *Br. J. Clin. Pharmacol.* 3 (Suppl. 3):757–761, 1976.
14. Antman, E., Miller, J., Golberg, S.: Nifedipine therapy for coronary artery spasm. *N. Engl. J. Med.* 302:1269–1273, 1980.
15. Aoki, K., Kondo, S., Mochizuki, A., Yoshida, T., Kato, S., Kato, K., and Takikawa, K.: Antihypertensive effect of cardiovascular Ca^2 + antagonist in hypertensive patients in the absence and presence of beta-adrenergic blockade. *Am. Heart J.* 96(2): 218–226, 1978.
16. Aoki, K., Sato, K., Kawaguchi, Y., and Yamamoto, M.: Acute and long-term hypotensive effects and plasma concentrations of nifedipine in patients with essential hypertension. *Eur. J. Clin. Pharmacol.* 23(3):197–201, 1982.
17. Atterhog, J. E., and Ekland, L. G.: Haemodynamic effects of intravenous verapamil at rest and during exercise in subjectively healthy middle-aged men. *Eur. J. Clin. Pharmacol.* 8:317–322, 1975.
18. Baber, N. S., and Lewis, J. A.: Confidence in results of beta-blocker post-infarction trials. *Br. Med. J.* 284:1749–1750, 1982.
19. Baber, N. S., Wainwright Evans, D., Howitt, G., Thomas, M., Wilson, C., Lewis, J. A., Dawes, P. M., Handler, K., and Tuson, R.: Multicentre post-infarction trial of propranolol in 49 hospitals in the United Kingdom, Italy and Yugoslavia. *Br. Heart J.* 44:96–100, 1980.
20. Bailey, R. R.: Labetalol in the treatment of a patient with phaeochromocytoma: A case report. *Br. J. Clin. Pharmacol.* 8 (Suppl. 2):141s–142s, 1979.
21. Balasubramanian, V., Mann, S., Raftery, E. B., Millar-Craig, M. V., and Altman, D.: Effect of labetalol on continuous ambulatory blood pressure. *Br. J. Clin. Pharmacol.* 8 (Suppl. 2):119s–123s, 1979.
22. Bartorelli, C., Magrini, F., Moruzzi, P., Olivari, M. T., Polese, A., Fiorentini, C., and Guazzi, M.: Haemodynamic effects of a calcium antagonistic agent (nifedipine) in hypertension. *Clin. Sci. Mol. Med.* 55:291S–292S, 1978.
23. Bateman, D. N., Dean, C. R., Mucklow, J. C., Bulpitt, C. J., and Dollery, C. T.: Atenolol and chlorthalidone in combination for hypertension. *Br. J. Clin. Pharmacol.* 7:357–363, 1979.
24. Bayley, S., Dobbs, R. J., and Robinson, B. F.: Nifedipine in the treatment of hypertension: Report of a double-blind controlled trial. *Br. J. Clin. Pharmacol.* 14:509–512, 1982.
25. Beer, N., Gallegos, I., Cohen, A., Klein, N., Sonnenblick, E., and Frishman, W.: Efficacy of sublingual nifedipine in the acute treatment of systemic hypertension. *Chest* 79:571–574, 1981.
26. Beevers, D. G., Johnston, J. H., Larkin, H., and Davies, P.: Clinical evidence that beta-adrenoceptor blockers prevent more complications than other anti-hypertensive drugs. *Drugs* 25 (Suppl. 2):326–330, 1983.
27. Bender, F.: Die Behandlung der tachycarden Arrhythmien und arteriellen Hypertonie mit Verapamil. *Arzneim. Forsch.* 20:1310, 1970.
28. Bengtsson, C.: Comparison between alprenolol and chlorthalidone as anti-hypertensive agents. *Acta Med. Scand.* 191:433–439, 1972.
29. Bengtsson, C.: Comparison between metoprolol and propranolol as anti-hypertensive agents. *Acta Med. Scand.* 199:71–74, 1976.

30. Bengtsson, C., Johnsson, G., and Regardh, C.-G.: Plasma levels and effects of metoprolol on blood pressure and heart rate in hypertensive patients after acute dose and between two doses during long-term treatment. *Clin. Pharmacol. Ther.* 17:400–408, 1975.
31. Berglund, G.: Anti-hypertensive effect of sotalol and propranolol: a double-blind crossover study. *Curr. Ther. Res.* 21:21–27, 1977.
32. Bertel, O., Conen, D., Radu, E. W., Muller, J., Lang, C., and Dubach, U. C.: Nifedipine in hypertensive emergencies. *Br. Med. J.* 286:19–21, 1983.
33. Beta-Blocker Heart Attack Trial Research Group: 1. Mortality results. A randomized trial of propranolol in patients with acute myocardial infarction. *JAMA* 247:1707–1714, 1982.
34. Birkenhager, W. H., Krauss, X. H., Schalekamp, M. A. D. H., Kolsters, G., and Kroon, B. J. M.: Anti-hypertensive effects of propranolol. Observations on predictability. *Folia Med. Neerlan.* 14:67–71, 1971.
35. Bolli, P., Waal-Manning, H. J., Wood, A. J., and Simpson, F. O.: Experience with labetalol in hypertension. *Br. J. Clin. Pharmacol.* 3 (Suppl. 3):765–771, 1976.
36. Braunwald, E.: Mechanism of action of calcium-channel-blocking agents. *N. Engl. J. Med.* 307(26):1618–1626, 1982.
37. Bravo, E. L., Tarazi, R. C., Dustan, H. P., and Lewis, J. W.: Dissociation between renin and arterial pressure responses to beta-adrenergic blockade in human essential hypertension. *Circ. Res.* Suppl. I:36–37, 1975.
38. Breckenridge, A.: Should every survivor of a heart attack be given a beta blocker? Part II: Evidence from a clinical pharmacological standpoint. *Br. Med. J.* 285:37–39, 1982.
39. Brogden, R. N., Speight, T. M., and Avery, G. S.: Timolol: A preliminary report of its pharmacological properties and therapeutic efficacy in angina and hypertension. *Drugs* 9:164–177, 1975.
40. Brown, J. J., Lever, A. F., Cumming, A. M. M., and Robertson, J. I. S.: Labetalol in hypertension. *Lancet* 1:1147, 1977.
41. Buhler, F. R., Laragh, J. H., Baer, L., Vaughan, E. D., and Brunner, H. R.: Propranolol inhibition of renin secretion. A specific approach to diagnosis and treatment of renin dependent hypertensive diseases. *N. Engl. J. Med.* 287:1209–1214, 1972.
42. Buhler, F. R., Burkart, F., Lutold, B. E., Kung, M., Marbet, G., and Pfisterer, M.: Anti-hypertensive beta blocking action as related to renin and age: A pharmacologic tool to identify pathogenic mechanisms in essential hypertension. *Am. J. Cardiol.* 36:653–669, 1975.
43. Buhler, F. R., Bertel, O., and Lutold, B. E.: Simplified and age-stratified anti-hypertensive therapy based on beta blockers. *Cardiovasc. Med.* 3:135–140, 144–148, 1978.
44. Burris, J. F., Notargiacomo, A. V., Papadmetriou, V., and Freis, E. D.: Acute and short-term effects of a new calcium antagonist in hypertension. *Hypertension* 4(3): (Suppl. II):II-32–II-35, 1982.
45. Cangiano, J. L., Ayala, J. M., Boksay, I. J. E., and Martinez-Maldonado, M.: Penbutolol: A new beta blocker in the treatment of moderate essential hypertension. *J. Clin. Pharmacol.* 19(7):334, 1979.
46. Carre, A.-G., Bertrand, M. E., Libersa, C.-C., and Lekieffre, J.-P.: Etude en double aveugle contre placebo de l'efficacite et de la tolerance du labétalol a 400mg/j. dans l'hypertension arterielle essentielle moderée de l'adulte. *Rev. Med. Interne* III:373–377, 1982.
47. Carruthers, S. G.: Cardiac dose response relationships of oral and intravenous pindolol. *Br. J. Clin. Pharmacol.* 13:193s–198s, 1982.

48. Castenfors, H.: Long term effects of timolol and hydrochlorthiazide or hydrochlorthiazide and amiloride in essential hypertension. *Eur. J. Clin. Pharmacol.* 12:97–103, 1977.
49. Chalmers, J., Horvath, J., Tiller, D., and Bune, A.: Effects of timolol and hydrochlorothiazide on blood pressure and plasma renin activity. Double blind factorial trial. *Lancet* 2:328–331, 1976.
50. Chu, D., and De Gori, D.: Antihypertensive effect of tiapamil, a calcium antagonist. *Cardiology* 69 (Suppl. 1):99–104, 1982.
51. Comerford, M. B., and Besterman, E. M. M.: A comparison of the effects of the slow release formulations of metoprolol and oxprenolol in hypertension. *Ann. Clin. Res.* 14:27–31, 1982.
52. Corris, P. A., Nariman, S., and Gibson, G. J.: Nifedipine in the prevention of asthma induced by exercise and histamine. *Am. Rev. Respir. Dis.* 128:991–992, 1983.
53. Cumming, A. M. M., Brown, J. J., Fraser, R., Lever, A. F., Morton, J. J., Richards, D. A., and Robertson, J. I. S.: Blood pressure reduction by incremental infusion of labetalol in patients with severe hypertension. *Br. J. Clin. Pharmacol.* 8:359-364, 1979.
54. Cumming, A. M. M., Brown, J. J., Lever, A. F., and Robertson, J. I. S.: Intravenous labetalol in the treatment of severe hypertension. *Br. J. Clin. Pharmacol.* 13 (Suppl. 1):93s–96s, 1982.
55. Dage, R. C., Cheng, H. C., and Woodward, J. K.: Cardiovascular properties of medroxalol, a new anti-hypertensive drug. *J. Cardiovasc. Pharmacol.* 3:299–315, 1981.
56. Dage, R. C., Hsieh, C. P., and Spedding, M.: Vasodilation by medroxalol mediated by beta-2 adrenergic receptor stimulation. *J. Cardiovasc. Pharmacol.* 5:143–150, 1983.
57. Dahr, A. S.: Use of hydralazine and selective cardiac adrenergic blockade in therapy of essential hypertension. *Circulation* Suppls. 45–46 (II):142, 1972.
58. Dal Palu, C., Pessina, A. C., Semplicini, A., Hlede, M., Morandin, F., Palatini, P., Sperti, G., and Rossi, G. P.: Intravenous labetalol in severe hypertension. *Br. J. Clin. Pharmacol.* 13:97s–99s, 1982.
59. Dale, J., Landmark, K. M., and Myhre, E.: The effects of nifedipine, a calcium antagonist, on platelet function. *Am. Heart J.* 105:103–105, 1983.
60. Dargie, H. J., Dollery, C. T., and Daniel, J.: Labetalol in resistant hypertension. *Br. J. Clin. Pharmacol.* 3 (Suppl. 3):751–755, 1976.
61. Dargie, H. J., Lynch, P. G., Krikler, D. M., Harris, L., and Krikler, S.: Nifedipine and propranolol: A beneficial drug interaction. *Am. J. Med.* 71:676–682, 1981.
62. Davidson, C., Thadani, U., Singleton, W., and Taylor, S. H.: Comparison of antihypertensive activity of beta-blocking drugs during chronic treatment. *Br. Med. J.* 2:7–9, 1976.
63. Davies, A. B., Balasubramanian, V., Gould, B., and Raftery, E. B.: Rapid reduction of blood pressure with acute oral labetalol. *Br. J. Clin. Pharmacol.* 13:705–710, 1982.
64. Day, G. M., and Prichard, B. N. C.: Hypotensive action from a combination of propranolol and other hypotensive drugs. *Br. J. Pharmacol.* 41:408P–409P, 1971.
65. Dean, S. and Kendall, M. J.: Nifedipine in the treatment of difficult hypertensives. *Eur. J. Clin. Pharmacol.* 24:1–5, 1983.
66. Decalmer, P. B. S., Chatterjee, S. S., Cruickshank, J. M., Benson, M. K., and Sterling, G. M.: Beta-blockers and asthma. *Br. Heart J.* 40:184–189, 1978.
67. Deitchman, D., LaBudde, J. A., and Seidehamel, R. J.: (1983). Bucindolol. In *New Drugs Annual: Cardiovascular Drugs*, edited by Scriabine, A., New York, Raven Press, 1983, pp. 1–18.

68. Dillon, N., Chung, S., Kelly, J., and O'Malley, K.: Age and beta adrenoceptor-mediated function. *Clin. Pharmacol. Ther.* 27(6):769–772.
69. Distler, A., Keim, H. J., Cordes, U., Philipp, T., and Wolff, H. P.: Sympathetic responsiveness and anti-hypertensive effect of beta-receptor blockade in essential hypertension. *Am. J. Med.* 64:446–451, 1978.
70. Dormois, J. C., Young, J. L., and Nies, A. S.: Minoxidil in severe hypertension: value when conventional drugs have failed. *Am. Heart J.* 90:360–368, 1975.
71. Douglas-Jones, A. P., and Cruickshank, J. M.: Once daily dosing with atenolol in patients with mild or moderate hypertension. *Br. Med. J.* 1:990–991, 1976.
72. Doyle, A. E.: Comparison of beta-adrenoceptor blockers and calcium antagonists in hypertension. *Hypertension* 5(II):103–108, 1983.
73. Duchin, K. L., Vukovich, R. A., Dennick, L. G., Groel, J. T., and Willard, D. A.: Effects of nadolol beta-blockade on blood pressure in hypertension. *Clin. Pharmacol. Ther.* 27:57–63, 1980.
74. Dunn, F. G., De Carvalho, J. G. R., and Frohlich, E. D.: Haemodynamic, reflexive and metabolic alteration induced by acute and chronic timolol therapy in hypertensive man. *Circulation* 57:140–144, 1978.
75. Edwards, R. C., and Raftery, E. B.: Haemodynamic effects of long-term oral labetalol. *Br. J. Clin. Pharmacol.* 3 (Suppl. 3):733–736, 1976.
76. Eggertsen, R., and Hansson, L.: Effects of treatment with nifedipine and metoprolol in essential hypertension. *Eur. J. Clin. Pharmacol.* 21:389–390, 1982.
77. Eliasch, H., Rosen, A., and Scott, H. M.: Systemic circulatory response to stress of simulated flight and to physical exercise before and after propranolol blockade. *Br. Heart J.* 29:671–683, 1967.
78. Erbel, R., Meyer, J., Brand, G., and Effert, S.: Emergency treatment of hypertensive crisis with sublingual nifedipine. *Postgrad. Med. J.* 59 (Suppl. 3):134–136, 1983.
79. Feltham, P. M., Watson, O. F., Peel, J. S., Dunlop, D. J., and Turner, A. S.: Pindolol in hypertension: A double-blind trial. *N. Z. Med. J.* 76:167–171, 1972.
80. Finnerty, F. A.: Diuretics as initial treatment for essential hypertension. *Br. J. Clin. Pharmacol.* 7 (Suppl. 2):185S–187S, 1979.
81. Fitzgerald, J. D.: Beta adrenergic blocking drugs. Present position and future developments. *Acta Cardiol.* Suppl. 15:199–216, 1972.
82. Fitzgerald, J. D.: The effect of beta-adrenoceptor antagonists on the morbidity and mortality in cardiovascular disease. *Postgrad. Med. J.* 52:770–781, 1976.
83. Fleckenstein, A.: Specific pharmacology of calcium in myocardium, cardiac pacemakers and vascular smooth muscle. *Annu. Rev. Pharmacol. Toxicol.* 17:149–166, 1977.
84. Floras, J. S., Jones, J. V., Hassan, M. O., and Sleight, P.: Ambulatory blood pressure during once-daily randomized double-blind administration of atenolol, metoprolol, pindolol and slow release propranolol. *Br. Med. J.* 285:1387, 1982.
85. Fox, K. M., Chopra, M. P., Portal, R. W., and Aber, C. P.: Long-term beta blockade: Possible protection from myocardial infarction. *Br. Med. J.* 1:117–119, 1975.
86. Franciosa, J. A., Freis, E. D., and Conway, J.: Antihypertensive and hemodynamic properties of the new beta adrenergic blocking agent timolol. *Circulation* 48:118–124, 1973.
87. Franciosa, J. A., Johnson, S. M., and Tobian, L. J.: Haemodynamic effects of oxprenolol and propranolol in hypertension. *Clin. Pharmacol. Ther.* 26(6):676–681, 1979.
88. Freeman, J. W., and Knight, L. W.: Oxprenolol and hydralazine in the treatment of hypertension. *Med. J. Aust.* 1 (Suppl. 1):12–13, 1975.
89. Frick, M. H., and Pörsti, P.: Combined alpha- and beta-adrenoceptor blockade with labetalol in hypertension. *Br. Med. J.* 1:1046–1048, 1976.

90. Frishman, W. H., Klein, N. A., Strom, J. A., Willens, H., LeJemtel, T. H., Jentzer, J., Siegel, L., Klein, P., Kirschen, N., Silverman, R., Pollack, S., Doyle, R., Kirsten, E., and Sonnenblick, E. H.: Superiority of verapamil to propranolol in stable angina pectoris: A double-blind randomized placebo-controlled crossover comparison. *Circulation* 65 (Suppl. I):152–159, 1982.
91. Frohlich, E. D., Tarazi, R. C., Dustan, H. P., and Page, I. H.: The paradox of beta-adrenergic blockade in hypertension. *Circulation* 37:417–423, 1968.
92. Furberg, C. and Michaelson, G.: Effect of Aptin, a beta-adrenergic blocking agent, in arterial hypertension. *Acta Med. Scand.* 186:447–450, 1969.
93. Gavras, I., Gavras, H., Sullivan, P. C., Tifft, C. P., Chobanian, A. V., and Brunner, H. R.: A comparative study of the effects of oxprenolol versus propranolol in essential hypertension. *J. Clin. Pharmacol.* 19:8–14, 1979.
94. Ghose, R. R., and Sampson, A.: Rapid onset of action of oral labetalol in severe hypertension. *Curr. Med. Res. Opin.* 5:147–151, 1977.
95. Gibson, D. G.: Pharmacodynamic properties of beta-adrenergic blocking drugs in man. *Drugs* 7:8–38, 1974.
96. Gibson, D. G.: Pharmacodynamic properties of beta-adrenergic blocking drugs in man. In *Beta-Adrenoceptor Blocking Drugs: Cardiovascular Drugs*, Vol. 2, edited by Avery, G. S., Sydney, Australia, Adis, 1977, pp. 1–40.
97. Gilmore, E., Weil, J. P., and Chidsey, C.: Treatment of essential hypertension with a new vasodilator in combination with beta-adrenergic blockade. *N. Engl. J. Med.* 282:521–527, 1970.
98. Giudicelli, J. F., Chauvin, M., Thuillez, C., Richer, G., Bianchetti, G., Gomeni, R., and Morselli, P. L.: Beta-adrenoceptor blocking effects and pharmacokinetics of betaxolol (SL 75212) in man. *Br. J. Clin. Pharmacol.* 10:41–49, 1980.
99. Gokal, R., Dornan, T. L., and Ledingham, J. G. G.: Peripheral skin necrosis complicating beta-blockade. *Br. Med. J.* 1:721–722, 1979.
100. Gomez, G., and Phillips, L. A.: Labetalol (Trandate) in hypertension: A multicentre study in general practice. *Curr. Med. Res. Opin.* 6(10):677–684, 1980.
101. Gonasun, L. M.: Anti-hypertensive effects of pindolol. *Am. Heart J.* 104(2, Pt. 2): 374–387, 1982.
102. Gottlieb, T. B., Katz, F. H., and Chidsey, C. A.: Combined therapy with vasodilator drugs and beta-adrenergic blockade in hypertension. A comparative study of minoxidil and hydralazine. *Circulation* 45:571–582, 1972.
103. Gould, B. A., Hornung, R. S., Mann, S., Balasubramanian, B., and Raftery, E. B.: Slow channel inhibitors verapamil and nifedipine in the management of hypertension. *J. Cardiovasc. Pharmacol.* 4 (Suppl. 3):S369–S373, 1982.
104. Grandjean, T., and Rivier, J. L.: Cardio-circulatory effects of beta-adrenergic blockade in organic heart disease. Comparison between propranolol and CIBA 39089-Ba. *Br. Med. J.* 30:50–59, 1968.
105. Guazzi, M., Olivari, M. T., Polese, A., Fiorentini, C., Magini, F., and Moruzzi, P.: Nifedipine, a new antihypertensive with rapid action. *Clin. Pharmacol. Ther.* 22: 528–532, 1977.
106. Guazzi, M. D., Fiorentini, C., Olivari, M. T., Bartorelli, A., Necchi, G., and Polese, A.: Short-term and long-term efficacy of a calcium-antagonistic agent (nifedipine) combined with methyldopa in the treatment of severe hypertension. *Circulation* 61(5):913–919, 1980.
107. Hampton, J. R.: The use of beta blockers for the reduction of mortality after myocardial infarction. *Eur. Heart J.* 2:259–268, 1981.
108. Hampton, J. R.: Should every survivor of a heart attack by given a beta blocker? Part I: Evidence from clinical trials. *Br. Med. J.* 285:33–36, 1982.
109. Hansson, B. G., Dymling, J. F., Hedeland, H., and Hulthen, U. L.: Long-term

treatment of moderate hypertension with the $beta_1$-receptor blocking agent metoprolol. *Eur. J. Clin. Pharmacol.* 11:239–245, 1977.

110. Hansson, L.: Beta-adrenergic blockade in essential hypertension. Effects of propranolol on haemodynamic parameters and plasma renin activity. *Acta Med. Scand.* 55 (Suppl. 1):1–40, 1973.
111. Hansson, L., and Hanel, B.: Labetalol, a new alpha- and beta-adrenoceptor blocking agent in hypertension. *Br. J. Clin. Pharmacol.* 3 (Suppl. 3):763–764, 1976.
112. Hansson, L., Olander, R., Aberg, H., Malmcrona, R., and Westerlund, A.: Treatment of hypertension with propranolol and hydralazine. *Acta Med. Scand.* 190: 531–534, 1971.
113. Hansson, L., Zweifler, A. J., Julius, S., and Ellis, C. N.: Propranolol therapy in essential hypertension. Observations on predictability of therapeutic response. *Int. J. Clin. Pharmacol.* 10:79–89, 1974.
114. Hansson, L., Aberg, H., Karlberg, B. E., and Westerlund, A.: Controlled study of atenolol in treatment of hypertension. *Br. Med. J.* 1:367–370, 1975.
115. Hansson, L., Berglund, G., Andersson, O., and Holm, M.: Controlled trial of acebutolol in hypertension. *Eur. J. Clin. Pharmacol.* 12:89–92, 1977.
116. Hansteen, V., Moinichen, E., Lorensten, E., Anderson, A., Strom, O., Soiland, K., Dyrbekk, D., Refsum, A.-M., Tromsdal, A., Knudsen, K., Eika, C., Bakken, J., Smith, P., and Hoff, P. I.: One year's treatment with propranolol after myocardial infarction; preliminary report of Norwegian Multicentre Trial. *Br. Med. J.* 284: 155–160, 1982.
117. Hartikainen, M., and Heikkila, J.: Twice-daily pindolol and alprenolol in essential hypertension of moderate severity. *Ann. Clin. Res.* 8:85–92, 1976.
118. Hauger-Klevene, J. H.: Treatment of severe essential hypertension with labetalol: Effect on active and inactive renin. *Pharmatherapeutica* 3:46–54, 1981.
119. Heel, R. C., Brogden, G. E., Speight, T. M., and Avery, G. S.: Nadolol: A review of its pharmacological properties and therapeutic efficacy in hypertension and angina pectoris. *Drugs* 20:1–23, 1980.
120. Heel, R. C., Brogden, R. N., Speight, T. M., and Avery, G. S.: Penbutolol: A preliminary review of its pharmacological efficacy in hypertension and angina pectoris. *Drugs* 22:1–25, 1981.
121. Henry, P. D.: Comparative pharmacology of calcium antagonists: nifedipine, verapamil and diltiazem. *Am. J. Cardiol.* 46:1047–1058, 1980.
122. Hjalmarson, A., Elmfeldt, D., Herlitz, J., Holmberg, S., Malek, I., Nyberg, G., Ryden, L., Swedberg, K., Vedin, A., Waagstein, F., Waldenstrom, A., Waldenstrom, J., Wedel, H., Wilhelmsen, L., and Wilhelmsson, C.: Effect on mortality of metoprolol in acute myocardial infarction. *Lancet* 2:823–827, 1981.
123. Hollenberg, N. K., Adams, D. F., McKinstry, D., Williams, G. N., Borucki, L. J., and Sullivan, J.: Beta-adrenoceptor blocking agents and the kidney: Effect of nadolol and propranolol on the renal circulation. *Br. J. Clin. Pharmacol.* 7 (Suppl. 2):219–226, 1979.
124. Hollifield, J. W., Sherman, K., Vander Zwaag, R., and Shand, D. G. (1976). Proposed mechanisms of propranolol's anti-hypertensive effect in essential hypertension. *N. Engl. J. Med.* 295(2):68–73, 1976.
125. Hornung, R. S., Gould, B. A., Jones, R. I., Tansukh, N., Sonecha, T. M., and Raftery, E. B.: Nifedipine tablets for systemic hypertension: a study using continuous ambulatory intra-arterial recording. *Am. J. Cardiol.* 51:1323–1327, 1983.
126. Hunyor, S. N., Bauer, G. E., Ross, M., and Larkin, H.: Labetalol and propranolol in mild hypertensives: comparison of blood pressure and plasma volume effects. *Aust. NZ J. Med.* 10:162–166, 1980.

127. Hurley, D. M., Vandongen, R., and Beilin, L. J.: Failure of labetalol to prevent hypertension due to clonidine withdrawal. *Br. Med. J.* 2:1122, 1979.
128. Ibsen, H., Rasmussen, K., Jensen, H. A., and Leth, A.: Changes in plasma volume and extracellular volume after addition of hydralazine to propranolol treatment in patients with hypertension. *Acta Med. Scand.* 203:419–423, 1978.
129. Jaillon, P., Weissenburger, J., Biour, M., Cheymol, G., Haegele, K., Schechter, P. J., and Koch-Wester, J.: Beta- and alpha-adrenoceptor antagonism by medraxolol in healthy volunteers: relationship to dose and plasma concentration. *J. Cardiovasc. Pharmacol.* 4:705–713, 1982.
130. Joekes, A. M., and Thompson, F. D.: Acute haemodynamic effects of labetalol and its subsequent use as an oral hypotensive agent. *Br. J. Clin. Pharmacol.* 3 (Suppl. 3):789–793, 1976.
131. Julian, D. G., Jackson, F. S., Prescott, R. J., and Szekely, P.: Controlled trial of sotalol for one year after myocardial infarction. *Lancet* 1:1142–1147, 1982.
132. Jurgensen, H. J., Frederiksen, J., Hansen, D. A., and Pederson-Bjergaard, O.: Limitation of myocardial infarct size in patients less than 66 years old treated with alprenolol. *Br. Heart J.* 45:583–588, 1981.
133. Kaltenbach, M., Schultz, W., and Kober, G.: Effects of nifedipine after intravenous and intracoronary administration. *Am. J. Cardiol.* 44:832–838, 1979.
134. Kane, J., Gregg, I., and Richards, D. A.: A double-blind trial of labetalol. *Br. J. Clin. Pharmacol.* 3 (Suppl. 3):737–774, 1976.
135. Kane, J., Gregg, I., and Stephens, M. D. B.: A long-term study of labetalol in general practice. *Br. J. Clin. Pharmacol.* 8 (Suppl. 2):167s–170s, 1979.
136. Karlberg, B., and Hornkvist, P. E.: Propranolol in the treatment of hypertension. *Opus Medica* 16:296–299, 1971.
137. Kaufman, L.: Use of labetalol during hypotensive anaesthesia and in the management of phaeochromocytoma. *Br. J. Clin. Pharmacol.* 8 (Suppl. 2):229s–232s, 1979.
138. Kelly, R. A., Wilcox, C. S., and Mitch, W. E.: Diuretics: an update. *J. Cardiovasc. Med.* 7:1153–1166, 1982.
139. Kincaid-Smith, P., MacDonald, I. M., Hua, A., Laver, M. C., and Fang, P.: Changing concepts in the management of hypertension. *Med. J. Aust.* 1:327–332, 1975.
140. Kloner, R. A., Fishbein, M. C., Cotran, R. S., Braunwald, E., and Maroko, P. R.: The effect of propranolol on microvascular injury in acute myocardial ischaemia. *Circulation* 55:872–880, 1977.
141. Koch, G.: Combined alpha- and beta-adrenoceptor blockade with oral labetalol in hypertensive patients with reference to haemodynamic effects at rest and during exercise. *Br. J. Clin. Pharmacol.* 3 (Suppl. 3):729–732, 1976.
142. Kostis, J. B., Frishman, W., Hosler, M. H., Thorsen, N. L., Gonasun, L., and Weinstein, J.: Treatment of angina pectoris with pindolol: the significnace of intrinsic sympathomimetic activity of beta blockers. *Am. Heart J.* 104 (2, Pt. II):496–504, 1982.
143. Krebs, R.: Adverse reactions with calcium antagonists. *Hypertension* 5 II (Suppl. 2):II-125–II-129, 1983.
144. Kristensen, B. O., and La Cour Petersen, E.: Effects of long-term high dose labetalol on blood pressure in patients with severe hypertension resistant to previous therapy. *Postgrad. Med. J.* 56 (Suppl. 2):57–59, 1980.
145. Kristensen, B. O., Brons, M., Christensen, C. K., Geday, E., Jacobsen, F. K., Jensen, S. N., and Linde, N. C.: Anti-hypertensive effect of atenolol (100 mg once a day) and methyldopa (250 mg thrice a day). *Acta Med. Scand.* 209:267–270, 1981.

146. Lancet: Long-term and short-term beta-blockade after myocardial infarction. *Lancet* 1:1159–1161, 1982.
147. Larochelle, P., Hamet, P., Hoffman, B., Kuchel, O., McKenzie, J., Mitenko, P., Ogilvie, R. I., and Ruedy, J.: Labetalol in essential hypertension. *J. Cardiovasc. Pharmacol.* 2:751–759, 1980.
148. Laver, M. C., Fang, P., and Kincaid-Smith, P.: Double-blind comparison of two beta-blocking drugs with previous therapy in the treatment of hypertension. *Med. J. Aust.* 1:174–176, 1974.
149. Lechi, A., Picotti, G. B., Covi, G., Pomani, S., Pedrolli, E., Cesura, A. M., Danti, G., and Mattioli, M.: Intravenous labetalol in severe hypertension: Effects on blood pressure, renin activity and catecholamines. *Arzneim. Forsch.* 33(I) 3:524–526, 1981.
150. Lehmann, H-U., Taegener-Torge, C., Witt, E., Beck, O. A., and Hochrein, H.: Wirkungsvergleich zwischen Gallopamil (D600) und Verapamil. *Angiocardiology* 2:103, 1979.
151. Lehmann, H-U., Hochrein, H., Witt, E., and Mies, H. W.: Hemodynamic effects of calcium antagonists: Review. *Hypertension* 5 (Suppl. II):II-66–II-73, 1983.
152. Leishman, A. W. D., Thirkettle, J. L., Allen, B. R., and Dixon, R. A.: Controlled trial of oxprenolol and practolol in hypertension. *Br. Med. J.* 4:342–344, 1970.
153. Leonetti, G., Mayer, G., Morganti, A., Terzoli, L., Zanchetti, A., Bianchetti, G., DiSalle, E., Morselli, P. L., and Chidsey, C. A.: Hypotensive and renin suppressing activities of propranolol in hypertensive patients. *Clin. Sci. Mol. Med.* 48:491–499, 1975.
154. Letac, B., Fillastre, J. P., and Wolf, L. M.: The treatment of essential hypertension with acebutolol (Sectral). *Clin. Trials J.* 11 (Suppl. 3):92–95, 1974.
155. Lewis, G. R. J., Morley, K. D., Lewis, B. M., and Bones, P. J.: The treatment of hypertension with verapamil. *N. Z. Med. J.* 87:351–354, 1978.
156. Lohmoller, G., and Frohlich, E. D.: A comparison of timolol and propranolol in essential hypertension. *Am. Heart J.* 89:437–442, 1975.
157. Lown, B. E.: Introduction: Symposium on nifedipine and calcium flux inhibition in the treatment of coronary arterial spasm and myocardial ischaemia. *Am. J. Cadiol.* 44:780–782, 1979.
158. Lund-Johansen, P.: Haemodynamic long-term effects of timolol at rest and during exercise in essential hypertension. *Acta Med. Scand.* 199:263–267, 1976.
159. Lund-Johansen, P.: Haemodynamic long-term effects of a new beta-adrenoceptor blocking agent, atenolol (ICI 66082) in essential hypertension. *Br. J. Clin. Pharmacol.* 3:445–451, 1976.
160. Lund-Johansen, P.: Long-term haemodynamic effects of penbutolol at rest and during exercise in essential hypertension. *Eur. J. Clin. Pharmacol.* 16:149–153, 1979.
161. Lund-Johansen, P., and Omvik, P.: Prizidilol in essential hypertension: Long-term effects on plasma volume, extracellular fluid volume and central haemodynamics at rest and during exercise. *J. Cardiovasc. Pharmacol.* 4:1012–1017, 1982.
162. McAinsh, J., Baber, N. S., Smith, R., and Young, J.: Pharmacokinetic and pharmacodynamic studies with long-acting propranolol. *Br. J. Clin. Pharmacol.* 6:115–121, 1978.
163. McCarron, D. A.: Diuretic therapy for mild hypertension: the "real" cost. *Am. J. Cardiol.* 53:9A–11A, 1984.
164. McDevitt, D. G.: The assessment of beta-adrenoceptor blocking drugs in man. *Br. J. Clin. Pharmacol.* 4:413–425, 1977.
165. McDevitt, D. G., Brown, C. H., Carruthers, S. G., and Shanks, R. G.: Influence of intrinsic sympathomimetic activity and cardioselectivity on beta-adrenoceptor blockade. *Clin. Pharmacol. Ther.* 21:556–566, 1977.

166. MacGregor, G. A., Banks, R. A., Markandu, N. D., Bayliss, J., and Roulston, J.: Lack of effect of beta-blocker on flat dose response to thiazide in hypertension: Efficacy of low dose thiazide combined with beta-blocker. *Br. Med. J.* 286:1535-1538, 1983.
167. McLeay, R. A. B., Stallard, T. J., Watson, R. D. S., and Littler, W. A.: The effect of nifedipine on arterial pressure and reflex cardiac control. *Circulation* 67(5): 1084-1090, 1983.
168. Magnani, B., Ambrosioni, E., Costa, F. V., Malini, P. L., and Magelli, C.: Comparison of antihypertensive activity of atenolol and methyldopa at rest and during exercise. *Int. J. Clin. Pharmacol. Ther. Toxicol.* 19:440-444, 1981.
169. Maharaj, R. J., Thompson, M., Brock-Utne, J. G., Williamson, R., and Downing, J. W.: Treatment of hypertension following endotracheal intubation: A study comparing the efficacy of labetalol, practolol and placebo. *S. Afr. Med. J.* 63:691-694, 1983.
170. Malini, P. L., Strocchi, E., and Ambrosioni, E.: Comparison of the anti-hypertensive efficacy of bucindolol and propranolol. *J. Hypertension* 1 (Suppl. 2):348-350, 1983.
171. Man In 't Veld, A. J., and Schalekamp, M. A. D. H.: How intrinsic sympathomimetic activity modulates the haemodynamic responses to beta-adrenoceptor antagonists. A clue to the nature of their antihypertensive mechanism. *Br. J. Clin. Pharmacol.* 13 (Suppl. 2):245S-257S, 1982.
172. Mann, S., Millar Craig, M., Balasubramanian, V., and Raftery, E. B.: Once daily beta-adrenoceptor blockade in hypertension: An ambulatory assessment. *Br. J. Clin. Pharmacol.* 12:223-228, 1981.
173. Maroko, P. R., and Braunwald, E.: Modification of myocardial infarction size after coronary occlusion. *Ann. Intern. Med.* 79:720-733, 1973.
174. Maroko, P. R., Kjekshus, J. K., Sobel, B. E., Watanabe, T., Covell, J. W., Ross, J., and Braunwald, E.: Factors influencing infarct size following experimental coronary artery occlusions. *Circulation* 43:67-82, 1971.
175. Marshall, A. J., Roberts, C. J. C., and Barritt, D. W.: Raynaud's phenomenon as side effect of beta-blockers in hypertension. *Br. Med. J.* I:1498-1499, 1976.
176. Marshall, A. J., Barritt, D. W., Pocock, J., and Heaton, S. T.: Evaluation of beta blockade, bendrofluazide and prazosin in severe hypertension. *Lancet* 1:271-274, 1977.
177. Materson, B. J., Oster, J. R., Michael, U. F., and Perez-Stable, E. C.: Anti-hypertensive effectiveness of oxprenolol administered twice daily. *Clin. Pharmacol. Ther.* 19:325-331, 1976.
178. Meekers, J., Missotten, A., Fagard, R., Demuynck, D., Harvengt, C., Pas, P., Billiet, L., and Amery, A.: Predictive value of various parameters for the anti-hypertensive effect of the beta blocker ICI 66082(1). *Arch. Int. Pharmacodyn. Ther.* 213:294-306, 1975.
179. Mehta, J., and Cohn, J. N.: Haemodynamic effects of labetalol, an alpha and beta adrenergic blocking agent, in hypertensive subjects. *Circulation* 55:370-375, 1977.
180. Meyer, H., Bossert, F., Wehinger, E., Towart, R., and Bellemann, P.: Chemistry of calcium antagonists. *Hypertension* 5 (Suppl. II):II-2-II-7, 1983.
181. Meyer-Sabellek, W. A., Schulte, K.-L., Thiede, H. M., and Gotzen, R.: Acute hypotensive response to the new anti-hypertensive agent BM 14190 in essential hypertensive patients. *J. Hypertension* 1 (Suppl. 2):351-352, 1983.
182. Midtbo, K., and Hals, O.: Verapamil in the treatment of hypertension. *Curr. Ther. Res.* 27(6):830-838, 1980.
183. Millar-Craig, M. W., Mann, S., Balasubramanian, V., Cashman, P., and Raftery, E. B.: Effects of oxprenolol on the intra-arterial blood pressure response to dynamic exercise in hypertensive men. *J. Cardiovasc. Pharmacol.* 3:468-476, 1981.

184. Moe, G. K. and Abildskov, J. A.: Antiarrhythmic drugs. In *The Pharmacological Basis of Therapeutics*, 5th ed., edited by Goodman, L. S., and Gilman, A., New York, Macmillan Co., 1975, pp. 683–704.
185. Morgan, T. O., Louis, W. J., Dawborn, J. K., and Doyle, A. E.: The use of pindolol (Visken) in the treatment of hypertension. *Med. J. Aust.* 2:309–312, 1972.
186. Morgan, T. O., Sabto, J., Anavekar, S. N., Louis, W. J., and Doyle, A. E.: A comparison of beta adrenergic blocking drugs in the treatment of hypertension. *Postgrad. Med. J.* 50:253–259, 1974.
187. Morgan, T. O., Roberts, R., Carney, S. L., Louis, W. J., and Doyle, A. E.: Beta adrenergic receptor blocking drugs, hypertension and plasma renin. *Br. J. Clin. Pharmacol.* 2:159–164, 1975.
188. Morganti, A. A., Terzoli, L., Sala, C., Bianchini, C., Leonetti, G., and Zanchetti, A. S.: Interactions between diuretics and propranolol in treatment of arterial hypertension. *Cardiovasc. Med.* 4:43–52, 1979.
189. Mueller, J., Byrne, M. J., Opie, L. H., and van Schalkwyk, J.: Renal impairment in hypertension not improved by nadolol when compared with atenolol. *Drugs* 25 (Suppl. 2):146, 1983.
190. Muiesan, G., Agabiti-Rosei, E., Castellano, M., Alicandri, C. L., Corea, L., Fariello, R., Beschi, M., and Romanelli, G.: Antihypertensive and humoral effects of verapamil and nifedipine in essential hypertension. *J. Cardiovasc. Pharmacol.* 4: S325–S329, 1982.
191. Multicentre International Study: Improvement in prognosis of myocardial infarction by long-term beta-adrenoceptor blockade using practolol. *Br. Med. J.* 3:735–740, 1975.
192. Murphy, M. B., Scriven, A. J. I., and Dollery, C. T.: Role of nifedipine in treatment of hypertension. *Br. Med. J.* 287:257–259, 1983.
193. Nabata, H.: Effects of calcium antagonistic coronary vasodilators on myocardial contractility and membrane potentials. *Jpn. J. Pharmacol.* 27:239–249, 1977.
194. Nayler, W. G.: The pharmacological protection of the ischaemic heart: The use of calcium and beta-adrenoceptor antagonists. *Eur. Heart J.* I (Suppl. B):5–13, 1980.
195. Nayler, W. G., and Ferrari, R.: The use of nifedipine in the protection of the ischaemic heart. *Excerpta Medica International Congress Series* 516:197–206, 1979.
196. New Zealand Hypertension Study Group: A multicentre open trial of labetalol in New Zealand. *Br. J. Clin. Pharmacol.* 8:(Suppl. 2) 179S–182S, 1979.
197. Nik-Akhtar, B., Rashed, M. A., and Khakpour, M.: Effect of beta-adrenergic blocking agents (alprenolol and propranolol) in essential hypertension. *Angiology* 26:339–343, 1975.
198. Norwegian Multicentre Study Group: Timolol-induced reduction in mortality and re-infarction in patients surviving acute myocardial infarction. *N. Engl. J. Med.* 304:801–807, 1981.
199. Ogilvie, R. I., Hamet, P., Kreeft, J. H., Larochelle, P., and Marquez-Julio, A.: Once-daily dosing of acebutolol in hypertension. *J. Cardiovasc. Pharmacol.* 5:157–161, 1983.
200. Olivari, M. T., Bartorelli, C., Polese, A., Fiorentini, C., Moruzzi, P., and Guazzi, M. D.: Treatment of hypertension with nifedipine, a calcium antagonistic agent. *Circulation* 59(5):1056–1062, 1979.
201. O'Malley, K., O'Callaghan, W. G., Laher, M. S., McGarry, K., and O'Brien, E.: Beta-adrenoceptor blocking drugs and renal blood flow with special reference to the elderly. *Drugs* 25 (Suppl. 2):103–107, 1983.
202. Opie, L. H.: Calcium antagonists. Mechanisms, therapeutic indications and reservations: a review. *Q. J. Med.* New Series LIII, 209:1–6, 1984.

203. Opie, L. H., Jee, L., and White, D.: Antihypertensive effects of nifedipine combined with cardioselective beta-adrenergic receptor antagonism by atenolol. *Am. Heart J.* 104(3):606–612, 1982.
204. Page, D. L., Caulfield, J. B., Kastor, J. A., De Sanctis, R. W., and Sanders, C. A.: Myocardial changes associated with cardiogenic shock. *N. Engl. J. Med.* 285;133–137, 1971.
205. Paget, G. E.: Carcinogenic action of pronethalol. *Br. Med. J.* 5367:1266–1267, 1963.
206. Papademetriou, V., Notargiacomo, A. D., Khatri, I. m., and Freis, E. D.: Treatment of severe hypertension with intravenous labetalol. *Clin. Pharmacol. Ther.* 32(4): 431–435, 1982.
207. Pearson, R. M., Bending, M. R., Bulpitt, C. J., George, C. F., Hole, D. R., Williams, F. M., and Breckenridge, A. M.: Trial of combination of guanethidine and oxprenolol in hypertension. *Br. Med. J.* 1:933–936, 1976.
208. Pedersen, L. O.: Dose verapamil have a clinically significant antihypertensive effect? *Eur. J. Clin. Pharmacol.* 13:21–24, 1978.
209. Pedersen, L. O.: Calcium blockade as a therapeutic principle in arterial hypertension. *Acta Pharmacol. Toxicol.* 49 (Suppl. II):1–31, 1981.
210. Pedersen, L. O., and Mikkelsen, E.: Acute and chronic effects of nifedipine in arterial hypertension. *Eur. J. Clin. Pharmacol.* 14:375–381, 1978.
211. Pedersen, L. O., Christensen, C. K., Mikkelsen, E., and Ramsch, K. D.: Relationship between the antihypertensive effect and steady-state plasma concentration of nifedipine given alone or in combination with a beta-blocking agent. *Eur. J. Clin. Pharmacol.* 18:287–293, 1980a.
212. Pedersen, L. O., Christensen, N. J., and Ramsch, K. D.: Comparison of acute effects of nifedipine in normotensive and hypertensive man. *J. Cardiovasc. Pharmacol.* 2:357–366, 1980b.
213. Pelides, L. J., Reid, D. S., Thomas, M., and Shillingford, J. P.: Inhibition by beta-blockade of the ST segment elevation after acute myocardial infarction in man. *Cardiovasc. Res.* 6:295–301, 1972.
214. Persson, I.: Combination therapy of essential hypertension with pindolol (Visken) and hydralazine. *Eur. J. Clin. Pharmacol.* 9:91–93, 1975.
215. Peter, T., Norris, R. M., Clarke, E. D., Heng, M. K., Singh, B. N., Williams, B., Howell, D. R., and Ambler, P. K.: Reduction of enzyme levels by propranolol after acute myocardial infarction. *Circulation* 57:1091–1095, 1978.
216. Pettinger, W. A., and Keeton, K.: Altered renin release and propranolol potentiation of vasodilatory drug hypotension. *J. Clin. Invest.* 55:236–243, 1975.
217. Pettinger, W. A., and Mitchell, H. C.: Minoxidil–an alternative to nephrectomy for refractory hypertension. *N. Engl. J. Med.* 289:167–171, 1973.
218. Prichard, B. N. C.: Hypotensive action of pronethalol. *Br. Med. J.* 1:1227–1228, 1964.
219. Prichard, B. N. C.: Beta-adrenergic receptor blocking drugs in angina pectoris. *Drugs* 7:55–84, 1974.
220. Prichard, B. N. C.: The combined effect of propranolol with bethanidine or methyldopa in hypertension. *Adv. Clin. Pharmacol.* 2:107–113, 1976.
221. Prichard, B. N. C.: Beta-adrenergic receptor blockade in hypertension, past, present and future. *Br. J. Clin. Pharmacol.* 5:379–399, 1978.
222. Prichard, B. N. C.: Mechanisms of myocardial infarct prevention with beta-adrenergic blocking drugs. *Drugs* 25 (Suppl. 2):295–302, 1983.
223. Prichard, B. N. C., and Boakes, A. J.: The use of sotalol in the treatment of hypertension. *Advances in Beta-adrenergic Blocking Therapy, Sotalol.* Amsterdam Excerpta Medica, 1974, IV, pp. 7–24.

224. Prichard, B. N. C., and Boakes, A. J.: Labetalol in long-term treatment of hypertension. *Br. J. Clin. Pharmacol.* 3:743–750, 1976.
225. Prichard, B. N. C., and Boakes, A. J.: The use of beta-adrenergic blocking drugs in hypertension: A review. *Curr. Med. Res. Opin.* 4 (Suppl. 5):51–76, 1977.
226. Prichard, B. N. C., and Gillam, P. M. S.: Use of propranolol (Inderal) in the treatment of hypertension. *Br. Med. J.* 2:725–727, 1964.
227. Prichard, B. N. C., and Gillam, P. M. S.: Propranolol in hypertension. *Am. J. Cardiol.* 18:387–391, 1966.
228. Prichard, B. N. C., and Gillam, P. M. S.: Treatment of hypertension with propranolol. *Br. Med. J.* 1:7–16, 1969.
229. Prichard, B. N. C., and Gillam, P. M. S.: Assessment of propranolol in angina pectoris. Clinical dose response curve and effect on electrocardiogram at rest and on exercise. *Br. Heart J.* 33:473–480, 1971.
230. Prichard, B. N. C., and Owens, C. W. I.: Drug treatment of hypertension. In *Hypertension*, 2nd ed., edited by Genest, J., Kuchel, O., Harnet, P., and Cantin, M., New York, McGraw-Hill Book Company, 1983, pp. 1171–1210.
231. Prichard, B. N. C., Aellig, W. H., and Richardson, G. A.: The action of intravenous oxprenolol, practolol, propranolol and sotalol on acute exercise tolerance in angina pectoris: The effect on heart rate and the electrocardiogram. *Postgrad. Med. J.* 46 (Suppl. Nov.):77–85, 1970.
232. Prichard, B. N. C., Gillam, P. M. S., and Graham, B. R.: Beta receptor antagonism in hypertension; comparison with the effect of adrenergic neurone inhibition on cardiovascular responses. *Int. J. Clin. Pharmacol.* 4:131–140, 1970.
233. Prichard, B. N. C., Shinebourne, E., Flemming, J., and Hamer, J.: Haemodynamic studies in hypertensive patients on oral propranolol. *Br. Heart J.* 32:236–240, 1970c.
234. Prichard, B. N. C., Boakes, A. J., and Day, G. M.: Practolol in the treatment of hypertension. *Postgrad. Med. J.* 47 (Suppl.):84–91, 1971.
235. Prichard, B. N. C., Boakes, A. J., and Graham, B. R.: A within patient comparison of bethanidine, methyldopa and propranolol in the treatment of hypertension. *Clin. Sci. Mol. Med.* 51 (Suppl. 3):567S–570S, 1976.
236. Prichard, B. N. C., Boakes, A. J., and Hernandez, R.: Long term treatment of hypertension with labetalol. *Br. J. Clin. Pharmacol.* 8 (Suppl. 2):171s–177s, 1979.
237. Rasmussen, S., and Nielsen, P. E.: Blood pressure, plasma volume, extracellular volume and glomerular filtration rate during treatment with labetalol in essential hypertension. *Postgrad. Med. J.* 56 (Suppl. 2):33–36, 1980.
238. Rasmussen, M. M., Reimer, K. A., Kloner, R. A., and Jennings, R. B.: Infarct size reduction by propranolol before and after coronary ligation in dogs. *Circulation* 56:794–798, 1977.
239. Reach, G., Thibonnier, M., Chevillard, C., Corvol, P., and Milliez, P.: Effect of labetalol on blood pressure and plasma catecholamine concentrations in patients with phaeochromocytoma. *Br. Med. J.* 280:1300–1301, 1980.
240. Richards, D. A., and Prichard, B. N. C.: Clinical pharmacology of labetalol. *Br. J. Clin. Pharmacol.* 8 (Suppl. 2):89s–93s, 1979.
241. Ronne-Rasmussen, J. O., Andersen, G. S., Bowal Jensen, N., and Andersson, E.: Acute effect of intravenous labetalol in the treatment of systemic arterial hypertension. *Br. J. Clin. Pharmacol.* 3 (Suppl. 3):805–808, 1976.
242. Rose, G.: Part III: Some conclusions (should every survivor of a heart attack be given a beta blocker?). *Br. Med. J.* 285:39–40, 1982.
243. Rosei, E. A., Brown, J. J., Lever, A. F., Robertson, A. S., Robertson, J. I. S., and Trust, R. M.: Treatment of phaeochromocytoma and of clonidine withdrawal hypertension with labetalol. *Br. J. Clin. Pharmacol.* 3:809–815, 1976.

244. Rosenthal, T., Rabinowitz, B., Boichis, H., Elazar, E., Brauner, A., and Neufeld, H. N.: Use of labetalol in hypertensive patients during discontinuation of clonidine therapy. *Eur. J. Clin. Pharmacol.* 20:237–240, 1981.
245. Russell, W. J., Kaines, A. H., Hooper, M. J., and Frewin, D. B.: Labetalol in the pre-operative management of phaeochromocytoma. *Anaesth. Intensive Care* 10: 160–162, 1982.
246. Salonen, J. T., and Palminteri, R.: Comparison of two doses of betaxolol and placebo in hypertension: A randomized double-blind crossover trial. *Eur. J. Clin. Pharmacol.* 23:491–494, 1982.
247. Sannerstedt, R., Stenberg, J., Vedin, A., Wilhelmsson, C., and Werko, L.: Chronic beta-adrenergic blockade in arterial hypertension. Haemodynamic influences of dihydralazine and dynamic exercise and clinical effects of combined treatment. *Am. J. Cardiol.* 29:718–723, 1972.
248. Saraste, K., Tarkiainen, A., Wennstrom, J., Harkonen, M., Gordin, A., and Sundberg, S.: A placebo-controlled study of the effects of carteolol in hypertensive patients. *Curr. Ther. Res.* 32:189–195, 1982.
249. Schechter, P. J., Tanskanen, A., Tuomilehto, J., and Koch-Weser, J.: Treatment of mild and moderate hypertension with medroxalol, an alpha- and beta-adrenergic antagonist. *J. Cardiovasc. Pharmacol.* 4:955–959, 1982.
250. Schutz, E., Riem, H., Buhler, F. A., and Follath, F.: Serum concentration and antihypertensive effect of slow release verapamil. *J. Cardiovasc. Pharmacol.* 4:S346–S349, 1982.
251. Scott, A. K., Rigby, J. W., Webster, J., Hawksworth, G. M., Petrie, J. C., and Lovell, H. G.: Atenolol and metoprolol once daily in hypertension. *Br. Med. J.* 284:1514–1516, 1982.
252. Sega, R., Mailland, F., Damiani, E., Groothold, G., and Libretti, A.: Indenolol in hypertension. *Clin. Pharmacol. Ther.* 33:289–293, 1983.
253. Semplicini, A., Pessina, A. C., Rossi, G. P., Hlede, M., and Morandin, F.: Alpha-adrenoceptor blockade by labetalol during long-term dosage. *Clin. Pharmacol. Ther.* 33(3):278–282, 1983.
254. Serlin, M. J., Orme, M. C. L. E., Maciver, M., Green, G. J., MacNee, M., and Breckenridge, A. M.: Rate of onset of hypotensive effect of oral labetalol. *Br. J. Clin. Pharmacol.* 7:165–168, 1979.
255. Shinebourne, E., Fleming, J., and Hamer, J.: Effects of beta-adrenergic blockade during exercise in hypertensive and ischaemic heart disease. *Lancet* 2:1217–1220, 1967.
256. Siitonen, L., Janne, J., Keyrilainen, O., Koskinen, P., Leskinen, O., Pitkajarvi, T., and Reinikainen, M.: Hydralazine and beta-adrenergic blockade in the treatment of hypertension. *Ann. Clin. Res.* 6:341–346, 1974.
257. Silke, B., Nelson, G. I. C., Ahuja, R. C., and Taylor, S. H.: Comparative haemodynamic dose response effects of propranolol and labetalol in coronary heart disease. *Br. Heart J.* 48:364–371, 1982.
258. Simon, G., Kiowski, W., and Julius, S.: Anti-hypertensive and beta-adrenoceptor antagonist action of timolol. *Clin. Pharmacol. Ther.* 23:152–157, 1978.
259. Singh, B. N., Nademanee, K., and Baky, S. H.: Calcium antagonists: clinical use in the treatment of arrhythmias. *Drugs* 25:125–153, 1983.
260. Sloan, P. J. M., and Beevers, D. G.: Nifedipine in combination therapy for resistant hypertension. *Pharmatherapeutica* 3(5):349–353, 1983.
261. Smith, C. D., and McKendry, R. J. R.: Controlled trial of nifedipine in the treatment of Raynaud's phenomenon. *Lancet* 2:1299–1301, 1982.
262. Stewart, I. McD. G.: Compared incidence of first myocardial infarction in hypertensive patients under treatment containing propranolol or excluding beta-receptor blockade. *Clin. Sci. Mol. Med.* 51 (Suppl. 3):509s–511s, 1976.

263. Stokes, G. S., and Weber, M. A.: Prazosin: Preliminary report and comparative studies with other anti-hypertensive agents. *Br. Med. J.* 2:298–300, 1974.
264. Stokes, G. S., Raftos, J., Lewis, R. G., Mitchell, A. S., Jeremy, D., Frost, G. W., and Thornell, I. R.: Combined use of prazosin and beta-blockers in hypertension. *J. Cardiovasc. Pharmacol.* 4:s172–s175, 1982.
265. Stoll, R. W., Cavanaugh, J. H., and MacLeod, C. M.: Beta-blocking effect of single oral doses of carteolol. *Clin. Pharmacol. Ther.* 30:605–610, 1981.
266. Stone, P. H., Antman, E. M., Muller, J. E., and Braunwald, E.: Calcium channel blocking agents in the treatment of cardiovascular disorders. Part III: Haemodynamic effects and clinical applications. *Ann. Intern. Med.* 93:886–904, 1980.
267. Svedmyr, N., Malmberg, R., and Haggendal, E.: The haemodynamic effects of sotalol (MJ 1999) and propranolol in man. *Pharmacol. Clin.* 2:82–85, 1970.
268. Svendsen, T. L., Hartling, O., and Trap-Jensen, J.: Immediate haemodynamic effects of propranolol, practolol, pindolol, atenolol and ICI 89406 in healthy volunteers. *Eur. J. Clin. Pharmacol.* 15:223–228, 1979.
269. Taggart, P., and Carruthers, M.: Suppression by oxprenolol of adrenergic response to stress. *Lancet* 2:256–258, 1972.
270. Taggart, P., Carruthers, M., and Somerville, W.: Electrocardiogram, plasma catecholamines and lipids and their modification when speaking before an audience. *Lancet* 2:341–346, 1973.
271. Takeda, T., Kaneko, Y., Omae, T., Yoshinga, K., Masuyama, Y., Nukada, T., and Shigiya, R. (1982). The use of labetalol in Japan: Results of multicentre clinical trials. *Br. J. Clin. Pharmacol.* 13 (Suppl. 1):49s–57s, 1982.
272. Takekoshi, N., Murakami, E., Murakami, H., Matsui, S., Masuya, K., Nomura, M., Fujita, S., Tsuji, S., Chatani, T., Emoto, J., Tsugawa, H., and Hashmoto, A.: Treatment of severe hypertension and hypertensive emergency with nifedipine, a calcium antagonistic agent. *Jpn. Circ. J.* 45:852–860, 1981.
273. Tarazi, R. C., and Dustan, H. P.: Beta-adrenergic blockade in hypertension. Practical and theoretical implications of long-term haemodynamic variations. *Am. J. Cardiol.* 29:633–640, 1972.
274. Tarazi, R. C., Dustan, H. P., Bravo, E. L., and Niarchos, A. P.: Vasodilating drugs: contrasting haemodynamic effects. *Clin. Sci. Mol. Med.* 51:575S–578S, 1976.
275. Taylor, S. H., and Meeran, M. K.: Different effects of adrenergic beta-receptor blockade on heart rate response to mental stress, catecholamines, and exercise. *Br. Heart J.* 4:257–259, 1973.
276. Taylor, S. H., and Meeran, M. K.: The cardiovascular response to some environmental stresses and their modification by oxprenolol. In *New Perspectives in Beta Blockade*, Horsham, CIBA, 1973, pp. 293–306.
277. Taylor, S. H., Silke, B., Lee, P. S., and Hilal, A.: Haemodynamic dose-response effects of intravenous beta-blocking drugs with different ancillary properties in patients with coronary heart disease. *Eur. Heart J.* 3:564–569, 1982a.
278. Taylor, S. H., Silke, B., Ebbutt, A., Sutton, G. C., Prout, B. J., and Burley, D. M.: A long-term prevention study with oxprenolol in coronary heart disease. *N. Engl. J. Med.* 307(21):1294–1301, 1982b.
279. Textor, S. C., Fouad, F. M., Bravo, E. L., Tarazi, R. C., Vidt, D. G., and Gifford, R. W.: Re-distribution of cardiac output to the kidneys during oral nadolol administration. *N. Engl. J. Med.* 307:601–604, 1972.
280. Thibonnier, M., Bonnet, F., and Corvol, P.: Antihypertensive effect of fractionated sublingual administration of nifedipine in moderate essential hypertension. *Eur. J. Clin. Pharmacol.* 17:161–164, 1980.
281. Tibblin, G., and Ablad, B.: Anti-hypertensive therapy with alprenolol, a beta-adrenergic receptor antagonist. *Acta Med. Scand.* 186:451–457, 1969.

282. Trust, P. M., Rosei, E. A., Brown, J. J., Fraser, R., Lever, A. F., Morton, J. J., and Robertson, J. I. S.: Effect on blood pressure, angiotensin II and aldosterone concentrations during treatment of severe hypertension with intravenous labetalol: Comparison with propranolol. *Br. J. Clin. Pharmacol.* 3:799–803, 1976.
283. Tuckman, J., Martin, R., and Hodler, J.: Hypertoniebehandlung mit hohen Dosen von oxprenolol, allein oder in Kombination mit dem vasodilator Dihydralazine. *Helv. Med. Acta* 36:243–244, 1972.
284. Tuckman, J., Messerli, F., and Hodler, J.: Treatment of hypertension with large doses of the beta-adrenergic blocking drug oxprenolol alone and in combination with the vasodilator dihydralazine. *Clin. Sci. Mol. Med.* 45:159s–161s, 1973.
285. Turi, Z. G., and Braunwald, E.: The use of beta-blockers after myocardial infarction. *JAMA* 249:12–16, 1983.
286. Ulrych, M., Frohlich, E. D., Dustan, H. P., and Page, I. H. (1968). Immediate haemodynamic effects of beta-adrenergic blockade with propranolol in normotensive and hypertensive man. *Circulation* 37:411–416, 1968.
287. Van Herwaarden, C. L. A., Binkhorst, R. A., Fennis, J. F. M., and Van't Laar, A.: Effects of propranolol and metoprolol on haemodynamic and respiratory indices and on perceived exertion during exercise in hypertensive patients. *Br. Heart J.* 41:99–105, 1979.
288. van Zwieten, P. A., van Meel, J. C. A., and Timmermans, B. M. W. M.: Pharmacology of calcium entry blockers: interaction with vascular alpha-adrenoceptors. *Hypertension* 5 II (Suppl. II):II-8–II-17, 1983.
289. Vater, W., Kroneberg, G., and Hoffmeister, F.: Zur pharmakologie von 4-2 (N′-triphenyl)-2-6-dimethyl-1-,4-dihydropridin-3-5 dicarbonsauredimethylester (nifedipine, Bay a 1040). *Arzneim. Forsch.* 22:1–14, 1972.
290. Velasco, M., Vizcarrondo, H., Urbina-Quintana, A., and Hernandez-Pieretti, O.: A comparative study between pindolol and nadolol on systemic and cardiac hemodynamics in hypertensive patients. *Curr. Ther. Res.* 32(5):663–668, 1982.
291. Vestal, R. E., Wood, A. J., and Shand, D. G.: Reduced beta-adrenoceptor sensitivity in the elderly. *Clin. Pharmacol. Ther.* 26(2):181–185, 1979.
292. Veterans Administration Cooperative Study Group on Anti-Hypertensive Agents.: Multi-clinic controlled trial of bethanidine and guanethidine in severe hypertension. *Circulation* 55:519–525, 1977.
293. Von Mollendorff, E., Huschka, C., Schröter, E., and Abshagen, U. (1981). BM 12343, a novel compound with vasodilating and beta-adrenoceptor blocking activitives. *Clin. Sci.* 61:477s–479s, 1981.
294. Waal-Manning, H. J.: Comparative studies on the hypotensive effects of beta-adrenergic receptor blockade. *Symposium on Beta-Adrenergic Receptor Blocking Drugs*, Auckland, CIBA, 1970, pp. 64–72.
295. Waal-Manning, H. J.: The antihypertensive action of several beta-adrenoceptor blocking drugs. *N. Z. Med. J.* 83:223–226, 1976.
296. Waal-Manning, H. J.: Atenolol and three nonselective beta-blockers in hypertension. *Clin. Pharmacol. Ther.* 25:8–18, 1979.
297. Waal-Manning, H. J., and Simpson, F. O.: Pindolol: A comparison with other antihypertensive drugs and a double-blind placebo trial. *N. Z. Med. J.* 80:151–157, 1974.
298. Waal-Manning, H. J., and Simpson, F. O.: Review of long-term treatment with labetalol. *Br. J. Clin. Pharmacol.* 13 (Suppl. i):65S–73S, 1982.
299. Wathen, C. G., Hannan, W. J., Turnbull, L. W., Roulston, J. E., and Muir, A. L.: The use of nifedipine in combination therapy for the management of hypertension. *Clin. Sci.* 66(2):66P, 1984.
300. Webster, J., Jeffers, T. A., Galloway, D. B., Petrie, J. C., and Barker, N. P.:

Atenolol, methyldopa and chlorthalidone in moderate hypertension. *Br. Med. J.* 1:76–78, 1977.
301. Weidmann, P., De Chatel, R., Ziegler, W. H., Flammer, J., and Reubi, F.: Alpha and beta adrenergic blockade with orally administered labetalol in hypertension. *Am. J. Cardiol.* 41:570–576, 1978.
302. Wikstrand, J., and Berglund, G.: Anti-hypertensive treatment with beta-blockers in patients aged over 65. *Br. Med. J.* 285:850, 1982.
303. Wilburn, R. L., Blaufuss, A., and Bennett, C. M.: Long-term treatment of severe hypertension with minoxidil, propranolol and furosemide. *Circulation* 52:706–713, 1975.
304. Wilcox, R. G., and Hampton, J. R.: Comparison between atenolol and nadolol in essential hypertension at rest and on exercise. *Br. J. Clin. Pharmacol.* 13:841–846, 1982.
305. Wilcox, R. G., and Mitchell, J. R. A.: Contribution of atenolol, bendrofluazide and hydralazine to the management of severe hypertension. *Br. Med. J.* 2:547–550, 1977.
306. Wilcox, R. G., Roland, J. M., Banks, D. C., Hampton, J. R., and Mitchell, J. R. A.: Randomised trial comparing propranolol with atenolol in immediate treatment of suspected myocardial infarction. *Br. Med. J.* 281:885–888, 1980.
307. Wilhelmsen, L., Wedel, H., and Tibblin, G.: Multivariate analysis of risk factors for coronary heart disease. *Circulation* 48:950–958, 1973.
308. Williams, L. C., Murphy, M. J., and Parsons, V.: Labetalol in severe and resistant hypertension. *Br. J. Clin. Pharmacol.* 8 (Suppl. 2):143s–147s, 1979.
309. Wilson, C., Scott, M. E., and Abdel-Mohsen, A.: Atenolol and methyldopa in the treatment of hypertension. *Postgrad. Med. J.* 53 (Suppl. 3):123–127, 1977.
310. Wilson, M., Morgan, G., and Morgan, T.: The effect on blood pressure of beta-adrenoceptor blocking drugs administered once daily and their duration of action when therapy is ceased. *Br. J. Clin. Pharmacol.* 3:857–861, 1976.
311. Yagil, Y., Kobrin, I., Leibel, B., Stessman, J., and Ben Ishay, D.: The combination of propranolol and nifedipine in the treatment of hypertension: acute and long-term effects. *Postgrad. Med. J.* 59 (Suppl. 2):114–118, 1983.
312. Yamakado, T., Oonishi, N., Kondo, S., Noziri, A., Nakano, T., and Takezawa, H.: Effects of diltiazem on cardiovascular responses during exercise in systemic hypertension and comparison with propranolol. *Am. J. Cardio.* 52(8):1023–1027, 1983.
313. Yusuf, S., Ramsdale, D., Peto, R., Furse, L., Bennett, D., Bray, C., and Sleight, P.: Early intravenous atenolol in suspected acute myocardial infarction. *Lancet* 2:273–276, 1980.
314. Zacest, R., Gilmore, E., and Koch-Weser, J.: Treatment of essential hypertension with combined vasodilation and beta-adrenergic blockade. *New Engl. J. Med.* 286: 617–622, 1972.
315. Zacharias, F. J., Cowen, K. J., Vickers, J., and Wall, B. G.: Propranolol in hypertension. A study of long-term therapy 1964–1970. *Am. Heart J.* 83:755–761, 1972.
316. Zacharias, F. J., Cowen, K. J., Cuthbertson, P. J. R., Johnson, T. B. W., Presst, J., Thompson, J., Vickers, J., Simpson, W. T., and Tuson, R.: Atenolol in hypertension: A study of long-term therapy. *Postgrad. Med. J.* 53 (Suppl. 3):102–110, 1977.
317. Zschiedrich, H., Neurohr, W., Luth, J. B., Philipp, T., and Distler, A.: sympathetic nervous activity and the pressor effect of noradrenaline under chronic alpha-beta-adrenoceptor blockade with labetalol in hypertension. *Klin. Wochenschr.* 61:661–667, 1983.

SUMMARY

Perspectives on Some Important Public Health Issues Related to Potassium Balance

W. GORDON WALKER and ANDREW WHELTON
The Johns Hopkins University School of Medicine and The Johns Hopkins Hospital, Baltimore, Maryland

PAUL K. WHELTON
The Johns Hopkins School of Hygiene and Public Health, The Johns Hopkins University School of Medicine, and The Johns Hopkins Hospital, Baltimore, Maryland

ANDREW WHELTON
The Johns Hopkins University School of Medicine and The Johns Hopkins Hospital, Baltimore, Maryland

This volume has considered in detail the diverse manifestations associated with pathophysiological alterations in both potassium deficits and excesses. Many of these manifestations have been well known for more than a half century, but others have only begun to receive attention within the past several years. It is not possible in the space of a single chapter to cover all of the issues of importance. It is reasonable to look at those issues that have not been adequately emphasized recently, as well as those that have important public health implications for all or for a significant subset of the population.

The acute and often life-threatening hazards associated with severe or rapidly developing hypokalemia and hyperkalemia, including the attendant electrolyte alterations, skeletal and smooth muscle abnormalities, and effects upon the myocardium are well recognized and in general are promptly diagnosed and effectively treated. Several chapters of this volume have summarized clinical features of these disturbances; they do not require repetition here. It is important, however, to address those aspects of potassium imbalance that have not received adequate emphasis. We will focus the attention of this final chapter on five issues recently recognized to have important pathophysiological and therapeutic implications:

1. The potential clinical importance of diuretic-induced hypokalemia
2. The catabolic response to potassium deficit
3. Potassium and blood pressure homeostasis
4. Hypokalemia and ventricular ectopy
5. The desirability of potassium supplementation

DIURETIC-INDUCED HYPOKALEMIA

The most common cause of hypokalemia is diuretic therapy. The use profile data summarized in Chapter 17 provide a reasonable estimate of the prevalence of this problem in the United States. If it is assumed that one individual on active and continuing therapy is likely to require four prescriptions per year, the 1985 projections that identify 124 million diuretic prescriptions annually would suggest that perhaps 30 million people in the United States alone are on maintenance therapy with diuretics. Even if this overestimates the point prevalence within the user population by a factor of two, one is left with a figure of 15 million people at risk, which is a very large fraction of the total population of this country. When the drug use profile data (Chapter 17, Table 2) and an estimate of the mean value for drug-category-related prevalence of hypokalemia (Chapter 17, Table 3) are evaluated in concert, they yield an estimate that more than 4 million of the population of the United States may be hypokalemic as a result of diuretic therapy. There seems little doubt that many such patients, representing the highest risk group for developing adverse clinical events as a consequence of hypokalemia, should be treated by potassium supplementation or addition of a potassium-sparing diuretic to their diuretic regimen. The most critical question for the clinician is the point at which one should introduce this modification of the treatment regimen. Most authorities recommend that one of these measures should be instituted when the serum potassium falls below 3.5, but significant deficits may accumulate in patients whose plasma values are above this level. The correlation between plasma values and balance data published by Sterns et al. (28) would indicate that decrease in serum potassium from an average value of, say, 4.2 to, say, 3.7 could be associated with a deficit of 200 or more mEq in total body potassium. Deficits as small as this may be associated with measurable physiological disturbances. This raises the question whether treatment should be instituted when serum potassium is decreased by 0.5 mEq/L even when the usual criteria for hypokalemia (serum potassium below 3.5 mEq/L) are not yet present. While a strong case cannot be made for such treatment as a routine, the apparent increased risk of cardiac arrhythmias and the attendant risk of increased morbidity and mortality forces consideration of such treatment under these circumstances.

CATABOLIC RESPONSE TO POTASSIUM DEFICIENCY

The relationship between potassium depletion and nitrogen balance has been discussed in considerable detail in Chapter 8 by Sapir. The adverse effect of a persisting potassium deficit upon nitrogen balance is reviewed principally within the context of patients undergoing a prolonged fast or starvation. However, the persistent nitrogen wasting that is associated with potassium deficits, and that may be sharply curtailed by providing an excess of potassium, is not limited to the starving state. In a study previously published from our laboratory, it was demonstrated that the same relationship could be identified in subjects in whom a potassium deficit had been created through the use of diuretic agents (29). Remarkably, loss of only a modest amount of potassium (a net negative balance of approximately 250 mEq of potassium) resulted in a sustained negative nitrogen balance. These individuals were maintained on a normal protein intake (0.75 g of protein per kilogram of body weight per day), and when furosemide was used to produce this modest potassium deficit, it created a sustained catabolic state with a mean net negative nitrogen balance of approximately 4 g per day. Although normal individuals achieve nitrogen balance within 3 days when placed on a nitrogen intake of 4 g per day, or roughly half the nitrogen intake employed in the study that we reported, these potassium-depleted subjects had a persistent catabolic state with a net loss of about 4 g of nitrogen per day for 9 days until potassium repletion was reinstituted. Following potassium repletion, nitrogen balance was achieved within 4 days. A significant fraction of this nitrogen loss represented increased ammonia excretion, but the increased ammonia excretion alone was not adequate to account for the total nitrogen loss. Ammonia loss of this magnitude should not have resulted in a net negative nitrogen balance in the face of what was a very liberal nitrogen intake. It would appear from these data that potassium deficiency has a catabolic effect that substantially exceeds the catabolic response necessary to sustain urinary ammonia excretion in potassium deficit states. While the clinical effects of such long-term protein catabolic states remain to be determined in individuals who are otherwise in reasonably good health, there certainly are circumstances under which such metabolic changes could accentuate existing risks. It may be that this could play a role in the arrhythmias that have been recognized during chronic maintenance diuretic therapy. At the least, the studies indicate that potassium deficits judged to be very modest by any reasonable standards can be documented to produce metabolic derangements that appear to be sustained for prolonged periods. They thus lend substantial credence to the proposition that modest potassium deficits may play an important clinical role in a number of disturbances.

POTASSIUM AND BLOOD PRESSURE HOMEOSTASIS

We reported in Chapter 26 of this volume that a correlation could be demonstrated between potassium and blood pressure in a sample that contained a sizable number of patients with elevated blood pressure. This same type of negative correlation, demonstrating that potassium output (and by inference, intake) is substantially lower in hypertensive subjects, has been subsequently reported by Berenson, Stamler, Khaw, Bulpitt, and others (3,4,8,13,14,26,27), but not by all. Page (22), in studies on Qash'gai nomads of southern Iran, failed to identify a relationship between potassium and blood pressure. He did demonstrate a significant correlation between blood pressure and sodium excretion in this relatively primitive tribal society with a high salt intake. Females of the tribe exhibited a significant correlation between sodium:potassium ratio and systolic blood pressure. These data are of particular interest insofar as they establish a correlation between excess sodium intake and hypertension within a single cultural unit; such an association had previously been supported mainly by epidemiological data from different cultures and social groups (20,21,23,24).

Experimental evidence identifies both sodium and potassium as being capable of contributing to the pathogenesis of elevated blood pressure. Meneely (17) and Dahl (5) both documented the importance of dietary potassium as a determinant of blood pressure in rats. Dahl provided quantitative characterization of the importance of the sodium:potassium ratio, demonstrating that when sodium was kept constant, progressive reduction of potassium in the diet was associated with a progressive rise in blood pressure. Langford and Watson (15) reported results of a study in young women that demonstrated that the sodium:potassium ratio of urine correlated positively with blood pressure.

Our data provide interesting results when the association between blood pressure and potassium excretion alone is compared with the relationship between blood pressure and the sodium:potassium ratio. Tables 1 and 2 present details of this analysis. For the purpose of this analysis, the subjects studied were grouped into four quartiles on the basis of their urinary potassium output (Table 1). Note that the prevalence of elevated blood pressure (here defined as a supine diastolic blood pressure exceeding 90 mm Hg) is, in general, higher the lower the potassium excretion, being highest (67%) in the first quartile. It drops successively in the second and third quartile but it is again high in the

Table 1 Prevalence of Hypertension in Each Quartile of Urinary Potassium

Urinary K	Number with diastolic BP ≤90 mm Hg	Number with diastolic BP >90 mm Hg	% with elevated BP
1st Quartile	47	96	67
2nd Quartile	72	71	50
3rd Quartile	87	56	39
4th Quartile	71	74	51

fourth, although not as high as in the first quartile. When the sodium:potassium ratio is substituted for potassium alone and this analysis repeated, the association is more impressive. The prevalence of hypertension increases from 38% in the first quartile to 80.5% in the fourth quartile, and the increase is a smooth and progressive one. It is of interest that over the range of sodium:potassium ratios observed in this study (Table 2), the risk of developing elevated blood pressure doubles between the first and fourth quartiles, a much greater and more sharply defined increase in risk, than is seen when the data are grouped by potassium excretion alone.

It is possible to propose a sequence of changes that assigns a central role to the potassium deficit as an important pathogenetic event in the development of hypertension. It is well known that potassium deficiency leads to increased tone in smooth muscle (10-12) and is associated with an increase in systemic vascular resistance and a reduction in renal blood flow (1,16). This reduction in renal blood flow can be expected to reduce the renal excretory capacity for sodium, or at least to impair sodium excretion. The "infinite gain principle" proposed by Guyton (9) as the mechanism for regulating the vascular volume and sodium load requires a normal renal blood flow and normally functioning kidneys. According to this schema, a rise in blood pressure yields a prompt natriuretic response in the normal kidney, which restores blood volume and pressure to its previous normal level. The capacity to respond in this fashion preserves a normal blood pressure and a constant vascular volume. A progressive increase in renal resistance that occurs in potassium depletion, as has been documented—at least in the dog—by Abbrecht (1), would disrupt this capacity to regulate body sodium, and consequently the capacity to maintain blood pressure in the normal range. The result would be a progressive elevation of blood pressure, which is then maintained at this higher level as a means of increasing filtration and excretion of sodium, thus permitting maintenance of normal volume and sodium balance despite an increase in sodium intake. The relationship between the sodium:potassium ratio and the prevalence of elevated blood pressure as indicated in Table 2 is at least

Table 2 Prevalence of Hypertension in Each Quartile Defined by Urinary Na/K

Urinary Na/K	Number with diastolic BP ≤90 mmHg	Number with diastolic BP >90 mm Hg	% Hypertensive
1st Quartile	88	55	38.4
2nd Quartile	80	64	44.4
3rd Quartile	73	71	49.3
4th Quartile	36	107	80.5

consistent with this postulated sequence of events. Moreover, it raises the possibility that in the "normal" nonobese state and perhaps in mild hypertension as well, the therapeutic maneuver that may be most effective in prevention of age-related increases in blood pressure and maintenance of blood pressure in the normal range may be an increase in potassium intake accompanied by reduction in sodium intake.

Data from different sources relating decreased potassium intake and elevated sodium intake to hypertension are sufficiently consistent (3,4,8,13,14,15,20,21.30) that clinical trials to test the hypothesis that a sharp reduction in the dietary sodium:potassium ratio represents an effective measure for prevention of hypertension should be pursued with sufficient vigor to define the role of dietary modification as a preventive maneuver.

HYPOKALEMIA AND VENTRICULAR ECTOPY

A causal association between severe hypokalemia or hyperkalemia and cardiac arrhythmias has been recognized for many years. Likewise, it has long been accepted that hypokalemia, even if mild, may be a precipitant of cardiac arrhythmias in patients being treated with digitalis. However, the suggestion that ventricular ectopic beats might occur purely as a consequence of mild hypokalemia is more recent and controversial. Much of the original data bearing on this issue is reviewed in Chapters 12-15 and 18-22.

On balance, the available information suggests that diuretic administration results in an increased rate of cardiac arrhythmias even in those who are not concurrently receiving digitalis. Although the situation is complex, hypokalemia probably plays a role in the genesis of diuretic induced ventricular ectopy. The proposition that diuretic-induced ventricular ectopy may occasionally take the form of ventricular fibrillation and lead to sudden death remains controversial. The most compelling data in favor of such a hypothesis has come from analyses of the Multiple Risk Factor Intervention Trial (MRFIT), such as those provided in Chapter 23 and elsewhere (18,19). The MRFIT findings, while troublesome, do not and cannot provide conclusive evidence of a relationship between diuretic administration and sudden death. Additional information from other data bases that will confirm or refute the proposed relationship between diuretic administration and sudden death is urgently needed. Likewise, clarification of the underlying mechanism and independent role of putative risk factors would provide clinicians with a firmer basis for prevention and treatment. The Medical Research Council trial of treatment in mild to moderate hypertension is the most likely source of useful information in the short term. However, clinicians should be aware that their decisions in this controversial area may have to be based on less than perfect data for some time to come.

Given the present uncertainty, what should we do? It is first relevant to note that recorded mortality from stroke and coronary heart disease has declined progressively in the United States during the same time period that antihypertensive—mainly diuretic—therapy has become increasingly common in the community (see Figure 1, Chapter 24). For this and other reasons, a recommendation to avoid the use of thiazide agents during antihypertensive drug therapy would be inappropriate at present. However, caution is in order. Diuretics should be administered in the lowest dose necessary to achieve the desired reduction in blood pressure. Likewise, hypokalemia should probably be prevented or treated with a sodium-restricted diet, potassium-sparing agents, or potassium chloride supplements. In selected patients, alternative forms of monotherapy should be considered. This is especially the case for those who are young, white, and/or have an unsatisfactory response to diuretics. Beta-blockers provide the best documented alternative, but monotherapy with receptor blockers centrally active agents, calcium-channel blockers, or angiotensin-converting enzyme inhibitors may be more appropriate in individual cases. It should be emphasized that none of the nondiuretic alternatives is a panacea, and none have been evaluated for the possibility of adverse effects as carefully as diuretics.

DESIRABILITY OF POTASSIUM SUPPLEMENTATION

General agreement exists respect to the desirability of recommending potassium supplements or potassium-sparing agents to certain patients being treated with thiazides or thiazidelike diuretics. This is particularly the case for older men, patients with known electrocardiographic abnormalities, those who are concurrently receiving digitalis therapy, and those with severe (serum potassium = 2.5–3.0 mEq/L) or symptomatic hypokalemia. The necessity to prevent or treat milder forms of hypokalemia in younger asymptomatic individuals remains controversial. However, such an approach has been advocated by many of the contributors to this book.

The desirability of increasing potassium intake in the general community is far more controversial, but such an increase could potentially result in a major public health benefit. Our traditional approach to the prevention of blood-pressure-related cardiovascular disease has been to recommend antihypertensive drug treatment for "high risk" hypertensive subjects at the upper end of the blood pressure distribution. As indicated in Figure 1, a major proportion of the cardiovascular complications that can be attributed to the effects of elevations in systolic and diastolic blood pressure occur below the level of blood pressure at which most physicians recommend antihypertensive drug therapy. Thus, any attempt to substantially reduce the current epidemic of blood-pressure-related cardiovascular disease can only be successful if our traditional "high-risk" treatment strategy is supplemented by a population-based "mass strategy" aimed at a slight downward shift in the entire distribution of blood pressure (Figure 2). As indicated in Chapter 33, a shift as small as 4 mm Hg in diastolic blood pressure could potentially provide lifesaving benefits greater than those currently being achieved by all antihypertensive drug therapy. It should be emphasized that the two treatment strategies are not mutually exclusive. Indeed, there is no reason to believe that any potential mass strategy would be effective enough to replace the more traditional drug-based approach for treatment of persons with established hypertension.

Few data exist on the efficacy of dietary modification in preventing mild potassium deficits in those patients whose serum potassiums are in the 3.5 to 4.0 range. Some of the data collected as a part of the HANES I study would indicate that much of the decrease in potassium content of foods available in general food markets in this country is the result of food-processing practices implemented by the food-marketing industry (2,6). Data on unprocessed fresh vegetables, fruits, and meats from the U.S. Department of Agriculture handbook (1984) indicate that the consumption of these foods without potassium loss during preparation would provide a total intake in excess of 150 mEq of potassium per day for the average adult! This is an approach that should be more carefully explored as a reasonable means of minimizing or preventing the development of potassium deficits in those segments of the population that are at increased risk for this abnormality. The alternative approach of supplementing an individual's "normal" diet with potassium-rich foods is less attractive. Such an approach not only would be more costly but would also increase the calorie content of the diet.

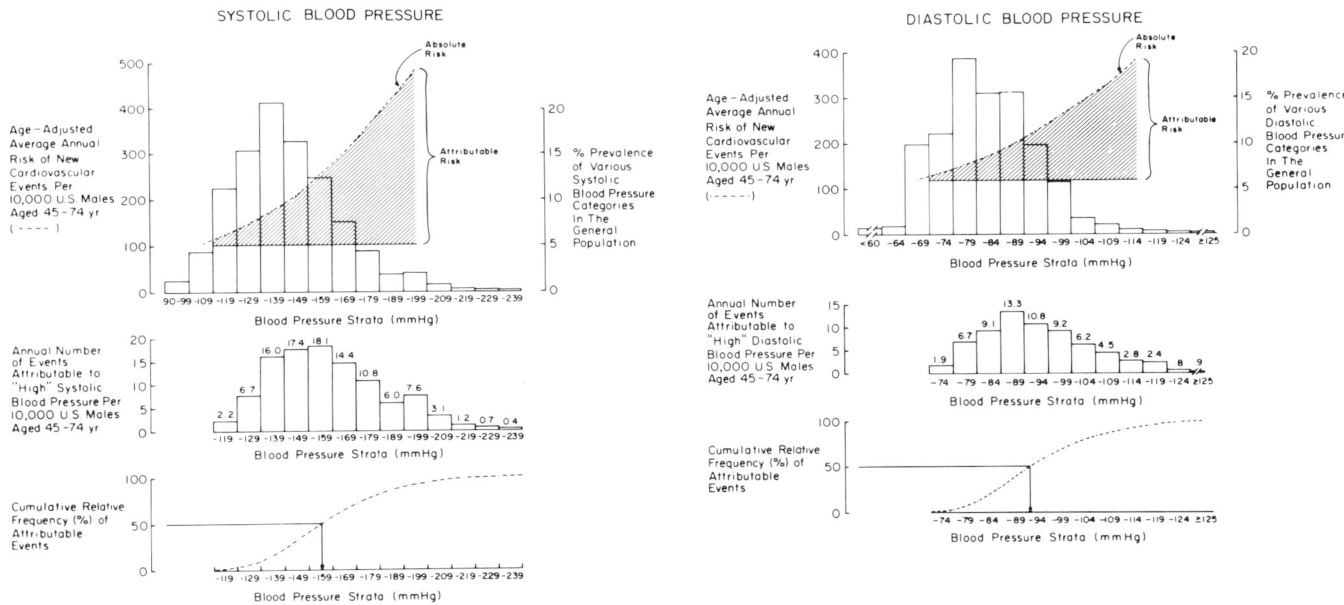

Figure 1 Risk of cardiovascular disease attributable to high blood pressure in U.S. men aged 45–74 years. The population attributable risk estimates (prevalence X attributable risk) presented are based on U.S. prevalence (7) and Framingham risk experience (25) at various levels of blood pressure. The estimates can serve only as a rough approximation of the true situation. However, they suggest that slight elevations of blood pressure, albeit still in the normotensive range, are responsible for many of the blood-pressure-related cardiovascular complications that occur in the general population.

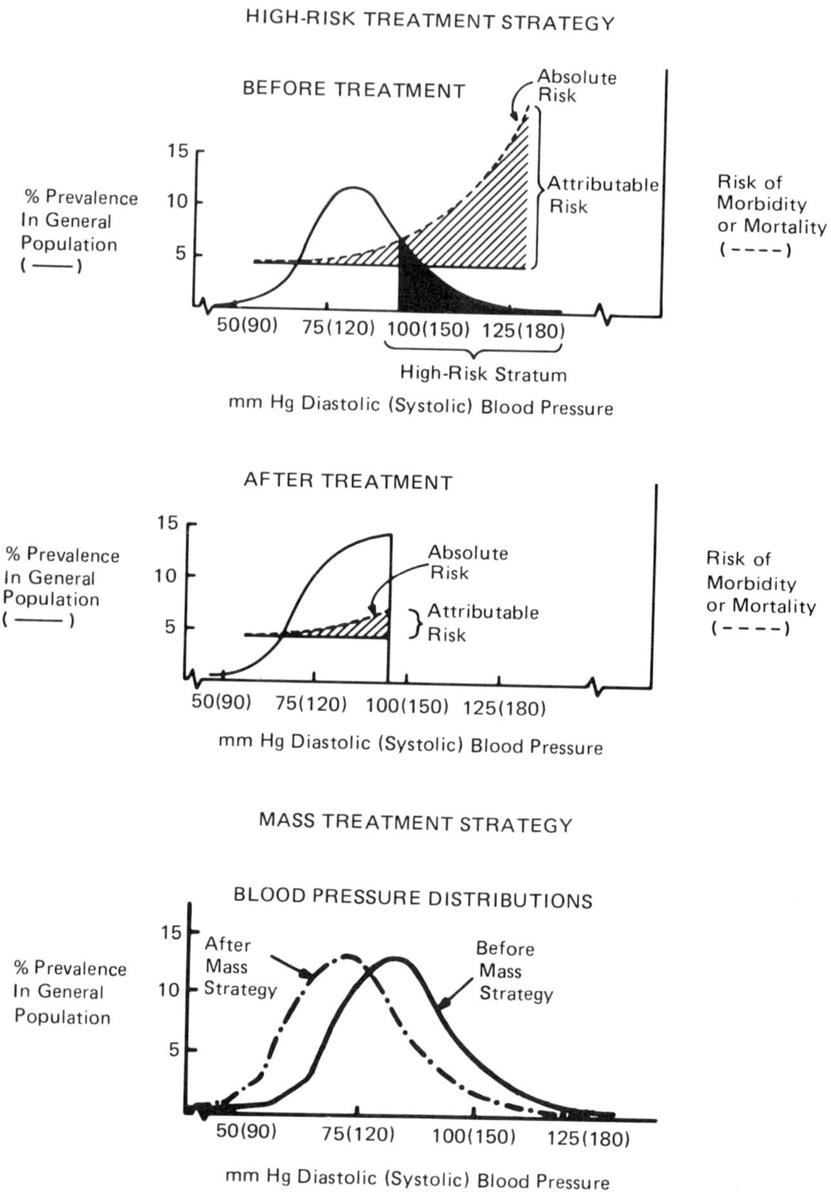

Figure 2 Objectives of "high-risk" and "mass" treatment strategies. In the traditional office-based high-risk approach to treatment, an attempt is made to lower blood pressure below an arbitrary cutoff point chosen to identify the presence of hypertension. In the less conventional mass-treatment strategy, an attempt is made to slightly lower the entire distribution of blood pressure. Risk estimates and treatment trial results suggest that a combination of high-risk and mass-treatment strategies would provide the greatest likelihood of substantially reducing our current epidemic of blood-pressure-related cardiovascular disease.

An increase in dietary potassium intake represents one of the most attractive options available as a mass strategy aimed at preventing blood-pressure-related cardiovascular morbidity and mortality. Such a diet would also tend to be lower in saturated fat and salt as well as higher in fiber content. Despite its attractiveness, more detailed information with respect to effectiveness, feasibility, and safety are needed before advocating increased potassium intake as a mass strategy.

ACKNOWLEDGMENTS

Data contained in this chapter represent work supported in part by NIH grants HL03303, RR35, RR722, plus support from the Jane Hilder Harris Foundation, the Irving Blum Memorial Fund, and the Milbank Fund. The technical assistance of Mrs. Judith Hermann and the secretarial help of Mrs. Sharon Manson are gratefully acknowledged.

REFERENCES

1. Abbrecht, P. H.: Cardiovascular effects of chronic potassium deficiency in the dog. *Am. J. Physiol.* 223:555, 1972.
2. Abraham, S., and Carroll, M. D.: *Fats, Cholesterol and Sodium Intake in the Diet of Persons 1-74 Years: United States,* Advanced Data 54, reissue, Washington, D.C., U.S. Department of Health Education and Welfare, 1981.
3. Berenson, G. S., Foster, T. A., Frank, G. C., Frevichs, R. R., Srinivassan, S. R., Voors, A. W., and Webber, L. S.: Cardiovascular disease risk factor variables at the pre-school age. The Bogaloosa Heart Study. *Circulation* 57:603, 1978.
4. Bulpitt, C., Shipley, M. J., and Semmence, A.: Blood pressure and plasma, sodium and potassium. *Clin. Sci.* 61:85s, 1981.
5. Dahl, L. K., Leitl, G., and Heine, M.: Influence of dietary potassium and sodium potassium molar ratios on the development of salt hypertension. *J. Exp. Med.* 136: 318, 1972.
6. Fregly, M. S., and Fregly, M. J.: The estimates of sodium intake by man. In *The Role of Salt in Cardiovascular Hypertension,* edited by Fregly, M. J., and Kare, M. R., New York, Academic Press, 1982.
7. Gordon, T.: *Blood Pressure of Adults by Age and Sex,* no. 1000, series 11, no. 4, Washington, D.C., National Center for Health Statistics, 1964.
8. Grim, C. E., Luft, F. C., Miller, J. Z., Meneely, G. R., Battarbee, H. D., Hames, C. G., and Dahl, L. K.: Racial differences in blood pressure in Evans County, Georgia: Relationship to sodium and potassium intake and plasma renin activity. *J. Chronic Dis.* 33:87, 1980.
9. Guyton, A. C., Lohmeier, T. E., Hall, J. E., Smith, M. J., and Kastner, P. R.: The infinite gain principle for arterial pressure control by the kidney-volume-pressure system. In *Fundamental Fault in Hypertension,* edited by Sambhi, M. P., Boston, Martinus Nijhoff PUblishers, 1984, pp. 35-61.
10. Haddy, F. J.: Potassium and blood vessels. *Life Sci.* 16:1489-1498, 1975.
11. Haddy, F. J., Pamnani, M. B., and Clough, D. L.: Humoral factors and the sodium-potassium pump in volume expanded hypertension. *Life Sci.* 24:2105-2118, 1979.
12. Haddy, F. J., Pamnani, M. B., and Clough, D. L.: The mechanism of sodium-dependent low renin hypertension. In *Fundamental Fault in Hypertension,* edited by Sambhi, M. P., Boston, Martinus Nijhoff Publishers, 1984, pp. 85-116.
13. Khaw, K. T., and Rose, G.: Population study of blood pressure and associated factors in Saint Lucia West Indies. *Int. J. Epidemiol.* 11:372, 1982.

14. Khaw, K. T., and Thorn, S.: Randomized double-blind crossover trial of potassium on blood pressure in normal subjects. *Lancet* 2:1127, 1982.
15. Langford, H. G., and Watson, R. L.: Electrolytes and hypertension. In *Epidemiology and Control of Hypertension,* edited by Paul, O., Miami Symposium Specialist, 1975, pp. 119–128.
16. Linas, S. L., and Dickmann, D.: Mechanism of the decreased renal blood flow in the potassium depleted conscious rat. *Kidney Int.* 21:752, 1982.
17. Meneely, G. R., and Ball, C. O. T.: Experimental epidemiology of chronic sodium chloride toxicity and the protective effect of potassium chloride. *Am. J. Med.* 25: 713, 1958.
18. Multiple Risk Factor Intervention Trial Research Group. Baseline rest electrocardiographic abnormalities, antihypertensive treatment, and mortality in the Multiple Risk Factor Intervention Trial. *Am. J. Cardiol.* 55:1–15, 1985.
19. Multiple Risk Factor Intervention Trial (MRFIT) Research Group: Multiple risk factor intervention trial. Risk factor changes and mortality results. *JAMA* 248:1465–1477, 1982.
20. Page, L. B.: Determinants of blood pressure in populations. In *Fundamental Fault in Hypertension,* edited by Sambhi, M. P., Boston, Martinus Mijhoff Publishers, 1984, pp. 69–82.
21. Page, L. B.: Epidemiologic evidence on the etiology of human hypertension and its possible prevention. *Am. Heart J.* 91:527, 1976.
22. Page, L. B., Vandevert, D. E., Nader, K., Lubin, N. K., and Page, J. R.: Blood pressure of Qash'gai Pastoral Nomads in Iran in relation to culture, diet, and body form. *Am. J. Clin. Nutr.* 34:527, 1981.
23. Sasaki, N.: The relationship of salt intake to hypertension in the Japanese. *Geriatrics* 19:735, 1964.
24. Shaper, A. G., Leonard, P. A., Jones, K. W., and Jones, M.: Environmental effects on the body build, blood pressure, and blood chemistry of nomadic warriors serving in the Army in Kenya. *E. Afr. Med. J.* 46:282, 1969.
25. Shurtleff, D.: Some characteristics related to the incidence of cardiovascular disease and death: Framingham Study, 18-year follow-up. In *The Framingham Study: An Epidemiological Investigation of Cardiovascular Disease,* section 30, edited by Kannel, W. B., and Gordon, T., Washington, D.C., U.S. Department of Health, Education and Welfare Publication (NIH), 1973, pp. 74–599.
26. Stamler, J., Berkson, D. M., Dyer, L., Lepper, M. H., Lindberg, H. A., Paul, O., McKean, H., Rhomberg, P., Schoenberger, J. A., Shekelle, R. B., and Stamler, R.: Relationship of multiple variables to blood pressure—findings from four Chicago Epidemiologic Studies. In *Epidemiology and Control of Hypertension,* edited by Paul, O., New York, Stratton Intercontinental Medical Book, 1975, pp. 307–356.
27. Stamler, J., Farinaro, E., Mojonnier, L. M., Hall, Y., Moss, D., and Stamler, R.: Prevention and control of hypertension by nutritional-hygienic means. *JAMA* 243: 1819–1823.
28. Sterns, R. H., Cox, M., Feig, P. U., and Singer, I.: Internal potassium balance in the control of the plasma potassium concentration. *Medicine* 60:339, 1981.
29. Walker, W. G., Sapir, D. G., Turin, M., and Cheng, J. T.: Potassium homeostasis and diuretic therapy. Inter. Congress Series No. 268, Modern Diuretic Therapy. In *The Symposium at Royal College of Physicians of London, May 8–9, 1972,* Excerpta Medica, Amsterdam, pp. 331–342.
30. Walker, W. G., Whelton, P. K., Saito, H., Russell, R. P., and Hermann, J.: Relation between blood pressure, and renin, renin substrate, angiotensin II, aldosterone, urinary sodium and potassium in 574 subjects. *Hypertension* 1:287, 1979.

Index